# Emerging Issues and Controversies in Infectious Disease

# Emerging Infectious Diseases of the 21st Century

**I.W. Fong**
*Professor of Medicine, University of Toronto*
*Infectious Diseases, St. Michael's Hospital*

For other titles in this series, go to:
www.springer.com/series/5903

A Continuation Order Plan is available for this series. A continuation order will bring delivery of each new volume immediately upon publication. Volumes are billed only upon actual shipment. For further information please contact the publisher.

I.W. Fong
Editor

# Emerging Issues and Controversies in Infectious Disease

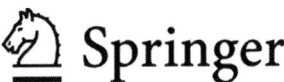 Springer

I.W. Fong
Professor of Medicine
University of Toronto
St. Michael's Hospital
30 Bond Street
Toronto ON M5B 1W8
Canada
fongi@smh.toronto.on.ca

ISBN 978-0-387-84840-2        e-ISBN 978-0-387-84841-9
DOI: 10.1007/978-0-387-84841-9

Library of Congress Control Number: 2008941665

© Springer Science+Business Media, LLC 2009

All rights reserved. This work may not be translated or copied in whole or in part without the written permission of the publisher (Springer Science+Business Media, LLC, 233 Spring Street, New York, NY 10013, USA), except for brief excerpts in connection with reviews or scholarly analysis. Use in connection with any form of information storage and retrieval, electronic adaptation, computer software, or by similar or dissimilar methodology now known or hereafter developed is forbidden. The use in this publication of trade names, trademarks, service marks and similar terms, even if they are not identified as such, is not to be taken as an expression of opinion as to whether or not they are subject to proprietary rights.
While the advice and information in this book are believed to be true and accurate at the date of going to press, neither the authors nor the editors nor the publisher can accept any legal responsibility for any errors or omissions that may be made. The publisher makes no warranty, express or implied, with respect to the material contained herein.

Printed on acid-free paper.

springer.com

*This book is dedicated to my wife, Cheryl,
and to our grandchildren, Miranda and Aiden.*

# Preface

The past decade has been highlighted by numerous advances in medical scientific knowledge, medical technology, and diagnostic techniques but there have been fewer dramatic changes or improvements in the management of medical conditions. This volume in the Emerging Infectious Disease of the 21st century series, addresses some of the emerging issues and controversies in Infectious Diseases.

The author has chosen these topics for review based on questions and contentions raised by medical residents, internists, emergency physicians, clinical infectious disease specialists, and family physicians. Hopefully the volume will provide guidance and answers to frequently asked questions in infectious disease to the generalists, specialists, and trainees in these areas, thus, facilitating improved patient care, prudent, and cost-effective management and investigation of these disorders.

This volume reviews the diagnosis and treatment of some common infections facing clinicians and family physicians such as sinusitis, otitis media, and pertussis. Recent studies and surveys have shown that these conditions are often over-diagnosed and treated unnecessarily with antibiotics. The approach and guidelines for diagnosis and management are reviewed in this volume. Other more complicated but less common conditions challenging internists, clinical infectious disease consultants, and other specialists are also reviewed (i.e., meningitis, ventilator associated pneumonia, sepsis, hepatitis C, B, etc.). This book discusses current guidelines provided by various medical societies for various infections, and analyzes the evidence to support those guidelines as well as contentious issues.

# Contents

**Section A: Bacterial and Fungal Infections**

**1 Issues in Central Nervous System Infections** .......................... 3
   1.1 Bacterial Meningitis ................................................... 3
      1.1.1 Introduction .................................................. 3
      1.1.2 Pathophysiology of Meningitis ............................... 3
      1.1.3 Clinical Issues in Meningitis ................................. 4
   1.2 Adjunctive Therapy in Tuberculous Meningitis ..................... 15
      1.2.1 Background ................................................... 15
      1.2.2 Treatment of Tuberculous Meningitis ....................... 17
   1.3 Adjunctive Therapy in Fungal Meningitis ............................ 18
      1.3.1 Background ................................................... 18
   1.4 Future Directions ..................................................... 20
   References .................................................................. 22

**2 Emerging Issues in Head and Neck Infections** .......................... 27
   2.1 Current Issues in Sinusitis ............................................ 27
      2.1.1 Background ................................................... 27
      2.1.2 Pathophysiology of Sinusitis ................................. 27
      2.1.3 Issues in Diagnosis of Bacterial Sinusitis .................... 28
      2.1.4 Microbiology of Sinusitis .................................... 30
      2.1.5 Treatment of Acute Bacterial Sinusitis ...................... 32
      2.1.6 Management of Chronic Sinusitis ........................... 35
      2.1.7 Issues in Acute Otitis Media ................................. 36
      2.1.8 Clinical Practice Guidelines ................................. 40
      2.1.9 Future Directions ............................................. 41
   References .................................................................. 43

**Section B: Emerging Trends in Pulmonary Infection**

**3 Current Issues in Ventilator-Associated Pneumonia** .................... 49
   3.1 Background ............................................................ 49
   3.2 Issues in the Diagnosis of VAP ....................................... 49
      3.2.1 Microbiological Techniques for Diagnosis .................. 51

|  |  | 3.2.2 | New Diagnostic Methods for VAP | 55 |
|---|---|---|---|---|
|  | 3.3 | Microbial Etiology of VAP | | 56 |
|  | 3.4 | Issues in Treatment of VAP | | 57 |
|  | 3.5 | Prevention of VAP | | 60 |
|  |  | 3.5.1 | Antibiotic Prophylaxis for Prevention of VAP | 61 |
|  |  | 3.5.2 | Maintaining Gastric Acidity to Prevent VAP | 63 |
|  |  | 3.5.3 | Methods to reduce Aspiration | 64 |
|  |  | 3.5.4 | Ventilator Circuit and VAP | 65 |
|  |  | 3.5.5 | Summary of Prevention | 65 |
|  | 3.6 | Future Directions | | 66 |
|  | References | | | 67 |
| 4 | **Emerging Issues in Pulmonary Infections of Cystic Fibrosis** | | | **75** |
|  | 4.1 | Introduction | | 75 |
|  | 4.2 | Pathobiology of Cystic Fibrosis | | 75 |
|  | 4.3 | Microbiology | | 78 |
|  |  | 4.3.1 | Pseudomonas aeruginosa | 79 |
|  |  | 4.3.2 | Late-Emerging Pathogens | 80 |
|  |  | 4.3.3 | Stentotrophomonas and Alcaligenes Species | 81 |
|  |  | 4.3.4 | Mycobacteria Species | 81 |
|  |  | 4.3.5 | Aspergillus Species and Other Fungi | 82 |
|  |  | 4.3.6 | Viral Infections | 83 |
|  | 4.4 | Management of Infections in CF | | 83 |
|  |  | 4.4.1 | Infants with CF | 84 |
|  |  | 4.4.2 | Antipseudomonal Therapy | 84 |
|  |  | 4.4.3 | Maintenance Therapy | 85 |
|  |  | 4.4.4 | Treatment of Pulmonary Exacerbation | 87 |
|  |  | 4.4.5 | Treatment of Other Emerging Pathogens | 89 |
|  | 4.5 | Prevention of Infections in CF | | 90 |
|  | 4.6 | Adjunctive Therapy for Pulmonary Exacerbation | | 90 |
|  |  | 4.6.1 | Anti-inflammatory Therapy | 91 |
|  | 4.7 | Future Directions | | 92 |
|  | References | | | 94 |
| 5 | **Re-Emergence of Childhood Respiratory Infections in Adults (RSV & Pertussis)** | | | **103** |
|  | **A: Respiratory Syncytial Virus infection in Adults** | | | **103** |
|  | 5.1 | Introduction | | 103 |
|  | 5.2 | Microbiology and Pathogenesis | | 103 |
|  |  | 5.2.1 | Immunity | 104 |
|  |  | 5.2.2 | Epidemiology | 105 |
|  |  | 5.2.3 | Management in Adults | 107 |
|  |  | 5.2.4 | Prevention | 108 |
|  |  | 5.2.5 | Future Directions | 109 |
|  | References | | | 109 |

Contents  xi

    **B: Pertussis in Adults** ............................................................ 113
    5.3  Introduction ................................................................... 113
          5.3.1  Microbiology and Pathogenesis ............................ 114
          5.3.2  Immunity .............................................................. 115
          5.3.3  Epidemiology ....................................................... 116
          5.3.4  Diagnosis and Management ................................. 118
          5.3.5  Prevention ............................................................ 119
          5.3.6  Future Directions .................................................. 120
    References ................................................................................ 121

**Section C:   New Concepts and Trends**

**6  New Concepts and Emerging Issues in Sepsis** ............................ 127
    6.1    Introduction ................................................................. 127
    6.2    Definitions ................................................................... 128
    6.3    Immune Response ...................................................... 128
    6.4    Pathogenesis ............................................................... 130
          6.4.1  Hemodynamics .................................................... 132
          6.4.2  Mechanisms ......................................................... 133
          6.4.3  Apoptosis of Immune Cells ................................. 135
          6.4.4  Immunoparalysis .................................................. 136
          6.4.5  Tissue Oxygenation .............................................. 137
          6.4.6  Coagulation .......................................................... 138
          6.4.7  Complement System ............................................ 139
          6.4.8  ARDS in Sepsis ................................................... 140
    6.5    Management in Sepsis ............................................... 141
    6.6    Early Goal-Directed Therapy .................................... 141
    6.7    Antimicrobial Therapy in Severe Sepsis ................... 142
    6.8    Activated Protein C .................................................... 144
    6.9    Corticosteroids in Severe Sepsis ............................... 145
    6.10  Intensive Insulin Therapy .......................................... 146
    6.11  Vasopressin and Vasopressors ................................... 147
    6.12  Blood Products in Sepsis ........................................... 147
    6.13  Ventilation and Other Adjunctive Therapy .............. 148
    6.14  Immunotherapies for Sepsis ...................................... 149
    6.15  Genetics and Sepsis ................................................... 150
    6.16  Future Directions ....................................................... 151
    6.17  Conclusion .................................................................. 154
    References ................................................................................ 154

**7  Febrile Neutropenia: Management Issues** ................................. 165
    7.1    Introduction .................................................................. 165
    7.2    Pathogenesis ................................................................ 166
    7.3    Febrile Neutropenia Definition .................................. 167
    7.4    Microbiology and Etiology ........................................ 168

|  |  | 7.4.1 | Initial Antibiotic Therapy | 169 |
|---|---|---|---|---|
|  |  | 7.4.2 | High-Risk Patients | 171 |
|  |  | 7.4.3 | Choice of Monotherapy | 173 |
|  | 7.5 | Duration of Therapy | | 174 |
|  | 7.6 | Empiric Antifungal Therapy | | 175 |
|  | 7.7 | Prevention | | 177 |
|  |  | 7.7.1 | Prophylactic Antibiotics | 177 |
|  |  | 7.7.2 | Colony-Stimulating Factors | 178 |
|  |  | 7.7.3 | Antifungal Prophylaxis | 179 |
|  | 7.8 | Future Directions | | 180 |
|  | References | | | 181 |

## 8 Emerging Issues and Trends in *Clostridium difficile* Colitis ... 189

|  | 8.1 | Introduction | | 189 |
|---|---|---|---|---|
|  | 8.2 | Microbiology | | 189 |
|  | 8.3 | Pathogenesis | | 190 |
|  |  | 8.3.1 | Binary Toxin and New Hypervirulent Strains | 192 |
|  | 8.4 | Clinical Aspects | | 194 |
|  |  | 8.4.1 | Antibiotic-Associated Diarrhea | 195 |
|  |  | 8.4.2 | Risk Factors for CDAD | 197 |
|  | 8.5 | Diagnosis | | 199 |
|  | 8.6 | Management | | 200 |
|  |  | 8.6.1 | Specific Therapy | 201 |
|  |  | 8.6.2 | Recurrences of CDAD | 204 |
|  |  | 8.6.3 | Prevention | 209 |
|  |  | 8.6.4 | Future Directions | 212 |
|  | References | | | 214 |

## 9 Probiotics in Infectious Diseases ... 227

|  | 9.1 | Introduction | | 227 |
|---|---|---|---|---|
|  | 9.2 | Background | | 228 |
|  | 9.3 | Mechanisms of Action | | 229 |
|  |  | 9.3.1 | Mucosal Integrity | 229 |
|  |  | 9.3.2 | Colonization Resistance | 231 |
|  |  | 9.3.3 | Inactivation of Microbial Toxins | 232 |
|  |  | 9.3.4 | Immunomodulation | 232 |
|  |  | 9.3.5 | Bacterial Translocation | 234 |
|  | 9.4 | Clinical Application of Probiotics | | 235 |
|  |  | 9.4.1 | Probiotics for Newborns and Children | 235 |
|  |  | 9.4.2 | Antibiotic-Associated Diarrhea | 238 |
|  |  | 9.4.3 | Urogenital Infections | 240 |
|  |  | 9.4.4 | Probiotics in Vaginitis | 245 |
|  |  | 9.4.5 | Miscellaneous Infections | 246 |
|  | 9.5 | Probiotics as Food Additives | | 249 |
|  | 9.6 | Adverse Effects of Probiotics | | 250 |

Contents                                                                     xiii

|        | 9.7    | Conclusion and Future Directions                              | 250 |
|--------|--------|---------------------------------------------------------------|-----|
|        |        | References                                                    | 251 |
| **10** | **Device-Related Infections**                                          | **261** |
|        | 10.1   | Introduction                                                  | 261 |
|        | 10.2   | Pathogenesis of Device-Related Infections                     | 263 |
|        |        | 10.2.1 Impairment of Local Defence                            | 264 |
|        |        | 10.2.2 Resistance to Antimicrobial Agents                     | 265 |
|        | 10.3   | Specific Device-Related Infections                            | 267 |
|        |        | 10.3.1 Intravascular Devices                                  | 267 |
|        |        | 10.3.2 Prevention of Central versus Catheter Infections       | 274 |
|        | 10.4   | Cardiovascular Device Infectious                              | 277 |
|        |        | 10.4.1 Cardiac Devices and Infections                         | 277 |
|        |        | 10.4.2 Trends in Prosthetic Valve Endocarditis                | 277 |
|        |        | 10.4.3 Infections of ICD, LVAD and Pacemakers                 | 280 |
|        | 10.5   | Vascular Grafts                                               | 285 |
|        | 10.6   | Future Directions                                             | 287 |
|        |        | References                                                    | 288 |
| **11** | **Current Concepts of Orthopedic Implants and Prosthetic Joint Infections** | **299** |
|        | 11.1   | Introduction                                                  | 299 |
|        | 11.2   | Microbiological Aspects                                       | 299 |
|        | 11.3   | Diagnosis                                                     | 302 |
|        | 11.4   | Clinical Presentation                                         | 304 |
|        | 11.5   | Management                                                    | 305 |
|        |        | 11.5.1 Basis of Medical Therapy                               | 305 |
|        |        | 11.5.2 Principles of Surgical Management                      | 308 |
|        |        | 11.5.3 Treatment Algorithm                                    | 312 |
|        |        | 11.5.4 Issues with Antimicrobial Therapy                      | 313 |
|        | 11.6   | Prevention of Orthopedic Device Infections                    | 316 |
|        | 11.7   | Future Directions                                             | 318 |
|        | 11.8   | Conclusion                                                    | 319 |
|        |        | References                                                    | 319 |
| **12** | **Combination Antimicrobial Therapies**                                | **327** |
|        | 12.1   | Introduction                                                  | 327 |
|        | 12.2   | Bacterial Infections                                          | 328 |
|        |        | 12.2.1 Bacterial Infective Endocarditis                       | 328 |
|        |        | 12.2.2 In Vitro Testing of Synergy                            | 329 |
|        |        | 12.2.3 Animal Models of Infective Endocarditis                | 330 |
|        |        | 12.2.4 Clinical Trials in Bacterial Endocarditis              | 332 |
|        |        | 12.2.5 Gram-Negative Bacilli Infections                       | 337 |
|        |        | 12.2.6 Community-Acquired Pneumonia                           | 338 |

- 12.3 Fungal Infections and Combination Therapy .................... 338
  - 12.3.1 In Vitro Antifungal Combination Assays ............... 339
  - 12.3.2 Antifungal Combinations for Candida species ......... 342
  - 12.3.3 Combination Therapy for Cryptococcal Meningitis ..... 344
  - 12.3.4 Combination Therapy for Invasive Aspergillosis ....... 345
- 12.4 Viral Infections ................................................. 347
  - 12.4.1 Chronic Hepatitis C Infections ......................... 347
  - 12.4.2 Chronic Hepatitis B Virus .............................. 351
- 12.5 Parasitic Infections ............................................. 355
  - 12.5.1 Antimalarial Combination Therapies .................... 355
  - 12.5.2 Filariasis Therapies .................................... 358
  - 12.5.3 Leishmaniasis .......................................... 360
  - 12.5.4 African Trypanosomiasis (Sleeping Sickness) .......... 361
- 12.6 Conclusion ..................................................... 362
- 12.7 Future Directions .............................................. 364
- References ........................................................... 364

**Index** ............................................................. 379

# Acknowledgment

I am very grateful to Winnie Yau for her secretarial and administrative assistance and to Maria Isabel Suarez, Bogusia Skucinska, and my wife (Cheryl) for their stenographic assistance in the preparation of this manuscript. I am also indebted to Carolyn Ziegler for her invaluable assistance in performing literature searches.

# Section A
# Bacterial and Fungal Infections

# Chapter 1
# Issues in Central Nervous System Infections

## 1.1 Bacterial Meningitis

### 1.1.1 Introduction

Bacterial meningitis is a serious, potentially fatal infection, which requires prompt diagnosis and immediate appropriate management. In the 20th century the annual incidence of bacterial meningitis ranges from approximately 3 per 100,000 population in the United States,[1] to 45.8 per 100,000 in Brazil,[2] to 500 per 100,000 in the "Meningitis belt" (sub-Sahara) of Africa.[3]

Despite the availability of effective antimicrobials the case fatality rate of bacterial meningitis remain high, with a 25% all-cause mortality rate between 1962 and 1988 for community-acquired meningitis in adults ($\geq 16$ years).[4] In the pediatric population although the case fatality rate is between 5% and 10%,[5] severe morbidity with long-term neurological sequelae occurs in 30% of newborn and young infants and 15–20% of older children.[5] These sequelae can result from parenchymal brain damage (causing cognitive deficits, seizure disorder, learning disabilities, behavior problems, paresis, spasticity), cranial nerve dysfunction (causing hearing deficit, visual impairment, ataxia), and increased intracranial pressure (ICP; causing hydrocephalus). Bacterial meningitis is one of the leading causes of acquired deafness in children in the United States,[6] with incidence of significant hearing deficit ranging from 5% to 20%.[7,8]

### 1.1.2 Pathophysiology of Meningitis

The brain is protected from infection by the skull, the pia, arachnoid, and dural meninges covering its surface; and the blood brain barrier. A breach in these barriers by a pathogen can lead to meningitis, but the exact mechanism by which community-acquired pathogens gain access to the subarachnoid space is not fully understood. Common bacterial pathogens associated with meningitis (*Neisseria meningococcus*, *Haemophilus influenzae* type B and *Streptococcus pneumoniae*) first bind and colonize the nasopharyngeal mucosa with local invasion (possibly precipitated by viral upper respiratory tract infection, or acquisition of a virulent bacterial strain in the absence of protective antibodies). This eventually leads to bacteremia and meningeal invasion with replication in the subarachnoid space, and release of bacterial components (cell wall, lipoprotein and, lipopolysaccharide). These products results in stimulation and recruitment of macrophages, neutrophils, endothelial and other central nervous system (CNS) cells with release of proinflammatory cytokines (tumor necrosis factor (TNF)α, interleukin (IL)-1, IL-6; chemokines (IL-8, monocyte chemotactic protein (MIP)-1α MIP-2) stimulating recruitment of leucocytes into the cerebrospinal fluid (CSF); adhesion molecules (integrins (CD18), and selections); prostaglandins ($PGE_2$, prostacyclin); and interferon γ. The effect of the medley of these molecules leads to subarachnoid space inflammation and increased permeability of the microvasculature endothelium, resulting in increased blood–brain barrier, vasogenic, and cytotoxic edema of the brain with increased intracranial pressure and sometimes cerebral vasculitis with cerebral infarction.

The clinical features of meningitis are a reflection of the underlying pathophysiologic process. Systemic infection results in constitutional symptoms of fever, myalgia, and rash often preceded by upper respiratory symptomatology. The inflammatory response within the cerebrospinal space progresses to increased intracranial pressure and cerebral edema resulting in alteration of mental status, headache, vomiting, seizures, nerve palsies, and coma. The resultant meningeal inflammation and irritation elicits a protective reflex to prevent stretching of the inflamed and hypersensitive nerve roots, which is detectable as neck stiffness, Kerring, or Brudzinski signs.[9,10]

## 1.1.3 Clinical Issues in Meningitis

### 1.1.3.1 Does this Patient have Acute Meningitis?

Early clinical recognition of meningitis is imperative to allow initiation of confirmatory tests to establish the diagnosis and start appropriate treatment. Not the least of which are identification and antimicrobial susceptibility of the offending pathogen.

The early manifestation of bacterial meningitis can be nonspecific and often mimic common benign viral infections. The clinical examination aids physicians in identifying patients with suspicion of meningitis requiring further diagnostic but invasive test with a lumbar puncture. Examination of the CSF is necessary to refute or establish the diagnosis and may help direct antimicrobial therapy. To avoid unnecessary invasive procedure, as early symptoms (fever and headache) are common in the population without meningitis, it is useful to identify clinical findings that can distinguish patients at high and low risk of meningitis. The classic triad of fever, neck stiffness, and change in mental status has been found only in 44%[11] to 66%,[4] with pooled sensitivity of 46% from three studies,[12] in adult patients with bacterial meningitis. In a large prospective study of 696 episodes of community-acquired acute bacterial meningitis, 95% of patients had at least two of the four symptoms of headache, fever, neck stiffness, and altered mental status.[11] Thus, on physical examination the absence of fever, neck stiffness, and altered mental status effectively eliminates meningitis (sensitivity, 99–100% for the presence of one of these findings).[12] Neck stiffness, the hallmark of meningeal irritation or inflammation, had a pooled sensitivity of 70% in retrospective series,[12] and was present in 83% in a large prospective study.[11]

There is little debate that patients presenting with only fever and altered mental state should have a lumbar puncture to exclude meningitis (after exclusion of intracranial mass lesion) but the presence of fever and headaches alone is another matter. Although the combination of fever and headache are very sensitive findings for acute meningitis, the specificity is very low. Other signs of meningeal irritation (Kernig and Brudzinski signs) have not been well-studied in large series, but the overall impression is that these signs are late manifestation of meningitis with sensitivity as low as 9%, but high specificity approaching 100% in one study.[13] Probably the most useful sign to determine further investigation to exclude meningitis in subjects presenting with fever and headaches is jolt accentuation of the headache. The patient is requested to turn his or her head horizontally (2–3 rotations per second) and worsening of the headache represents a positive sign.[13] In a review of symptoms and signs for acute meningitis from 10 studies, jolt accentuation of headaches was found to have a sensitivity of 100%, specificity of 54%, and a negative likelihood ratio of 0 for the diagnosis of meningitis.[12] However, only one of the studies assessed this sign in 97 episodes.[13]

In summary all adults with fever and altered mental status should probably have a lumbar puncture if there are no contraindications. This should be considered in clinical context with each individual subject as the elderly frequently manifest confusion and altered mental status with significant fever. Alert patients with headache and fever can be observed without a lumbar puncture if jolt accentuation of headache is absent. Fever is not always present with meningitis (especially in the elderly) and was noted on initial assessment in only 77% of 680 episodes in a prospective study.[11] Thus, lumbar puncture should be considered in the absence of fever for an unexplained altered mental status, neck stiffness, or jolt accentuation of headache (especially in the presence of leucocytosis).

In a review of bacterial meningitis in children, fever (94%), vomiting (82%), and nuchal rigidity (77%) were the most common (presenting symptoms in 1–4 years of age), with many experiencing lethargy, irritability, anorexia, and photophobia.[14] Neck stiffness is generally less prominent the younger the child, and headaches are seen in almost all older children.

### 1.1.3.2 Should CT of the Head be Performed?

A frequent misconception and practice by some physicians is to perform a computed tomography (CT) scan of the head before lumbar puncture in patients with suspected meningitis. The fear of missing an intracranial mass lesion that may precipitate brain herniation, and litigation concerns have been the driving force behind this practice. After a lumbar puncture there is normally a mild, transient lowering of the lumbar CSF pressure, and in the presence of increased intracranial pressure with a space-occupying lesion the relative pressure gradient with downward displacement of the cerebrum and brainstem can be increased, thus precipitating coning.

In studies before the advent of CT imaging physicians relied on the presence of papilledema to assess the risk of brain herniation. In an earlier study of 129 patients with elevated intracranial pressure, 1.2% of patients with papilledema and 12% without papilledema had unfavorable complications within 48 h after the procedure.[15] However, in infants and children with bacterial meningitis the prevalence of brain herniation was 6% of 302 episodes, within 8 h after lumbar puncture.[16] In more recent times a study of 301 adults with bacterial meningitis found that low-risk patients rarely had CT abnormalities (3 of 96 patients), with a negative predictive value of 97%.[17] Moreover, of the three patients with CT abnormalities only one had a mild mass effect and all three underwent lumbar puncture without brain herniation. Specific guidelines for adult patients who should undergo CT before lumbar puncture have been developed (Table 1.1). In the most recent prospective study of adult bacterial meningitis[11] only 63% of patients fulfilling these guidelines underwent CT before lumbar puncture, and a large number of patients without these indications also underwent CT first. Unfortunately this report did not provide information on the prevalence of coning post-lumbar puncture.

### 1.1.3.3 Should Antimicrobials be Given Before Lumbar Puncture?

An important clinical and medicolegal issue is the urgency for starting antimicrobial therapy in bacterial meningitis, or the effect of delay in treating on the outcome by waiting for the analysis of CSF or CT of the head. Theoretically it appears plausible that any delay in treatment may be detrimental but there is lack of good evidence to support this, and it would be impossible to design a randomized study to answer this question because of ethical concerns. Also the question of how long a

**Table 1.1** Criteria of CT prior to lumbar puncture in adults (From Turkel et al.[18] With permission of the publisher)

| Criterion | Comments |
|---|---|
| Immunocompromized state | HIV or AIDS, transplantation, immunosuppressive therapy |
| History of CNS disease | Mass lesion, stroke, or focal infection |
| New onset seizure | Within 1 week of presentation, prolonged seizures |
| Papilledema | Presence of venous pulsations against inter-cranial hyperemia |
| Abnormal level of consciousness | Moderate to severe impairment (inability to answer two consecutive questions correctly, or to follow two consecutive commands) |
| Focal neurologic deficit | Dilated nonreactive pupil, abnormal ocular motility, or visual fields, gaze palsy, arm, or leg drift |

delay is significant would be hard to answer, i.e., 30 min, 1–2 h, etc. The earlier literature on this issue examined the relationship between duration of patient's symptoms before starting treatment and patient outcome. However, this may not be accurate as there may be a preceding nonspecific illness phase before actual meningitis phase. Thus distinction has to be made between duration of patients' symptoms versus duration of meningitis. Moreover, the progression of the disease process can be rapid (hours) or insidious (days), and this may depend on host factors and virulence of the specific strain of bacteria.

In an earlier review of this topic, 25 studies (7 of which were prospective cohort) correlated duration of symptoms with an outcome of bacterial meningitis.[19] Many of the studies reviewed were not of high quality and as a consequence no firm conclusion could be drawn as the reports were discordant and conflicting. In a subsequent retrospective study of 269 patients with community-acquired bacterial meningitis, proven within 24 h of presentation to the emergency, delay in therapy was associated with adverse clinical outcome when the patient's condition advance from a low risk to the highest prognostic severity before the initial antibiotic dose was given.[20] Three baseline clinical features (hypotension, altered mental status, and seizures) were independently associated with adverse clinical outcome and were used to create the prognostic model. Patients were stratified into low risk (stage I), intermediate risk (stage II), and high risk (stage III). The outcome was worst when patients in stage I or II at arrival in the emergency department advanced to stage III before administration of antibiotics. For patients (227) who remained in a given prognostic stage the median delay of initiation of antibiotic therapy was 4 h and did not significantly differ between patients with and without adverse outcome. Patients in the low-risk groups (stage I) with an adverse outcome showed a trend toward longer median delay in antibiotic therapy (13.6 h) compared with those without an adverse outcome (6.0 h), but the difference was not statistically significant ($p = 0.08$) because of small numbers in this subgroup.[20] Similar observations were made in more recent but smaller retrospective studies. In Taiwan the timing of appropriate antimicrobial therapy, as defined by consciousness level, was a major determinant of survival and neurological outcomes for community-acquired bacterial meningitis.[21] It also indicated that the first dose of therapy should best be given before the level of consciousness deteriorates to a Glasgow coma scale lower than 10 (confusion, clouding of consciousness, stupor, or coma). In another study of 171 cases of community-acquired bacterial meningitis, the mortality rate for patients receiving antibiotics in the emergency department was 7.9% (with a mean time to receive antibiotics of 1.08 h ± 13 min), in those that received the antibiotics as inpatients the mortality rate was 29% (with a mean time to receive antibiotics of 6 ± 9 h).[22]

There are several drawbacks, however, in administering antibiotics before diagnostic investigations (i.e., lumbar puncture), including affecting the CSF culture sensitivity and the ability to confirm the diagnosis of bacterial meningitis or identify the specific organism. This may lead to an inappropriate course of antibiotics and prolong hospitalization for aseptic meningitis. This is a dilemma when there are predominantly neutrophils in the CSF pleocytosis with normal or borderline low

CSF glucose and negative gram stain and culture (a situation not uncommonly seen with early viral meningitis). Moreover, it is the author's experience that most patients who receive the initial dose of antibiotics before lumbar puncture in the emergency department do not have meningitis (no CSF pleocytosis), and that those who do predominantly have aseptic meningitis. Thus the majority of patients receiving empirical antibiotics for meningitis in the emergency department are exposed to expensive, unnecessary drugs with potential adverse events. Similar observations have also been made in other reports. In a prospective study of 301 adults with suspected meningitis, only 80 patients (27%) had objective evidence of meningitis (defined as >5 white cells for milliliter of CSF), and only 20 patients (7%) had confirmed bacterial meningitis (combined CSF analysis and blood culture).[17] In another prospective study of 297 adults with suspected meningitis only 80 patients (27%) had evidence of meningitis and only 3 patients had confirmed bacterial meningitis (1.0%).[23] However, unfortunately neither of these studies indicated the number of patients receiving antibiotics before lumbar puncture or before results of CSF analysis.

In children similar results have been found. For example, of 709 children who underwent lumbar puncture because of suspicion of meningitis in 1970 only 16% were found to have abnormal CSF.[24] Again in more recent times from 1989 to 1991 at the Boston City Hospital only 40 of 529 (7.6%) children undergoing lumbar puncture had evidence of meningitis.[25]

### 1.1.3.4 Guidelines for Empiric Antimicrobial Therapy

Based on the available evidence the Infectious Disease Society of America (IDSA) concluded that there is inadequate data to delineate specific guidelines on the interval between the initial physician encounter and the administration of the first dose of antimicrobial therapy.[18] However, antimicrobial therapy should be instituted as soon as possible after the diagnosis is considered to be likely (leaving the decision on the clinician's judgment for the probability of bacterial meningitis). Other recommendations include obtaining CSF examination within 30 min after physician encounter for suspected bacterial meningitis and initiating antimicrobial therapy based on results of the CSF characteristics and gram stain.[26] For cases where lumbar puncture cannot be performed promptly, or there are contraindications to this procedure, or need for CT of head (as outlined in Table 1.1) then blood cultures should taken (preferably 2–3 sets) and appropriate antimicrobial therapy started promptly before lumbar puncture. This would also apply to critically ill patients presenting with hypotension (septic shock). IDSA guidelines for treatment of specific bacterial pathogens are shown in Table 1.2. Although vancomycin is recommended for initial therapy, this is mainly indicated in areas where highly resistant *S. pneumoniae* (penicillin MIC $\geq 4.0$ µg/mL) is fairly common or prevalent, as up to 25% of these strains are resistant to ceftriaxone. Where these strains are exceedingly rare in invasive pneumococcal disease (as in most of Canada), then vancomycin as initial therapy is not necessary.

## 1.1 Bacterial Meningitis

**Table 1.2** Recommendations for antimicrobial therapy in adult patients with presumptive pathogen identification by positive gram stain (Adapted from Tunkel et al.[18] With permission of the publisher)

| Microorganism | Recommended therapy | Alternative therapies |
|---|---|---|
| Streptococcus pneumoniae | Vancomycin plus a third-generation cephalosporin[a,b] | Meropenem (C-III), fluoroquinolone[c] (B-II) |
| Neisseria meningitides | Third-generation cephalosporin[a] | Penicillin G, ampicillin, chloramphenical, fluoroquinolone, aztreonam |
| Listeria monocytogenes | Ampicillin[d] or penicillin G[d] | Trimethoprim-sulfamethoxazole, meropenem (B-III) |
| Streptococcus agalactiae | Ampicillin[d] or penicillin G[d] | Third-generation cephalosporin[a] (B-III) |
| Haemophilus influenzae | Third-generation cephalosporin[a] (A-I) | Chloramphenicol, cefepime (A-II), meropenem (A-I), fluoroquinolone |
| Escherichia coil | Third-generation cephalosporin[a] (A-II) | Cefepime, meropenem, aztreonam, fluoroquinolone, trimethoprim-sulfamethoxazole |

All recommendations are A-III, unless otherwise indicated. In children, ampicillin is added to the standard therapeutic regimen of cefotaxime or ceftriaxone plus vancomycin when *L. monocytogenes* is considered and to an aminoglycoside if a gram-negative enteric pathogen is of concern.
[a] Ceftriaxone or cefotaxime
[b] Some experts would add rifampin if dexamethasone is also given (B-III)
[c] Gatifloxacin or moxifloxacin
[d] Addition of an aminoglycoside should be considered

### The Value of Corticosteroids in Bacterial Meningitis

Interest in the role of steroids in bacterial meningitis has existed for many decades, but it was not until 1988 that a prospective randomized trial in children was reported that the value began to be appreciated. Steroids as an anti-inflammatory agent to dampen the inflammatory response mediated by cytokines and chemokines, thus limiting CNS pathology and resultant sequelae, was biologically plausible for treatment. The results of animal studies indicated efficacy of dexamethasone in reducing brain water content, CSF pressure, pleocytosis, lactate concentration, TNF activity, and other indices of meningeal inflammation.[27] Dexamethasone was not recommended for routine use in childhood meningitis (especially for *H. influenzae*) until the early 1990s.[28,29]

The initial prospective double-blind controlled trail with dexamethasone (0.15 mg/kg every 6 h for 4 days) involved 200 children (2 months to 15 years old); with 77% of the cases due to *H. influenzae* type b.[30] Significant decrease in the frequency of sensorineural hearing loss in children who received dexamethasone was identified. One year after the acute illness 3 of 81 (3.7%) steroid treated and 9 of 75 (12%) placebo-treated children had neurological sequelae ($p = 0.052$). The percentages of children with one or more neurologic and one or more audiologic abnormalities after 1 year were 6.5% and 24%, respectively ($p = 0.003$). Only two of the children in the dexamethasone group developed gastrointestinal bleeding (during the acute illness) that required transfusion.

A large open randomized prospective study of dexamethasone in 429 children and adults (ages 3 months to 60 years) with bacterial meningitis was subsequently reported from Egypt.[31] The pathogens isolated were *N. meningitidis* in 62% of the patients, *S. pneumoniae* in 25% and *H. influenzae* type b in 13%. The mortality and permanent sequela were lower in dexamethasone-treated patients with pneumococcal meningitis (13.5% vs 40.7%, $p < 0.002$); fewer deaths occurred in the steroid-treated patients with meningococcal meningitis but the number with permanent sequelae was not reduced; no significant differences were noted in the children with *H. influenzae* meningitis due to small number of cases. All patients in this study received ampicillin and chloramphenicol, which was not considered a standard regimen in developed countries.

A subsequent meta-analysis of two randomized controlled trials of dexamethasone in childhood bacterial meningitis (from 1988 to 1996) was reported in 1997.[33] As the incidence of severe hearing loss differed significantly by organisms among control subjects, organism-specific estimates were made. In *H. influenzae* type b meningitis, dexamethasone reduced severe hearing loss overall (combined odds ratio [OR], 0.31, 95% confidence interval [CI], 0.14–0.69. There was no change in the results when analyzed for timing of administration of dexamethasone (before, with, or after initiating antibiotics). In pneumococcal meningitis, only studies in which dexamethasone was given early suggested protection, significant reduction of severe hearing loss (combined OR, 0.09, 95% CI, 0.0–0.71), and approached significance for any neurological deficit (combined OR, 0.23, 95% CI, 0.04–1.05). For all organisms combined, the pooled OR suggested protection against neurological deficits other than hearing loss but was not significant (OR, 0.39; 95% CI, 0.34–1.02). Outcomes were similar in studies that used 2 versus more than 2 days of dexamethasone. The incidence of gastrointestinal bleeding was increased with longer duration of dexamethasone (3.0% with 4 days of therapy), but was not significantly increased with 2 days of treatment, 0.8% versus 0.5% in controls. Since then a recent double-blind placebo-controlled randomized trial in children in Malawi[33] showed no benefit of adjunctive dexamethasone, with similar mortality (31% in both groups) and sequelae at final outcome (28% in both groups). This discrepancy in results from previous studies may be explained by the severe illness in these Malawi children presenting late in the course after delay in seeking therapy, high incidence of malnutrition, and HIV infection.[34]

Despite the variability in outcome from randomized trials the evidence supports the use of adjunctive dexamethasone in children with *H. influenzae* meningitis, and is sanctioned by the committee on Infectious Disease of the American Academic of Pediatrics.[28] Although corticosteroids have not shown a clear benefit in pneumococcal or meningococcal meningitis in children, the use is reasonable and biologically plausible, as the pathogenic mechanisms does not appear to be different among the bacterial agents of community-acquired meningitis. Experts vary in recommending dexamethasone in these types of meningitis, and for pneumococcal meningitis in children, the guidelines state: "adjunctive therapy with dexamethasone maybe considered after weighing the potential benefits and possible risk."[35] Both *H. influenzae* and pneumococcal meningitis in children has decreased dramatically since the advent of HIB vaccine and the seven valent pneumococcal conjugate vaccines, and further studies in developed countries will unlikely occur to provide definitive answers. When corticosteroids is being used in bacterial meningitis in children it is ideal and preferable to administer dexamethasone 0.15 mg/kg every 6 h for 2–4 days starting 10–20 min prior to, or at least concomitant with the first antimicrobial dose. Although, the IDSA[18] guidelines recommend not administering dexamethasone to children who have already received antimicrobial therapy, as this is unlikely to improve outcome, this statement is debatable. The meta-analysis by Mc Intyre et al.[32] showed no difference in outcome when results were analyzed for timing of administration of dexamethasone to the initial antimicrobial therapy. Moreover, when the clinician encounters a critically ill child with bacterial meningitis, knowing that the risk of 2 days dexamethasone is no greater than placebo, there is argument in favor of a prudent short course of corticosteroids when weighing the risk/benefit ratio.

Adults

There have been three earlier randomized and placebo-controlled trails with dexamethasone in adults with bacterial meningitis[36–38] and one randomized but not placebo-controlled study.[31] Although the results of three of the studies were inconclusive for definitive recommendations (due to small sample size) for use of corticosteroids, benefit was suggested.[31] However, a large multicentre double-blind, placebo-controlled trial confirmed the benefit of adjunctive dexamethasone in adult bacterial meningitis.[38] A total of 301 patients were enrolled in the study to receive dexamethasone 10 mg every 6 h for 4 days or placebo, administered 15–20 min before or with the first dose of antibiotic. Treatment with dexamethasone was associated with a reduction of an unfavorable outcome (relative risk (RR) 0.59; 95% CI, 0.37–0.94, $p = 0.03$). Also there was a reduction in the mortality (RR of death, 0.48; 95% CT, 0.24–0.96, $p = 0.04$) in the dexamethasone-treated group. Among the patients with pneumococcal meningitis, there were significant reductions in unfavorable outcome (52–26%, RR 0.50, $p = 0.006$), death (34–14%, RR 0.41, $p = 0.04$) with dexamethasone therapy, but not hearing loss (21–14%, RR 0.67, 0.55).[38] Whilst in patients with meningococcal meningitis none of the outcome measures significantly improved with dexamethasone, the risk reduction of unfavorable outcome ($RR = 0.75, p = 0.74$), focal neurological abnormalities ($RR = 0.57, p = 0.48$), and hearing loss ($RR = 0.57, p = 0.48$) somewhat improved with corticosteroids. This may well be due to the low complication rates and better prognosis with meningococcal meningitis (mortality rate 2–4%, versus up to 35% with pneumococcal meningitis).[38] Thus this would require a much larger sample size to prove a 25% reduction in outcome with dexamethasone in meningococcal meningitis. In all groups (total population studied) dexamethasone was most beneficial in those with moderate to severe disease. In this study dexamethasone did not increase the risk of gastrointestinal bleeding (2 in the dexamethasone versus 5 in the placebo group[38]).

There have been two recent RCT-assessing corticosteroids in adult bacterial meningitis conducted in developing countries.[39,40] A double-blind, placebo-controlled trial of dexamethasone in 435 patients over 14 years of age with suspected bacterial meningitis in Vietnam was recently reported.[39] Bacterial meningitis was confirmed in 300 patients (69.0%), of whom 143 received dexamethasone (0.4 mg/kg every 12 h for 4 days) and 157 placebo. Streptococcus species (including *S. suis*, *S. pneumoniae*, and others) accounted for the major proportion of isolates (42.5–44.5%), with *N. meningitides* only in 4.1–4.6%. In patients with confirmed bacterial meningitis there was a significant reduction in mortality at 1 month (RR = 0.43) and risk of death or disability at 6 months (OR, 0.56, CI 0.32–0.98). Results of multivariate analysis did not show benefit in patients without confirmation of acute bacterial meningitis.[39] The second recent RCT published at the same time, enrolled 465 adults with bacterial meningitis (90% of whom were HIV-positive) from Malawi (Sub-Saharan Africa).[40] Bacterial meningitis was confirmed in 325 (70%) of patients, and *S. pneumoniae* was isolated in 68–72%, and *N. meningitides* in 4%. There was no significant difference in mortality at 40 days or disability between dexamethasone (16 mg twice daily for 4 days) and placebo-treated patients in the entire groups or those with proven pneumococcal meningitis.[40] The results of this study and the previous report in children from Malawi indicate that corticosteroids are neither beneficial nor indicated in patients with bacterial meningitis and coinfection with HIV.

One concern with the concomitant use of dexamethasone and vancomycin for possible highly penicillin-resistant *S. pneumoniae* is the reduction of vancomycin concentration in the CSF, as shown in animal models.[41] However, vancomycin concentration in CSF can be increased with larger doses in the presence of corticosteroids.[42] In a small study of children with bacterial meningitis vancomycin concentration was not reduced by corticosteroids when compared to historical controls.[43]

Thus the question arises: should dexamethasone be used for all adults with bacterial meningitis? Predicated on evidence-based medicine the answer would be no, as recommended by IDSA guidelines[18] and the editorial by Turkel and Scheld,[26] where dexamethasone is advised only for pneumococcal meningitis in adults. However, lack of proof does not mean lack of benefit and clearly further studies are needed in moderate to severe meningococcal meningitis. This is unlikely to be accomplished in developed countries but trials could be conducted in the "meningitis belt" of Africa (Sub-Sahara), where epidemics of meningococcal meningitis occur relatively frequently and in Saudi Arabia during the religious observation of the Hajj, when outbreaks commonly occur. In the meantime should dexamethasone be avoided in meningococcal meningitis as advised by current guidelines? It could be argued that the use of dexamethasone for 2 days in moderate to severe meningococcal meningitis is not unreasonable in view of the extremely low risk of adverse event, and the fact that there is no evidence to suggest that there are differences in biological mechanisms and pathogenesis between *N. meningococcus* and *S. pneumoniae* or *H. influenzae* meningitis. Therefore in the meantime the decision in these circumstances should be judged on an individual basis by the clinician.

## 1.1 Bacterial Meningitis

**Table 1.3** Pooled data for meningococcal meningitis

| Total | Placebo<br>N = 236 | Dex<br>N = 230 | P-Valve<br>Fisher's<br>Exact Test | Relative Risk<br>(95% CI) |
|---|---|---|---|---|
| Deaths | 13(5.5%) | 11(4.8%) | 0.8349 | 0.8616 (0.3778–1.9647) |
| Deafness | 15(6.4%) | 8(3.5%) | 0.1995 | 0.5309 (0.2207–1.2775) |
| Permanent Sequelae | 14(5.9%) | 9(3.9%) | 0.3938 | 0.6596 (0.2739–1.5228) |
| Combined death/ unfavorable outcome | 42(17.8%) | 28(12.2%) | 0.0936 | 0.6403 (0.3817–1.0739) |

To achieve a more accurate estimate of the value of corticosteroids in meningococcal meningitis I have pooled the data from five more recent larger randomized (with or without placebo) trials[30,31,33,34,36] in both adults and children, as there are insufficient numbers to analyze according to adult status only. The main criteria for inclusion are: (i) prospective, randomized, studies using dexamethasone versus placebo, or no adjunctive therapy (one study); (ii) sufficient information to assess response according to individual pathogens. Types of antibiotics were not assessed as *N. meningococci* are generally susceptible to all first-line therapy used in bacterial meningitis. Timing of dexamethasone was not assessed as this would affect the power of the analysis by having subgroups.

The results are shown in Table 1.3. This analysis suggests that dexamethasone may have some benefit in reducing deafness and permanent sequelae in meningococcal meningitis, and future studies would require more than 600 cases per arm to prove or disprove the value of corticosteroids. However, a smaller sample size maybe sufficient, if future studies assess the benefit of dexamethasone in moderate to severe disease only.

Although it is ideal and the aim should be to administer dexamethasone just before or at the time of empiric antimicrobial therapy, it is still reasonable to use corticosteroids in moderate to severe bacterial meningitis if there was an oversight in giving the first dose of antibiotic a few hours before. Even though the guidelines by IDSA recommends otherwise and the largest prospective randomized study in adults supports their recommendation, no randomized controlled study was specifically designed to address this issue. A recent prospective uncontrolled study of a large cohort on community bacterial meningitis attempted to answer this question as part of a tertiary analysis. In a recent report by van de Beek et al.[11] when corticosteroids were administered before antibiotics an unfavorable outcome was less likely than in episodes of bacterial meningitis where corticosteroids were administered after antibiotics (3 of 24 (12%) versus 48 of 94 (51%)), $p = 0.001$. However, only 118 episodes (17%) of the cohorts received corticosteroids and these patients overall had the worst outcome (including bias for severely ill with advanced disease receiving corticosteroids). Thus there is lack of proof that delayed corticosteroids (after antimicrobial initiation) is of no benefit in bacterial meningitis.

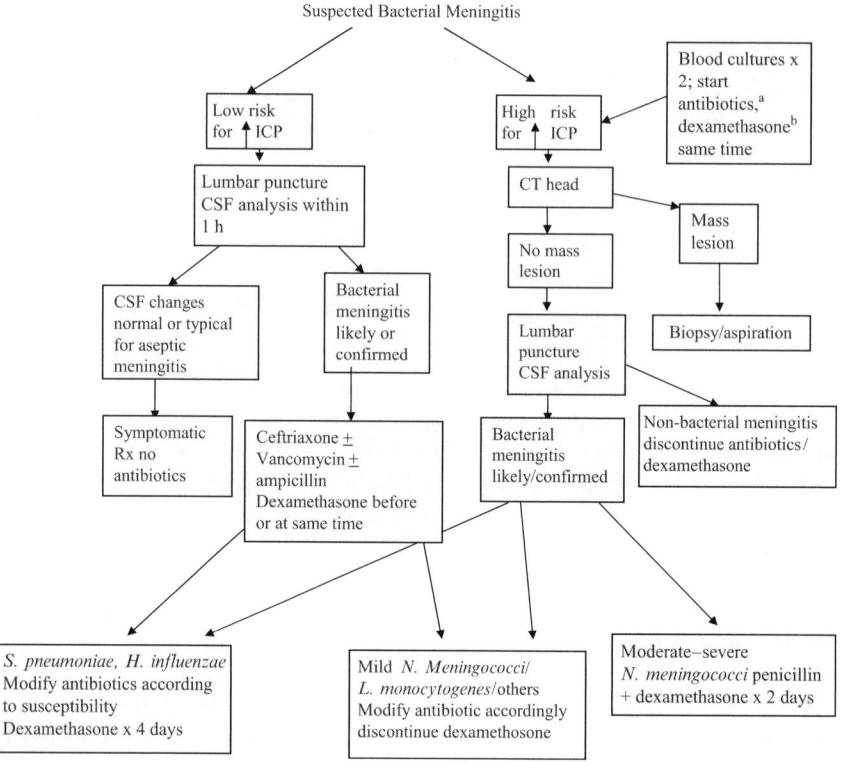

**Fig. 1.1** An algorithm for the diagnosis and management of suspected bacterial meningitis is shown above. CSF = cerebrospinal fluid; CT computerized tomography ICP = increased intracranial pressure A – choice of antibiotics may depend on age, immunological state, incidence of highly penicillin-resistant *S. pneumoniae* in the specific region. B – for adults dexamethasone is given at 10 mg every 6 h; for children 0.15 mg/kg every 6 h

Figure 1.1 outlines an algorithm for the investigation and management of suspected bacterial meningitis; my recommendation also differs from the IDSA guidelines for choice of antimicrobial agents in certain areas. When *N. meningitis* is isolated penicillin G should be the drug of choice for fully susceptible strains. Although penicillin-resistant *N. meningitides* are extremely rare there have been increasing reports in several countries of decreased penicillin-susceptible (low level resistant) strains with MIC of >0.125 to <1.0 μg/mL. Moreover, clinical experience in children with meningococcal meningitis in Spain demonstrated higher mortality and sequelae in children with relative penicillin resistance (9/15 = 60%) as compared to those with full penicillin susceptibility (69/215 = 32%) ($p = 0.04$).[44] Hence, progressive reductions of susceptibility to penicillin among *N. meningitis* isolates in several countries have resulted in ceftriaxone being used as initial antimicrobial choice. Table 1.4 shows areas where decreased penicillin-susceptible *N. meningococci* are reported.[45–55] The other area of difference or contention is the

**Table 1.4** *N. Meningococci* with reduced penicillin susceptibility (>0.125 μg/mL)

| Country | No. isolates | Prevalence | MIC | Reference |
|---|---|---|---|---|
| France 1999–2002 | 2167 | 31.2% | >0.125 <1.0 μg/mL | Antignar et al.[43] |
| Portugal 2000–2001 | 116 | 11.2% | | Canica et al.[44] |
| Italy 199–2001 | 270 | 3% | 0.09–0.19 μg/mL | Mastrantonio et al.[45] |
| Turkey 2000–2001 | 30 | 43% | 0.09–1.0 μg/mL | Punar et al.[46] |
| Poland 1995–2000 | 166 | 27% 0.6% (1) | 0.1–<1.0 μg 2.0 μg | Gozybowska and Tyski[47] |
| Croatia 1996–1999 | 19 | 16% | 0.12 | Boras et al.[48] |
| North America 1998–1999 | 53 | 30.2% | 0.09–0.25 μg/mL | Richter et al.[49] |
| Spain 1986–1997 | 498 | 9.1–71.4% | ≤0.5 μg/mL | Latorre et al.[50] |
| Venezuela 1994 | 29 | 86.2% | >0.12 μg/mL | Toro et al.[51] |
| Thailand 1994–1999 | 36 | 16.6% | 0.125 μg/mL | Pancharoen et al.[52] |
| Senegal 1999 | 22 | 0 | – | Sow et al.[53] |
| Ontario, Canada 2000–2006 | 363 | △ 8% | ≥0.25 μg/mL | Unpublished* |

*Personal communication with Dr. Frances Jamieson and colleagues (Ontario Public Health Laboratory)

routine use of vancomycin for all *S. pneumoniae* meningitis until susceptibility is available. Although this is a reasonable recommendation for some areas (usually countries with high rate of high penicillin-resistant strains), it is an overkill in most other countries and have contributed to overuse and possible increase in vancomycin-resistant enterococci and *Staphylococcus aureus*. In fact, in our institution most patients receiving vancomycin for meningitis do not even have a bacterial infection (unpublished data). In the province of Ontario, Canada, the rates of all penicillin-resistant *S. pneumoniae* was about 12–13% in the past 3 years (2003–2005), but highly penicillin-resistant strains accounted for just over 4%. During the same time period the rate of Ceftriaxone resistance (>2 μg/mL) was just about 2% (Canadian Bacterial Surveillance Network, http://microbiology.mtsinai.on.ca(. However, of 5,599 isolates collected during 1988–2005 from normally sterile sites (CSF, blood, pleural effusion, etc.) only 80 (1.43%) were resistant to ceftriaxone (by the meningitis concentration cut-off level).

## 1.2 Adjunctive Therapy in Tuberculous Meningitis

### 1.2.1 Background

Tuberculous meningitis is a relatively uncommon condition in developed countries, but in developing nations it is a significant clinical problem with high morbidity and mortality despite effective chemotherapy. In Sub-Saharan Africa, mainly because of the burden of the Acquired Immunodeficiency Syndrome (AIDS) epidemic, tuberculosis has become the predominant bacterial cause of meningitis. In countries with high incidence of tuberculosis this complication usually occurs in young children 3–6 months after primary infection. Whereas, in countries with low incidence of tuberculosis, tuberculous meningitis most commonly occurs from reactivation of dormant subcortical or meningeal focus in adults. In developed countries most cases of tuberculous meningitis are seen in immigrants from high incidence areas, patients with AIDS or other immunosuppression, drug abusers, and alcohol dependency.

Early studies on the pathogenesis of tuberculous meningitis in animals[56] indicated that the meninges was not easily infected by hematogenous spread. In postmortem studies there was always a subcortical or meningeal focus which released organisms in the subarachnoid space,[57] presumably from reactivation of dormant granulomas due to local or systemic decrease in immunity. This rupture of granulomatous material with bacilli in the subarachnoid space results in a dense gelatinous exudate. This dense granulomatous reaction was most pronounced in the interpendular fossa and suprasellar region anteriorly, and could extend throughout the prepontive cistern and surround the spinal cord.[57] The thick envelop of exudates surrounding arteries and cranial nerves, could block the flow of CSF at the tentorial opening causing hydrocephalus. Moreover, direct invasion of the vessels could lead to infective vasculitis resulting in infarctions of vertebrobasilar vessels, and the perforating branches of the middle cerebral artery. Hence the consequences of tuberculous meningitis may include hemiplegia, quadriplegia, cranial nerve palsies, and chronic hydrocephalus.

The clinical features of tuberculous meningitis most commonly are gradual and insidious in onset, with fluctuating fever, headaches, personality changes, weight loss, malaise, vomiting, and eventually convulsions and coma if undetected for sometime. The typical CSF changes include lymphocytic or mononuclear cell pleocytosis, high protein, and hypoglycorrhachia. The organisms are rarely seen on fluorescent auramine rhodamine or Ziehl-Neelsen stain, and although molecular techniques (polymerase chain reaction [PCR]) are more sensitive, cultures of a large volume of CSF (10–30 mL) is the most sensitive diagnostic technique. Hence, treatment is often instituted based on the typical clinical picture, exclusion of fungal, or other meningitis and a positive Mantoux test. The Mantoux test can be negative in severely ill or immunosuppressed subjects, and the chest radiograph may show changes compatible with active or remote tuberculosis in 50–80%.[58] In a minority of cases the clinical picture can be more acute with rapid progression (presumably from release of large amount of organisms and caseous material in the subarachnoid space or from immunosuppression), and the CSF changes may resemble other pyogenic bacterial meningitis, with predominant neutrophils with or without a low CSF glucose. In 10–20% of early cases the CSF glucose concentration can be normal (>2.2 mmol/L) and the protein less than 0.8 gm/L or less than 0.45 gm/L and typically the CSF cell count is <300 cells/μL.

## *1.2.2 Treatment of Tuberculous Meningitis*

Treatment of suspected tuberculous meningitis is often started before confirmation of the diagnosis to prevent complications and progression, as CSF cultures may take 4–8 weeks to confirm or exclude the diagnosis. The management includes standard antituberculous chemotherapy with isoniazid, rifampin, pyrazinamide, and ethambutol or streptomycin for the initial 2 months, until susceptibility is available. For patients with coma or stupor, medications are given via nasogastric tube and parenteral agents such as streptomycin or kanamycin should be considered. In some countries, including Canada, isoniazid and rifampin parenteral preparations can be obtained through special access program of the Health Protection Branch, Federal Government. For *M. tuberculosis* fully susceptible to the first-line agents isoniazid and rifampin would be continued for at least 4 more months (World Health Organization recommendation), but other guidelines (including IDSA and American Thoracic Society) recommend continuation for 6–8 months.[58] Hydrocephalus is most often noncommunicating and if symptomatic is best managed by ventricular-peritoneal shunt. Occasionally, hydrocephalus is communicating and medical management with furosemide and acetazolamide maybe tried first for 2 weeks.

Death or severe neurological deficits have been reported in more than half of those affected despite antituberculous.[59,60] Attenuation of the inflammatory response to improve outcome have been considered and used for decades. Early studies suggested that corticosteroids could reduce CSF inflammatory changes and time to recovery, but were too small to show survival benefit.[61–63] Randomized trials conducted in Egypt[64] and South Africa[65] showed that corticosteroids improved survival and reduced neurological sequelae in severe disease of children.

A subsequent meta-analysis of randomized controlled trials of corticosteroid for tuberculous meningitis was reported.[66] In this analysis 595 cases (158 adults) met the inclusion criteria in six trials, and the results suggested that corticosteroids reduced the risk of death in children (RR 0.77; 95% CI, 0.62–0.96), but not in patients over 14 years of age (RR 0.96; 95% CI, 0.50–1.84). Moreover, there was no data on patients coinfected with HIV infection, thus further studies in adults were recommended.

In a recent randomized, double blind, placebo-controlled trial[67] in Vietnam, 545 adolescents and adults were enrolled to study the adjunctive value of dexamethasone in tuberculous meningitis. Forty-four (16.1%) in the corticosteroid group and 54 (19.9%) in the placebo group were HIV-infected. Patients were stratified on entry according to a severity of illness grading (modification of the British Medical Research Council criteria; Grade I representing milder disease, Grade II moderate, and Grade III more severe disease). Patients with Grade II or III disease received intravenous dexamethasone for 4 weeks (0.4 mg/kg/day for 1 week, 0.3 mg/kg/day for week 2, 0.2 mg/kg/day for week 3, and 0.1 mg/kg/day for week 4), and then oral treatment for 4 weeks, starting at 4 mg/day and decreasing by 1 mg per week. Patients with grade I disease received 2 weeks of intravenous dexamethasone

(0.3 mg/kg/day for week 1 and 0.2 mg/kg/day for week 2), then 4 weeks of oral therapy (0.1 mg/kg/day for week 3, then 3 mg/day decreasing by 1 mg each week). Treatment with dexamethasone was associated with reduced risk of death (RR, 0.69; 95% CI, 0.52–0.92, $p = 0.01$).[67] The treatment effect was consistent across subgroups by disease severity grade, and by HIV status, there were fewer serious adverse events in the corticosteroid group (9% versus 16.6%, $p = 0.02\%$); surprisingly, steroids did not reduce the morbidity or proportion of severely disabled in the survivors (18.2% versus 13.8% in the placebo arm, $p = 0.27$).[67] Thus, dexamethasone should be used in all cases of tuberculous meningitis despite age, severity of illness, and HIV status.

## 1.3 Adjunctive Therapy in Fungal Meningitis

### *1.3.1 Background*

Fungal meningitis are very rare in the normal population and *Cryptococcus neoformans* is the most common form of fungal meningitis. Before the AIDS epidemic, cryptococcal meningitis was seen occasionally in patients on chronic corticosteroids, organ transplantations, lymphoma, leukemias, and rarely in elderly subjects without these conditions. Since the advent of AIDS 80–90% of cryptococcal meningitis occurred in HIV-infected subjects, and before highly active antiretroviral therapy (HAART) approximately 5–10% of the patients developed disseminated cryptococcus in developed countries.[68] The incidence has declined dramatically in developed countries with the use of effective HAART, and the majority of cases are in advanced AIDS with CD4 lymphocyte count of <50 cell/μL.

Most patients with cryptococcal meningitis present a subacute clinical picture with fever, malaise, and headache, with photophobia and neck stiffness occurring in only one fourth to one third of patients. Encephalopathic symptoms (altered level of consciousness, personality changes, and lethargy) were seen in some patients with advanced disease. Although classically cryptococcal meningitis CSF changes are identical to tuberculous meningitis, in AIDS patients the changes are less prominent with mildly elevated protein and lymphocytes, normal or slightly low glucose and on occasion normal parameters but with numerous organisms seen on India ink stain (80% positive in HIV subjects), or positive cryptococcal antigen. The cryptococcal antigen in blood (90% sensitive) or CSF (>95% sensitive) is the most sensitive and rapid diagnostic test.

Cryptococcal meningitis is frequently associated with elevated intracranial pressure, and the opening pressure in the CSF is often elevated above 200 mm of water in up to 75% of patients. Elevated ICP of >250 mm $H_2O$ correlate with higher pathogen burden, greater incidence of cranial neuropathies, and decreased survival.[69] Initial CSF pressure correlated with papilledema, impaired hearing, pathological reflexes, delayed clearance of the organism from the CSF, and

## 1.3 Adjunctive Therapy in Fungal Meningitis

increased mortality at 2 weeks and long-term clinical outcome.[69] Treatment of elevated ICP is aimed at decompressing the fluid, either by ventricular drainage or by medical means, such as treatment with acetazolamide, mannitol, or corticosteroids. Although dexamethasone has proven benefits in acute bacterial and tuberculous meningitis there is no good evidence of benefit in cryptococcal meningitis. In the nonranomdized observational study[69] patients receiving methylprednisone or dexamethasone (for reasons other than suppression of amphotericin B infusion reaction), had lower successful clinical response (27/41 or 66%) at 2 weeks, versus 86% of 191 patients not receiving high-dose steroids ($p = 0.001$). Moreover, 20% of the patients treated with corticosteroids died within 2 weeks versus 3% not receiving steroids, $p < 0.001$. The mycological failure rate (positive CSF culture at 2 weeks) was also higher in the patients treated with corticosteroids, 59% versus 38%, $p = 0.001$.[69] However, inherent biases exist in this type of study, such as patients with more severe disease were likely to have received corticosteroids. As a result of this observational study, large-volume (unspecified) CSF drainage was recommended (by repeated lumbar puncture or lumbar drainage) in patients with opening pressures >250 mm $H_2O$, and avoidance of high doses of corticosteroids.[70] It should be noted that there was insignificant number of patients treated with acetazolamide, furosemide, or mannitol to assess alternate medical management of high ICP.

Since these recommendations, adopted by the IDSA practice guidelines for management of cryptococcal meningitis, have been published,[70] the adherence have been very variable with less compliance in North America than in Asia. In two hospitals in Washington DC, of 26 patients with cryptococcal meningitis only 13 (50%) had CSF opening pressure measured, and major deviations from the IDSA guidelines were observed in 14 (54%).[71] In contrast Thai investigators have been consistent in managing elevated ICP in cryptococcal meningitis along IDSA guidelines.[72] Furthermore, a recent study in Thailand demonstrated no benefit with the use of acetazolamide for management of increased ICP in patients with cryptococcal meningitis.[73] Similarly, in Taiwan a standardized protocol for management of cryptococcal meningitis have been adopted since 1994.[74] Patients with initial CSF opening pressure ≥350 mm $H_2O$ had lumbar puncture daily to drain 20–30 mL of CSF until the pressure was <350 mm $H_2O$. Later lumbar puncture was performed every 2–3 days until the pressure measured <200 mm $H_2O$, followed by one lumbar puncture a week until the patients discharged from hospital.

The patients underwent multiple lumbar punctures and received glycerol or mannitol for increased ICP. Nine of 35 patients had extremely high ICP, a lumbar drain was placed in one and another underwent ventriculoperitoneal (VP) shunt. The median number of lumbar punctures performed was 6 (range 1–29). Except for two who died from increased ICP and the patient with VP shunt placement, in the remaining patients ICP decreased to <350 mm $H_2O$ after a median of 3.5 lumbar punctures.[74] Only one of these patients had a relapse after treatment with amphotericin B and oral flucytosine. See Tables 1.5 and 1.6 for IDSA guidelines of management of cryptococcal disease in HIV-infected subjects.

**Table 1.5** Treatment options for cryptococcal disease in HIV-infected patient (Adapted from Saag et al.,[70] With permission of the publisher)

| Cryptococcal disease, treatment regimen | Reference | Class |
|---|---|---|
| Pulmonary | | |
| Mild to moderate symptoms or culture positive specimen from this site[a] | | |
| Fluconazole, 200–400 mg/day, lifelong | 15 | AII |
| Itraconazole, 200–400 mg/day, lifelong[b] | 9 | CII |
| Fluconazole, 400 mg/day plus flucytosine 100–150 mg/kg/day for 10 weeks | 15 | CII |
| CNS | | |
| Induction/consolidation: amphotericin B, 0.7–1 mg/kg/day plus flucytosine, 100 mg/kg/day for 2 weeks, then fluconazole, 400 mg/day for a minimum | 11,32 | AI |
| Amphotericin B, 0.7–1 mg/kg/day plus 5 flucytosine 100 mg/kg/day for 6–10 weeks | 13,18,29 | BI |
| Amphotericin B, 0.7–1 mg/kg/day for 6–10 weeks | 13 | CI |
| Fluconazole, 400–800 mg/day for 10–12 weeks | 13,18,36,37 | CI |
| Itraconazole, 400 mg/day for 10–12 weeks[b] | 9,33 | CII |
| Fluconazole, 400–800 mg/day plus flucytosine, 100–150 mg/kg/day for 6 weeks | 16,28 | CII |
| Lipid formulation of amphotericin B, 3–6 mg/kg/day for 6–10 weeks[c,b] | 12,19,20 | CII |
| Maintenance: | | |
| Fluconazole, 200–400 mg po q.d., lifelong[d] | 17,23,24 | AI |
| Itraconazole, 200 mg po bid, lifelong[d] | 9,17 | BI |
| Amphotericin B, 1 mg/kg iv 1–3 times/week, lifelong[d] | 24 | CI |

Among patients receiving prolonged (>2 weeks) or flucytosine therapy, renal function should be monitored frequently and dose adjustment should be made via use of a nomogram, or preferably, through monitoring of serum flucytosine levels. Serum flucytosine levels should be measured 2 h after dose with optimal levels between 30 and 80 μg/mL.

[a] The clinician must determine whether to follow lung therapeutic regimen or CNS (disseminated) regimen for treatment of infection in other body sites. When other disseminated sites of infection are noted or the patient is at risk for disseminated infection, it is important to rule out CNS disease.
[b] Not formally approved by the US Food and Drug Administration for use in cryptococcal disease.
[c] Experience with lipid preparations of amphotericin B are limited in treatment of cryptococcal meningitis with HIV infection, but with present experience, AmBisome 4 mg/kg would be the choice for amphotericin B substitution in this infection.
[d] Unclear whether secondary prophylaxis may be discontinued in patients with prolonged success with highly active antiretroviral therapy.

## 1.4 Future Directions

Adjunctive therapy has proven effective in acute pyogenic, tuberculous, and fungal meningitis. However, further research is needed to refine the indications and timing of administration in some areas. In community-acquired meningitis such as in *S. pneumoniae* and *H. influenzae* infections, dexamethasone for 2–4 days starting before or at the initial dose of antimicrobial is the accepted standard. However, in

## 1.4 Future Directions

**Table 1.6** Management of elevated intracranial pressure in HIV-infected patients with cryptococcal disease (Adapted from Saag et al.[70] With permission of the publisher)

| Assessment | Management | Class |
| --- | --- | --- |
| Before treatment | | |
| Focal neurological signs, obtunded | Radiographic imaging before lumbar puncture to identify mass lesions that may contraindicate | B-II |
| Normal opening pressure | Initiate medical therapy, with follow-up lumbar puncture at 2 weeks | A-I |
| Opening pressure >250 mm $H_2O$ | Lumbar drainage sufficient to achieve closing pressure $\leq 200$ mm $H_2O$ or 50% of initial opening pressure | A-II |
| Follow-up for elevated pressure | Repeated drainage daily until opening pressure is stable | A-II |
| If elevated pressure persists: | Lumbar drain | B-II |
| | Ventriculoperitoneal shunt | B-II |
| | Corticosteroids: not recommended for HIV-infected patients, and evidence of benefit for HIV-negative patients is not established | C-III |

many cases antimicrobials are started first either by another referring center or inadvertently by emergency physicians, and the value of later initiation of corticosteroids need to be defined in future trials. As discussed earlier, further studies are needed in moderate to severe meningococcal meningitis as to the benefit of dexamethasone in survival and sequelae. Although corticosteroids should now be considered standard adjunctive therapy in tuberculous meningitis (children and adults), areas for further evaluation include duration of steroid therapy (i.e., 1 versus 2 months), and the need for intravenous versus oral dexamethasone in the first month.

Oral glycerol (a trivalent alcohol and osmotic diuretic) has previously been used to reduce raised tissue pressure in neurosurgery and neurology and may be useful in bacterial meningitis. Oral glycerol as adjunctive therapy in acute bacterial meningitis needs further assessment in larger trials in developing countries, as a recent randomized trial in Latin America showed significant reduction of neurological sequelae and death with oral glycerol alone or combined with dexamathasone in children.[75] This is important since steroids have not been shown to be beneficial in subjects in developing nations, with high rates of malnutrition and AIDS and acute bacterial meningitis.

In cryptococcal meningitis attempts should be made to standardize the volume of CSF to be removed and frequency of lumbar puncture for increased ICP (as in the Taiwan protocol), as there is unlikely to be any definitive randomized trail; however, future randomized trials could compare the utility and efficacy of repeated lumbar puncture versus temporary lumbar drainage for control of ICP.

# References

1. Turkel, A. R., Scheld, W. M. (1993). Pathogenesis and pathophysiology of bacterial meningitis. Clin. Microbiol. Rev. 6:118–136.
2. Bryan, J. P., de Silva, H. R., Tavares, A., Rocha, H., Scheld, W. M. (1991). Etiology and mortality of bacterial meningitis in North Eastern Brazil. Rev. Infect. Dis. 12:128–135.
3. Scheld, W. M. (1990). Meningococcal diseases. In: Warren, K. S., Mahmoud A. A. F. (eds). Tropical and Geographical Medicine, 2nd ed. New York: McGraw-Hill, pp. 798–814.
4. Durand, M. L., Calderwood, S. B., Weber, D. J., Miller, S. I., Southwick, F. S., Caviness, V. S., Swartz, M. N. (1993). Acute bacterial meningitis in adults – a review of 493 episodes. N. Engl. J. Med. 328:21–28.
5. Klein, J., Feigin, R., Mc Cracken, G. (1993). Report of the task force on diagnosis and management of meningitis. Pediatr. Infect. Dis. J. 326:42–47.
6. Wolff, A., Brown, S. (1987). Demographics of meningitis induced hearing impairment: Implications for immunization of children against *Haemophils influenzae* type B. Am. Ann. Deaf. 131:26–31.
7. Finitzo-Hieber, T., Simhadri, R., Gieber, J. (1981). Abnormalities of the auditory brainstem response in post-meningitic infants and children. Int. J. Pediatr. Otorhinolaryngol. 3:275–286.
8. Dodge, P., Davis, H., Feigin, R. D. Holmes, S. J., Kaplan, S. L., Jubeliner, D. P., Stechenberg, B. W., Hirsch, S. K. (1984). Prospective evaluation of hearing impairment as a sequelae of acute bacterial meningitis. N. Engl. J. Med. 311:869–874.
9. O'Connell, J. E. A. (1946). The clinical signs of meningeal irritation. Brain 69:9–21.
10. Brody, I. A., Wilkins, R. H. (1969). The signs of Kernig and Brudznski. Arch. Neurol. 21: 215–218.
11. Van de Beek, D., de Gans, J., Spanjaard, L., Weisfeldt, M., Reitsma, J. B., Vermeulen, M. (2004). Clinical features and prognostic factors in adults with bacterial meningitis. N. Engl. J. Med. 351:1849–1859.
12. Altia, J., Hatala, R., Cook, D. J., Wong, J. G. (1999). Does this adult patient have acute meningitis? JAMA 282:175–181.
13. Uchihara, T., Tsukagoshi, H. (1991). Jolt accentuation of headache: the most sensitive sign of CSF pleocytosis. Headache 31:167–171.
14. Ashwal, S., Perkin, R. M., Thompson, J. R., Schneider, S., Tomasi, L. G. (1994). Bacterial meningitis in children: current concepts of neurologic management. Curr. Problems Pediatr. 24:267–284.
15. Korein, J., Cravisto, H., Leicach, M. (1959). Reevaluation of lumbar puncture: a study of 129 patients with papilledema or intracranial hypertension. Neurology 9:290–297.
16. Horwitz, S. J., Boxerbaum, B., O'Bell, J. (1980). Cerebral herniation in bacterial meningitis in childhood. Ann. Neurol. 7:524–528.
17. Hasbun, R., Abrahams, J., Jekel, J., Quagliarello, V. J. (2001). Computed tomography of the head before lumbar puncture in adults with suspected meningitis. N. Engl. J. Med. 345:1727–1733.
18. Tunkel, A. R., Hartman, B. J., Kaplan, S. L. Kaufman, B. A., Roos, K. L., Scheld, W. M. (2004). Practice guidelines for the management of bacterial meningitis. Clin. Infect. Dis. 39:1267–1284.
19. Bonadio, W. A. (1997). Medical-legal considerations related to symptom duration and patient outcome after bacterial meningitis. Am. J. Emerg. Med. 15:420–423.
20. Aronin, S. I., Peduzzi, P., Quagliarello, V. J. (1998). Community acquired bacterial meningitis. Risk stratification for adverse clinical outcome and effect of antibiotic timing. Ann. Intern. Med. 129:862–869.
21. Lu, C. H., Huang, C. R., Chang, W. N., Chang, C. J., Cheng, B. C., Lee, P. Y., Lin, M. W., Chang H. W. (2002). Community acquired bacterial meningitis in adults: the epidemiology,

# References

timing of appropriate antimicrobial therapy, and prognostic factors. Clin. Neurol. Neuro. Surg. 104:352–358.
22. Miner, J. R., Heegaard, W., Mapes, A., Biros, M. (2001). Presentation, time to antibiotics, and mortality of patients with bacterial meningitis at an urban county medical center. J. Emerg. Med. 21:387–392.
23. Thomas, K. E., Hasbun, R., Jekel, J., Quagliarello, V. J. (2002). The diagnostic accuracy of Kernig's sign, Brudzinski sign and nuchal rigidity in adults with suspected meningitis. Clin. Infect. Dis. 35:46–52.
24. Gururaj, V. J., Russo, R. M., Allen, J. E., Herszkowicz, R. (1973). To tap or not to tap – what are the best indicators for performing a lumbar puncture in an out patient child? Clin. Pediatr. 12:488–493.
25. Feigin, R. D., McCracken, G. H., Klein, J. O. (1992). Diagnosis and management of meningitis. Pediatr. Infect. Dis. J. 11:785–814.
26. Turkel, A. R., Scheld, W. M. (1995). Acute bacterial meningitis. Lancet 346:1675–1680.
27. Saez-Llorens, X., Ramilo, O., Manstafa, M. M., Mertsola, J., McCracken, G. H. (1990). Molecular pathophysiology of bacterial meningitis: current concepts and therapeutic implications. J. Pediatr. 116:671–684.
28. American Academic of Pediatrics committee on Infectious Diseases. (1990). Dexamethasone therapy for bacterial meningitis in infants and children. Pediatrics 86:130–133.
29. The meningitis working party of the British Pediatric Immunology and Infectious Disease Group. (1992). Should we use dexamethasone in meningitis? Arch. Dis. Child. 67:324–326.
30. Lebel, M. H., Freij, B. J., Syrogiannopoulos, G. A., Chrane, D. F., Hoyt, M. J., Stewart, S. M., Kennard, B. D., Olsen, K. D., McCraken, G. H. (1998). Dexamethasone therapy for bacterial meningitis: results of two double-blind placebo controlled trials. N. Engl. J. Med. 319: 964–971.
31. Girgis, N. I., Farid, Z., Mikhail, I. A., Farrag, I., Sultan, Y., Kilpatrick, M. E. (1989). Dexamethasone treatment for bacterial meningitis in children and adults. Pediatr. Infect. Dis. J. 8:848–851.
32. McIntyre, P. B., Berkey, C. S., King, S. M., Schaad, U. B., Kilpi, T., Kanra, G. Y., Odio Perez, C. M. (1997). Dexamethasone as adjunctive therapy in bacterial meningitis. A meta-analysis of randomized clinical trials since 1988. JAMA 278:925–931.
33. Molyneuz, E. M., Walsh, A. L., Forsyth, H., Membo, M., Mwenechanya, J., Kayira, K., Bwanaisa, L., Njobvu, A., Rogerson, S., Molenga, G. (2002). Dexamethasone treatment in childhood bacterial meningitis in Malawi: a randomized controlled trial. Lancet 360:211–218.
34. McCracken, G. H. Jr., (2002). Rich nations, poor nations, and bacterial meningitis. Lancet 360:183.
35. American Academic of Pediatrics. (2003). Pneumococcal infections. In: Pickering LK (ed). Red book: 2003 report of the committee on Infectious Disease, 26th ed., Elk Grove Village, IL: American Academic of Pediatrics, pp. 490–500.
36. Thomas, R., Le Tulzo, Y., Bouget, J., Camus, C., Michelet, C., Le Corre, P., Bellissant, E., and the Adult Meningitis Steroid Groups (1999). Trial of dexamethasone treatment for severe bacterial meningitis in adults. Intens. Care Med. 8:848–851.
37. Gijwani, D., Kumhar, M. R., Singh, V. B., Chadda V. S., Soni, P. K., Nayak, K. C., Gupta, B. K. (2002). Dexamethasone therapy for bacterial meningitis in adults: a double blind placebo controlled study. Neurol. India 50:63–67.
38. de Gans, J., van de Beek, D., for the European Dexamethasone in Adulthood bacterial meningitis study investigators. (2002). Dexamethasone in adults with bacterial meningitis. N Engl. J. Med. 347:1549–1556.
39. Mai, N. T. H., Chau, T. T. H., Thwaites, G., Chuong, C. V., Sinh, D. X., Nghia, H. D. T., Tuan, P. Q., Phong, N. D., Phu, N. H., Diep, T. S., Chau, N. V. V., Duong, N. M., Campbell, J., Schultsz, C., Parry, C., Torok, M. E., White, N., Chinh, N. T., Hien, T. T., Stepniewska, K., Farrar, J. J. (2007). Dexamethasone in Vietnamese adolescents and adults with bacterial meningitis. N. Engl. J. Med. 357:2431–2440.

40. Scarborough, M., Gordon, S. B., Whitty, C. J. M., French, N., Njalale, Y., Chitani, A., Peto, T. E. A., Lalloo, D. G., Zijlstra, E. E. (2007). Corticosteroids for bacterial meningitis in adults in Sub-Saharan Africa, N. Engl. J. Med. 357:2441–2450
41. Cabellos, C., Martinez-Lucasa, J., Martos, A., Tubau, F., Fernandez, A., Viladrich, P. F., Gudiol, F. (1995). Influence of dexamethasone on efficacy of ceftriaxone and vancomycin therapy in experimental pneumococcal meningitis. Antimicrob. Agents Chemother. 39:2158–2160.
42. Ahmed, A., Jafri, H., Lustar, I., McCoig, C. C., Trujillo, M., Wubbel, L., Shelton, S., McCracken, G. H. (1999). Pharmacodynamics of vancomycin for the treatment of experimental penicillin and cephalosporin – resistant pneumococcal meningitis. Antimicrob. Agents Chemother. 43:876–881.
43. Klugman, K. P., Fried-land, I. R., Bradley, I. S. (1995). Bactericidal activity against cephalosporin-resistant *Streptococcus pneumoniae* in cerebrospinal fluid of children with acute bacterial meningitis. Antimicrob. Agents Chemother. 39:1988–1992.
44. Luaces Cubells, C., Garcia Garcia, J., Roca Martinez, J., Latorre, O. T. (1997). Clinical data in children with meningococcal meningitis in a Spanish hospital. Acta Pediatr. 86:26–29.
45. Antijnac, A., Ducos-Galand, M., Guiyoule, A., Pires, R., Alonso, J. M., Taha, M. K. (2003). *Neisseria meningitidis* strains isolated from invasive infections in France (1999–2002). Phenotypes and antibiotic susceptibility patterns. Clin. Infect. Dis. 37:912–920.
46. Canica, M., Dias, R., Ferreira, E., and Meningococci Study Group. (2004). *Neisseria meningitidis*, 2b: P1.25 with intermediate resistance to penicillin; Portugal. Emerg. Infect. Dis. 10:526–529.
47. Mastrantonio, P., Stefanelli, P., Fazio, C., Sofia, T., Neri, A., La Rosa, G., Marianelli, C., Muscillo, M., Caporali, M. G., Salmaso, S. (2003). Serotype distribution, antibiotic susceptibility, and genetic relatedness of *Neisseria meningitidis* strain recently isolated in Italy. Clin. Infect. Dis. 36:422–428.
48. Punar, M., Eraksoy, H., Cagatay, A. A., Ozsut, H., Kaygusus, A., Calongu, S., Dilmener, M. (2002). *Neisseria meningitidis* with decreased susceptibility to penicillin in Istanbul, Turkey. Scand. J. Infect. Dis. 34:11–13.
49. Grzybowska, W., Tyski, S. (2001). Characteristics of *Neisseria meningitidis* strains isolated from patients with symptoms of meningococcal meningitis in Poland in 1995–2000. Meddycyna Doswiadczalna: Mikrobiolgia. 53:117–132.
50. Boras, A., Popovic, T., Bozinovic, D. (2001). *Neisseria meningitidis* with a decreased sensitivity to penicillin in the Zagreb District. Lijecnicki Vjesnik 123:231–233.
51. Richter, S. S., Gordon, K. A., Rhomberg, P. R., Pfaller, M. A., Jones, R. N. (2001). *Neisseria meningitidis* with decreased susceptibility to penicillin: Report from the sentry antimicrobial surveillance program, North America, 1998–99. Diagn. Microbiol. Infect. Dis. 41:83–88.
52. Latorre, G., Gene, A., Juncosa, T., Munoz, C., Gonzalez-Cuevas, A. (2000). *Neisseria meningitidis*: evolution of penicillin resistance and phenotype in a children's hospital in Barcelona, Spain. Acta Paediat. 89:661–665.
53. Toro, S., Berron, S., de La Fuente, L., Fernandez, S., Franco, E., Leon, L., Vazquez, J. A. (1997). A clone of *Neisseria meningitidis* serogroup C was responsible in 1994 of an unusual high rate of strains with a moderate resistance to penicillin in Caracas (Venezuela). Enfermedades Infect. Microbiol. Clin. 15:414–417.
54. Pacharoen, C., Hongiriwon, S., Swasdichai, K., Puthanakit, T., Tangsathapornpong, A., Lolekha, S., Punpanich, W., Tarunotai, U., Warachit, B., Mekmullica, J., Kosalaraksa, P., Chokephaibulkit, K., Kerdpanuh, A. (2000). Epidemiology of invasive meningococcal disease in 13 government hospitals in Thailand, 1994–1999. Southeast Asian J. Trop. Med. Publ. Health 3:708–711.
55. Sow, A. I., Caugant, D. A., Cisse, M. F., Hoiby, E. A. Samb, A. (2000). Molecular characteristics and susceptibility to antibiotics of serogroup A *Neissearia meningitidis* strains isolated in Senegal in 1999. Scand. J. Infect. Dis. 32:185–187.

# References

56. Rich, A. R., McCorduck, H. A. (1929). An enquiry concerning the role of allergy, immunity and other factors of importance in the pathogenesis of human tuberculosis. Bull. Johns Hopkins Hosp. 44:273–382.
57. Idem. (1993). The pathogenesis of human tuberculosis meningitis. Bull. Johns Hopkins Hosp. 52:5–37.
58. Donald, P. R., Schoeman, J. F. (2004). Tuberculous meningitis (Perspective). N. Engl. J. Med. 351:1719–1720.
59. Girgis, N. I., Sultan, Y., Farid, Z., Mansour, M. M., Erian, M. W., Hanna, L. S., Mateczun, A. J. (1998). Tuberculous meningitis, Abassia Fever Hospital-Naval Research Unit No. 3 – Cairo, Egypt, from 1976 to 1996. Am. J. Trop. Med. Hyg. 58:28–34.
60. Hosoghu, S., Geyik, M. F., Balik, I. (2002). Predictors of outcome in patients with tuberculous meningitis. Int. J. Tuber. Lung Dis. 6:64–70.
61. Shane, S. J., Riley, C. (1953). Tuberculous meningitis: combined therapy with cortisone and antimicrobial agents. N. Engl. J. Med. 249:829–834.
62. Ashby, M., Grant, H. (1955). Tuberculous meningitis treated with cortisone. Lancet 268: 65–66.
63. O'Toole, R. D., Thornton, G. F., Mukherjee, M. K., Nath, R. L. (1969). Dexamethasone in tuberculous meningitis: relationship of cerebrospinal fluid effects to therapeutic efficacy. Ann. Intern. Med. 70:39–48.
64. Girgis, N. I., Farid, Z., Vilpatrick, M. E., Sultan, Y., Mikhail, I. A. (1991). Dexamethasone adjunctive treatment for tuberculous meningitis. Pediatr. Infect. Dis. 10:179–183.
65. Schoeman, J. F., VanZyl, L., E., Laubscher, J. A., Donald, P. R. (1997). Effect of corticosteroids on intracranial pressure computed tomography findings and clinical outcome in young children with tuberculous meningitis. Pediatrics 99:226–231.
66. Prasad, K., Volmink, J., Menon, G. R. (2002). Steroids for treating tuberculous meningitis. Cochrane Database Syst. Rev. 3: CD00224.
67. Thwaites, G. E., Bang, N. D., Dung, W. H., Quy, H. T., Tuong Oanh, D. T., Cam Thoa, N. T., Hien, N. Q., Lan, N. N., Duc, N. H., Tuan, V. N., Hiep, C. H., Hong Chau, T. T., Farrar, J. J. (2004). Dexamethasone for treatment of tuberculous meningitis in adolescents and adults. N. Engl. J. Med. 351:1741–1751.
68. Mirza, S. A., Phelan, M., Rimland, D., Graviss, E., Hamill, R., Brandt, M. E., Gardner, T., Saltah, M., Pone de Leon, G., Baughman, W., Hajjeh, R. A. (2003). The changing epidemiology of cryptococcosis: an update from population based active surveillance in 2 large metropolitan areas, 1992–2000. Clin. Infect. Dis. 36:789–794.
69. Graybill, J. R., Sobel, J., Saag, M., vander Horst, C., Powderly, W., Cloud, G., Riser, L., Hamil, R., Dismukes, W., and the NIAID Mycoses Study Group and AIDS Cooperative Treatment Groups. (2000). Diagnosis and management of increased inracrainal pressure in patients with AIDS and cryptococcal meningitis. Clin. Infect. Dis. 30:47–54.
70. Saag, M. S., Graybill, R. J., Larsen, R. A., Pappas, P. G., Perfect, J. R., Powderly, W. G., Sobel, J. D., Dismukes, W. E. (2000). Practice guidelines for the management of cryptoccal disease. Clin. Infect. Dis. 30:710 717.
71. Shoham, S., Cover, C., Donegan, N., Fulnecky, E., Kumar, P. (2005). *Cryptococcus neoformans* meningitis at 2 hospitals in Washington, D. C. Adherence of health care providers to publish practice guidelines for the management of cryptococcal disease. Clin. Infect. Dis. 40:477–479.
72. Pappas, P. G. (2005). Managing cryptococcal meningitis is about handling the pressure. Clin. Infect. Dis. 40:480–482.
73. Newton, P. N., Thai, L. H., Tip, N. Q. Short, J.M., Chierakul, W., Rajanuwong, A., Pitisuttithum, P., Chasombat, S., Phonrat, B., Meek-A-Nantawat, W., Teaunadi, R., Lalloo, D.G., White, N.J. (2002). A randomized, double-blind, placebo-controlled trail of acetazolamide for the treatment of elevated intracranial pressure in cryptococcal meningitis. Clin. Infect. Dis. 35:769–772.

74. Sun, H. Y., Hung, C. C., Chang, S. C. (2004). Management of cryptococcal meningitis with extremely high intracranial pressure in HIV infected patients. Clin. Infect. Dis. 38:1791–1792.
75. Peltola, H., Roine, I., Fernandez, J., Zavala, I., Ayala, G., Mata, A.G., Arbo, A., Bologna, R., Mino, G., Goyo, J., Lopez, E., de Andrade, S.D., Sarna, S. (2007). Adjuvant glycerol and/or dexamethazone to improve the outcomes of childhood bacterial meningitis; a prospective, randomized, double – blind, place-controlled trial. Clin. Infect Dis. 45:1277–1286.

# Chapter 2
# Emerging Issues in Head and Neck Infections

## 2.1 Current Issues in Sinusitis

### 2.1.1 Background

Sinusitis is a common disorder that is frequently diagnosed in clinical practice and has been diagnosed in more than 30 million people each year in the United States.[1] Inflammation of the nasal and sinus mucosa can arise from various causes and leads to different sequelae. The term rhinosinusitis is more accurate than sinusitis as the nasal and sinus mucosae are contiguous but the latter is more commonly used and entrenched in medical parlance, thus will be used in this chapter. The three most common inciting factors or causes of sinus inflammation (sinusitis) are viral infections, allergies, and bacterial infections. Accumulating evidence over the past decade has indicated that most children and adults with symptoms of sinusitis are treated unnecessarily with antibiotics, as most cases are due to viral infection. This has contributed to the global increase in antibacterial resistance and exposes subjects to unnecessary side effects.

### 2.1.2 Pathophysiology of Sinusitis

The maxillary, frontal, ethmoid, and sphenoid sinuses all drain into the nasal cavity though the ostia (1–3 mm in diameter), see Fig. 2.1. The paranasal sinuses are lined with ciliated epithelium, which produce mucus and actively propels it into the nasal cavity via the ostia. Viral or allergic rhinitis typically precedes sinusitis and sinusitis without rhinitis is rare.[2,3]

A preceding viral upper respiratory tract infection or allergy can increase local inflammatory reaction in the nasopharynx and surrounding contiguous mucosa of the sinuses, from local production of cytokines and other inflammatory mediators. This can result in excessive mucus production, edema, and swelling of the mucosal lining and damage or impairment of the ciliated epithelium, thus, leading to obstruction of the narrow ostia draining the sinuses, which then predispose to

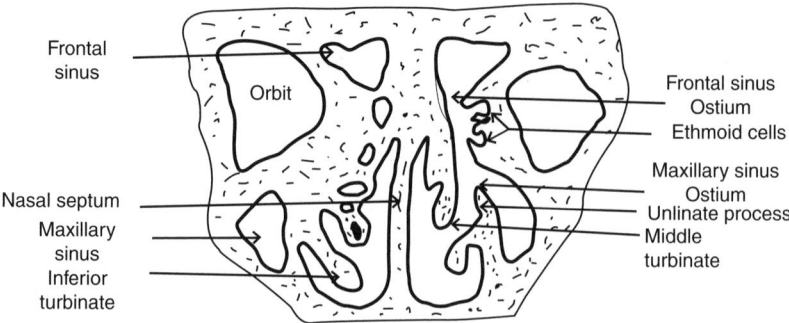

**Fig. 2.1** Paranasal sinuses are shown in the above diagram. The ciliated respiratory epithelium of the nasal passages and the paranasal sinuses are continuous

secondary bacterial infection. Viral upper respiratory tract infection also can decrease function of the macrophages and lymphocytes and allow subsequent bacterial infection of colonizing pathogens of the nasopharynx, such as *Streptococcus pneumoniae* and *Haemophilus influenzae*. Respiratory tract viral infection may enhance bacterial attachment to the mucosa by upregulation of expression of epithelial cell surface receptors, including cell adhesion molecules.[4]

Allergy can lead to reactive rhinosinusitis (as in hay fever) and may predispose to acute bacterial sinusitis. Release of mediators from mast cells during an allergic reaction can cause increased transudation of fluid, and increased proliferation of bacteria, by affecting ciliary transport to clear bacteria and expose epithelial receptors for binding pathogens. In a mouse model, sinusitis allergy augments infection and inflammation when *S. pneumoniae* is instilled.[5]

The symptoms of sinusitis (irrespective of cause) are the consequences of activation of the inflammatory pathways and the parasympathetic nervous system. In a viral upper respiratory tract infection (URTI), symptoms of fever, myalgia, and pharyngitis usually resolve in 5–7 days. But nasal congestion, postnasal drainage, and cough may persist for 2–3 weeks. A change in the color of nasal discharge to yellowish-green indicating purulence does not necessarily indicate bacterial sinusitis.[4] Thus, the clinical determination of when to diagnose and treat an acute bacterial sinusitis has become a diagnostic dilemma. Once bacterial superinfection occurs numerous cytokines and proinflammatory mediators including interleukin (IL) Iβ, IL-2, IL-6, IL-8, TNF-α, histamine, prostaglandins, and leukotriene C4 are upregulated,[6] with worsening of the inflammatory reaction (recurrent fever, pain and pressure, nasopharyngeal stuffiness and increased mucopurulent secretion).

### 2.1.3 Issues in Diagnosis of Bacterial Sinusitis

Sinusitis maybe classified as acute or chronic depending on the duration of symptoms. Acute sinusitis is defined as infection of one or more paranasal sinuses with a bacteria lasting from 1 day to 3–4 weeks. The symptoms are characterized by pain over the affected sinus(es), nasal congestion or obstruction, purulent nasal discharge, and fever. However, there is a great deal of overlap with viral and bacterial infection in symptoms and signs, and imaging of the sinuses such as x-rays and computerized tomography (CT) usually cannot distinguish between viral, allergic, or bacterial sinusitis. Plain film radiographs are valuable for visualizing the frontal and maxillary sinuses but not ethmoid, and have better negative predicative value (in excluding sinusitis) than positive results. Thus radiography only have moderate sensitivity and specificity (76–79%) for sinusitis and since it cannot distinguish between bacterial and viral infection (as only 50% will yield a bacterial pathogen from a sinus tap despite abnormal radiographs),[6] routine x-rays are not recommended for the diagnosis of sinusitis. To exclude ethmoid sinusitis, where the index of suspicion is high, would require CT scan, but this modality is more commonly used for anatomic consideration, i.e., obstruction, polyps, or masses. A clinical diagnosis of acute bacterial sinusitis maybe made when symptoms of nasal congestion, facial pain, or pressure (especially unilateral) and postnasal drip or nasal discharge worsen after 5–7 days or do not improve after 10–14 days,[4] with or without fever and leucocytosis. However, no specific signs or symptoms can reliably predict bacterial infection.[4]

According to the Task Force on Rhinosinusitis or the American Academic of Otolaryngology – Head and Neck Surgery[7], diagnosis of acute sinusitis depends on the presence of at least two major diagnostic factors or one major and two minor factors. The number of diagnostic factors correlates with the likelihood that a bacterial infection is present. However, even the above guidelines would include many cases of viral URTI or influenza, and would be best considered of diagnostic value after 7–14 days of illness. Lindback et al.[8] found four symptoms and signs associated with a CT diagnosis of acute sinusitis to be: (1) second phase in the illness history, (2) purulent rhinorrhea, (3) purulent secretion in the nasal cavity, (4) an erythrocyte sedimentation rate greater than 10 mm. If three of these four signs and symptoms were present, the diagnosis had a specificity of 81% and a sensitivity of 66%. The gold standard used for diagnosis (CT scan) is not specific and cannot distinguish between viral and bacterial infection, and these criteria have not been validated by any large study. Although visualization of purulent drainage on examination is suggestive of acute sinusitis, purulence does not differentiate between viral and bacterial infection.

The diagnosis of acute bacterial sinusitis is even more difficult in children than adults, as some of the chronic features found in adults (facial pain and headaches) are rare in children.[9] The most common complaints are cough and nasal discharge, nonspecific symptoms that are common in viral URTI and allergic rhinitis. Transillumination of the sinuses has limited diagnostic value and depends on the clinicians skill,[10,11] and ultrasound has limited diagnostic usefulness to confirm or exclude sinusitis.[12] Imaging studies are not recommended for the routine diagnosis of uncomplicated sinusitis, but for atypical cases and treatment failures. The diagnostic value of sinus radiographs is limited by poor sensitivity and specificity. Radiologic evidence of sinusitis is common with viral rhinitis.[13] Although opacification or air fluid is suggestive of bacterial infection, it is seen in only 60% of patients with acute sinusitis.[14] Mucosal thickening of the sinuses is a nonspecific finding with specificity as low as 36%.[15]

Chronic sinusitis is defined as symptoms and signs of sinus inflammation lasting longer than 12 weeks, with documented sinus inflammation by imaging techniques at least 4 weeks after appropriate therapy with no intervening acute infection.[16] CT scanning is recommended to identify the sinuses involved and any complications that may exist or predispose to chronic sinusitis (i.e., polyps or obstruction). Table 2.2 summarizes important clinical features and investigations for acute sinusitis.

## 2.1.4 Microbiology of Sinusitis

In acute bacterial sinusitis the causative organisms include *S. pneumoniae* (30–40% of isolates), *H. influenzae* (20–30%), *Moraxella catarrhalis* (12–20%), and *S. pyogenes* (up to 3%).[12] Other pathogens that are found much less frequently include other *Streptococcus* species, *Staphylococcus aureus*, *Neisseria species*, and gram-negative bacilli (coliforms and *Pseudomonas* species are seen in critical care patients with nasopharyngeal catheters or tubes). Fungi are most commonly seen in the immunocompressed hosts or diabetic subjects with ketoacidosis and present more subacutely. These are most commonly due to mucormycosis or aspergillosis.

Sinus puncture with aspiration and culture, under aseptic technique, is the reference standard for identifying etiological agents, but it is mainly a research tool. Nasopharyngeal cultures are not considered reliable and are prone to contamination and misinterpretations. Rigid nasal endoscopes have been used most commonly to obtain cultures from the maxillary sinus in chronic sinusitis, but a recent study in acute sinusitis compared the value to sinus puncture and aspiration.[17] After preparation with decongestant and topical anesthesia a rigid nasal endoscope is advanced to the middle meatus adjacent to the maxillary ostium, where a swab or aspirate could be obtained. When compared to sinus puncture and aspiration endoscopy cultures demonstrated a sensitivity of 85.7%, specificity of 90.6%, positive predictive value of 80%, negative predictive value of 93.5%, and accuracy of 89.1% in 46 patients.[17] Thus, this technique could be used more often for clinical investigations and in clinical practice for unresponsive and complicated cases.

### 2.1.4.1 Chronic Sinusitis

The etiology of chronic sinusitis is more complex and there is a lack of consensus of the pathogenesis. Multiple factors may predispose to chronic sinusitis, and allergy appears to play a prominent role with or without polyps. Other factors include structural abnormalities (outflow obstruction, retention cyst, trauma, previous surgery), irritants (smoke) mucociliary abnormalities, immunodeficiencies (genetic and acquired), aspirin hypersensitivity, and rarely autoimmune disorders (e.g., Wegener's granulomatosis). The role of infectious agents have not been well-defined (although antimicrobials are most commonly used), but may involve bacterial or viral superinfection with exacerbation of inflammatory edema and secretion (synonymous to exacerbation of chronic bronchitis) or through allergy, as in most fungal chronic sinusitis.[18] Bacterial colonization may also enhance the inflammatory process through an allergic process. Bacteria-specific IgE has been identified in 57% of patients with chronic sinusitis as compared to only 10% in subjects with allergic rhinitis.[19] It has also been hypothesized that bacterial superantigens may contribute to chronic sinusitis,[20] but there is little evidence to support this theory.

There are only a few studies that have investigated the microbiological etiology of chronic sinusitis, however, they are often flawed because of recent antibiotic therapy or surgery. Many studies of bacterial flora in chronic sinusitis report a mixed flora of anaerobes and aerobes, including gram-positive and gram-negative organisms, but the results have varied with technique, age, and selection criteria.[18] In general these studies have reported higher prevalence of *S. aureus*, gram-negative coliforms or *Pseudomonas species* (especially in patients with previous surgery or with irrigation), anaerobes, and low virulent organisms such as coagulase-negative staphylococci and *S. viridan* compared to studies in subjects with acute sinusitis. It is very likely that many of these bacteria (such as *S. viridan*, coagulase-negative staphylococci and even *Pseudomonas* species) represent colonization or contamination from adjacent middle meatus and irrigation fluids as studies of healthy adults report similar colonizing bacteria of the middle meatus.[21]

The prevalence of anaerobes in chronic sinusitis has varied from 5% to 67%,[22,23] and this variance may largely be due to techniques in obtaining specimens and culture methods. The prevalence may also be related to the site of the affected sinus. In one study high rates of anaerobes were obtained from maxillary sinus, whereas none were obtained from the ethmoid sinuses (using the same techniques).[24] The results of a recent multicenter study of 150 patients, with properly defined criteria for chronic sinusitis, appropriate sampling by aspiration, assiduous transportation and culture methods for anaerobes, was reported from an internationally renowned laboratory.[25] In this study of adults with maxillary sinusitis 70 (52.2%) aerobic and 64 (47.8%) anaerobic pathogens were recovered at baseline before therapy.[25] The most common isolated anaerobes were *Prevotella* species (31.1%), anaerobic streptococci (21.9%) and *Fusobacterium* species (15.6%). The aerobes most frequently recovered included *Streptococci* species (21.4%), *H. influenzae* (15.7%), *Pseudomonas aeruginosa* (15.7%), and *S. aureus* and *M. catarrhalis* (10.0% each). Recurrences of signs or symptoms of bacterial sinusitis associated with anaerobes were twice as frequent as those associated with aerobes (when anaerobic counts were $\geq 10^3$ cfu/ml).[25] Another study using PCR techniques to analyze aerobic bacteria found that routine culture grew aerobic bacteria in 50% of 64 specimens from 32 patients (maxillary and ethmoid sinuses), whereas PCR detected 62% aerobic bacteria.[26] However, *Staphylococcus epidermidis* was recovered in 39% by PCR which may represent skin contamination or colonization.

There is little debate of the role of bacteria in acute sinusitis, but the function of bacteria in the pathogenesis of chronic sinusitis still remains unresolved. Although there is some evidence that patients with chronic sinusitis treated with antimicrobials have improvements in symptoms, similar to chronic bronchitis or chronic obstructive lung disease, the data are scant. Moreover, occasionally patients develop more serious infectious complications such as brain abscess, osteomyelitis, or extra-dural empyema. However, there is lack of randomized, prospective, placebo-controlled studies.

## 2.1.5 Treatment of Acute Bacterial Sinusitis

The issues facing clinicians with respect to treatment of acute sinusitis include when to initiate antimicrobial therapy, and the most appropriate choice. The point at which viral UTI becomes superinfected with pathogenic bacteria has been determined by a few studies with repeated sinus aspiration. Although duration of symptoms beyond 7 days is a moderate sensitive predictor of acute bacterial sinusitis, it is relatively nonspecific and cannot reliably distinguish from viral infection.[27] In sinus aspiration studies in adults significant bacterial growth occurs in about 60% of patients with URTI symptoms for 10 days or more.[28] In general, treatment for acute bacterial sinusitis is recommended when symptoms suggestive of sinusitis (combination of symptoms and signs listed in Table 2.1) persists beyond 10 days or worsen after 5 to 7 days (fever, facial erythema, swelling, and severe pain). It should be noted that cough with mild congestion and postnasal drip can commonly persists for 3 weeks in viral URTI.

The guidelines for choice of antimicrobial agents have changed somewhat over the past decade, and will continue to change with emerging resistance of respiratory

**Table 2.1** Useful clinical and laboratory parameters in acute sinusitis

History
- URT symptoms >7–10 days
- Fever >3 days
- Mucopurulent discharge >7 days
- Pain in upper teeth (in absence dental disease)
- Lack of response to decongestants

Signs
(Most useful after 7 days of symptoms)
- Unintended tenderness of sinus or mid-face
- Intranasal pus (especially unilateral)
- Postnasal purulent mucus in pharynx

Diagnostic tests
Anterior rhinoscopy
Sinus puncture and aspiration (when indicated)
Rigid endoscopy for culture (when indicated)
Plain radiograph with air fluid level (low sensitivity)
Computed tomography (in chronic sinusitis/complications)

bacteria from extensive overuse of antibiotics. Since resistance patterns vary from country to country, so too are the current guidelines. In a recent report from an international surveillance network of the susceptibility of respiratory pathogens in adults (from 26 countries, the worldwide prevalence of *S. pneumoniae* resistance to penicillin [MIC $\geq$2 mg/l] was 18.2%) and resistance to macrolides (erythomyin $\geq$1 mg/l) was 24.6%.[29] In the United States, 37% of 2432 *S. pneumoniae* isolates were resistant to penicillin,[29] but strains with low to moderate penicillin resistance (<4 mg/l) may still respond to amoxicillin. In this surveillance study lactam-producing *H. influenzae* and *M. catarrhalis* isolates were 16.9% and 92.1%, respectively. Resistance to fluoroquinolones was very low among all isolates.

Guidelines for selection of antimicrobial therapy are usually based on the results of large controlled, prospective, randomized studies, or the results of meta-analysis of several studies, changing microbial resistance patterns and experts' opinion. The agency for health care policy and research 1999 guidelines[30] identified only six studies that met the criteria for a meta-analysis evaluating antimicrobials versus placebo or no antibacterials for treatment of acute bacterial sinusitis. A previous meta-analysis by the Cochrane collaboration was also published in 1997.[31] Both these reviews concluded that antibiotics are more effective than placebo in eliminating symptoms at 10 and 14 days, but the clinical benefit was small, and most untreated patients improve without antibiotic therapy. For instance, 81% of antibiotic treated patients and 66% of controls were considered to be either cured or improved at 10–14 days follow-up. However, some of these trials may have had methodologic limitations such as diagnostic criteria, comparators, endpoints, and outcome measures. Furthermore, trends in antimicrobial resistance have changed dramatically in the past decade. Although previous meta-analyses had concluded that newer broad-spectrum antibiotics are not more effective than narrow-spectrum agents,[30–32] Current Sinus and Allergy Health Partnership (SAHP) guidelines in 2004[4] considered changes in antimicrobial resistance patterns. The approach of current SAHP treatment guidelines are based on use of a mathematical model (the Poole therapeutic outcomes model), that predicts the bacteriological and clinical efficacy of antibacterials according to pathogen distribution, rates of spontaneous resolution without symptoms, in vitro antimicrobial activity, and pharmacodynamic parameters.[4] The 2004 SAHP guidelines divided patients with mild disease into those receiving antimicrobials within the past 4–6 weeks, and those not treated with previous antibacterials, and patients with moderate–severe disease, regardless of recent antibiotic exposure. For adults with mild disease and no recent antimicrobial exposure, the recommended choices initially include amoxicillin (1.5–4 g/day), amoxillin/clavalanate (clavilin), second-generation oral cephalosporin (cefuroxime axetil), or third-generation cephalosporin (cefdinir or cefpodoxime proxetil) (see Table 2.2). For patients with moderate to severe penicillin or β-lactam allergies alternate choices include trimethoprim-sulfamethoxazole (TMP-SMZ), doxycycline, macrolides-azalides (azithromycin, clarithromycin). If there is no improvement after 72 h, treatment maybe changed to higher dose amoxicillin/clavulanate, a respiratory fluoroquinolone, or a combination of agents. Adjunctive therapy includes topical and/or oral decongestants to ameliorate nasal symptoms and reduce

**Table 2.2** Recommended antibiotic therapy for adults with acute bacterial sinusitis

| Initial therapy | Calculated clinical efficiency (%) | Worsening/No improvement >72 h with therapy |
|---|---|---|
| Mild Disease: No Recent Antibacterial use (4–6 weeks) | | |
| Amoxicillin (1.5–4 g/day) | 87–88 | Levofloxacin or moxifloxacin |
| Amoxicillin – clavulanate (clavulin – 500 tid, 875 bid) | 90–91 | Amoxicillin-clavulanate Dose (clavulin – 875 2 bid) |
| Cefuroxime axetil, cefdinir or cefpodoxime proxetil | 83–87 | Ceftriaxone (in hospital), or combination therapy[a] |
| β-lactam allergic | | |
| TMP/SMX | 83 | Fluoroquinolones alone, or clindamycin + TMP/SMX |
| Doxycycline | 81 | |
| Erythromycin, azithromycin, clarithromycin | 77 | |
| Moderate disease or mild disease with antibacterial use | | |
| Amoxicillin-clavulanate (Clavulin 875 2 bid | 91 | Reevaluate/consult ENT or ID specialist, culture via rigid endoscope, CT scan should be considered |
| Moxifloxacin or levofloxacin | 92 | |
| Ceftriaxone intravenous, or combination therapy | 91 | |
| β-lactam allergic, above fluoroquinolones, or clindamycin/TMP-SMX | 92 | |

= 3 times/day
bid = 2 times/day
TMP/SMX = trimethoprim – sulfamethoxazole
This table is a modification of guidelines by Anon et al.[4] The dosage for amoxicillin-clavunate has been changed for more practical usage.
[a]Combinations cited included high-dose amoxicillin (4 g/day), or cefixime combined with clindamycin or rifampin. This author does not agree with the use of rifampin in sinusitis.
Rifampin have not been studied in sinusitis, may cause several drug interaction, and increase the risk for mycobacterial tuberculosis resistance to rifampin in the community.

mucosal swelling and promote mucus clearance, and analgesics for pain control. However, results of eight randomized trials of symptomatic therapy in adults with sinusitis have been inconclusive.[27]

In adults previously treated with antimicrobials (within 4–6 weeks) or with more severe disease (moderate to severe not defined by the guidelines), maybe treated with high-dose amoxicillin-clavulanate or fluoroquinolone (levofloxacin or moxifloxacin). Severely ill patients requiring hospital admission maybe treated with intravenous ceftriaxone or a combination of agents. It should be noted that these guidelines have not been validated by large well-controlled, prospective clinical trials. Although high cure rates or improvement have been found in controlled trials with recommended respiratory fluoroquinolones (88–96%) in acute bacterial sinusitis, they were not superior to the comparator agents (including amoxicillin-clavulanate, cefuroxime axetil, or clarithromycin).[6]

It is also surprising that the guidelines did not include the newer oral cephalosporin (cefdinir, cefpodoxime proxetil, or cefixime) as alternative for moderate disease or mild disease with previous antimicrobial exposure). At present the fluoroquinolones are recommended as second-line therapy for acute bacterial sinusitis, but should not be used if patients have received these agents in the past 3 months, situation where quinolone-resistant *S. pneumoniae* may occur. Overuse of these agents may compromise the value of this class of compound for the future. In general it is best to avoid similar class of agents used in the recent 6–12 weeks. The combination therapy recommended in the guidelines includes high-dose amoxicillin (4 g/day) or clindamycin plus cefixime, or clindamycin plus rifampin, or TMP/SMX plus rifampin.[4] However, there is no clinical trials to support these combinations and this author have major reservations about these guidelines. These include increased adverse events such as *Clostridium difficile* colitis, hepatitis, drug interactions, and potentially increasing rifampin-resistant *Mycobacterium tuberculosis* in the community. The recommendation for pediatric patients are similar to adults, except for dosage adjustment for weight and avoidance of the fluoroquinolones, even in moderate to severe disease or in previous antimicrobial experience in children.[4] These agents are routinely avoided in children because of potential cartilage toxicity during the growing period. For more severe disease or recent antimicrobial use (past 4–6 weeks) amoxicillin-clavulanate is considered the agent of choice; for those with β-lactam allergies, TMP/SMX, macrolides—azalides or clindamycin are alternate choices. Ceftriaxone should be reserved for the very ill patients admitted to hospital. A concern with respect to the use of macrolide—azalides for moderate–severe disease is the rising *S. pneumoniae* macrolide resistance in many areas of the world, with resistant rates of 20–30% in the United States.[29] Since these strains remain susceptible to the ketalides,[33] telithromycin would be a better choice. However, telithromycin is no longer approved for use in sinusitis because of recent reports and concerns of liver toxicity.

On the most recent Cochrane Review in 2005,[34] of 49 trials, involving 13, 660 participants with acute maxillary sinusitis, the conclusion was that current evidence is limited but supports the use of penicillin or amoxicillin for 7–14 days (moderate benefits). However, comparisons between classes of antibiotics showed no significant differences, but there were fewer adverse events with cephalosporins compared to amoxicillin – clavulanate.[33]

## 2.1.6 Management of Chronic Sinusitis

The treatment of chronic sinusitis is challenging as there are multiple etiological factors to consider, and there is no general consensus or recently published guidelines. Moreover there is a lack of properly conducted prospective or randomized clinical trails in this area. Medical management often includes repeated or longer courses of antibacterial (3–4 weeks) for acute exacerbation, which is best guided by sinus cultures (by puncture or endoscopy guided). For presurgical cases empiric antimicrobials should be effective against *S. pneumoniae*, *H. influenzae*, other streptococcal species and anaerobes.[25,35] Amoxicillin-clavulanate would be a suitable choice and for β-lactam allergic patient, a newer fluoroquinolone with enhanced anaerobic activity, moxifloxacin, or gatifloxacin may be used. Adjunctive therapy would include topical and systemic decongestants, antihistamines, and topical or short-course systemic steroids. Failure to respond to medical management usually requires surgical intervention with functional endoscopy sinus surgery (FESS) replacing traditional surgery. This procedure has allowed more limited resection, preserving mucosa and reestablishing ventilation and drainage through the natural ostia of the diseased sinuses with short-term improvement of 85%.[36] As recurrences are common nasal and sinus lavage with sterile saline have been used to help control exacerbations. The decrease in response to treatment over time may be correlated with predisposing factors such as inhalant sensitivities (allergy in up to one third of cases), inhaled irritants (tobacco smoke), nasal polyps, aspirin hypersensitivity, immune deficiencies, and more resistant bacteria. Nasal endoscopy is the most reliable predictor of early recurrence of sinus disease with subsequent nasal/sinus symptoms, purulent discharge, and deterioration of quality of life measures, and radiographic changes.[18] With previous surgical intervention and saline irrigation the bacteriology change to involve more gram-negative coliforms, *Pseudomonas* species, *S. aureus*, and anaerobes. Treatment should be guided in these cases by direct sinus cultures. Ciprofloxacin and metronidazole or a newer quinolone (moxifloxacin) may be needed for acute purulent exacerbations. However, the role of these superinfecting organisms causing disease is very questionable.

Allergic fungal sinusitis is an emerging disease described about two decades ago. The typical patient is an immunocompetent adult with bilateral nasal polyps and areas of intranasal hyperdense area on CT scan. Hypersensitivity or allergy to the colonized fungus (frequently *Aspergillus* species) is the believed etiology, and this maybe associated with eosinophilia (or increased eosinophils in nasal secretion), and raised serum IgE antibodies directed against the fungi.[37] Bony expansion and erosion may be seen secondary to pressure necrosis and remodeling rather than fungal invasion. Occasionally, documented fungal invasion can be seen by biopsy down to the submucosal tissue, and orbital and intracranial spread can rarely occur in non-immunosuppressed subjects. Antifungal agents are not indicated except for the rare cases of histologically proven tissue invasion. Endoscopy surgery to remove inspissated mucous, fungus ball, and polyps, is usually necessary for management of chronic fungal sinusitis.

### 2.1.7  *Issues in Acute Otitis Media*

More than half of all children experience at least one bout of acute otitis media (AOM) before the age of 3 years. Although less common in adults acute otitis media may lead to life-threatening pneumococcal meningitis in this age group. Acute otitis media is defined as a history of acute onset of signs and symptoms, the presence of middle-ear effusion, and signs and symptoms of middle-ear inflammation. Persistent middle-ear effusion may follow AOM in children, which can sometimes lead to hearing loss; effects on speech, language, and learning; physiologic sequelae; health utilization and quality of life. AOM is one of the most common infectious disease of children and the leading cause of office visits and antibiotic prescription for this population.

### 2.1.7.1 Pathogenesis of Otitis Media

The pathogenesis of AOM is very similar to that of acute sinusitis. The middle ear is lined by ciliated, mucous-secreting goblet cells of the respiratory epithelium that is continuous with the nares, nasopharynx, and eustachian tube medially and anteriorly, and the mastoid air cells posteriorly. Disturbance in the anatomy (i.e., obstruction) or functions of the eustachian tube results in accumulation of effusion in the middle ear, which predispose to secondary bacterial infection and purulent AOM. Thus preceding viral URTI with mucosal congestion is present in most cases, and chronic sinusitis predisposes to recurrences. However, unlike sinusitis the role of allergy is less well-defined. Otitis media with effusion (OME) is a related but separate condition which should be distinguished from AOM, as the treatment may be different. OME is defined as the presence of fluid in the middle ear without signs or symptoms of acute ear infection. The fluid in OME is not purulent and is usually serous or mucoid.

### 2.1.7.2 Microbiology of Acute Otitis Media

Viral upper respiratory infections are strongly associated with AOM by virologic and epidemiological studies. Narrowing of the opening of the eustachian tube from mucosal edema and congestion, and dysfunction of the ciliated epithelium predispose to impaired drainage, and thus bacterial superinfection. Also, viral otitis media with serous effusion is commonly mistreated with antibiotics for AOM. Respiratory viruses or viral antigen have been recovered from almost a quarter of middle-ear fluid in children with AOM.[38,39] The most common viruses found in middle-ear fluid include respiratory syncytial virus, influenza virus, enteroviruses, and rhinoviruses. The bacteriology of AOM with cultures of middle aspirates have consistently demonstrated *S. pneumoniae* (average 39%), *H. influenzae* (mean 27%, predominantly non-typable strains), *M. catarrhalis* (mean 10%), and others (less than 5%), including *S. pyogenes* and *S. aureus*.[40] The microbiology is remarkably similar to that of acute bacterial sinusitis. Occasional causes of otitis media include *Mycoplasma pneumoniae* and *Chlamydia pneumoniae*.

### 2.1.7.3 Diagnosis of Otitis Media

There is a general consensus that AOM is overdiagnosed by family physicians and pediatricians. Symptoms are neither sensitive nor specific for the diagnosis of

AOM; fever and ear pain are present in only one half of patients.[41] Undue reliance on redness of the tympanic membrane and failure to assess tympanic membrane motility with pneumatic otoscopy contribute to inaccurate diagnoses. Adequate visualization of the tympanic membrane is essential, and distinguishing AOM from OME is clinically important (and not reliable with regular otoscope), because antibiotics are not usually indicated for the latter correlation. A key differentiating feature is the position of the tympanic membrane; it is usually bulging in AOM and in a neutral or retracted position in OME.[41] Selective use of tympanocentesis in cases of refractory of recurrent middle-ear disease can help guide therapy and avoid unnecessary medication. Tympanometry or acoustic reflectometry can be used as adjunctive techniques to confirm middle-ear effusion.

In a recent review of the precision or accuracy of history and physical examination for the diagnosis of AOM in children, 397 studies were identified but only 6 were suitable for analysis.[42] Ear pain was the most useful symptom with calculated likelihood ratio (LR, 3.0–7.3); whilst fever, URT symptoms, and irritability were less useful. A cloudy (adjusted LR, 34), bulging (adjusted LR 51), or distinctly immobile (adjusted LR 31) tympanic membrane on pneumatic otoscopy were the most useful signs.[42] A distinctly red tympanic membrane was helpful (adjusted LR, 8.4), and a normal color makes AOM very unlikely (adjusted LR, 0.2). Thus, a cloudy, bulging, or clearly immobile tympanic membrane is most helpful in diagnosing AOM, and a distinctly red membrane increases the likelihood significantly.

### 2.1.7.4 New Concepts in the Treatment of Acute Otitis Media

The use of antimicrobials in the treatment of AOM remains a controversial issue in medical practice. Systematic reviews of the literature have reached the conclusion that antibiotics play a small role in resolving symptoms of AOM. There is no doubt that since the widespread use of antibiotics there has been dramatic reductions in the complications of otitis media (meningitis, brain abscess, mastoiditis, and deafness), as compared with the pre-antibiotic era. But this has been associated with widespread development of antibacterial resistance in the world to many antimicrobial agents.

Spontaneous cure and recovery in children without antibiotics with the diagnosis of AOM is common, as shown by several meta-analyses of placebo-controlled trials. The reason for this may be partly due to dilution of the trials by inclusion of viral otitis media or OME cases, because of clinical difficulty in diagnosing purulent AOM, or from lax entry criteria. It is also possible that even with bacterial superinfection, symptoms may resolve spontaneously with time or by drainage via patent eustachian tube or perforated tympanic membrane. In an earlier study of documented bacterial infection of the middle ear and sequential aspirates 2–7 days apart with no antibacterial therapy, 19% of pneumonococcal infection became sterile and 48% of *H. influenzae* became sterile spontaneously.[43] This indicated that the host immune response was more effective in eradicating *H. influenzae* more frequently than *S. pneumoniae*.

Placebo-controlled trials of AOM over the past 30 years have consistently shown that without antibacterial therapy most children do well without adverse sequelae. It has been estimated that between 7 and 20 children must be treated with antibiotics to derive benefit in one child.[44–46] Sixty-one percent of children will have decreased symptoms by 24 h irrespective of placebo or antibiotics, and by day 7, 75% will have resolution of symptoms.[47] Compared to placebo or observation antibiotics (ampicillin or amoxicillin) will improve resolution of symptoms (within 7 days) by only 12.3%.[48]

Since 1990 Dutch practitioners have adopted a conservative approach to the management of AOM in children; symptomatic therapy would be instituted without antibiotics for 24 h (for those 6–24 months old) or 72 hs (for those older), and in the revised guidelines of 1999 antibiotics were recommended only if there were no improvement or worsening after reassessment after 3 days in all ages.[49] These guidelines, widely adopted in the Netherlands, were based on previous studies by van Buchen et al.,[50,51] which found that only 2.7% of 4,860 Dutch children (older than 2 years) given only symptomatic treatment developed severe illness (persistent fever, pain, or ear discharge) after 3–4 days. Only two of the children developed mastoiditis, one present at initial presentation, and the other evolved after a week but responded promptly to antibiotics.

Since then there have been a few randomized trials of observation with symptomatic therapy. In one such study in the United Kingdom in children aged 6 months to 10 years, immediate antibacterial therapy was compared to delaying antibiotics until reassessment in 72 h.[52] Seventy-six percent of children in the delayed-treatment group never required antibiotics. Although the immediate treatment group was symptomatically better at 3 days more frequently (86%) compared to the delayed-treatment group (70%), the earlier use of antibiotics was associated with only 1 day shorter illness.[52] Limitations of this study included imprecise criteria for diagnosis of AOM, and lack of dose adjustment of amoxicillin for weight (125 mg three times a day for 7 days). Further analysis of this trial[53] and a previous earlier study[54] had found that the likelihood of recovery without antibacterial therapy may depend on the severity of symptoms and signs on initial assessment. For instance children with more severe illness with fever, severe pain, and vomiting were more likely to have persistent or worst distress in 3–4 days on placebo (21–23.5%) then those with initial milder symptoms (3.8–4%).[53,54]

Previous reports had also suggested that younger children less than 2 years were at greater risk for failure of observational symptomatic therapy. For instance Kaleida et al.[54] showed a greater clinical failure rate (9.8%) in children less than 2 years than in older children (5.8%) who were treated with placebo. In a randomized trial in the Netherlands in children with AOM 6–24 months of age, amoxicillin led to resolution of more symptoms after 4 days of treatment; but after 11 days amoxicillin did not differ from placebo.[55] A recent trial[56] conducted in Canada randomized 512 children 6 months to 5 years of age to receive amoxicillin or placebo with AOM; 415 (81%) had moderate disease. Children who received placebo had more pain in the first 2 days. At 14 days 84.2% of the children receiving placebo and 92.8% of those receiving amoxicillin had clinical resolution of symptoms (absolute difference − 8.6% (95% CI − 14.4–3.0%).[56] Subgroups analysis according to age showed that children 6–23 months of age had lower clinical resolution rates 79.3% with placebo and 85.4% with amoxicillin than older children who had rates of 87.2% and 96.9%, respectively. However, the benefits of antibacterial therapy in both age groups were modest and do not support initial widespread use of antibiotics for AOM.[57]

Concerns have been raised that restricted use of antibiotics in AOM may lead to increased rates of mastoiditis. However, pooled data from six randomized trials and two cohort studies showed comparable rates of mastoiditis in children (0–59%) who received placebo or observation.[48] The incidence rates of mastoiditis were compared in different countries from 1991 to 1998 for children 14 years of age or younger.[58] Despite initial use of antibacterial agents more than the Netherlands, mastoiditis rates in all three countries were comparable. Although the incidence of mastoiditis were lower in North America, Australia, and United Kingdom (where initial antibiotics are prescribed more often [96% of uses]), the potential increase is only two cases per 100,00 person-years with observation.[58]

Another issue with delaying antibiotic therapy for AOM is the risk of bacteremia and the development of acute meningitis (especially from *S. pneumoniae*).

In the previous Dutch study[51] of 4,860 children with AOM not treated with antibiotics, no cases of bacterial meningitis occurred. In one report positive blood cultures were equally common in children with bacterial meningitis regardless of treatment with antibacterial for AOM (77% and 78%).[59] Moreover, there has been a decline in invasive pneumococcal disease in children less than 2 years between 1999 and 2001, since introduction of the pneumococcal conjugate vaccine (69% decline).[60] Overall, the incidence of bacterial meningitis is unlikely to be influenced by the initial treatment of AOM with antibiotics.

## 2.1.8 Clinical Practice Guidelines

A subcommittee on management of AOM sanctioned by the American Academy of Pediatrics and American Academy of Family Physicians recently published their guidelines in 2004.[61] The guidelines included seven recommendations:

1. To diagnose AOM the clinician should confirm a history of acute onset, identify signs of middle-ear effusion, and evaluate for the presence of signs and symptoms of inflammation.
2. Management should include treatment to reduce pain when present. These may include acetaminophen, ibuprophen, and topical anesthetic for mild to moderate pain, and narcotic analgesia with codeine for more severe pain.
3. Observation without use of antibacterial agent, in selected children with uncompleted AOM based on diagnostic certainty, age, illness severity, and assurance of follow–up (within 48–72 h).
4. For treatment with antibacterial agent, amoxicillin 80–90 mg/kg/day should be used for most children. For patients with severe illness (severe otalgia or fever

>39°C) therapy may be initiated with high-dose amoxicillin-clavulanic acid (90–6.4 mg/kg/day) for broader coverage of β-lactamase positive *H. influenzae* and *M. catarrhalis*.
5. Failure to respond to initial management within 48–72 h requires reassessment to confirm the diagnosis of AOM and exclude other illnesses. Patients managed with symptomatic therapy should begin antibiotics (as per 4). Failure of initial amoxicillin should result in changing to high-dose amoxicillin-clavulate. A patient who fails amoxicillin-clavulate should be treated with 3 days of parenteral ceftriaxone. Tympanocentesis should be considered at this stage to confirm the microbiology. Alternatives for penicillin-allergic patients include cephalosporins (cefadinivir, cefpodoxime, or cefuroxime) for mild non-type 1 allergic reaction. In cases of Type 1 allergic or more severe reactions, alternatives include azithromycin, clarithromycin, erythromycin-sulfisoxazole, or TMP-SMX.
6. Encourage the prevention of AOM through reduction of risk factors. These include breast-feeding for at least 6 months, immunoprophylaxis with pneumococcal conjugate vaccine (only 6% reduction in incidence of AOM), intranasal live attenuated influenza vaccine (30% efficiency in prevention of AOM).
7. No recommendations for complementary and alternative medicine were made. It is hopeful that those guidelines will encourage physicians to use antibacterial agents more judiciously, and even if antibiotics rates for AOM were reduced by 50%, this would be a step forward in reducing antibiotic resistance. A Finnish study has shown that a reduction of 50% in prescribed antibiotics resulted in 50% decrease of resistant bacteria.[62] A recent randomized-controlled trial was conducted in 283 children with diagnosis of AOM aged 6 months to 12 years seen in an emergency department.[63] A "wait-and-see prescription" (WASP, N = 138) for antibiotics (not to be filled unless the child is worse in 48 h) was compared to a "standard prescription" (SP, N = 145). Follow-up by structured phone interviews were performed at regular intervals up to 30–40 days after enrollment. There was no significant difference in the two groups with respect to outcome, unscheduled visits for medical care, subsequent fever, or otalgia. Within the WASP group, both fever (60%) and persistent or worsening otalgia (34%) were associated with filling the prescription. The WASP approach substantially reduced unnecessary use of antibiotics with AOM, almost by 50%.[63] Since there are no guidelines or significant controlled trials in adults with AOM, it would be reasonable to adopt these principles in the management of adults presenting with AOM. An algorithm for the management of AOM is shown in Fig. 2.2.

## 2.1.9 Future Directions

The greatest impediment to appropriate management of acute bacterial sinusitis and acute bacterial otitis media is the lack of a simple reliable diagnostic test. This is an area for further research to identify tools that could be used in an office setting to differentiate viral from bacterial infections. Additional studies in the meantime should be conducted to validate the standard definition of AOM, new or improved

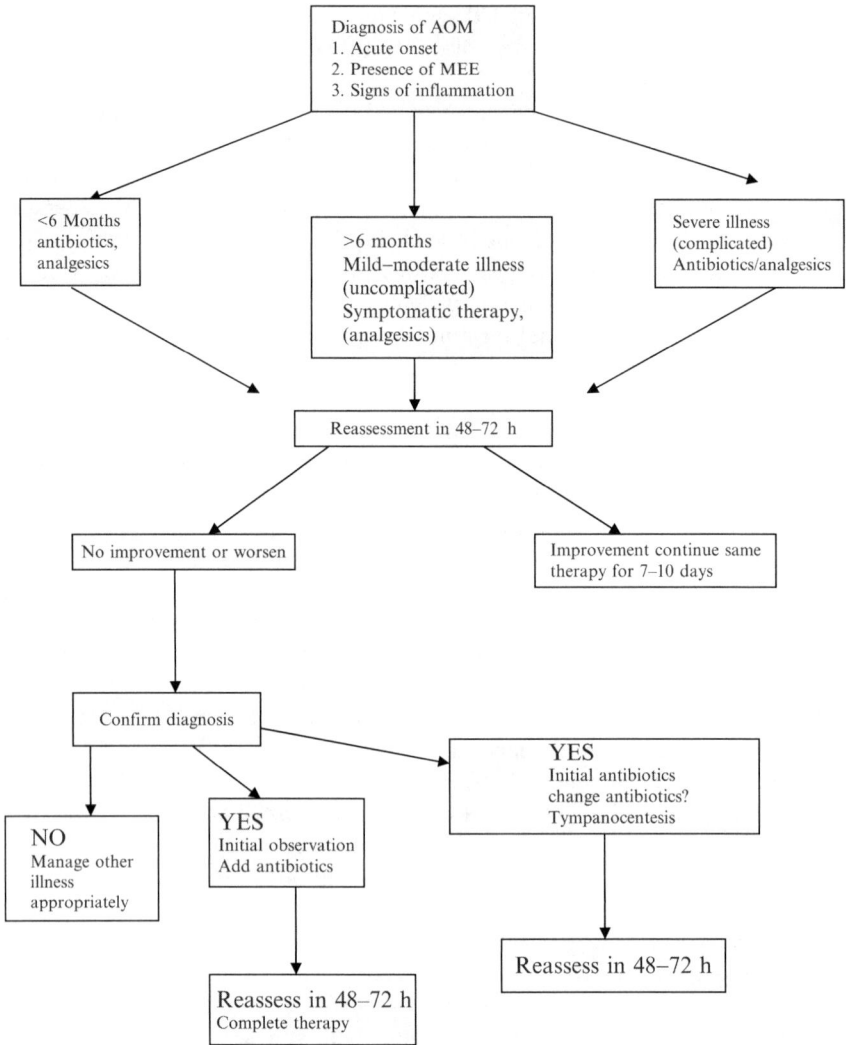

**Fig. 2.2** This figure shows the algorithm for the management of acute otitis media (AOM) in children, but could be applied to adults also. This algorithm was developed from principles published from review articles including references [45, 46, 61]. MEE = middle ear effusions

technologies for the objective diagnosis of middle-ear effusion should be developed.

In acute sinusitis further multicenter, controlled prospective studies are needed to test the Poole therapeutic outcome model and proposed guidelines. In chronic sinusitis placebo-controlled studies are still needed to define the benefit of antimicrobial therapy, and the role of bacterial infection or colonization.

In AOM further clinical studies should address the utility of delayed antibiotics and observation in children less than 6 months of age. Prevention of bacterial AOM by maximizing utilization of vaccines needs further study. Since the introduction of the heptavalent conjugate pneumococcal vaccine has been reported to reduce the incidence of AOM by 6% and pneumococcal episodes by 34%[64] in healthy infants and toddlers, but not in children with recurrent AOM.[65] With the advent of the heptavalent conjugate pneumococcal vaccine there has been a shift from vaccine to non-vaccine-type strains of *S. pneumoniae* in the nasopharynx and infected cases,[64–68] combination of the conjugate vaccine and the polysaccharide pneumococcal vaccine did not seem to be of benefit in children 1–7 years of age.[65] Future research is needed on the development of a higher-valent conjugate vaccine, similar to the 23-valent polysaccharide vaccine.

# References

1. United States Department of Health and Human Services. (1987) National Health survey. Prevalence of Selected Chronic conditions, United States; 1983–85, Hyattsville, MD, US Department of Health and Human Services.
2. Kaliner, M.A., Osguthorpe, J.D., Fireman., O., Anon. J., Georgitis. J., Davis, M.L., Naclerio. R., Kennedy, D. (1997), Sinusitis: bench to bedside, Current findings, future directions. J. Allergy Clin. Immnol. 99(Suppl.): S829–S848.
3. Lusk, R.P., Stankiewiez, J.A. (1997), Pediatric Rhinosinusitis: Report of the Rhinosinusitis Task Force committee meeting. Otolaryngol. Head Neck Surg. 117(Suppl.): S53–S57.
4. Anon, J.B., Jacobs, M.R., Poole, M.D., Ambrose, P.G., Benninger, M.S., Hadley, J.A., Craig, W.A., Allergy Health Partnership. (2004), Antimicrobial treatment guidelines for acute bacterial rhinosinusitis. Otolaryngol. Head Neck Surg. 130(Suppl 1): 1–45.
5. Blair, C., Nelson, M., Thompson, K., Boonlayangoor, S., Haney, L., Gabr, U., Baroody, F.M., Naclerio, R.M. (2001), Allergic inflammation enhances bacterial sinusitis in mice. J. Allergy Clin. Immnol. 108: 424–429.
6. Anon, J.B. (2005) Current management of acute bacterial rhinosinusitis and the role of moxiflaxacin. Clin. Infect. Dis. 41(Suppl.): S167–S176.
7. Lanza, D.C., Kennedy, D.W. (1997), Adult rhinosinusitis defined. Report of the Rhinosinusitis Task force Committee Meeting. Otolaryngol. Head Neck Surg. 117 (Suppl.): S1–S7.
8. Lindbeck, M., Hjortdahl, P., Johnson, U. (1996), Use of symptoms, signs and blood tests to diagnose acute sinus infections in primary care: Comparison with computed tomography. Fam. Med. 28: 183–188.
9. Dowell, S.F., Schwartz, B., Phillips, W.R. (1998), Appropriate use of antibiotics for URI's in children. Part I. Otitis media and acute sinusitis, Am. Fam. Physician 58: 1113–1118.
10. Williams, J.W. Jr., Simel, D.L., Roberts, L, Samsa, G.P. (1992), Clinical evaluation for sinusitis. Making the diagnosis by history and physical examination. Ann Intern. Med. 117: 705–710.
11. Williams, J.W. Jr., Simel, D.R. (1993), Does this patient have sinusitis? Diagnosing acute sinusitis by history and physical examination. JAMA 270: 1242–1246.
12. Brook, I., Gooch, W.M., Reiner, S.A., Jenkins, S.G., Sher, L., Pichichero, M.E., Yamauchi, T. (2000), Medical management of acute bacterial sinusitis. Recommendations of a clinical advisory committee on pediatric and adult sinusitis. Ann. Otol. Rhinol. Laryngol. 109: 2–20.
13. Gwaltney, J.M., Jr., Phillis, C.D., Miller, R.D., Riker, D.K. (1994), Computed tomographic study on the common cold: N. Engl. J. Med. 330: 25–30.
14. The Institute for Clinical Systems Integration, (1998), Acute sinusitis in adults. Postgrad. Med.103: 154–156.

15. Willet, L.R., Carson, J.L., Williams, J.W. Jr. (1994), Current diagnosis and management of sinusitis. J. Gen. Intern. Med. 9: 38–45.
16. International Rhinosinusitis Advisory Board, (1997), Infectious rhinosinusitis in adults: Classification, etiology and management. Ear Nose Throat J. 76(Suppl 72): 1–19.
17. Talbot, G.H., Kennedy, D.W., Schild, W.M., Gramto, K., for the Endoscopy Study Group. (2001), Rigid nasal endoscopy versus sinus puncture and aspiration for microbiologically documentation of acute bacterial maxillary sinusitis. Clin. Infect. Dis. 33: 1668–1675.
18. Benninger, M.S., Ferguson, B.J., Hadley, J.A., Hamilos, D.L., Jacobs, M., Kennedy, D.W., Lanza, D.C., Marysle, B.F., Osguthorpe, J.P., Stankiewicz, J.A., Anon, J., Denneny, J., Emanuel, I., Levine, H. (2003), Adult Chronic rhinosinusitis: Definition diagnosis, epidemiology, and pathophysiology. Otolaryngol. Head Neck Surg. 129(Suppl 3): SI–S32.
19. Calenoff, E., McMahan, J.T., Herzon, G.D., Kern, R.C., Ghadge, G.D., Hanson, D.G. (1993), Bacterial allergy in nasal polyposis; a new method for identifying specific Ig E. Arch. Otolaryngol. Head Neck Surg. 119: 830–836.
20. Schubert, M.S. (2001), A superantigen hypothesis for the pathogenesis of chronic hypertrophic rhinosinusitis, allergic fungal sinusitis, and related disorders. Ann. Allergy Asthma Immunol. 81: 181–188.
21. Gordts, F., Halewyck, S., Pierard, D., Clement, P.A.R., Kaufman, L. (2000), Microbiology of the middle meatus: a comparison between normal adults and children. J. Laryngol. Otol. 114: 184–188.
22. Frederick, J., Braude, A.I. (1974), Anaerobic infection of the paranasal sinuses. N. Engl. J. Med. 290: 135–140.
23. Brook, I. (2002), Anaerobic bacteria in upper respiratory tract and other head neck infection. Ann. Otol. Rhinol. Laryngol. 111: 430–440.
24. Doyle, P.W., Woodham, J.D. (1991), Bacterial flora in acute and chronic sinusitis. J. Clin. Neurol. 29: 2396–2399.
25. Finegold, S.M., Flynn, M.J., Rose, F.K., Jousimies-Somer, H., Jukielaszek, C., McTeague, M., Wexler, H.M., Bekowitz, E., Wynne, B. (2002), Bacteriologic findings associated with chronic bacterial maxillary sinusitis in adults. Clin. Infect. Dis. 35: 428–433.
26. Keech, D.R., Romadan, H., Mathers. P. (2000), Analysis of aerobic bacterial strains found in chronic rhinosinusitis using the polymerase chain reaction. Otolaryngol. Head Neck Surg. 123: 363–367.
27. Hickner, J.M., Barlett, J.G., Besser, R.E., Gonzales, R., Hoffman, M.A., Sande, M.A., American Academy of Family Physicians; American College of Physicians-American Society of Internal Medicine; Centers for Disease Control; Infectious Diseases Society of America. (2001), Principles of appropriate antibiotic use for acute rhinosinusitis in adults: background. Ann. Intern. Med. 134: 498–505.
28. Gwaltney, J.M., Scheld, W.M. Jr., Sande, M.A., Sydnor, A. (1992), The microbial etiology and antimicrobial therapy of adults with acute community-acquired sinusitis: a fifteen-year experience at the University of Virginia and review of other selected studies. J. Allergy Clin. Immunol. 90: 457–461.
29. Jacobs, M.R., Felmingham, D., Appelbaum, P.C., Gruneberg, R.N. (2003), The Alexander project 1998–2000: susceptibility of pathogens isolated from community-acquired respiratory tract infection to commonly used antimicrobial agents. J. Antimicrobial. Chemother. 52: 229–246.
30. Zucher, D.R., Balk, E., Engels, E., Barza, M., Lau, J., Agency for Healthcare Research. (1999), Diagnosis and treatment of acute bacterial rhino-sinusitis. Evidence report /technology assessment no. 99-E016. Available at: www.ahrq.gov./chemi/sinussum.htm
31. Williams, J.W., Aguilar, C. Jr., Makela, M., Cornell, J., Hollman, D., Chiquette, E.: Cochrane Acute Respiratory Infections Group. (1997), Antibiotic therapy for acute sinusitis: a systemic literature review. In: Douglas, R., Bridges-Webb, C., Glasziou, P., Lozano, J., Steinhoff, M., Wang, E. (eds), Acute Respiratory Infections Module of the Cochrane Database of Systematic Reviews. The Cochrane Library, Oxford. Updates software.

# References

32. deBock, G.H., Dekker, F.W., Stolk, J., Springer, M.P., Kiwit, J., van Houwelingen, J.C. (1997), Antimicrobial treatment of acute maxillary sinusitis: a meta-analysis. J. Clin. Epidemiol. 50: 881–890.
33. Karchmer, A.W. (2004), Increased antibiotic resistance in respiratory tract pathogen: PROTECT US- an update Clin. Infect Dis. 39(Suppl.): S142–S150.
34. Williams, J.W., Aguilar, C. Jr., Cornell, J., Chiquette, E., Dolor, R.J., Makela, M., Holleman, D.R., Simel, D.L., Cochrane Acute Respiratory Infections Group. (2005), Antibiotics for acute maxillary sinusitis. Cochrane database Systematic Reviews. 4.
35. Winther, B., Vickery, C.L., Gross, C.W., Hendley, J.O. (1996), Microbiology of the maxillary sinus in adults with chronic sinus disease. Am. J. Rhino. 10: 347–350.
36. Kennedy, D.W., (1992), Progrnostic factors, outcome and staging in ethmoid sinus surgery. Laryngoscope 102: 1–18.
37. Thakar, A.W., Sanker, C., Dhiwaker, M., Bahadur, S., Dahiya, S. (2004), Allergic fungal sinusitis: Expanding the clinicopathologic spectrum. Otolaryngol. Head Neck Surg. 130: 209–216.
38. Chonmaitree, T., Howie, V.M., Truant, A.L., (1986), Presence of respiratory viruses in middle ear fluids and nasal wash specimens from children with acute otitis media. Pediatrics 77: 698–702.
39. Klein, B.S., Dallette, E.R., Volken, R.H. (1982), The role of respiratory syncytial virus and other viral pathogens in acute otitis media. J. Pediater. 101: 16–20.
40. Klein J.O., (2000), Otitis externa, Otitis media and mastoditis. In: Mandell, G.L., Bennett, J. E., Dolin, R. (eds), Principles and Practice of Infectious Diseases, Fifth Edition, Churchill Lewingstone, Philadelphia, pp. 669–675.
41. Pichichero, M.E. (2000), Acute otitis media: part I, Improving diagnostic accuracy. Am. Fam. Phys. 61: 2051–2056.
42. Rothman, R., Owens, T., Simel, D.L. (2003), Does this child have acute otitis media? JAMA 290: 1633–1640.
43. Howie, V.M., Ploussard, J.H. (1969), Bacteriology of middle ear exudates during antimicrobial therapy in otitis media. Pediatrics: 44: 940–944.
44. Rosenfeld, R.M., Vertrees, J.E., Carr, J., Cipolle, R.J., Urden, D.L., Giebink, G.S., Canafax, D.M. (1994), Clinical efficacy of antimicrobial drugs for acute otitis media: meta-analysis of 5400 children from thirty three randomized trials. J. Pediatr. 124: 355–367.
45. Del Mar, C., Glasziou, P., Hayem, M. (1997), Are antibiotics indicated as initial treatment for children with acute otitis media? A meta-analysis. BMJ. 314: 1526–1529.
46. Glasziou, P.P., Delmar, C.B., Hayem, M., Sanders, S.L. (2006), Antibiotics for acute otitis media in children. Cochrane Database Sys. Rev. 4: CD000219.
47. Rosenlfeld, R.M., Kay, D. (2003), Natural history of untreated otitis media, In: Rosenfeld, R. M., Bluestone C.D. (eds). Evidence Based Otitis Media, 2nd edition/BC Decker, Hamilton, ON, pp. 180–198.
48. Marcy, M., Takata, G., Chan, L.S., Shekelle, P., Mason, W., Wachsman, L., Ernst, R., Hay, J. W., Corley, P.M., Morphew, M.S., Ramieone, F., Nicholson, C. (2001), Management of acute otitis media. Evidence report/technology assessment no. 15. Rockville, MD, Agony for Healthcare Research and Quality, AHRQ Publication.no. 01-E010
49. Appleman, C.L., Van Balen, F.A., Vandelisdonk, E.H., van Weert, H.C., Eizenga, W.H. (1999), Otitis media acute, NHG- standaard Eerste herziening [in Dutch]. Huisarts Wet. 42: 362–366.
50. van Buchem, F.L., Dunk, J.H., van't Hof., M.A. (1981), Therapy of acute otitis media: myrngotomy, antibiotics or neither? A double blind study in children. Lancet 2: 882–887.
51. van Buchem, F.L., Peeters, M.F., van't Hof, M.A. (1985), Acute otitis media: a new treatment strategy. Br Med. J. (Clin. Res. Ed) 290: 1033–1037.
52. Little, P., Gould, C., Williamson, I., Moore, M., Warner, G., Dunleavey, J. (2001), Pragmatic randomized controlled trail of two prescribing strategies for childhood acute otitis media. BMJ 322: 336–342.

53. Little, P., Gould, C., Moore, M., Warner, G., Dunleavey, J., Williamson, I., (2002), Predictors of poor outcome and benefits from antibiotics in children with acute otitis media: pragmatic randomized trial. BMJ 325: 22.
54. Kaleida, P.H., Casselbrant, M.L., Rockette, H.E., Paradise, J.L., Bluestone, C.D., Blatter, M. M., Reisinger, K.S., Wald, E.R, Supance, J.S. (1991), Amoxicillin or myringotomy or both for acute otitis media: Results of a randomized clinical trial. Pediatrics 87: 466–474.
55. Damoiseaux, R.A., van Balen F.A., Hoes, A.W., Verhey, T.J., de Melker, R.A. (2000), Primary care based randomized double blind trail of amoxicillin versus placebo for acute otitis media in children aged under 2 years. BMJ 320: 350–354.
56. Le Saux, N., Gaboury, I., Baird, M., Klassen, T.P., MacCormick, J., Blanchard, C., Pitters, C., Sampson, M., Moher, D. (2005), A randomized, double-blind, placebo-controlled non-inferiority trial of amoxicillin for clinically diagnosed acute otitis media in children 6 months to 5 years of age. CMAJ 172: 335–341.
57. Damoiséaux, R.A.M.J. (2005), Antibiotic treatment for acute otitis media: time to think again (editorial). CMAJ 172: 657–658.
58. van Zuijlen, D.A., Schilder, A.G., van Balen, F.A., Hoes, A.W. (2001), National differences in acute mastoiditis; relationship in prescribing patterns of antibiotics for acute otitis media? Pediatr. Infect. Dis. 20: 140–144.
59. Kilpi, T., Anttila, M., Kallio, M.J., Peltola, H. (1991), Severity of childhood bacterial meningitis: duration of illness before diagnosis. Lancet 338: 406–409.
60. Black, S., Shinefield, H., Fireman, B., Lewis, E., Ray, P., Hansen, J.R., Elvin, L., Ensor, K.M., Haikell, J., Siber, G., Malinoski, F., Madove, D., Chang, I., Kohberger, R., Watson, W., Austrian, R., Edwards, K. (2000), Efficacy, safety and immunogenicity of heptavalent pneumococcal conjugate vaccine in children. Pediatr. Infect. Dis. 19: 187–195.
61. American Academy of Pediatrics and American Academy of Family Physicians. (2004), Diagnosis and management of acute otitis media. Pediatrics 113: 1451–1465.
62. Seppälä, H., Klaukka, T., Vuopio-Varkila, J., Muotiala, A., Helemus, H., Lager, K., Huovinen, P., For the Finnish Study Group for Antimicrobial Resistance. (1997), The effect of changes in the consumption of macrolide antibiotics on erythromycin resistance in group *A. Streptococci* in Finland. N. Engl. J. Med. 337: 441–446.
63. Spiro, D.M., Tay, K.-Y., Arnold, D.H., Dziura, J.D., Baker, M.D., Shapiro, E.D. (2006) Wait-and-see prescription for the treatment of acute otitis media. JAMA 296: 1235–1241.
64. Eskola, J., Kilpi, T., Palma, A., Jokinen, J., Haapakoski, J., Herva, E., Takala, A., Käythy, H., Karma, P., Kohberger, R., Siber, G., Mäkelä, H., For the Finnish Otitis Media Study Group. (2001), Efficacy of a pneumococcal conjugate vaccine against acute otitis media. N. Engl. J. Med. 344: 403–409.
65. Veenhoven, R., Bogaert, D., Uniterawal, C., Brouwer, C., Kiezebrink, H., Bruin, J., Ijzerman, E., Hermans, P., de Groot, R., Zegers, B., Kuis, W., Rifkers, G., Schilder, A., Sanders, E. (2003), Effect of conjugate vaccine followed by polysaccharide pneumococcal vaccine on recurrent otitis media. Lancet 361: 2189–2195.
66. Veenhoven, R.H., Bogaert, D., Schilder, A.G.M., Rifkers, G.T., Uiterwaal, C.S.P.M., Kiezebrink, H.H., Van Kempen, M.J.P., Dhooge, I. J., Bruin, J., IJzeerman, E.P.F., de Groot, R., Kuis, W., Hermans, P.W.M., Sanders, E.A.M. (2004), Nasopharyngeal pneumococcal carriage after combined pneumococcal conjugate and polysaccharide vaccination in children with a history of recurrent acute otitis media. Clin. Infect. Dis. 39: 911–919.
67. Ghaffer, F., Barton, T., Lozano, J., Muniz, L.S., Huks, P., Gan, V., Ahmad, N., McCracken Jr., G.H. (2004), Effect of the 7-valent pneumococcal conjugate vaccine on nasopharyngeal colonization by *Streptococcus pneumoniae* in the first 2 years of life. Clin. Infect. Dis. 39: 930–938.
68. McEllistrem, M.C., Adams, J.A., Patel, K., Mendelsolm, A.B., Kaplan, S.L., Brodley, J.S., Schitze, G.E., Kim, K.S., Mason, E.O., Wald, E.R. (2005), Acute otitis media due to penicillin-nonsusceptible *Streptococcus pneumoniae* before and after introduction of the pneumococcal conjugate vaccine. Clin. Infect. Dis. 40: 1738–1744.

# Section B
# Emerging Trends in Pulmonary Infection

# Chapter 3
# Current Issues in Ventilator-Associated Pneumonia

## 3.1 Background

Infections in critically ill patients account for a major proportion of the mortality, morbidity, and cost associated with their care. Infection rate in critically ill patients are about 40% and may be 50–60% in those remaining in the intensive care unit (ICU) for more then 5 days.[1,2] Pneumonia acquired in the ICU (after 48 h intubation) ranges from 10% to 65%,[3,4] and respiratory infections account for 30–60% of all infections acquired in the ICU.[5,6] Mortality rates of ventilator-associated pneumonia (VAP) have been very high (30–70%) and may account for 15% of all deaths in the ICU. [7–9] When controlled for severity of underlying disease and other factors the attributable mortality of VAP range from 0% to 50% absolute increase, and prolonged length of ICU stay (range 5–13 days).[10] In a recent review of the clinical and economic consequences of VAP from analysis of studies published after 1990, the findings were: 10–20% of ICU-ventilated patients will develop VAP, and are twice as likely to die compared to patients without VAP, with 6 extra days in the ICU and an additional US$10019 hospital cost per case.[11]

Empiric broad-spectrum antimicrobials in the ICU for presumed pneumonia has contributed substantially to the worldwide increase in antibiotic-resistant bacteria in hospitals. This has compounded the problem of increasing morbidity, mortality, and cost because of the challenge posed by these difficult-to-treat microorganisms, particularly the use of expensive drugs and need for isolation.

This chapter will address emerging issues in VAP such as diagnosis, appropriate management, and prevention.

## 3.2 Issues in the Diagnosis of VAP

Confirming a diagnosis of VAP is a most challenging and difficult task, but is crucial for appropriate management. The criteria used for diagnosing VAP are controversial with some studies relying on clinical and radiological findings and others on microbiological specimens. Differing criteria may largely account for the variable rates of VAP reported from different centers – 5–85%. The standard clinical criteria such as new or progressive infiltrates on chest radiographs, together with fever, leukocytosis or leucopenia, and purulent tracheobronchial secretion are of limited diagnostic accuracy. In studies using histologic analysis and culture of lung samples immediately after death for confirmation of the diagnosis, the presence of new or progressing chest infiltrate with two of three clinical criteria had a sensitivity of 69% and a specificity of 75% for the diagnosis of VAP.[12] This is quite understandable considering that there are several common causes of pulmonary infiltrates in critically ill patients (i.e., pulmonary edema, ARDS, atelectasis, and pulmonary hemorrhage) that can mimic pneumonia; and many intubated patients have tracheobronchitis with purulent respiratory secretions, and may develop fever and leucocytosis from a number of sources (such as urinary tract infection, venous, or arterial catheter infections, *Clostridium difficile* colitis, drugs, blood products, etc.).

Alternative clinical criteria such as the "clinical pulmonary infection score (CPIS)" (a composite of clinical, microbiologic, and oxygenation-related criteria) have not been consistently superior, even with addition of analysis of tracheobronchial secretion.[12,13] The use of CPIS or Pugin score of >6 as recommended by Pugin et al.[14] resulted in a sensitivity of 77% and a specificity of 42%. Although analysis of qualitative culture of tracheobronchial secretion is helpful in identification of the underlying pathogen, it is not specific for the diagnosis of VAP. A common abuse and overuse of antibiotics that we have observed in the ICU by physicians is treatment of potential pathogens from purulent respiratory secretions (tracheobronchitis), with no evidence of pneumonia (personal observation). There is no evidence that antibiotics in these situations are of value and treatment of tracheobronchitis in the ICU is not justified. On the other hand prompt and appropriate treatment of VAP is beneficial and may have a major impact on mortality and morbidity. Although appropriate antibiotics may improve survival in VAP, empiric broad-spectrum antibiotics without clinical infection is potentially harmful, increasing the risk for colonization and superinfection with multiresistant bacteria, fungi (candidiasis), *C. difficile* colitis, and potential adverse events. Numerous studies have documented the increase in multiresistant gram-negative bacilli and gram-positive bacteria in hospital-acquired infection worldwide,[5,15] and the ICU have been deemed "factories for creating, disseminating and amplifying resistance to antibiotics."[16] The presence of methicillin-resistant *Staphylococcus aureus* (MRSA), vancomycin-resistant enterococci (VRE), multiresistant *Pseudomonas aeruginosa*, multiresistant *Acinetobacter baumannii*, extended-spectrum beta lactamase (ESBL) producing coliforms (*Escherichia coli*, *Klebsiella* species, *Enterobacter* species, *Serratia marcescens*, etc.) have become common isolates in many tertiary ICUs.[16] In the United States data from the National Nosomial Infection Surveillance (NNIS) System from 2003 found that *S. aureas* was the most common pathogen in VAP (27.8%), followed by *P. aeruginosa* (18.1%), *Enterobacter* species (10%), *Klebsiella pneumoniae* (7.2%), and *Acinetobacter* species (6.9%).[17]

## 3.2.1 *Microbiological Techniques for Diagnosis*

While qualitative cultures of endobronchial aspirates yield a higher rate of false-positive results (from tracheobronchial colonization), efforts were made to study the role of quantitative analysis of cultures of respiratory secretions to aid in the diagnosis of VAP in the past two decades. These techniques include simple endobronchial aspiration (EA), use of bronchoscopic techniques with or without protected devices, such as protected specimen brush (PSB), or protected catheter to retrieve distal respiratory secretions by lavage (BAL).

Quantitative cultures of EAs with use of cutoff points between $>10^5$ and $>10^7$ CFU/ml have been used, and is simple and practical to perform at anytime in any ICU without fiberoptic bronchoscopy. Although some studies showed favorable results with PBB cultures, with slightly higher sensitivity (82% vs 64%) and lower specificity (83% vs 96%)[17]; others found this technique was only modestly accurate with sensitivity of 70% and relative specificity of <72% in diagnosing pneumonia.[18,19] Most of the studies also used a standard clinical or microbiological criteria as the reference for diagnosing VAP, which as mentioned before lacks accuracy. In one study which compared results of EA quantitative cultures (using $>10^7$ CFU/ml) with those of postmortem lung biopsy quantitative cultures, only 53% of the microorganism isolated in EA samples were also found in lung tissue cultures,[20] Thus indicating poor specificity.

Some investigators have found that quantitative cultures of BAL correlate well with VAP diagnosis, but others have found mixed results and poor specificity especially in patients with tracheobronchial colonization.[7]

Also there is a lack of consensus on the cutoff point for diagnosis; some investigators use $10^4$ and others $10^5$ CFU/ml of at least one microorganism for interpretative threshold. An International Consensus Conference in 1992 had recommended $\geq 10^4$ CFU/ml as the best threshold.[21] To overcome the problem of contamination present in the proximal airways, use of a protected transbronchoscopic balloon-tipped catheter to obtain BAL for quantitative culture has been used. One study of 13 patients with pneumonia and 33 controls, with a threshold of $10^4$ CFU/ml, yielded a diagnostic sensitivity of 97% and a specificity of 92%.[22] Samples obtained by the protected BAL can also be examined directly by Giemsa stain or the gram stain immediately after the procedure to enable intervention with antimicrobial therapy before obtaining culture results. Several studies found that if the Giemsa or gram stain was positive, where >3% or 5% BAL cells contained intracellular bacteria, this correlated with most patients with pneumonia and negative for patients without pneumonia.[13,23,24] Furthermore, the morphological findings on the stained specimens closely correlated with the bacterial cultures.

Other studies used the combination of the BAL procedures sampling and PSB technique to try and improve the diagnostic accuracy. But the PSB by itself has been extensively studied for quantitative cultures (using a special double-catheter brush system with a distal occluding plug to reduce contamination). The PSB is done with a fiberoptic bronchoscope, with cutoff threshold set at $10^3$ CFU. Since

0.01–0.001 ml of secretion is collected with PSB technique, $>10^3$ CFU of bacteria represents $10^5$–$10^6$ CFU/ml of secretion.

Comparison of quantitative BAL and PSB microbiological findings has been noted to have high correlation. In one study[25] the quantitative agreement was 83% of the organisms isolated, and the qualitative results were significantly correlated (rho = 0.46, $p < 0.0001$). Numerous studies have been done in patients with VAP to assess quantitative BAL and PSB. Most of these studies were limited by small sample size and use of clinical or microbiological criteria as the "gold standard" for diagnosis. In studies evaluating both techniques a meta-analysis of 11 studies in 435 ICU patients found the overall accuracy BAL to be close to that of PSB.[26]

Blind-protected telescoping catheter (PTC) (or blind-protected brush PTB) without bronchoscopy has been compared to quantitative BAL via bronchoscope to diagnose VAP. Although blind PTC and PTB specimens have been reported to show very good correlation with BAL in some studies,[27,28,29] provided the sample containing visible secretions expelled from the catheter and both lungs are sampled, other studies showed low concordance between blind and directed PSB samples (53%).[30]

Although there are numerous studies assessing quantitative cultures of various respiratory samples (EA, BAL, blind, and directed PSB or PTC) for diagnosis of VAP they have several shortcomings. Most of the studies involved small sample size with pneumonia; there were frequent flaws and design-related biases,[31] and most important, the "gold standard" for diagnosis of VAP used is controversial and not well-established. The "gold standard" for diagnosis of VAP in several studies included autopsy or histopathology and cultures from open or percutaneous biopsies of lungs immediately after death. The correlation of the various sampling techniques with histology and biopsy culture results is summarized in Table 3.1. Eleven studies performed between 1984 and 2001, were reviewed,[12,32–41] involving 378 subjects from the ICU with 209 (55%) with confirmed VAP. Seventy-two percent of the cases received antibiotics within 48 h of the postmortem studies, thus potentially affecting the accuracy of quantitative cultures in the majority of studies. The sensitivity of quantitative PSB ranged from 15% to 100% (mean 54.6%) and the specificity ranged from 50% to 100% (mean 74.6%), similar to the results of BAL (bronchoscopic and mini-BAL combined) with mean sensitivity and specificity of 51.3% and 79.8%, respectively. Unfortunately only five of the studies assessed the clinical criteria for pneumonia compared to the gold standard, and the mean sensitivity was 81% (range 69–100%) and the mean specificity 62.8% (range 42–85%). Thus, the clinical criteria for pneumonia were not inferior to more invasive investigations and may be somewhat more sensitive. However, it is very likely that prior antibiotics treatment before the quantitative cultures (within 48 h) was responsible for the low sensitivity of these techniques.

There were a few studies assessing the accuracy of these invasive techniques for diagnosis of VAP in animal models. In a canine model of *S. pneumoniae* infection of 18 ventilated dogs quantitative cultures 24 h after infection from transbronchial biopsy, protected-catheter brush, and percutaneous needle aspiration yielded sensitivity of 100%, and specificity of 88% for needle aspiration, and 72% for both catheter brush and transbronchial aspirations specimens.[42] Fiberoptic bronchial

**Table 3.1** Diagnosis techniques for VAP:Histology as "Gold Standard" Sensitivity/Specificity (%) of quantitative

| Source | Year | Total no. patients | No. (%) with pneumonia | No. (%) receiving antibiotics | PSB | BAL | Clinical criteria | Method of Validation | Shortcomings |
|---|---|---|---|---|---|---|---|---|---|
| Chastre et al.[33] | 1984 | 26 | 6(23) | 14(54) | 100/42–87 | — | — | Open lung (L) biopsy 1 cm³ immediately after death. | Pneumonia sample size small. |
| Rouby et al.[34] | 1992 | 83(33 had quantitative cultures) | 43(52) | 67(81) | — | 70/69 (Protected mini-BAL) | — | Pneumonectomy 30 min after death. | Most patients received antibiotic. |
| Torres et al.[35] | 1994 | 30 | 18(60) | 30(100) | 36/50 | 50/45 | 70/45 | Lung Biopsies <1 h after death. | All received antibiotics. |
| Chastre et al.[36] | 1995 | 20 | 11(55) | 18(90) | 82/89 | 91/78 | — | Open lung biopsy PM 2 × 5 cm³ <1 h after death. | Used bacterial burden in lung tissue, not histology as gold standard. |
| Papazian et al.[37] | 1995 | 38 | 18(47) | 16(43) <48 hr | 33/95 | 50/95 | 72/85(CPIS) | Pneumonectomy 30 min after death | — |
| Marquette et al.[38] | 1995 | 28 | 19(68) | 15(54) | 57/88 | 77/58 | — | Lungs at autopsy | Clinical criteria for VAP not analyzed. |
| Kirtland et al.[39] | 1997 | 39 | 9(23) | 38(97) | 15–50/50–77 | 11–14/80 | — | Open lung biopsy <1 h after death | Most patients received antibiotics. |
| Fabregas et al.[12] | 1999 | 25 | 23(92) | 17(68) | 62/75 | 77/58 | 69/75 77/42 (CPIS) | Multiple lung biopsies (2 cm³) immediately after death. | Most patients received antibiotics. |

(*continued*)

**Table 3.1** (continued)

| Source | Year | Total no. patients | No. (%) with pneumonia | No. (%) receiving antibiotics | PSB | BAL | Clinical criteria | Method of Validation | Shortcomings |
|---|---|---|---|---|---|---|---|---|---|
| Bregeon et al.[40] | 2000 | 27 | 14(52) by histology 9, (33) by culture + histology | 13(48) | (PDA) Histo-criteria 57/100 Combined-criteria 67–71/ 75–87 | (Mini BAL) 50/86 78/86 | 100/61 100/69 (CPIS) | Pneumonectomy within 30 min of death. | Two different criteria for pneumonia: lower cut off threshold than others. |
| Torres et al.[41] | 2000 | 25 | 23(92) | 17(68) | Histo-criteria 24–28/50–54 Combined-criteria 67–71/75–87 | PBAL 16–19/ 75–77 43–63/83–91 | 80/– | Bilateral open lung biopsies (2 cm$^3$) <90 min after death | Clinical criteria not assessed for specificity; criteria for pneumonia. |
| Balthazar et al.[42] | 2001 | 37 | 20(54) | Not given | – | 90/94 | – | Open lung biopsy <1 h after death | Antibiotic treatment not mentioned clinical criteria not assessed. |
| Total 11 studies: | 1984–2001 | 378 | 209(55) | 245/341(72) | 54.6/74.6 (mean) | 51.3/79.8 (mean) | 81/62.8 (mean) | – | – |

aspirations specimens were found to be unreliable, and unfortunately quantitative cultures were not performed.

In a baboon model of VAP (ventilated for 7–10 days), BAL recovered 74% of all species present in lung tissue compared to 41% by PSB and 56% for needle aspirates.[43] Although false-positive rates for the three techniques were similar, the specificity was not provided. Tracheal aspirations revealed 78% of the organism but 40% of the species were not present in lung tissue.

In summary, quantitative cultures from BAL (with or without protected catheter) or PSB have not been proven superior to clinical criteria for diagnosis of VAP. This is reflected in the most recent consensus conference on VAP in 2001,[44] when it was acknowledged that there is no accepted "gold standard" for diagnosis, and no superiority of any specific diagnostic method. The diagnosis of VAP was still defined as the presence of new, persistent pulmonary infiltrates not otherwise explained, appearing on chest radiograph (not present before intubation); and the presence of at least two of the following criteria: (1) temperature $>38°C$, (2) leukocytosis $>10,000$ cells/mm$^3$, and (3) purulent respiratory secretions.[44] A recent multicenter randomized trial of 740 patients in 28 ICUs in Canada and the United States have confirmed these opinions.[46] There were no differences in outcome and overall use of antibiotics when two diagnostic strategies for VAP were compared, BAL with quantitative culture and EA with nonquantitative culture.[46]

### 3.2.2 New Diagnostic Methods for VAP

Several biological markers have been studied to improve the diagnostic accuracy of VAP but with disappointing results. These include serum and bronchial procalcitonin levels,[47,48] C-reactive protein,[48] tumor necrosis factor alpha (TNFα),[49] and other proinflammatory cytokines concentrations.[49,50] The most promising investigative tool to date appears to be the measurement of soluble triggering receptor expressed on myeloid cells (sTREM-1) from BAL fluid.

TREM-1 is a member of the immunoglobulin super family[51] that is important in the acute inflammatory response to infections,[52] and the expression is up-regulated on phagocytes on exposure to bacterial and fungal products. Neutrophils and monocytes in tissues infected with bacteria express high levels of TREM-1, whereas noninfectious inflammatory disorders weakly express TREM-1 on those calls.[52] TREM-1 can be measured in body fluids in the soluble form as it is shed by the membrane of activated phagocytes.

In a study of 76 patients admitted to the ICU with suspected infection and fulfilling at least two criteria for the systemic inflammatory response syndrome (SIRS) sTREM-1 plasma levels were measured.[53] Sepsis or septic shock was diagnosed in 47 (62%) patients, and a plasma level of $>60$ ng/ml of sTREM-1 was more accurate than any other clinical or laboratory findings for indicating infection (sensitivity 96%, specifically, 89%).[53] The same investigators also assessed sTREM-1 in BAL fluid in patients admitted to the ICU with and without pneumonia.[35] In a prospective study of 148 patients receiving mechanical ventilation a rapid immunoblot technique (also available from R & D systems, with the entire procedure taking less than 3 h), was used to measure sTREM-1 in BAL fluid (sensitivity 5 pg/ml),[54] obtained by mini-BAL technique. Forty-six patients were diagnosed with VAP (clinical criteria similar to the consensus conference in 2001),[44] 38 patients had community-acquired pneumonia, and 68 patients had no pneumonia. A sTREM-1 cutoff value of 5 pg/ml had a sensitivity of 98% and specificity of 90% for presence of any pneumonia; and was the strongest predictor of pneumonia, with an odds ratio of 41.5.[55] The best clinical predictor of pneumonia was a CPIS of >6 (odds ratio, 3.0).

In a more recent study from the Netherlands, BAL fluid and plasma were collected sequentially on alternate days (from start of ventilatory support until complete weaning) for measurement of sTREM-1 levels by enzyme-linked immunosorbent assay (ELISA) in 9 patients who developed VAP and 19 controls without pneumonia.[55] Plasma levels of sTREM-1 did not change significantly in either patient group, while BAL fluid levels increased towards significance with the diagnosis of VAP but not in controls.[55] A cutoff value of 200 pg/ml in BAL fluid for sTREM-1 on the day of pneumonia diagnosis had a sensitivity of 75% and specificity of 84%.

## 3.3 Microbial Etiology of VAP

The causes of VAP can vary considerably by geographic location, local epidemiology, patient characteristics, length of hospital stay, and duration of mechanical ventilation. Most studies of VAP, however, find a predominance of gram-negative bacilli and staphylococci that normally colonize the oropharynx and gut. The most common pathogens include *S. aureus*, *P. aeruginosa*, *Klebsiella* species, *Enterobacter* species, *Acinetobacter* species, and *S. marcescens*, but the relative frequency will vary from center to center. In early-onset VAP, soon after admission and <7 days on mechanical ventilation, *S. pneumoniae*, *Haemophilus influenzae*, and more susceptible gram-negative bacilli, maybe the etiological agents.[44] Polymicrobial infections with mixed bacteria have also been reported in up to 48% of all cases of VAP.[57] The importance of anaerobes is unknown due to inadequate studies and is likely underestimated. The rates of isolation of anaerobes in VAP have been low in most studies (1–3.5%),[44] but has been higher (23%) in one study.[58] This suggests that other studies may be using inadequate techniques for obtaining (oxygen administration), transporting, and culturing respiratory secretions for anaerobes. Atypical bacteria (*Legionella pneumophila*, *Chlamydia pneumoniae*, viruses (i.e., respiratory syncytial virus), and fungi have also been implicated at times, but these pathogens have not been studied systematically and their role is presently unclear.[58]

The method of obtaining specimen to confirm the etiology has been contentious, with, advocates of deep endotracheal aspirates citing simplicity, easy to perform by any ICU nurses, versus advocates of more invasive bronchoscopy techniques.

However, recent studies have found similarities in obtaining clinically significant pathogens from four procedures used (blind endotracheal aspiration, PSB, bronchoscopic BAL, or directed brushings).[59,60] Although, initial prospective studies showed improved outcomes (mortality) with invasive versus noninvasive diagnostic management for suspected VAP,[61,62] more recent studies have not.[63,64] In the most recent review and meta-analysis of this topic it was concluded that the invasive strategies do not alter mortality in VAP, but affect antibiotic use and prescribing.[65,66] Although most investigators favored a more invasive approach,[44] others recommended initial endotracheal aspiration for diagnosis, and reserve invasive methods for patients not responding to initial empirical antibiotic treatment.[64,67] The latter course is reasonable and may allow more rapid intervention, as a precise bacteriologic diagnosis is of paramount importance for therapeutic success and cultures should be obtained before initiating therapy. Other areas where initial invasive diagnostic procedures are warranted include immunocompromised hosts (i.e., acquired immune deficiency syndrome [AIDS]), and BAL samples should be sent for viral studies, mycobacterial and fungal smears and cultures, cytology, and stain for *Pneumocystis carinii*.

## 3.4 Issues in Treatment of VAP

Treatment of VAP should be started in a timely manner with appropriate antibiotics once the diagnosis is made. The results of cultures should not delay starting empirical therapy, usually a broad-spectrum agent (or combination) to cover *S. aureus* and gram-negative bacilli. There is some data to indicate that starting therapy early in VAP lowers the mortality (trend) than delaying therapy for >48 h after the diagnosis was considered.[67,68] Treatment may be guided by gram stain of respiratory samples to assist in choice of antimicrobial agents, as the overall accuracy in diagnosing VAP for any organism was 88% in one retrospective study.[69] A combination of gram stain and bacterial adenosine triphosphate (ATP) assay have also been used for rapid diagnosis of BAL samples, with sensitivity of 95.3%, specificity of 54.9%, and negative predictive value of 97.6%.[70] Thus a negative result may allow use of narrow spectrum antimicrobial agents or withholding empiric therapy for suspected VAP.[70] Assaying for endotoxin from BAL samples have also been used to diagnose gram-negative bacterial VAP as a rapid test, but this is not generally available in most centers and appears to provide the same accuracy as a gram stain (which is cheaper and easier to perform in any clinical laboratory).[71]

There is no consensus as to the initial empiric therapy for VAP, as this should depend on the individual center's experience with the prevalence and pattern of antimicrobial-resistant bacteria. Factors that should be taken into consideration in selecting an antibiotic include onset of pneumonia after ventilation, duration of hospitalization, previous antimicrobial therapy, and underlying disease. Early onset of VAP (<7 days of ventilation) in patients not previously treated with antibiotics may be due to more sensitive bacteria, such as in *S. pneumoniae, H. influenzae*, methicillin-susceptible *S. aureus*, and enteric gram-negative bacilli. In this situation it is recommended to use a single agent that has no anti-pseudomonal activity such as ampicillin-sulbactam, -ceftriaxone, or -cefotaxime, newer fluoroquinolones, or ertapenem.[44]

In cases of VAP occurring >7 days after ventilation, or previously treated with antibiotics or hospitalized for prolonged periods, more resistant bacteria may be responsible for pneumonia such as MRSA, *P. aeruginosa*, *Acinetobacter* species, and multiresistant organisms. However, it would appear that the duration of ventilation before development of pneumonia is less important than the duration of hospitalization and previous antibiotic therapy in predisposing to *Pseudomonas* or more resistant bacterial infection.[72] Initial therapy under these circumstances may include a broad-spectrum coverage (such as imipenem or meropenem, piperacillin-tazobacterum, or combination of agents) to cover the most prevalent bacteria circulating in the ICU. Empiric therapy for MRSA is usually not necessary unless the patient is known to be colonized or in close contact with a subject with MRSA, and the respiratory sample shows gram-positive cocci in clusters. In a consensus conference most investigators preferred to use a combination of an aminoglycoside or a fluoroquinolone with an anti-pseudomonal, extended-spectrum β-lactam or a carbapenem plus an aminoglycoside in late onset VAP, until cultures and susceptibility are available, but there are no clinical trials available to support these guidelines.[44] Intuitively it seems rational that selection of an antimicrobial regimen should be effective against recent pathogens that colonize the patient's respiratory tract. However, serial routine microbial cultures result in the initial management of VAP has been found to be of limited value.[73]

Does *P. aeruginosa* pneumonia require a combination therapy? It has been standard practice in many centers and recommendation by most investigators to use a combination of anti-pseudomonal, extended-spectrum β-lactam with an aminoglycoside or with a fluoroquinolone (i.e., ciprofloxacin) for *P. aeruginosa* pneumonia.[74] However, the concept that dual therapy is superior to monotherapy or less likely to develop antibacterial resistance is unproven. Despite this, since *P. aeruginosa* pneumonia carries a poor prognosis with mortality rate that exceeds 40%[8] and the variable resistance pattern to extended-spectrum β-lactam agents and ciprofloxacin (which is increasing in many centers)[75] it is a reasonable recommendation to use a combination of two agents.

The most common advocated practice for VAP is to maximize empirical antimicrobial coverage with subsequent streamlining of therapy once culture and sensitivity data are available.[76,77] This appears to be a successful strategy but studies using historical controls may suffer from significant bias. It has been suggested that computer-assisted antibiotic prescription in ICUs may supplement or replace such strategies in the future.[76]

Duration of therapy for VAP was often variable and empirical with a tendency for overtreatment. A recent randomized multicenter study of 402 patients with VAP showed no difference in outcome between 8-day versus 15-day course of antibiotic therapy and the recurrence rate was similar (28.9% and 26.0%), except

*P. aeruginosa* was associated with higher recurrence in the shorter course group (40.6% vs 25.4%).[78] Thus shorter course of therapy may lead to less antibiotic exposure and possible help reduce antimicrobial resistance in the ICU. Another approach to limit antibiotic overuse in the ICU for low-risk patients with pulmonary infiltrates with suspected pneumonia is to initiate monotherapy then stop antibiotic therapy at 3 days for those with a CPIS < 6.[79] In this randomized, unblinded, controlled study of 81 patients, the outcome was similar but patients receiving earlier discontinuation of antibiotics had lower incidence of antimicrobial resistance or superinfection, and lower mean antibiotic costs.[79]

In the past when less active anti-pseudomonal β-lactam (carbenicillin) was available and aminoglycosides were used by multiple dosing, there was concern about inadequate endobronchial concentration of aminoglycoside for severe *Pseudomonas* or gram-negative pneumonia. Interest was generated by a few studies to administer the aminoglycoside endobronchially via endotracheal tube or tracheostomy to complement combined systemic therapy. In a double-blind randomized study of gram-negative VAP, all patients received systemic tobramycin plus piperacillin or cefazolin and half the patients were randomized to receive 40 mg tobramycin every 8 h or placebo instilled enotracheally.[80] *P. aeruginosa* was the main pathogen in 41% of 41 assessable cases. Although the causative pathogens were eradicated from respiratory tract more frequently in those receiving endotracheal tobramycin, there was no difference in the clinical outcome of the two groups.[80] In a more recent study of 38 VAP patients with a similar design half the patients were randomized to receive either additional nebulized tobramycin (6 mg/kg/day) or placebo, once daily for 5 days.[81] Extubation by day 10 was achieved in 35% of patients receiving nebulized tobramycin and 18.5% of those in the placebo group but the difference was not statistically significant.

Of growing concern in the past three decades is the emergence of *Acinetobacter* nosocomial infection worldwide, especially in ICUs. This is alarming in view of the ability of this gram-negative bacteria to accommodate diverse mechanisms of resistance, with multiresistant strains to all available antibiotics occurring in local outbreaks.[82] *A. baumannii*, the most important of the three commonly isolated species (including *A. calcoaceticus*, and *A. lwoffi*), has shown dramatic increased resistance to carbapenem from 9% in 1995 to 40% in 2004 in surveillance of 300 US hospitals.[83] These nosocomial strains of *Acinetobacter* commonly demonstrate extended-spectrum beta-lactamases (ESBL), alterations in cell-wall channels (porins), antibiotic efflux pumps, aminoglycoside-modifying enzymes, mutations in the genes gyrA and par C (conferring quinolone resistance), and serine or metallo-β-lactamases conferring resistance to carbapenems.[82] The most frequent clinical manifestation of *Acinetobacter* infection are VAPs and bacteremias (often from vascular catheters).

VAP due to *Acinetobacter* occurs later in the ICU stay in patients on prolonged ventilation, often previously treated with broad-spectrum β-lactams (third-generation cephalosporins and quinolones). The clinical effect of *Acinetobacter* VAP on outcome has been variable. The major impact has been on longer ICU stays and hospitalization when matched for severity of underlying illness, suggesting that coexisting conditions were the major predictors of outcome.[82] Treatment of multi-drug-resistant *Acinetobacter* VAP is a challenge with limited options. Recent reports have been mostly small retrospective case series on the use of colistin alone or in combination with rifampin (with success of 25–50%).[81] Tigecycline, a new glycylcycline antibiotic, has in vitro activity against some *A. baumannii* resistant strains but there is evidence of increased resistance.[81] Susceptible strains can be treated with sulbactam, imipenem, third-generation cephalosporins, or aminoglycosides depending on in vitro susceptibility.

## 3.5 Prevention of VAP

There are several issues and areas of contention in the approach to prevent pneumonia in the mechanically ventilated patients. Obviously this would be worthwhile as it should save lives, reduce mortality, decrease duration of ventilation and hospitalization, and reduce costs. It would appear evident that the best way to prevent VAP is to avoid intubation and mechanical ventilation but this is not feasible in most instances. There has been much interest in the use of noninvasive positive-pressure ventilation (NPPV) to prevent intubation and manage patients with respiratory failure. In a recent review and meta-analysis of 12 studies, NPPV showed a strong benefit in reducing pneumonia compared to standard ventilation (relative risk 0.31, 95% CI 0.16 to 0.57, $p = 0.0002$).[84] However, the strongest evidence to support use of NPPV in patients with acute respiratory failure is in patients with exacerbation of underlying chronic obstructive pulmonary disease.[85] Patients with cardiogenic pulmonary edema and pulmonary contusion have also been found to require lower intubation rates, whereas patients with a higher severity score, an older age, ARDS or pneumonia, or fail to improve after 1 h of treatment, the risk of failure with NPPV is higher.[86] Thus in hypoxic acute respiratory failure management with NPPV can be successful in selected patients.

Rotational beds, prone position and semi-recumbent position have been proposed and investigated as simple measures to prevent VAP. These measures as preventative techniques have recently been reviewed by Hess.[87] Rotational therapy uses a special kinetic bed designed to turn continuously, or nearly continuously, the patient from side to side. A meta-analysis of studies evaluating the effect of rotational bed therapy shows a decrease in risk of pneumonia but no effect on mortality.[88] Considering increased cost of these kinetic beds ($200/day), potential for an advertent disconnection of intravenous catheters, they are not routinely recommended but may be useful in select patients with neurologic problems or surgical patients.[88]

Prone positioning has been shown to increase alveolar oxygenation ($PaO_2$) in patients with ARDS and lung injury but no survival benefit.[87] Two randomized studies on prone positioning (4–8 h/day) compared to supine position has been performed. One small study showed reduction in VAP (not statistically significant), and a larger study in 21 ICUs found just significant lower VAP with prone positioning (20.6% vs 24.1%) but no improvement in mortality in both studies.[89,90] Thus prone positioning is not recommended as technical considerations preclude its use and it is associated with increased complications such as pressure ulcers and obstruction of the endotracheal tube.[89]

Studies have shown that radiolabeled enteral feeding in mechanically ventilated patients are more likely to be aspirated in the supine position compared to the semi-recumbent position (head elevated at a 45 degree angle).[87] One randomized study have found that semi-recumbent position was associated with lower VAP compared to the supine position (RRO.22, 95%, CI 0.05–0.92, $p$ = 0.04).[91] Since semi-recumbent positioning is a low-cost, low-risk approach to preventing VAP it has been recommended for routine positioning in the ICU by the Centers for Disease Control and Prevention[92] and the Canadian Critical Care Society,[10] despite the fact that mortality was not improved in the randomized study.[89] However, in a more recent randomized, prospective study 109 patients were assigned supine position (with backrest elevation of 10 degrees), and 112 to the semi-recumbent position (target backrest elevation of 45 degrees) was not achieved 85% of the study time. The achieved difference in the treatment position (28 degrees vs 10 degrees) did not prevent the development of VAP.[93]

In a small pilot study 35 patients on mechanical ventilation received continuous lateral rotational therapy (CLRT) for 5 days, compared to 35 control patients matched for age, gender, cause of respiratory failure, admission APACHE score, received routine positional change.[94] The patients receiving CLRT had improved oxygenation and reduced incidence of VAP compared to controls. Thus a large, randomized, prospective study is warranted to confirm this observation. In another small study 60 ventilated patients were randomized to receive chest physiotherapy or sham physiotherapy, VAP occurred in 39% of the controls and 8% of the treated group, $p$ = 0.02.[95] However, there were no differences in duration of stay or ICU mortality. It is surprising that larger randomized control trials have not been reported since this report in 2002 to confirm these results.

### 3.5.1 Antibiotic Prophylaxis for Prevention of VAP

Interest in the use of antibiotic prophylaxis for prevention of nosocomial pneumonia has existed from the early 1970s. Although a randomized study in 1974 had shown that gentamicin administered endotracheally could prevent gram-negative pneumonia in patients with tracheotomies,[96] this method was not widely adopted due to fears of antimicrobial-resistant bacteria developing.

The gastrointestinal tract is believed to play an important role in the pathogenesis of VAP, and gram-negative enteric bacteria colonizing the stomach and oropharynx are the same bacteria isolated from respiratory secretions in VAP. Interventions used to reduce the bacterial colonization and hence VAP include selective decontamination of the digestive tract (SDD) with antimicrobials (topical with or without systemic therapy), use of sucralfate for stress ulcer prophylaxis, and external feeding strategies that preserve gastric acidity, or lessen pooling of oropharyngeal secretions.

Numerous studies have been published on antibiotic prophylaxis or SDD to prevent VAP in the past two decades. In the most recent Cochrane Review of 36 trials involving 6,922 patients, 17 trials ($N = 4,295$ patients) tested a combination of topical and systemic antibiotics, the average rate of respiratory tract infections and mortality in the control group were 36% and 29%, respectively.[97] There was a significant reduction of both VAP (OR 0.35, 95% CI 0.29–0.41) and mortality (OR 0.78, 95% CI 0.68–0.89) and on average required 5 patients to be treated to prevent one VAP, and 21 patients to prevent one death. In 17 trials ($N = 2,664$) that tested topical antimicrobial alone, there was a significant reduction in VAP (OR 0.52, 95% CI, 0.43–0.63) but not in total mortality in the treated group.[97] However, only one of the trials explored the consequences of antibiotic resistance and superinfection as a result of prophylaxis. With accumulating evidence of increasing antimicrobial resistance in the ICU, and evidence that SDD promotes gram-positive bacterial infections, most guidelines do not recommend routine antibiotic prophylaxis in the ICU.[10,92,97–100]

Efforts to reduce heavy colonization of oropharyngeal bacteria by improving oral hygiene and use of topical antiseptics have received little attention in the scientific literature as a means of prevention of VAP. Oral hygiene is compromised in ICU patients by the presence of intubations tube, nasogastric catheter, heavy sedation, anticholinergic drugs, and mouth breathing all impair salivation and normal swallowing mechanism and allow bacterial overgrowth. Unfortunately, little is known about the efforts of oral care interventions in ICU patients on mechanical ventilation and development of VAP.[101]

Chlorhexidine is a broad-spectrum antibacterial agent (bactericidal for both gram-negative and gram-positive bacteria), that is not absorbed through mucosa or skin, and is the recommended antiseptic of choice for preoperative preparations. It is also available as an oral rinse to prevent and treat gingivitis. An advantage of chlorhexidine is the absence of any significant bacterial resistance and good safety profile when used topically. Two previous randomized, placebo-controlled studies were performed before intubating and continued therapy throughout the ICU stay in patients undergoing elective cardiac surgery.[102,103] Both studies showed a reduction in nosocomial pneumonia, but was significant only for one study,[102] and for a subgroup of those at highest risk of pneumonia in the other.[103]

In a prospective, nonrandomized, controlled study in a surgical ICU patient's intubated for mechanical ventilation for the 5 months were given standard care with ventilator weaning protocol (controls).[104] During the following 5 months 0.12% chlorhexidine gluconate oral rinse was added twice daily to all intubated patients ($N = 95$ for both groups). The addition of chlorhexidine led to a significant reduction and delay in the occurrence of VAP (37% overall, 75% for late VAP, $p < 0.05$). The median duration of mechanical ventilation and length of stay in the ICU or hospital, between the groups were no different.[104] This type of design, however, may lead to biases that could influence results.

A recent randomized, placebo-controlled multicenter trial on the value of antiseptic oral decontamination in 228 nonedentulous patients on mechanical ventilation has been reported.[105] A 0.2% chlorhexidine gel or placebo gel on gingival and dental surfaces was applied three times daily during the entire ICU stay. No difference was observed in the incidence of VAP, duration of ventilation, mortality, or length of stay, but the number of positive dental plaque cultures was significantly lower in the treated group (29% vs 66%, $p < 0.05$).[105]

### 3.5.2 Maintaining Gastric Acidity to Prevent VAP

It is a routine practice in ICUs to give stress ulcer prophylaxis to prevent upper gastrointestinal hemorrhage. However, gastric colonization with potentially pathogenic bacteria increases with decreasing acidity, and these enteric pathogens are the potential causes of VAP from aspiration. Medications used for stress ulcer prophylaxis that alter gastric pH include antacids, H2 antagonists, and proton pump inhibitors, which increase bacterial colonization of the stomach and may increase the risk for VAP. Sucralfate, which is a gastric cytoprotective agent that enhances natural mucosal barrier, is an alternative prophylactic agent that may reduce VAP. Seven meta-analysis of 20 randomized trials on the benefit of sucralfate therapy compared to H2 antagonists have been reported.[10] Four of the seven meta-analysis found a significant decrease in VAP with sucralfate, and three also found a reduction of mortality with sucralfate.[93] Three other meta-analyses found similar but insignificant trends in reduction of VAP with use of sucralfate. Thus sucralfate has been recommended for stress ulcer prophylaxis in patients with low to moderate risk for gastrointestinal bleeding (absence of bleeding tendency or need for prolong mechanical ventilation).[10,92]

In patients at high risk for gastrointestinal bleeding H2 antagonists or a proton pump inhibitor are preferred for stress ulcer prophylaxis. In these circumstances other methods to reduce gastric enteric bacterial overgrowth are needed. A recent pilot study has examined the benefit of acidifying feeding formula using potassium sorbate to reduce bacterial burden.[106] Sixteen patients on mechanical ventilation were randomized to receive acidified formula (PH 4.25) and 14 controls received standard formula. The number of organisms isolated in each patient per week and the quantity of bacteria (colony forming units/ml) of gastric aspirates were significantly higher in the controls.[106]

There was no difference in gastrointestinal bleeding between the two groups. Thus large, randomized clinical trials to assess prevention of VAP and bleeding risk in patients requiring H2 antagonists or proton pump inhibitor are warranted with this acidified feeding formula. A previous randomized study of acidified feeding formula used hydrochloric acid added to the formula in critically ill patients, all on sucralfate with 120 enrolled but 95 analyzed with primary outcome measure being bacterial colonization of gastric contents, and secondary outcome VAP.[107] Bacterial colonization was significantly less in the acidified treatment group 2% versus 43%; VAP was less than half in the acid feeds (6.1%) versus control group (15%) but sample size was too small to show any significant difference.

### 3.5.3 Methods to reduce Aspiration

Pooling of oropharyngeal secretions above the endotracheal tube cuff may play a role in aspiration of bacteria-laden fluid and subsequent VAP. Thus methods to reduce or drain subglottic secretions require use of specially designed endotracheal tube with a separate dorsal lumen that opens into the subglottic region.

In a recent meta-analysis of five randomized studies with 896 patients enrolled, subglottic secretions drainage reduced the incidence of VAP by nearly half ($RR = 0.51$, 95% CI 0.37–0.71), mainly within 7 days of intubation.[108] Secretion drainage shortened the duration of mechanical ventilation by 2 days and the length of ICU stay by 3 days and delayed the onset of pneumonia by almost 7 days. Thus subglottic secretion appears effective in preventing early-onset VAP in patients requiring mechanical ventilation for >3 days. Although no beneficial effect on mortality was reported, it would be cost-effective even though the specialized endotracheal tubes cost about 25% more than standard endotracheal tubes, and there is no significant harm reported with this technique. This method for prevention of VAP has been recommended by the CDC and other guidelines.[10,89,92]

Few other methods to reduce oropharyngeal or gastric content aspiration have been examined in randomized studies. One approach is to use gel lubrication of the tracheal tube cuff to reduce pulmonary aspiration. In a small pilot study of 36 anesthetized patients and 9 ICU patients with tracheostomies, lubricated cuffs were compared to non-lubricated cuffs leakage of dye placed in the subglottic space[109]. Dye leakage was 11% in the lubrication group and 83% in the non-lubrication group of anesthetized patients, $p < 0.001$. In the ICU patients with lubricated cuff tracheostomy tubes leakage first occurred after a mean of 48 h (range 24–120 h). Thus for patients with prolonged intubation/ventilation changing or reinserting the tube with fresh lubrication every 48 h would be a practical limitation.

Use of large-bore nasogastric tube may promote gastroesophageal reflux and pulmonary aspiration in ICU patients. In a pilot study of 30 patients on mechanical ventilation 16 received external feeding through a small-bore tube and 14 received no tube feeding, all in the semi-recumbent position, and aspiration of gastric contents was assessed by radioisotope technique.[110] There were no gastric contents aspirations in both groups, but patients with large bore nasogastric tubes should have been assessed as well. This hypothesis has not been tested in any large, randomized clinical trials.

The mere presence of a nasogastric tube is considered a risk factor for development of VAP. Alternatively, gastrostomy can be used for administration of external feedings. A previous randomized study had found no benefit of small-bowel feeding versus gastric feeding, when the nasoenteric tube was placed in the duodenum versus the stomach.[111] Two recent meta-analysis reviewed the evidence from randomized control trials comparing gastric with post-pyloric feeding (3 studies). Heyland et al.[112] found a significant reduction in VAP with post-pyloric feeding (OR 0.76, 95% CI 0.59–0.99), while Marick and Zaloga[113] found a nonsignificant trend in reduction of VAP with post-pyloric feeding.

In a recent small, randomized study in patients mechanically ventilated for stroke or head injury, 20 subjects were allocated for gastrostomy and 21 for nasogastric tube (controls) for 3 weeks.[114] VAP developed in 12.5% of patients with gastrostomy and 44.4% with nasogastric tube, but the overall duration of hospitalization and mortality were no different. This study needs to be confirmed by larger studies, and the result is suggestive that for patients with central nervous system deficit on ventilation, gastrostomy feeding is preferable to nasogastric feeding when prolong ventilatory support is needed.

### 3.5.4 Ventilator Circuit and VAP

In recent years, the relationship of respiratory care equipment and VAP has been undergoing scrutiny by several studies. Several randomized, controlled studies have examined the effect of antibacterial humidification strategies, such as the replacement of heated humidifiers by heat and moisture exchangers, in preventing VAP. In a meta-analysis of eight studies conducted between 1990 and 2003 revealed a reduction in a relative risk of VAP (0.7) with heat and moisture exchanges particularly in patients on mechanical ventilation for 7 days (RR0.57).[115] Also, those heat and moisture exchangers do not need to be changed more than every 5 days. However, for wider applicability further studies were recommended because of patient selection and exclusion for patients with high risk of airway occlusion.

There is potential for cross-infection in the ICU of multiresistant bacteria, or contamination of the patients' airway by extrinsic microorganism during the traditional suction of the airway by disconnection from the ventilator (open system). In the past several years there have been several randomized, prospective studies of VAP pneumonia in patients using closed versus open suction system. Most of the studies enrolled insufficient number of patients to demonstrate a significant difference (<100 patients), and as yet no meta-analysis have been published. However, two large studies are worthwhile reviewing. Combes et al.[116] enrolled 54 patients to closed suction and 50 to open suction, and the rate of VAP was lower with the closed suction group, 7.32 versus 15.89/1,000 patient days, $p = 0.07$. A much larger randomized study of 443 patients, recently found no difference in mortality or VAP between open or closed suctioning, 17.59 versus 15.94/1,000 ventilation-days but the cost per day for the closed suction was more expensive.[117]

### 3.5.5 Summary of Prevention

Several methods are available that have been shown by randomized, controlled studies to reduce the incidence of VAP. Surprisingly, most of these techniques have not resulted in improved survival.

Before intubation and mechanical ventilation attempts should be made to give a trial of NPPV for at least an hour in selected patients (exacerbation of COPD, cardiogenic pulmonary edema, and pulmonary contusion). The available evidence suggests that semi-recumbent position should be used routinely, rotational therapy should be considered in selected patients, and prone position should not be used as a technique to reduce VAP. Sucralfate rather than H2 antagonists in patients at low to moderate risk for gastrointestinal tract bleeding should be used for prophylaxis. Aspiration of subglottic secretions should be routinely practiced to decrease VAP, but closed tracheal suctioning is not superior to an open system. Small bowel feeding rather than gastric feeding for patients requiring prolonged mechanical ventilation (>7 days) may be considered but the value is still controversial.

Selected patients with low risk of airway occlusion (tenacious secretions etc.), intubation for >7 days can benefit from heat and moisture exchangers, which may not be changed more than every 5 days. Although selective decontamination of the upper digestive tract is of proven value, it is not routinely recommended as the risk of widespread antimicrobial resistance is a major concern.

## 3.6 Future Directions

A noninvasive method of confirming VAP or a clinical "gold standard" for the diagnosis is still elusive. The most promising technique to date is to measure BAL fluid s-TREM-1 concentration. Further large prospective studies are needed to confirm its utility with autopsy/open lung biopsies as "gold standard" for VAP. Moreover, controls without VAP should include septic patients from other sources; patients with lung cancers and tracheobronchitis without pneumonia to confirm the specificity.

New innovative methods to prevent VAP should be investigated. Development of substances to block adhesion of bacteria to oropharyngeal and gastric mucosa may be of benefit to prevent VAP, rather than antimicrobial prophylaxis. For example, cranberry juice (or its metabolite) can prevent adhesion of enteric coliform bacteria to the uroepithelium and has been shown to decrease recurrent urinary tract infections.

A recent study on the long-term prognosis of VAP has shown that the in-hospital mortality was 42.3%, but also the estimated after discharge mortality was substantial at 1, 3, and 5 years, 25.9%, 33.6%, and 44.7%, resperctively.[118] The 5-year estimated mortality of the survivors is just less than 50%. Thus, there should be great impetus for clinicians and intensivists to try and prevent VAP.

Rapid methods to identify and determine antibiotic susceptibility to the organisms causing VAP are needed and should be studied. A recent prospective, randomized study over 2 years in Spain demonstrated the utility of direct E-test (AB Biodisk) of respiratory samples in VAP.[119] In 250 patients with VAP, 167 were enrolled in the direct E-test and 83 in the standard methods of susceptibility, results were available to the clinicians with a mean of 1.4 days by direct E-test versus 4.2 days by the standard method. This method of rapid antimicrobial susceptibility resulted in decreased antibiotic consumption, *C. difficile* colitis, and fewer days on mechanical ventilation with significant cost savings.[119] One of the limitations of this method is the unreliability of direct E-test with polymicrobial infection.[120] Novel molecular technologies, using real-time PCR and peptide nucleic acid fluorescent in situ hybridization (PNA-FISH), are now available that can provide rapid identification of resistant bacteria such as MRSA in 1 h.[121] These techniques need to be studied in respiratory secretions of VAP and would facilitate more targeted therapy, less utilization of unnecessary agents such as vancomycin. This would likely improve outcome with less superinfection and predisposition to proliferation of resistant bacteria.

Should a newer macrobide be used in combination with other antimicrobials for VAP with sepsis? Atypical microorganisms are rare causes of VAP or nosocomial pneumonia, except for the occasional case and local mini-outbreaks of legionella pneumonia and, thus, macrolides are not routinely used for VAP. However, there is evidence that some macrolides (e.g., clarithromycin) have anti-inflammatory properties by inhibiting the biosynthesis of proinflammatory cytokines in mononuclear cells in vitro an in vivo. In a recent randomized, blinded, multicenter trial clarithromycin 1 g/day for 3 days was compared to placebo in 200 patients with VAP.[122] Clarithromycin accelerated the resolution of VAP (5.5 days earlier, $p = 0.011$) and weaning from mechanical ventilation (6.5 days earlier, $p = 0.049$) but did not improve survival. Thus larger RCTs are warranted to confirm these results.

New endotracheal tubes silver coated internally and externally may be of value to prevent VAP, as the silver ion microdispersed in the proprietary polymer exert sustained antimicrobial effect that can block biofilm formation at the surface. In a recent prospective, randomized, single-blind controlled study of 9417 adults intubated for 24 h the prevalence of VAP declined from 7.5% in controls versus 4.8% in the silver-coated endotracheal tube group, $p = 0.005$.[123] There were a few limitations of this trial including not blinding the investigators, and imbalance of patients with chronic obstructive lung disease favoring the study group.[124] Thus further blinded larger studies with cost-effective analysis are needed; moreover, this trial did not demonstrate decrease in mortality, ICU or hospital stay and duration of intubation.

# References

1. Bueno-Cavanillas, A., Delgado- Rodriguez, M., Lopez-Luque, A., Schaffinocano, S., Galvez-Vargas, R., (1994), Influence of nosocomial infection on mortality rate in intensive care unit. Unit Core Med. 22:55–60.
2. Ginou, E., Stephen, F., Novara, A., Safor, M., Fagon, J.Y., (1998), Risk factors and outcome of nosocomial infections: results of a matched case-control study of ICU patients. Am. J. Respir. Crit. Care. Med. 157:1151–1158.
3. Rello, J., Quintana, E., Ausina, V., Castella, J., Luquin, M., Net., A., Prats, G., (1991), Incidence, etiology and outcome of nosocomial pneumonia in mechanically ventilated patients. Chest 100:439–444.
4. Fagon, J.Y., Chastre, J., Vuagnat, A., Trouillet, J.L., Novora, A., Gilbert, C., (1996), Nosocomial pneumonia and mortality among patients in intensive care unit. JAMA 275:866–869.

5. Vincent, J.L., Bihari, D.J., Suter, P.M., Bruining, H.A., White, J., Nicholas-Chanoin, M.H., Wolff, M., Spencer, R.C., Hemmer, M., (1995), The prevalence of nosocomial infection in intensive care units in Europe. Results of the European Prevalence of Infection in Intensive Care (EPIC) Study. EPIC International Advisory Committee.JAMA 274:639–644.
6. Potgieter, P.D., Linton, D.M., Oliver, S., Forder, A.N., (1987), Nosocomial infections in a respiratory intensive care unit. Crit. Care. Med. 15:495–498.
7. Chastre, J., Fagon, J.Y., Trouillet, J.L., (1995) Diagnosis and treatment of nosocomial pneumonia in patients in intensive care units. Clin. Infect. Dis. 21(Suppl. 3):S226–S237
8. Fagon, J.Y., Chastre, J., Hance, A.J., Montravers, P., Novara, A., Gilbert, C., (1993), Nosocomial pneumonia in ventilated patients: a cohort study evaluating attributable mortality and hospital stay. Am. J. Med. 94:281–288.
9. Crouch, B.S., Wunderink, R.G., Jones, C.B., Leeper, K.V.J., (1996) Ventilator associated pneumonia due to *Pseudomonas aeruginosa*. Chest 109:1019–1029.
10. Dodek, P., Keenan, S., Cook, D., Heyland, D., Jacka, M., Hand, L., Muscedere, J., Foster, D., Mehta, N., Hall, R., Bun-Buisson, C., For the Canadian Critical Care Trials Group and The Canadian Critical Care Society, (2004), Evidence based clinical practice guideline for the prevention of ventilator associated pneumonia. Ann. Intern. Med 141:305–313.
11. Safdar, N., Dezfulian, C., Collard, H.R., Saint, S., (2005), Clinical and economic consequences of ventilator associated pneumonia: a systematic review. Crit. Care. Med. 33:2184–2193.
12. Fabregas, N., Ewig, S., Torres, A., El-Ebiary, M., Ranirez, J., dela Bellacusa, J.P., Bauer, T., Cabello, H., (1999), Clinical diagnosis of ventilator associated pneumonia revisited: comparative validation using immediate post-mortem lung biopsies. Thorax 54:867–873.
13. Torres, A., Ewig, S., (2004), Diagnosing ventilator associated pneumonia. N. Engl. J. Med. 350:433–435.
14. Pugin, J., Anckenthaler, R., Mili, N., Janssens, J.P., Lew, P.D., Suter, P.M, (1991), Diagnosis of ventilator associated pneumonia by bacteriologic analysis of bronchoscopic and non-bronchoscopic "blind" bronchoalveolar lavage fluid. Am. Rev. Respir. Dis. 143:1121–1129.
15. Richards, M.J., Edwards, J.R., Culver, D.H., David, H., Gaynes, R., (1999), Nosocomial infection in medical intensive care unit in the United States. National Nosocomial Infections Surveillance System. Crit. Care Med. 27:887–892.
16. Carlet, J., Ben Ali, A., Chalfine, A., (2004), Epidemiology and control of antibiotic resistance in the intensive care unit. Curr. Opin. Infect. Dis. 17:309–316.
17. Gaynes, R., Edwards, J.R., (2005), Overview of nosocomial infections caused by gram-negative bacilli. Clin. Infect. Dis. 41:848–854.
18. Marquette, C., Georges, H., Wallet, F., Ramon, P., Saulnier, F., Neviere, R., Mathieu, D., Rime, A., Tonnel, A.B., (1993), Diagnostic efficiency of endotracheal aspirates with quantitative bacterial cultures in intubated patients with suspected pneumonia. Am. Rev. Respir. Dis. 148:138–144.
19. el Ebiary, M., Torre, A., Gonzales, J., dela Bellacasa, J.P., Garcia, C., Jimenez de Anta, M.T., Ferrer, M., Rodriguez-Roisin, R., (1993), Quantitative cultures of endobronchial aspirates for the diagnosing of ventilator associated pneumonia. Am. Rev. Respir. Dis. 148:1552–1557.
20. Mondi, M.M., Chang, M.C., Bowton, C.L., Kiglo, P.D., Meredith, J.W., Miller, P.R., (2005), Prospective comparison of bronchial-alveolar lavage quantitative deep –tracheal aspirate in the diagnosis of ventilator associated pneumonia. J. Trauma-Injury Infect. Crit. Care. 59:891–895.
21. Borderon, E., Leprince, A., Guevelier, C., Borderon, J., (1981), Valeirs des examenes barteriologiques des secretions tracheales. Rev. Fr. Mal. Resp. 9:229–239.
22. Meduri, G.U., Chastre, J., (1992), The standardization of bronchoscopic techniques for ventilator-associated pneumonia. Chest 102(Suppl. 1):5575–5645.
23. Meduri, G.U., Beals, D.H., Maijub, A.G., Baselski, V.L., (1991), Protested bronchoalveolar lavage: a new bronchoscopic technique to retrieve uncontaminated distal airway secretions. Am. Rev. Respir. Dis. 143:855–864.

# References

24. Chastre, J., Fagon, J.Y., Soler, P., Bornet, M., Domart, Y., Trouillet, J.L., Gibert, C., Hance, A. J., (1988), Diagnosis of nosocomial bacterial pneumonia in intubated paitents undergoing ventilation: comparison of the usefulness of bronchoalveolor lavage and the protected specimen brush. Am. J. Med. 85:499–506.
25. Chastre, J., Fagon, J.Y., Soler, P., Domart, Y., Pierre, J., Dombret, M.C., Gibert, C., Hance, A. J., (1989), Quantitation of BAL cells containing intracellular bacteria rapidly identifies ventilated patients with nosocomial pneumonia. Chest 95(Suppl.):190S–192S.
26. Jourdain, B., Jolly-Guillou, M.L., Dombret, M.C., Calvat, S., Trouillet, J.L., Gibert, C., Chastre, J., (1993), Usefullness of quantitative cultures of BAL fluid for diagnosing nosocomial pneumonia in ventilated patients. Chest 103:1017–1022.
27. de Jaeger, A., Litalien, C., Lacroix, J., Guertin, M.C., Infante-Rivard, C., (1999), Protected specimen brush or bronchoalveolar lavage to diagnose nosocomial pneumonia in ventilated adults: a meta-analysis, Crit. Care Med. 27:2548–2560.
28. Brun-Buisson, C., Fartoukh, M., Lechapt, E., Honore, S., Zahar, J.R., Cerf, C., Maitre, B., (2005), Contribution of blinded, protected quantitative specimens to the diagnosis and therapeutic management of ventilator associated pneumonia. Chest 128:533–544.
29. Mentec, H., May-Michelangeli, L., Rabbat, A., Varon, E., Le Turdu, F., Bleichner, G., (2004), Blind and bronchoscopic sampling methods on suspected ventilator associated pneumonia. A multicentre prospective study. Inten. Care Med. 30:1319–1326.
30. Wood, A.Y., Dovit, A.J. 2nd, Ciraulo, D.L., Ays, N.W., Richart, O.M., Maxwell, R.A., Baxer, D.E., (2003), A prospective assessment of diagnostic efficacy of blind protective bronchial brushings compared to bronchoscope-assisted lavage, bronchoscope-directed brushing, and blind and endotracheal aspirates in ventilator associated pneumonia. J. Trauma-Injury Infect. Crit. Care: 55:825–834.
31. Butler, K.L., Best, I.M., Oster, R.A., Katon-Benitez I., Lyn Weaver, W., Bumpers, H.L., (2004), Is bilateral protected specimen brush sampling necessary for the accurate diagnosis of ventilation-associated pneumonia. J. Trauma-Injury Infect. Crit. Care: 57:316–322.
32. Michaud, S., Suzuki, S., Harlarth, S., (2002), Effect of design-related bias in studies of diagnostic tests for ventilated pneumonia. Am. J. Respir. Crit. Care Med. 166:1320–1325.
33. Chastre, J., Viau, F., Brum, P., Pierre, J., Dauge, M.C., Bouchama, A., Akesbi, A., Gibert, C., (1984), Prospective evaluation of the protected specimen brush for the diagnosis of pulmonary infections in ventilated patients. Am. Rev. Respir. Dis. 130:924–929.
34. Rouby, J.J., De Lassale, E.M., Poete, P., Nicolas, M.H., Bodin, L., Jarlier, V., Le Carpentier, Y., Grosset, J., Viars, P., (1992), Nosocomial bronchopneumonia in the critically ill. Histologic and bacteriologic aspects. Am. Rev. Respir. Dis. 146:1059–1066.
35. Torres, A., el-Ebiary, M., Padro, L., Gonzalez, J., De La Bellacasa, J.P., Ramirez, J., Xaubet, A., Ferrer, M., Rodriguez-Roisin, R., (1994), Validation of different techniques for the diagnosis of ventilator-associated pneumonia. Am. J. Respir. Crit. Care Med. 149:324–331.
36. Chastre, J., Fagon, J.Y., Barnet-Lecso, M., Calvat, S., Dombret, M.C., Al Khani, R., Basset, f., Gibert, C., (1995), Evaluation of broncoscopic techniques for the diagnosis of nosocomial pneumonia. Am. J. Respir. Crit. Care Med. 152:231–240.
37. Papazian, L., Thomas, P., Garbe, L., Guignon, I., Thirion, X., Charrel, J., Bollet, C., Fuentes, P., Gouin, F., (1995), Bronchoscopic or blind sampling techniques for the diagnosis of ventilator-associated pneumonia. Am. J. Respir. Crit. Care Med. 152:1982–1991.
38. Marquette, C.H., Copin, M. C., Wallet, F., Neviere, R., Saulnier, F., Mathieu, D., Dirocher, A., Ramon, P., Tonnel, A.B., (1995), Diagnostic tests for pneumonia in ventilated patients: Prospective evaluation of diagnostic accuracy using histology as a diagnostic gold standard. Am. J. Respir. Crit. Care Med. 151:1878–1888.
39. Kirtland, S.H., Corley, D.E., Winterbauer, R.H., Springmeyer, S.C., Casey, K.R., Hampson, N.B., Dreis, D.E., (1997), The diagnosis of ventilator associated pneumonia: a comparison of histologic, microbiologic, and clinical criteria. Chest 112:445–457.

40. Bregeon, F., Papazian, L., Thomas, P., Corret, V., Garbe, L., Saux, P., Drancourt, M., Auffray, J.P., (2000), Diagnostic accuracy of protected catheter sampling in ventilator associated bacterial pneumonia. Eur. Respir. J. 16:969–975.
41. Torres, A., Fabregas, N., Ewig, S., de la Bellacasa, J.P., Bauer, T.T., Ramirez, J., (2000), Sampling methods for ventilator associated pneumonia: validation using different histologic and microbiological references. Crit. Care Med. 28:2799–2804.
42. Balthazor, A.B., Von Nowakonski, A., De Copitani, E.M., Bottini, P.V., Terzi, R.G.G, Araujo, S., (2001), Diagnostic investigation of ventilator associated pneumonia using bronchoalveolar lavage: comparative study with a postmortem lung biopsy. Brazilian J. Med. Biolog. Res. 34:993–1001.
43. Moser, K.M., Maurer, J., Jassy, L., Kremsdorf., R., Konopka, R., Share, D., Hurrell, J.H., (1982), Sensitivity, specificity, and risk of diagnostic procedures in a canine model of *Sreptocousl pneumoniae* pneumonia. Am. Rev. Respir. Dis. 125:436–442.
44. Johanson, W.G.Jr, Seidenfeld, J.R., Gomez, P., De Los Santos, R., Coalson, J.J., (1988), Bacteriologic diagnosis of nosocomial pneumonia following prolonged mechanical ventilation. Am. Rev. Respir. Dis. 137:259–264.
45. Rello, J., Paiva, J.A., Baraibor, J., Barcenilla, F., Bodi, M., Castander, D., Correa, H., Diaz, E., Garnacho, J., Llorio, M., Rios, M., Rodriguez, A., Sol-Violan, J., (2001), International Conference for the Development of Consensus on the Diagnosis and Treatment of Ventilator associated pneumonia. Chest 120:955–970.
46. The Canadian Critical Care Trials Group, (2006), A randomized trial of diagnostic techniques for ventilator-associated pneumonia. N, Engl. J. Med. 335:2619– 2630.
47. Duflo, E., Debon, R., Monneret, G, Bienvenu, J., Chassard, D., Allaouchiche, B., (2002), Alveolar and serum procalcitonin: diagnostic and prognostic value in ventilator-associated pneumonia. Anesthesiology 96:74–79.
48. Brunkhorst, F.M., Al-Nawas, B., Krummenauer, F., Forycki, Z.F., Shah, P.M., (2002), Procalcitonin, C – reactive protein, APACHE II Score for risk evaluation in patients with severe pneumonia. Clin. Microbiol. Infect. 8:93–100.
49. Fukushuma, R., Alexander, J.W., Gianotti, L., Ogle, C.K., (1994), Isolated pulmonary infection acts as a source of systemic tumor necrosis factor. Crit. Care Med. 22:114–120.
50. Wu, C.L., Lee, L.Y., Chang, K.M., King, S.L., Chiang, C.D., Niederman, M.S., (2003), Bronchoalveolar interleukin I β: a marker of bacterial burden in mechanically ventilated paitents with community acquired pneumonia. Crit. Care Med. 31:812–817.
51. Bonten, M.J., Froon, A.H., Gaillard, C.A., Greve, J.W., Drent, M., Stobberingh, E.E., Buurman, W.A., (1997), The systemic inflammatory response in the development of ventilator associated pneumonia. Am. J. Respir. Crit. Care Med. 156:1105–1113.
52. Bouchon, A., Dietrich, J., Colonna, M., (2000), Inflammatory responses can be triggered by TREM-1, a novel receptor expressed in neutrophils and monocytes. J. Immunol. 164:4991–4995.
53. Bouchon, A., Facchetti, F., Weigand, M.A., Colonna, M., (2001), TREM-1 amplifies inflammation and is a critical mediator of septic shock. Nature 410:1103–1107.
54. Gibot, S., Kolopp-Sarda, M.N., Béné, M.C., Cravoisy, A., Levy, B., Faure, G.C., Bollaert, P. E., (2004), Plasma level of a triggering receptor expressed on myeloid cells-1: Its diagnostic accuracy in patients with suspected sepsis. Ann. Intern. Med. 141:9–15.
55. Gibot, S., Cravoisy, A., Levy, B., Béné, M.C., Faure, G., Bollaert, P.E., (2004), Soluble triggering receptor expressed on myeloid cells and the diagnosis of pneumonia. N. Engl. J. Med. 350:451–458.
56. Determann, R.M., Miller, J.L., Gibot, S., Korevaar, J.C., Vroom, M.B., van der Poll, T., Garrard, C.S., Schultz, M.J., (2005), Serial changes in soluble triggering receptor expressed on myeloid cells in the development of ventilator-associated pneumonia. Intern. Care Med. 31:1495–1500.

57. Combes, A., Figliolini, C., Trouillet, J.L., Kasis, N., Wolff, M., Gibert, C., Chastre, J., (2002), Incidence and outcome of polymicrobial ventilator-associated pneumonia. Chest 121:1390–1391.
58. Dor, P., Robert, R., Grollier, G., Rouffineau, J., Languetot, H., Charries, J.M., Fauchere, J.L., (1996), Incidence of anaerobes in ventilator-associated pneumonia with use of a protected specimen brush. Am. J. Respir. Crit. Care Med. 153:1292–1298.
59. Park, D.R., (2005), Microbiology of ventilator-associated pneumonia. Respir. Care 50: 742–763.
60. Woody, A.Y., Davit, A.J. 2nd, Ciraulo, D.L., Arp, N.W., Richart, C.M., Maxwell, R.A., Barker, D.E., (2003), A prospective assessment of diagnostic efficacy of blind protective bronchial brushings compared to bronchoscope assisted lavage, bronchoscope-directed brushings, and blind endotracheal aspirates in ventilator-associated pneumonia. J. Trauma-Injury Infect. Crit. Care 55:825–834.
61. Elatrous, S., Boukef, R., Ouanes Besbes, L., Marghli, S., Noonan, S., Nouira, S., Abroug, F., (2004), Diagnosis of ventilator-associated pneumonia: agreement between cultures of endotracheal aspiration and plugged telescoping catheter. Intern. Care Med. 30:853–858.
62. Heyland, D.K., Cook, D.J., Marshall, J., Heule, M., Guslits, B., Lang, J., Jaeschke, R., (1999), The clinical utility of invasive diagnostic techniques in the setting of ventilator associated pneumonia. Canadian Critical Care Trial Groups. Chest 115:1076–1084.
63. Fagon, J.Y., Chastre, J., Wolff, M., Gervais, C., Parer-Aubas, S., Stephan, F., Similowski, T., Mercat, A., Diehl, J.L., Sollet, J.P., Tenaillon, A., (2000), Invasive and non-invasive strategies for management of suspected ventilator-associated pneumonia. A randomized trial. Ann Interm. Med. 132:621–630.
64. Ruiz, M., Torres, Ewig, S., Marcos, M.A., Alcon, A., Lledo, R., Asenjo, M.A., Maldonaldo, A., (2000), Non-invasive versus invasive microbial investigation in ventilator-associated pneumonia. Am. J. Respir. Crit. Care Med. 162:119–125.
65. Ioanas, M., Ferrer, R., Angrill, J., Ferrer, M., Torres, A., (2001), Microbial investigation in ventilator-associated pneumonia. Europ. Respir. 17:791–801.
66. Shorr, A.F., Sherner, J.H., Jackson, W.1., Kollef, M.H., (2005), Invasive approaches to the diagnosis of ventilator-associated pneumonia: a meta-analysis. Crit. Care Med. 33:46–53.
67. Luna, C.M., Vujacich, P., Niederman, M.S., Vay, C., Gherardi, C., Matera, J., Jolly, E.C., (1997), Impact of BAL data on therapy and outcome of ventilator-associated pneumonia. Chest 111:676–685.
68. Ibrahim, E.H., Sherman, G., Ward, S., Fraser, V.J., Kollef, M.H., (2000), The influence of inadequate antimicrobial treatment of bloodstream infections on patient outcomes in the ICU setting. Chest 118:146–155.
69. Davis, K.A., Eckert, M.J., Reed, R.L., 2nd, Esposito, T.J., Santaniello, J.M., Poulakidas, S., Luchette, F.A., (2005), Ventilator-associated pneumonia in injured patients: do you trust your Gram's-stain? J. Trauma-Injury Infect. Crit. Care 58:462–466.
70. Laupland, K.B., Church, D.L., Gregson, D.B., (2005), Validation of a rapid diagnostic strategy for determination of significant bacterial counts in bronchoalveolar lavage samples. Arch. Pathol. Lab. Med. 129:78–81.
71. Flanagan, P.G., Jackson, S.K., Findlay, G, (2001), Diagnosis of gram negative, ventilator-associated pneumonia by assaying endotoxin in bronchial lavage fluid. J. Clin. Pathol. 54:107–110.
72. Ibrahim, E.H., Ward, S., Sherman, G., Kollef, M.H., (2000), A comparative analysis of patients with early-onset vs late onset nosocomial pneumonia in the ICU setting. Chest 117:1434–1442.
73. Hayon, J., Figliolini, C., Combes, A., Trouillet, T.L., Kassis, N., Dombret, M.C., Gibert, C., Chastre, J., (2002), Role of serial routine microbiologic culture results in the initial management of ventilator-associated pneumonia. Am, J. Respir. Crit. Care Med. 165:41–46.

74. American Thoracic Society, Infectious Disease Society of America, (2005), ATS/IDSA: guidelines for the management of hospital-acquired, ventilator-associated, and healthcare-associated pneumonia. Am. J. Respir. Crit. Care Med. 171:388–416
75. National Nosocomial Infection Surveillance, (2004), System report: data summary from January 1992 thorough June 2004, issue October 2004. Am. J. Infect. Control 41:848–854
76. Beardsley, J.R., Williamson, J.G., Johnson, J.W., Ohl, C.A., Karehmer, TB, Bowton, D.L., (2006), Using local microbiologic data to develop institution-specific guidelines for the treatment of hospital-acquired pneumonias. Chest 130:787–793.
77. Peterson, D.L., Rice, L.B., (2003), Empirical antibiotic choice for the seriously ill patient: are minimization of selection of resistant organisms and maximization of individual outcome mutually exclusive? Clin Infect. Dis. 36:1006–1012.
78. Chastre, J., Wolff, M., Fagon, J.Y., Chevret, S., Thomas, F., Wermert, D., Clementi, E., Gonzalez, J., Jusserand, D., Asfar, P., Perrin, D., Fieux, F., Aubas, S., (2003), Comparison of 8 vs 15 days of antibiotic therapy for ventilator-associated pneumonia in adults: a randomized trial. JAMA 290:2588–2598.
79. Singh, N., Rogers, P., Atwood, C.W., Wagener, M.M., Yu, V.L., (2000), Short-course empiric antibiotic therapy for patients with pulmonary infiltrates in the intensive care unit. A proposed solution for indiscriminate antibiotic prescription. Am. J. Respir. Crit. Care Med. 162: 205–211.
80. Brown, R.B., Kruse, J.A., Counts, G.W., Russell, J.A., Christou, N.V., Sards, M.L, and The Endobronchial Tobramycin Study Group. (1990), Double-blind study of endobronchial tobramycin in the treatment of gram-negative bacterial pneumonia. Antimicrob. Agents Chermother. 34:269–272.
81. Le Conte, P., Potel, G., Clementi, E., Legras, A., Villars, D., Bironneau, E., Cousson, J., Baron, D., (2000), Administration d'aerosols de tobramycine chez des patients ayant une pnemopathie nosocomiale: etcide preliminaire. RESSE Med. 29:76–78.
82. Munoz-Price, L.S., Weinstein, R.A., (2008), Acinetobacter infection. N. Engl. J. Med. 358: 1271–1281.
83. Carey, R.B., Banerjee, S.N., Srinivasan, A., (2006), Multidrug-resistant acinetobacter infection. 1995–2004. 46th Intersc. Conf. Antimicrob. Agents Chemother, San Francisco Calif. Sept. 27–30, Abstract.
84. Hess, D.R., (2005), Noninvasive positive-pressure ventilation and ventilator-associated pneumonia. Respir. Care; 50:924–929.
85. Sinciff, T., Cook, D.J., (2003), Health technology assessment in the ICU: noninvasive positive pressure ventilation for acute respiratory failure. J. Crit. Care 18:59–67.
86. Antonelli, M., Conti, G., Moro, M.L., Esquinas, A., Gonzalez-Diaz, G., Confalonieri, M., Proietti, R., Passariello, M., Meduri, G.U., (2001), Predictors of failure of noninvasive positive pressure ventilation in patients with acute hypoxic respiratory failure: a multi-centre study. Intern. Care Med. 27:1718–1728.
87. Hess, D.R., (2005), Patient positioning and ventilator-associated pneumonia. Respir. Care 50:892–898.
88. Choi, S.C., Nelson, LD., (1992), Kinetic therapy in critically ill patients: combined results based on meta-analysis. J. Crit. Care 7:57–62.
89. Collard, H.R., Saint, S., Matthay, M.A., (2003), Prevention of ventilator-associated pneumonia: an evidence-based systemic review. Ann. Intern. Med. 138:494–501.
90. Guerin, C., Gaillard, S., Lemasson, S., Ayzac, L., Girord, R., Beuret, P., Palmier, B., Le, Q.U., Sirodot, M., Rosselli, S., Cadiergue, V., Sainty, J.M., Barbe, P., Combourieu, E.O., Renault, A., Sibille, J.P., Kaidomar, M., (2004), Effects of systematic prone positioning in hypoxic acute respiratory failure: a randomized controlled trial. JAMA 292:2379–2387.
91. Drakulovic, M.B., Torres, A., Bauer, T.T., Nicolas, J.M., Nogue, S., Ferrer, M., (1999), Supine body position as a risk factor for nosocomial pneumonia in mechanically ventilated patients: a randomized trial. Lancet 354:1851–1858.

# References

92. Tablan, O.C., Anderson, L.J., Bescer, R., Bridges, C., Hajjeh, R., CDC. Healthcare Infection Control Practices Advisory Committee, (2003), Guidelines for preventing health-care-associated pneumonia: recommendations of CDL and the Healthcare Infection Control Proactive Advisory Committee. M.M.W.R 53:1–36.
93. van Nieuwenhoven, C.A., Vandenbroucke-Grauls, C., van Tiel, F.H., Joone, H.C., van Schijndel, R.J., van der Tweel, I., Ramsay, G., Bonten, M.J., (2006), Feasibility and effects of the semirecumbent position to prevent ventilator-associated pneumonia: a randomized study. Crit. Care Med. 34:559–561.
94. Wang, J.Y., Chuang, P.Y., Lin, C.J., Yu, C.J., Yang, P.C., (2003), Continuous lateral rotational therapy in the medical intensive care unit. J. Formosan Med. Assoc. 102:788–792.
95. Ntoumenopoulos, G., Presneill, J.J., McElholum, M., Code, J.F., (2002), Chest physiotherapy for the prevention of ventilator-associated pneumonia. Intern. Care Med. 28:850–856.
96. Klastersky, J., Huysmans, E., Weerts, D., Hensgens, C., Daneau, D., (1974), Endotracheally administered gentamicin for the prevention of infections of the respiratory tract in patients with tracheotomy: a double blind study. Chest 65:650–654.
97. Libérati, A., D'Amico, R., Pifferi, Torri, V., Brazzi, L., (2004), Antibiotic prophylaxis to reduce respiratory tract infections and mortality in adults receiving intensive care. Cochrane Database Systemic Reviews CD000022: PMID 14973945.
98. Bonten, M.J., Kullberg, B.J., van Dalen, R., Girbes, A.R., Hoepelman, I.M., Hustrix, W., van der Meer, J.W., Speelman, P., Stobberingh, E.E., Verbrugh, H.A., Verhoef, J., Zwaveling, J. H., (2000), Selective digestive decontamination in patients in intensive care. The Dutch Working Group on Antibiotic Policy. J. Antimicrob. Chemother 43:351–362.
99. Kollef, M.H., (2003), Selective digestive decontamination should not be routinely employed. Chest 123(Suppl. 5):4645–4685.
100. Kallet, R.H., Quinn, T.E., (2005), The gastrointestinal tract and ventilator-associated pneumonia. Respir. Care 50:910–921.
101. Munro, C.L., Grap, M.L., (2004), Oral health and care in the intensive care unit: state of the science. Am. J. Crit. Care 13:25–33.
102. DeRiso, A.J., Jr Ladowski, J.S., Dillon, T.A., Justice, J.W., Peterson, A.C., (1996), Chlorhexidine gluconate 0.12% oral rinse reduces the incidence of total nosocominal respiratory infection and nonprophylactic systematic antibiotic use in patients undergoing heart surgery. Chest 109:1556–1561.
103. Houston, S., Hougland, P., Anderson, J.J., LaRocco,M., Kennedy, V., Gentry, L.O., (2002), Effectiveness of 0.12% chlorhexidine gluconate oral rinse in reducing prevalence of nosocominal pneumonia in patients undergoing heart surgery. Am. J. Crit. Care 11:567–570.
104. Genuit, T., Bochicchio, G., Napolitano, L.M., McCarter, R.J., Roghman, M.C., (2001), Prophylactic chlorhexidine oral rinse decreases ventilator-associated pneumonia in surgical ICU patients. Surg. Infect. 2:5–18.
105. Fourrier, F., Dubios, D., Pronnier, P., Herberg, P., Leroy, O., Desmettre, T., Potier-Cau, E., Boutigny, H., Di Pompeo, C., Durocher, A., Roussel-Delvallez, M., PIRAD Study Group, (2005), Effect of gingival and dental plague antiseptic decontamination on nosocomial infections acquired in the intensive care unit: a double-blind placebo-controlled multicentre study. Crit. Care Med. 33:1867–1868.
106. Tulamait, A., Laghi, F., Mikrut, K., Carey, R.B., Budinger, G.R., (2005), Potassium sorbate reduces gastric colonization in patients receiving mechanical ventilation. J. Crit. Care 20:281–287.
107. Heyland, D.K., Cook, D.J., Schoenfeld, P.S., Frietag, A., Varon, J., Wood, G., (1999), The effect of acidified enteral feeds on gastric colonization in critically ill patients: results of a multicentre randomized trial. Canadian Critical Care Trials Group. Crit. Care Med. 27: 2399–2406.
108. Dezfulian, C., Shojania, K., Collard, H.R., Kim, H.M., Matthay, M.A., Saint, S., (2005), Subglottic secretion drainage for preventing ventilator-associated pneumonia: a meta-analysis. Am. J. Med. 118:11–18.

109. Blunt, M.C., Young, P.J., Patil, A., Haddock, A., (2001), Gel lubrication of the tracheal cuff reduces pulmonary aspiration. Anesthesiology 92:377–381.
110. Ibanez, J., Penafiel, A., Morse, P., Jorcla, R., Raurich J.M., Mata, F., (2000), Incidence of gastroesophageal reflux and aspiration in mechanically ventilated patients using small-bore nasogastric trials. J. Parenteral Enteral Nutr. 24:103–106.
111. Kearns, P.J., Chin, D., Mueller, L., Wallace, K., Jensen, W.A., Krisch, C.M., (2000), The incidence of ventilator-associated pneumonia and success in nutrient delivery with gastric versus small intestinal feeding: a randomized clinical trial. Crit. Care Med. 28:1742–1746.
112. Heyland, D.K., Drover, J.W., Dhaliwad, R., Greenwood, J., (2002), Optimizing the benefits and minimizing the risks of enteral nutrition in the critically ill: role of small bowel feeding. J. Parenter. Enteral. Nutr. 26:551–555.
113. Marik, P.E., Zaloga, G.P., (2003), Gastric versus post-pyloric feeding: a systematic review. Crit. Care Med. 7:46–51.
114. Kostadima, E., Kaditis, A.G., Alexopoulos, E.I., Zakynthinos, E., Sfyras, D., (2005), Early gastrostomy reduces the rate of ventilator-associated pneumonia in stroke or head injury patients. Eur. Respir. J. 26:106–111.
115. Kola, A., Eckmanns, T., Gastmeier, P., (2005), Efficacy of heat and moisture exchangers in preventing ventilator-associated pneumonia: meta-analysis of randomized controlled studies. Intern. Care Med. 31:5–11.
116. Combes, P., Fauvage, B., Oleyer, C., (2000), Nosocominal pneumonia in mechanically ventilated patients, a prospective randomized evaluation of the stericath closed suctioning system. Intern. Care Med. 26:878–882.
117. Lorente, L., Lecuona, M., Martin, M.M., Garcia, C., Mora, M.L., Siera, A., (2005), Ventilator-associated pneumonia using closed versus an open tracheal suction system. Crit. Care Med. 33:115–119.
118. Ranes, J.L., Gordon, S.M., Chen, P., Fatica, C. Hammel, J., Gonzales, J.P., Arroliga, A.C., (2006), Predictors of long-term mortality in patients with ventilator-associated pneumonia. Am. J. Med. 119:897.e13–19.
119. Bouza, E., Torres, M.V., Radice, C., Cercenado, E., deDiego, R., Sánchez-Carrillo, C., Munoz, P., (2007), Direct e-test (AB Biodisk) of respiratory samples improves antimicrobial use in ventilator-associated pneumonia. Clin. Infect. Dis. 44:382–387.
120. Kollef, M.H., (2007), Moving towards real-time antimicrobial management of ventilator associated pneumonia. Clin. Infect. Dis. 44:388–390.
121. Tenover, F.C., (2007), Rapid detection and identification of bacterial pathogens using novel molecular technologies, Infection control and beyond. Clin. Infect. Dis. 44:418–423.
122. Giamarellos-Bourboulis, EJ, Pechére. J-C, Routsi, C, Plachouras, T, Kollias, S, Raftogiannis, M, Zeruakis, D, Baziaka, F, Koronaios, A, Antonopoulou, A, Markaki, V, Koutoukas, P, Papadomichelakis, E, Tsaganos,T, Armaganidis, A, Koussoulas, V, Kotanidou, A, Roussos, C, Giamarellou, H, (2008), Effect of clarithromycin in patients with sepsis and ventilator-associated pneumonia. Clin. Infect. Dis. 46:1157–1164.
123. Kollef, A.H., Afessa, B., Anzueto, A., Veremakis, C., Kerr, K.M., Margolis, B.D., Craven, D.E., Roberts, P.R., Arroliga, A.C., Hubmayr, R.D., Restrepo, M.I., Auger, W.R., Schinner, R., for the NASCENT Investigation Group, (2008), Silver-coated endotracheal tubes and incidence of ventilator-associated pneumonia. JAMA: 300:805–813.
124. Chastre, J., (2008), Preventing ventilator-associtaed pneumonia. Could silver-coated endotracheal tube be the answer? JAMA; 300:842–844.

# Chapter 4
# Emerging Issues in Pulmonary Infections of Cystic Fibrosis

## 4.1 Introduction

Pulmonary infections are the leading cause of morbidity and mortality in patients with cystic fibrosis. Empiric broad-spectrum antibiotics are often used for prolonged periods and repeatedly for exacerbation of bronchiectasis. Hence, as a consequence this select group of patients has the highest incidence of multi-resistant bacteria causing respiratory colonization or infection second to none. It is estimated that 25–45% of adults with cystic fibrosis are chronically infected with multi-resistant bacteria in their airways.[1]

Moreover, these bacteria usually cannot be eradicated and persist in the respiratory tract despite cycles of different combination of antibiotics.

There is no doubt that current management of the complications of cystic fibrosis, including antimicrobial therapy, has improved the lifespan of these patients. More than 38% of subjects with cystic fibrosis are now adults, although only 7% are diagnosed in adulthood, and the mean survival now exceeds 32 years.[2] A dramatic turnabout in the past 3 decades, as before children with cystic fibrosis rarely survived to adulthood. This chapter will deal with the emerging issues in the management of the infectious complications and the underlying pathobiology.

## 4.2 Pathobiology of Cystic Fibrosis

Cystic fibrosis is a common autosomal recessive inherited disorder in Caucasians, with an incidence of one in 2,500 live births. The primary defect is a dysfunction or decrease in a glycosylated membrane of glycoprotein that functions as a cyclic-AMP-regulated chloride channel, caused by a mutation in the cystic fibrosis transmembrane conductance regulator (CFTR) gene, located on the long arm of the chromosome.[3] Over 1,000 unique mutations have been described but a deletion of phenylalanine in the amino acid position 508 is responsible for the defect in 70%

of patients in the United Kingdom.[3] At birth the lungs are anatomically normal and progression of lung disease is insidious, and many patients do not have symptoms until 10 months of age. Cough and pulmonary infection may be the first manifestation of disease, with inflammation in bronchoalveolar fluid (elevated neutrophils and interleukin (IL)-8), and bacterial overgrowth. In the early years pulmonary infection was usually due to *Haemophilus influenzae*, *Staphylococcus aureus*, and subsequently *Pseudomonas aeruginosa* after multiple antibiotic courses. Early infections with *P. aeruginosa* can be transient and may clear spontaneously in half the patients.[4] Most patients, however, will have colonization persistently as teenagers.[5] However, in a longitudinal study of 56 children from birth to 16 years, 29% acquired non-mucoid *P. aeruginosa* in the first 6 months of life.[6] Mucoid *P. aeruginosa* increased markedly from age 4 to 16. Non-mucoid and mucoid *P. aeruginosa* were acquired at medium ages of 1 and 13, respectively.[6]

The mechanism for the high incidence of early bacterial infection in cystic fibrosis is unclear. It is postulated that mutation in the CFTR gene product may affect innate immunity through decreased bacterial clearance, intrinsic hyperinflammation, and decreased bacterial killing (see Fig. 4.1).[5]

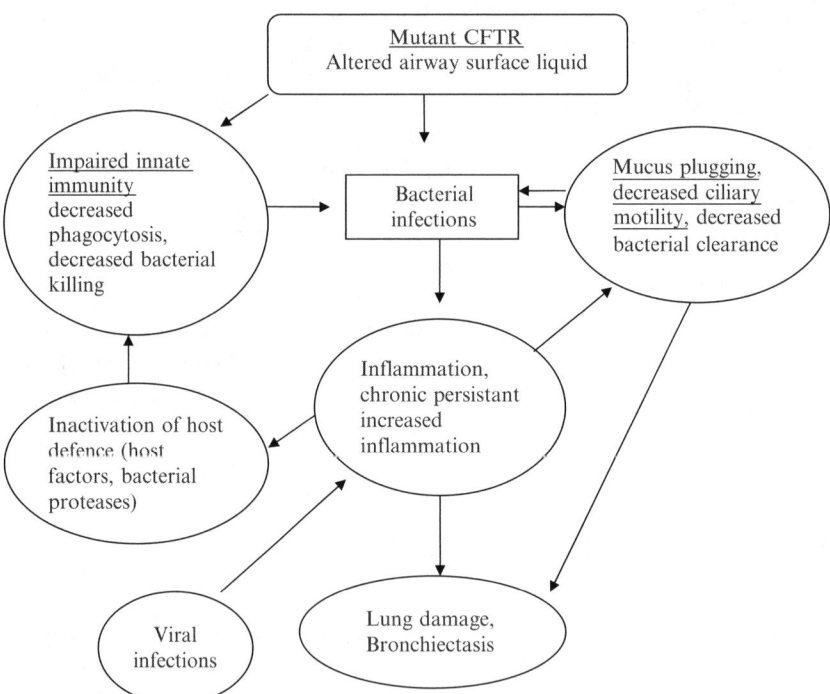

**Fig. 4.1** Pathogenesis of lung disease in cystic fibrosis is outlined above: several interconnected cycles and events result in impairment of host defense, leading to recurrent and persistent bacterial infections with progressive lung damage. CFTR = cystic fibrosis transmembrane conductance regulator

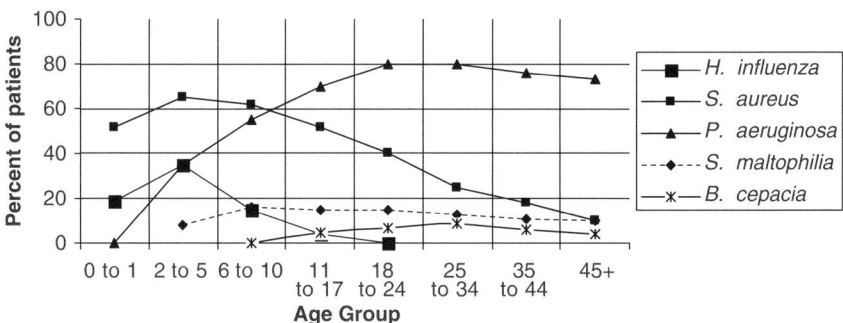

Fig. 4.2 The above figure outlines respiratory infections with specific bacteria according to age in cystic fibrosis. Overall percentage in 2004: *S. aureus* (51.7%), *P. aeruginosa* (57.3%), *H. influenza* (16.2%), *S. maltophilia* (11.6%), MRSA (14.6%), *B. cepacia* (2.9%) (Data obtained from Cystic Fibrosis Foundation Registry: Annual Data Report 2004, Cystic Fibrasis Foundation, Washington, Dc)

The CFTR mutation leads to defective chloride transport across the apical surface of the airway epithelial cells. In the normal airway, the airway surface liquid (ASL) is hypotonic and it is proposed that salt content increases in cystic fibrosis which may cause desiccated mucus and reduces ciliary function.[3] The possibility that salt sensitive antimicrobial peptides (β-defensin 1) are inactivated in ASL in cystic fibrosis (CF) have been raised.[7] Furthermore, ASL from normal patients but not from cystic fibrosis killed *P. aeruginosa* in vitro.[8] The defensins have broad antimicrobial activity and does not explain the predominance of *P. aeruginosa*. Moreover, a later study found no evidence that liquids lining airway surfaces were hypotonic or that salt concentration differed between CF and normal.[9] In this study CF airway epithelia exhibited abnormally high rates of airway surface liquid absorption, which depleted the periciliary liquid layer and abolished mucus transport. This failure to clear thickened mucus in the airway likely initiates infection.[9]

Decreased bacterial clearance may result from defective CFTR by increasing bacterial adherence through altered epithelial cell glycosylation[10] or by increasing the availability of receptors, such as asialo-GMI.[11] Asialo-GMI and fucosylated oligosaccharides have been shown to be receptors for some strains of *P. aeruginosa*, with pili and flagella mediating binding. Binding to asialo-GMI is enhanced in regenerating respiratory epithelium,[12] and damage from previous viral or bacterial infection could enhance susceptibility to *P. aeruginosa* by this mechanism. Once infection sets in there is a cycle of increased inflammation, increased neutrophils in the airway with leucocytic proteases, and oxygen radicals gradually destroying lung tissue.

Normal clearance of *P. aeruginosa* from the airway may include internalization into the respiratory epithelium by binding to CFTR as a receptor on the plasma membrane. The epithelial cells then desquamate to eliminate the bacteria. Internalization of *P. aeruginosa* could also lead to transcription of genes that encode cytokines and other mediators of innate immunity.[1] Mutation of the CFTR gene may reduce this mechanism of internalization, and allow persistence of

*Pseudomonas* in the airway. Transgenic mice either lacking CFTR in the lungs or homozygous for the F508 CFTR allele had decreased internalization of *P. aeruginosa* in the lung, resulting in increased levels of the microorganism in lung tissue.[13]

Other defects in the local immunity in the lungs hypothesized include impaired nitric-oxide activation; intrinsic hyperinflammation (some studies found decreased anti-inflammatory cytokines and increased inflammatory damage to infection); reduced airway surface liquid glutathione levels, which may enhance oxidant injury.[5] Reduced airway nitric oxide in the CF lung may increase susceptibility to *P. aeruginosa* and other infection, as nitric oxide is cytolytic and cytostatic against viruses and bacteria.[14]

The CFTR mutation lead to glycosylation changes in mucin and there is evidence of mucin hyperproduction and accumulation.[3] By 4 months of age infants with CF have hyperplasia and significantly dilated submucosal gland acini.[15] The demonstration that the predominant sites of expression of the CF gene in normal lungs are the submucosal glands, together with histological evidence of hyperplasia of these glands and mucin occlusion of the gland ducts, which are the earliest signs of disease in the CF lung, indicate that malfunction of the submucosal glands is a major contributing factor in the pathophysiology.[16] Moreover, excessive thick mucin will impair muco-ciliary clearance.

Although neutrophils of CF patients from bronchoalveolar fluid express and produce bactericidal permeability-increasing (BPI) protein, the function may be hampered by autoantibodies, as the majority of CF subjects have antineutrophil cytoplasmic antibodies directed against BPI, resulting in chronic infection.[17]

## 4.3 Microbiology

It has been considered for many years that the spectrum of microorganisms infecting CF subjects was limited to a few bacteria, but that may be changing. In the early years *S. aureus* and *H. influenzae* (usually nonencapsulated) are frequently isolated from sputa and are believed to play a role in exacerbation of respiratory symptoms. *S. aureus* may appear as three different phenotypes: mucoid, nonmotile and small colony variants, and methicillin-resistant stains (MRSA) has emerged as a problem since the early 1980s.[3]

*S. aureus* continues to be isolated in approximately 50% of children with CF, and small colony variants accounts for 50% of these isolates. However, selective medium with mannitol salts should be used for recovery of these auxotrophic strains.[18]

In the United States approximately 6% of *S. aureus* isolates recovered from CF patients are MRSA, and as high as 20% in some areas.[19]

Although *S. aureus* is frequently the initial bacterium isolated from young CF subjects, its role in disease progression has not been well-defined. The reason for the increased *S. aureus* colonization/infection of the airways of CF patients is also not well understood. This organism may evade the normal clearance as *S. aureus* escapes more efficiently from the phagosome of CF bronchial epithelial cell line than from its normal counterpart, and this may explain the propensity of *S. aureus* to cause chronic lung infection in this population.[20]

## 4.3.1 Pseudomonas aeruginosa

*P. aeruginosa* is the most important pathogen of CF lung disease with about 80% of adolescent and adults with CF colonized or infected in the lung, and approximately 60% of the entire CF population.[21] The initial strains of *P. aeruginosa* that infect young children from infancy are non-mucoid or "planktonic" strains. These mobile prototrophs, with smooth lipopolysaccharide are more susceptible to antimicrobial treatment, and thus more easily eradicated. Hence, this stage is considered "a window of opportunity to eradicated" *P. aeruginosa* from CF respiratory tract with aggressive treatment.[5] After a median of 13 years most patients develop chronic infection with a mucoid phenotype of *P. aeruginosa*. These isolates are nonmotile, auxotrophic (requires special growth factors), have rough lipopolysaccharide, usually multiresistant to many antibiotics and become permanent residents.[22] The mucoid strains of *P. aeruginosa* grow in biofilm in which the cells are surrounded by very large expanses of matrix material composed of polysaccharide polymer or alginate. The bacterial cells in biofilm grow as stationary sessile micro-colonies enclosed and protected from hostile environment by the matrix alginate.

Structural examination of biofilms show that the micro-colonies are composed of cells ($\wedge$15% by volume) embedded in matrix material ($\wedge$85% by volume), bisected by water channels that carry bulk fluid in the community by convective flow.[23] Microbial biofilms constitute the most "defensive" strategy that can be adopted by the organism. Thus, the mucoid *P. aeruginosa* are refractory to clearance by the immune system, and there is increasing evidence that the lung pathology that occurs during the chronic *P. aeruginosa* infection is due predominantly to the immune response directed against pseudomonal biofilm.[18] These bacteria in biofilm are not only protected against phagocytes and complement but also against antibiotics. Micro-colonies in biofilm can survive antibiotic concentration as much as 1,000-fold higher than the same bacteria in free-living, planktonic state.[24] Thus, even with a combination of antibiotics and endobronchial aerolization, the antibiotic concentration may not be adequate to clear biofilm infection, allowing bacterial persistence, spread, and further antibacterial resistance. Local hypoxia within mucus plaque in the airways may increase biofilm production, and antimicrobial-resistance phenotype may also enhance the ability to form biofilms.[25] Moreover, *P. aeruginosa* isolated from CF airway have larger genomes than the usual laboratory strain, and a higher frequency of hypermutability, which may be due to a combination of factors.[25,26] Recent studies also indicate that *P. aeruginosa* express neuramidases that can cleave alpha, 2,3-linked sialic acid from glycoconjugates (present on epithelials surfaces), contributing to the formation of biofilms.[27] Viral neuramidase inhibitors in clinical use (e.g., oseltamivir for influenza) blocked

*P. aeruginosa* biofilm production in vitro.[27] Biofilm formation is a complex phenomena probably controlled by a hierarchy of regulatory mechanisms operating at multiple levels. There is also new evidence that nitrate sensing, response regulation, and metabolism are directly linked to biofilm and virulence factors of *P. aeruginosa*.[28] The microenvironment present in CF lungs (thick mucus), the nitrate and nitrite levels in the mucus (generated by inflammatory response), support anaerobic metabolism of *P. aeruginosa*, which promotes nitrate dissimilation (via quorum sensing and nitrate-sensor-response regulator gene upregulation), and modulates motility and biofilm formation. Furthermore, there is evidence that *P. aeruginosa* (even non-mucoid isolates) secretes a protein (Cif) that reduces the apical membrane expression of CFTR protein, facilitating the colonization of the CF lung by this microbe.[29]

## 4.3.2 Late-Emerging Pathogens

*Burkholderia cepacia* includes nine genomic species, referred to as *B. cepacia* complex, which has been recognized as a serious pathogen in CF since 1984.[30] Two genomovars *Burkholderia multivorans* (II) and *Burkholderia cenocepacia* (III) account for 85% of the *B. cepacia* complex recovered from CF patients with *B. cenocepacia* representing ~50%.[31] The prevalence of *B. cepacia* in CF varies between centers and countries and is ~3% in the United States and ~15% in Canada.[18] Colonization or infection with this group of organisms can cause different clinical patterns of the disease. Some patients become chronically colonized without clinical deterioration or remain with the usual pattern of intermittent exacerbation. Others develop a progressive deterioration over several months, with recurrent fever and progressive weight loss (the "cepacia syndrome"). These patients may experience a rapid decline in respiratory function, develop bacteremia and subsequently die from pulmonary failure. It has been estimated that about 20% of CF patients with *B. cepacia* complex colonization present with the "cepacia syndrome".[18] Moreover, person-to-person transmission among CF patients within centers, regionally and intercontinentally has been demonstrated.[32] Thus, isolation of *B. cepacia* complex may have adverse consequences on patients, including isolation in centers and socially, and patients may be rejected for potential lung transplant due to perceived poor outcomes.[33] However, poor prognosis post-transplantations is mainly associated with *B. cenocepacia* (genomovar III),[34] and only patients with these subspecies should be excluded from lung transplantations. Thus, it is very important that laboratory identification of *B. cepacia* complex from CF patients' respiratory secretion be accurate with subspecies or genomovar speciation. Selective media has been used to improve *B. cepacia* complex isolation and studies have shown that the *B. cepacia* selective agar (BCSA) is the preferred medium.[35]

Commercial identification systems are inadequate for differentiation among *B. cepacia* genomovars, and definitive identification relies on molecular analysis.[18]

*B. cepacia* complex is frequently multiresistant to most antimicrobial agents, including cephalosporins and aminoglycosides. Initial isolates may be susceptible to piperacillin, ceftazidime, chloramphenicol, trimethoprim-sulfamethoxazole, with variable susceptibility to imipenem or meropenem. After multiple antibiotic exposures the isolates often become resistant to all available antibiotics. High-level antimicrobial resistance may involve a combination of mechanisms, including selective cell wall permeability, cellular target alterations, enzymatic inactivation of antibiotics, and drug efflux pumps. Hence, eradication of *B. cepacia* is extremely difficult or impossible, and aggressive infection control measures are important to limit the spread in CF units. Also, it is important for the laboratory to identify CF patients with *B. cepacia* colonization with selective medium, as failure to identify infected or colonized subjects may permit transmission among the CF population. High transmissibility of *B. cepacia* causing CF center epidemics have been related to the CblA pilin subunit gene, which encodes the expression of a novel cable (Cbl) pili that bind to CF mucin.[36] Strong affinity for mucin binding allows braiding and intertwining of pili from adjacent bacteria, making it difficult for cilia and host clearance mechanisms to remove *B. cepacia* from the lung. Patient segregation and infection control measures can prevent transmission of *B. cepacia* complex among CF patients.

### *4.3.3 Stentotrophomonas and Alcaligenes Species*

*Stentotrophomonas maltophilia* and *Alcaligenes xylosoxidans* are seen with increased frequency in adult CF patients with advanced lung disease.[37,38] The role of these organisms in CF lung disease is not well established, as with *B. cepacia* complex. Epidemiological studies have not demonstrated any association between infection with these organism and the outcomes of morbidity and mortality in CF patients.[39,40] The identification of *S. maltophilia* and *Alcaligenes* spp can be problematic in respiratory secretion of CF patients, as misidentification as *B. cepacia* has been reported.[41] Both *S. maltophilia* and *Alcaligenes* spp are often multi-resistant to a wide variety of antibiotics. Susceptibility testing of *S. maltophilia* is not reliable with the disk diffusion method, and *trimethoprim-sulfamethoxazole* is usually the most effective antimicrobial agent.

Overall, *S. maltophilia* and *alkaligenes* spp appear to be less virulent (in CF patients) than *P. aeruginosa* and *B. cepacia*, and person-to-person spread is rarely documented.[42]

### *4.3.4 Mycobacteria Species*

There is no evidence that *Mycobacterium tuberculosis* is increased in CF patients and their risk of infection would be similar to the normal population.

However, there are increasing reports of non-tuberculosis mycobacteria recovered from CF patients. In one case series in the early 1990s, *Mycobacteria avium* complex and rapidly growing mycobacterial species were recovered from as many as 20% of CF patients.[43] In a more recent prospective study conducted at 21 CF centers in the United States, 13% of patients had non-tuberculosis mycobacteria in their sputa.[44] *M. avium* complex was the most frequent isolate (72%), and *Mycobacterium abscessus* (16%) was the next most frequent. However, another prospective study of 298 CF patients found *M. abscessus* was by far the most prevalent nontuberculous mycobacteria recovered.[45] Furthermore, whereas *M. avium* has been mainly isolated in CF patients over age 15, *M. abscessus* was isolated in all ages.[46]

There was evidence of geographical variation in the prevalence of nontuberculous mycobacteria colonization. Boston had a prevalence rate of 7% with New Orleans 24% and most of the centers with greater than 15% were in the coastal states.[44] Nontuberculous mycobacteria tend to be recovered more frequently in older CF subjects with a lower frequency of *P. aeruginosa* colonization. In a substudy of 60 CF subjects with nontuberculous mycobacteria colonization there was no significant decline in pulmonary infection over 15 months compared to controls without colonization.[47]

However, patients with higher organism burden, indicated by positive smear or multiple positive cultures, were more likely to have changes on high-resolution chest computed tomography (HRCT). Patients with changes on HRCT (peripheral pulmonary nodules) were more likely to show progression and may benefit from anti-mycobacterial therapy.[47] Overgrowth of sputum by *P. aeruginosa* may lead to underestimation of atypical mycobacterial infection colonization. Sputum samples treated with chlorhexidine decontamination improves the recovery of nontuberculous mycobacteria in CF patients.[48]

## 4.3.5 Aspergillus *Species and Other Fungi*

Colonization of respiratory secretions from CF patients with fungi is common due to recurrent exposures to broad spectrum antibiotics. Most of the times these are not clinically significant, and represent oropharyngeal colonization such as those seen with *Candidal albicans*. However, *Aspergillus* spp (especially *Aspergillus fumigatus*) has been isolated from up to 25% of CF patients.[49] The presence of *Aspergillus* spp. in sputum can represent contamination even in the laboratory, colonization as a commensal organism, invasive disease (which is rare in the immunocompetent CF subject) and may be seen post-lung-transplantation, or allergic bronchopulmonary aspergillosis. There is no evidence that the CF patients without systemic immunosuppression require specific antifungal therapy. Thus, the presence of filamentous fungi is of limited value in this population.[18] Hence, there is insufficient evidence to recommend treatment for *Aspergillus* spp or other filamentous fungi in the sputum of CF patients.[50] However, allergic bronchopulmonary aspergillosis is a noninvasive disease, due to sensitization against allergens from aspergillosis colonization of the airway can be seen in 2–8% of the CF population.[51,52] This occurs in patients with atopy or asthma and exposure to fungal spores or hyphae can lead to production of specific IgE and $CD_4$ $Th_2$ cell response to organisms, with bronchospasm (wheezing), fleeting pulmonary infiltrates, and eosinophilia or eosinophils in the sputum.

Other filamentous fungi that can be isolated from respiratory secretions of CF patients include *Scedosporium apiospermium* (8.6% in one study),[53] *Wangiella dermatitidis*,[54] *Penicillium emersonii*,[55] but their significance is unknown and may represent colonization or commensals without causing disease.

## 4.3.6 Viral Infections

Respiratory viruses have been implicated in exacerbations of pulmonary symptoms and in the long-term cause of respiratory dysfunction in CF patients.[56] Both influenza and respiratory syncytial viruses have been implicated in pulmonary exacerbation in CF patients,[57] but the impact of viral infections on large cohorts of CF subjects has not been well defined. In a prospective study from a single center over a 3-year span, acute respiratory illnesses during a 6-month respiratory viral season were similar between CF infants and controls.[57] However, CF infants were four times more likely to develop lower respiratory tract infections than controls ($p < 0.05$).[57] Despite the fact that controls showed twice as many documented viral infection (by culture, fourfold rise in titer, or both) none of the controls were hospitalized, but 7 of 30 CF infants were hospitalized for acute lower respiratory tract infections. Respiratory syncytial virus (RSV) was cultured in three CF infants and picornavirus in one. Deterioration in lung function persisted for months (mean 3.2 months) after the acute illness (especially with RSV and adenovirus).

## 4.4 Management of Infections in CF

The morbidity and progression of lung disease in CF are largely related to repeated infections and inflammation of the airways; hence much of the treatment is targeted to these areas. Since the microbial pathogens change over the lifespan of the CF subject, the choice of antimicrobial should be based on the periodic isolation and identification of the pathogens from sputum, with characterization of the susceptibility pattern.

Indiscriminate use of antibiotics for protracted periods and suppressive therapy have been practiced widely in CF centers, but the data to support them are mainly retrospectively obtained and this practice have contributed to the multiresistant bacterial colonization commonly seen in CF patients.

## 4.4.1 Infants with CF

In the first year of life, initial respiratory infections causing exacerbation of pulmonary symptoms are predominantly due to *S. aureus*, nontypeable stains of *H. influenzae*, and viruses. Antibiotics should not be used for viral exacerbations with nonpurulent respiratory secretions. The role of antiviral agents in CF has not been systematically assessed but aerolized ribavirin for RSV infection in infants may be of benefit.

Methicillin-sensitive *S. aureus* (MSSA) are usually treated with semisynthetic penicillin (nalficillin, methicillin, or cloxacillin) or a first-generation cephalosporin (cefazolin, cephalexin); MRSA infection in hospitalized patients usually require vancomycin therapy but outpatient cases could be treated with *trimethoprim-sulfamethoxazole* if susceptible.

Continuous maintenance antistaphylococcal antibiotic therapy was thought to improve the morbidity and mortality of young CF patients, and was a common practice for decades.[58] However, this approach may lead to colonization or superinfections with more resistant organisms (such as MRSA and *P. aeruginosa*) and has no proven benefit in the long term. In a large database retrospectively reviewed continuous versus intermittent antistaphylococcal therapy resulted in no better outcome but high acquisition of *P. aeruginosa* colonization.[59] A multicenter randomized, placebo-controlled study of 209 children with CF, comparing continuous cephalexin or placebo with 119 completing a 5-year course confirmed these results.[60] There was no difference in clinical outcome or pulmonary function, but higher rates of *P. aeruginosa* colonization in the cephalexin group. Thus, antibiotics should be used intermittently for exacerbations due to staphylococcal infections and not for prophylaxis or suppression. *H. influenzae* may be treated with amoxicillin for β-lactamase negative stains, amoxicillin-clavulanic acid, or cefuroxime/cefixime for β-lactamase-producing strains.

## 4.4.2 Antipseudomonal Therapy

*P. aeruginosa* is considered the most important respiratory pathogen responsible for progressive lung damage, increased morbidity, and mortality in the CF population. In the early years CF subjects may have transient, intermittent pseudomonal colonization without much respiratory symptoms. It is during this period that the organism is non-mucoid and antibiotic-sensitive and may be more susceptible for eradication. During the later stages when there is heavy persistent colonization, increased airway inflammation, or appearance of the mucoid strains of *Pseudomonas*, eradication is usually not possible and ultimately repeated treatments leads to multi-antimicrobial resistance. Thus, advocates of eradication therapy recommend elimination of bacteria at the first detection of *P. aeruginosa* to break the vicious cycle of infection, inflammation, and irreversible airway damage.[5] Eradication strategies was first used in Denmark[61] and several methods have been implemented (or combination of methods) with some success, including oral, inhaled and intravenous antibiotics. A compilation of nine eradication trials have been reviewed by Starner et al.[5] (with different antibiotics, dosages, and methods of delivery) in the short term: 138 of 161 treated patients (86%) and 31 of 72 untreated controls (43%) become culture-negative for *P. aeruginosa*. The rate of transition to chronic infection was significantly reduced (or delayed) but the rate of intermittent colonization of *P. aeruginosa* was unaffected. A previous study using DNA genotyping had found that 50% of *P. aeruginosa* transient colonization was due to multiple genotypes.[62]

Only two of the eradication trials had used DNA genotyping for verification of elimination in the longitudinal monitoring of *P. aeruginosa* isolates.[63,64] Recurrence of the same genotypes were found in 20–25% of CF children after treatment. The limitations of these trials include small sample size, limited follow-up, unclear effect of selection for other pathogens and development of antibiotic resistant *P. aeruginosa*; and lack of consensus of an optimal regimen and duration of therapy. The experience in Denmark over the past 20 years with the eradication program, however, has been very encouraging. The prevalence of chronic *P. aeruginosa* respiratory colonization in the CF population has steadily decreased over the years from 60% in 1980 to 45% in 1995 and 36% in 2000.[65,66] As a result of their agenda CF children under 14 years rarely experience chronic colonization of *P. aeruginosa* since 1990 in Denmark.[67] The data on the impact of eradication of *P. aeruginosa* of the lungs of CF subjects with respect to long-term morbidity and mortality is not available yet. However, eradication of *P. aeruginosa* has been correlated with improved lung function,[4] and it is known that persistent infection is associated with increased pro-inflammatory cytokines in the airway which is associated with heightened inflammation and further damage.[68] Ongoing studies in Europe[69] and the United States[70] should provide further important information on the long-term benefit of *P. aeruginosa* eradication.

## *4.4.3 Maintenance Therapy*

Maintenance therapy to suppress *P. aeruginosa* infection in CF subjects chronically colonized has also varied from combined intravenous anti-pseudomonal antibiotics, to inhaled antibiotics, to oral quinolones or macrolides. Although most of the data on effectiveness is based on retrospective and observational studies there are a few randomized trials. Inhalation of aerosolized antimicrobials (especially tobramycin) has become popular as a form of suppressive therapy. The advantages are direct delivery of high concentrations to the airways with little or no systemic toxicity, thus overcoming the unfavorable environment in CF endobronchial tree and increasing the bioactivity of the aminoglycoside. Well-conducted pharmacokinetic studies, however, are lacking for most antimicrobials administered by aerolization. Only about 10% of the administered drug is deposited in the lung and the remainder is swallowed or lost to the environment.[71] A great variability has been noted with respect to drug delivered to patients. In one study of 250 CF patients tobramycin 300 mg twice daily delivered by a nebulizer/compressor produced sputum concentrations ranging from <20 to >8,000 ug/g (10 min after dosing) and serum levels (1 h after dosing) from <0.18 to 3.62 ug/ml.[72] No data on the drug half-life in lungs are available. Factors that may affect lung concentrations between individuals include tidal volume, respiratory rate, mucus volume, inflammation, and pre-treatment with bronchodilators. Moreover, the drug may not be equally distributed throughout lung fields because of underlying pathology or anatomic abnormalities or variation.

Efficacy trials in CF subjects colonized or infected with *P. aeruginosa* include a large randomized two-phase study of 520 patients.[73] In the first phase of the study patients were randomized to receive either 300 mg of aerolized tobramycin or placebo twice a day for 28 days, in three cycles interrupted by 28 days without therapy in between. Tobramycin treatment resulted in improved lung function over baseline (10% relative increase in FEVI) and compared with placebo over the 24-week study period.[73] Also, patients treated with tobramycin were 36% less likely to require intravenous antibiotics and 26% less likely to be hospitalized compared to the placebo group $p < 0.05$. In the second phase of the study, patients completing the initial phase, were all given inhaled tobramycin at the same dose for another 45 weeks.[74] A total of 242 patients completed the entire 96-week period (including the initial phase), and patients with initial improvement in lung function maintained this effect throughout the study period. Antibiotic susceptibility of the bacterial isolates did not predict clinical response. However, in the initial phase of the study tobramycin-resistant *P. aeruginosa* isolates ($\geq 8$ µg/ml) increased from 25% at baseline to 32% at week 24 in the tobramycin group, and decrease from 20% at baseline to 17% at week 24 in the placebo group.[73] In 2001, 60.8% of all CF pseudomonal colonized patients in the United States received maintenance therapy with aerolized tobramycin[75] and this increased to 67.5% by 2004.[76]

In Europe, aerolized polymixin/colistin has been used widely in uncontrolled studies in doses of 500,000 to 1 million IU twice daily for several months.[61,77] This form of therapy has been associated with decreased recovery of *P. aeruginosa* in CF sputum and possible slowing of the decline in forced vital capacity (FVC). In a randomized, unblinded trial between inhaled tobramycin (300 mg twice daily) and colistin (80 mg twice daily) for 28 days in 109 CF patients demonstrated 6.7% greater improvement in the tobramycin.[78] There was a comparable reduction of the *P. aeruginosa* burden in the sputum of both groups. Inhaled colistin also may cause bronchoconstriction in CF patients.[79]

Other inhaled antibiotics used in CF include aztreonam, a monobactam, active against *P. aeruginosa*. In a preliminary study of 19 CF patients treated with inhaled aztreonam (500 mg to 1 gm twice daily) for up to 18 months, several patients had improved pulmonary function and 15 of 16 patients who completed the trial had decreased *Pseudomonas* density.[80] However, resistance to aztreonam developed in ten (52%) of the patients. Phase I and II trials with inhaled aztreonam lysinate in the United States showed the drug was well-tolerated (similar to placebo), and two Phase III clinical trials have been started to assess the effectiveness of a 28-days treatment in CF subjects who do not use antibiotics regularly, and the other in subjects who utilize inhaled tobramycin frequently.[81]

Oral antibiotics have also been used for chronic suppressive or maintenance therapy in CF. Although ciprofloxacin has good *Pseudomonas* activity with very good bioavailability in airway secretion of CF subjects,[82] the emergence of resistance in *P. aeruginosa* and *S. aureus* is a concern after 3–4 weeks of therapy.[83] The development of arthropathy in children has been a concern with the quinolones, but over 3,000 children treated with ciprofloxacin has been associated with a very low incidence of arthropathy.[84] However, ciprofloxacin is best used for exacerbation of pulmonary infection in CF patients for short periods, but after 3–4 cycles of therapy resistance is likely to develop.

Although the macrolides (erythromycin, clarithromycin, and azithromycin) have little in vitro activity against *P. aeruginosa* they have been used in maintenance therapy of chronic infection with this organism in CF. Proposed mechanism of action include anti-inflammatory effect,[85] excellent biofilm penetration and intracellular accumulation in *P. aeruginosa* to inhibit protein synthesis and production of virulence factors, and alter the structure and architecture of biofilm.[86,87] Macrolides also accumulate in neutrophils and may ameliorate the inflammatory effect including oxygen radicals production, apoptosis, macrophage-activation complex-I expression, and pro-inflammatory cytokine production.[88] In phase II randomized controlled trials in children[89] and adults,[90] azithromycin resulted in improved lung function ($FEV_1$) and fewer respiratory exacerbations than controls, and demonstrated an anti-inflammatory effect in adults (reduced C-reactive protein levels).[90] In a recent larger phase III, randomized controlled trial in 185 CF subjects (6 years or older) colonized with *P. aeruginosa*, subjects received 6 months of twice weekly azithromycin (250–500 mg depending on weight) or placebo.[91] The azithromycin-treated groups had decreased rate of pulmonary exacerbations, increased weight, relative increase in FEVI of 6.2%, and half as many hospitalization as those on placebo. Since then the use of macrolides (particularly azithromycin) for maintenance therapy in CF subjects greater than 6 years have risen to 49.3% in the United States in 2004.[76]

### 4.4.4 Treatment of Pulmonary Exacerbation

There is no standard criteria for pulmonary exacerbation of CF but the symptoms may include a combination of increased cough with increased or new production of sputum; or change in color, new onset, or increased hemoptosis; increased shortness of breath; and decreased exercise tolerance, fatigue, malaise, fever, and poor appetite.[25] Pulmonary exacerbation may be secondary to various conditions including bacterial infection, viral infection, pollutants, and reactive airway disease. Only in patients where bacterial endobronchial infection is likely (with increased purulent sputum) are antibiotics of proven benefit. Pulmonary exacerbation may vary in severity from mild to severe, and milder exacerbations can be treated with oral antibiotics (such as ciprofloxacin) or inhaled antibiotics depending on the sputum culture results. More severe exacerbations usually require hospitalization for intravenous therapy, and choice of antibiotics should be selected based on recent or current cultures of respirations secretions. It is a common practice in most CF centers to initiate a combinations of two antibiotics (most often an anti-pseudomonal β-lactam agent and an aminoglycoside) in hospital, to complete intravenous therapy for 2–3 weeks at home (or switch to oral agent if susceptible). In a recent meta-analysis of eight trails comparing single versus combination antibiotic therapy for people with CF exacerbation, however, the results were inconclusive.[92] Overall the meta-analysis did not demonstrate any significant differences between monotherapy and combination therapy, in terms of lung function, symptoms score, or bacteriological outcome measures. However, six of the trials were performed between 1977 and 1988, had small sample sizes, and were of poor methodological quanlity.[92] Clinical efficacy is usually measured by improved pulmonary function, reduction in symptoms, improved quality of life measures, and reduction in bacterial density.[25] In patients with chronic *P. aeruginosa* colonization eradication is not usually possible. Since many CF patients with chronic *P. aeruginosa* or *B. cepacia* complex infection/colonization develop multi-resistant strains (resistant to anti-pseudomonal β-lactams, quinolones, and aminoglycosides), CF units have been using specialized centers to perform in vitro multiple combination susceptibility testing (MCBT) to guide combination therapy. However, the value of this approach over standard methods of susceptibility testing to guide therapy has not been proven to be more effective. In a recent multicenter, randomized controlled trail of 251 CF patients with chronic infection with gram negative bacteria, therapy directed by MCBT did not improve clinical or bacterial outcomes compared to standard techniques.[93] Even routine susceptibility testing in chronic *P. aeruginosa* infection in CF patient is not predictive of clinical response to antibiotic therapy. In a recent study from an adult CF unit over a 6-month period reduced number of susceptibility testing by 56% had no impact on clinical outcomes.[94] However, infection with multiple-antibiotic-resistant *P. aeruginosa* is associated with accelerated progression of cystic fibrosis in a 4-year period study in a cohort of 75 consecutive adult CF patients.[95] Once-daily aminoglycoside parenteral administration in CF patients is considered equally efficacious and potentially safer than multiple daily dosing. However, the most suitable pharmacodynamic index (maximum concentration/minimal inhibitory concentration [Cmax/MIC] versus area under the curve in 24 h/MIC [$AUC_{24}$/MIC]) to ensure optimal clinical outcome is not clear. In a recent study 33 adult CF patients were treated with intravenous tobramycin (10 mg/Kg/day) for 14 days given as a single once a day (17 patients) or as three doses every 8 h (16 patients).[96] For equal values of $AUC_{24}$/MIC once daily treatment provided better improvement in lung function than multiple daily dosing, but Cmax/MIC did not show any dosing dependence. Thus, the most important pharmacodynamic parameter for clinical outcome in CF patients was Cmax/MIC, whereas $AUC_{24}$/MIC outcome prediction was dependent on the regimen. Increase in *P. aeruginosa* resistance was significantly greater with once-daily dosing and was linked to a long dosing interval.[96]

## 4.4.5 *Treatment of Other Emerging Pathogens*

*B. cepacia* complex are usually highly resistant to multiple antibiotics. They are intrinsically resistant to the aminoglycosides, most β-lactam antibiotics, except the carbapenems (meropenem, imipenem) and the quinolones have variable activity but resistance is readily induced.[97] Although in vitro combinations have been used to test for synergy, 49% of isolates inhibited by chloramphenicol plus minocycline and 26% of isolates by chloramphenicol plus ceftazidime,[98] their clinical value have not been proven. Thus a carbapenem is most commonly used if resistance has not already occurred.

Treatment of *S. maltophilia* and *A. xylosoxidans* are also limited because of multi- resistance to many antibiotics. They are often resistant to the aminoglycosides with variable susceptibility to the quinolones and β-lactams agents.[25] *S. maltophilia* is most consistently susceptible to sulfamethoxazole/trimethoprim (about 80%) which can be used orally as the bioavailability is excellent and it is considered the drug of choice. Ticarcillin/clavulanate is active in vitro as well and may be useful clinically, often in combination empirically with sulfamethoxazole/trimethoprim for severe infections. Although, minocycline has very good in vitro activity against *S. maltophilia* there is limited clinical experience in treatment.[99] Strains of *A. xylosoxidans* may be susceptible to sulfamethoxazole/trimethoprim, ureidopenicillins, imipenem, ceftazidime, cefoperazone, and β-lactamase inhibitors combinations.[99] They are usually resistant to the aminoglycosides, aztreonam and most and were resistant to the quinolones. In a multicenter study of 106 strains of *A. xylosoxidans* from 78 CF patients, 11% were misidentified.[100] Minocycline (51%), imipenem (59%), piperacillin-tazobactam (55%) were the most active agents.[100] Combination of chloramphenicol with minocycline and ciprofloxacin with imipenem showed additive affect in 40% and 32%, respectively. Thus treatment should be guided by the susceptibility results.

The recovery of nontuberculosis mycobacteria from CF patients appears be increasing. The distinction between active lung infection and colonization is often difficult because of overlap in symptoms and radiological appearance. Patients with repeatedly positive acid fast smears of sputum and peripheral pulmonary nodules on HRCT are more likely infected than colonized and may benefit from specific therapy.[47] Treatment varies according to the mycobacterial species and multiple antimycobacterial drugs for a year is often used. Multidrug regimens include clarithromycin, ethambutol, and rifamycin and drug monitoring of serum levels is useful (when available) because of potential drug interaction and altered pharmakinetics in patients with CF.[101] *M. abscessus* is usually chemotherapy-resistant and in vitro the organism is most consistently susceptible to clarithromycin (or azithromycin), amikacin, tigecycline, and linezolid, with variable susceptibility to cefoxitin and imipenem.[102] Empiric regimen for pulmonary *M. abscessus* has been a combination of intravenous amikacin and cefoxitin for 2 weeks and oral clarithromycin for 6 months.

## 4.5 Prevention of Infections in CF

Patients with CF should receive the standard immunization recommended for children by the American Academy of Pediatrics. They should also receive the annual influenza virus vaccine in the fall. Attempts to prevent *P. aeruginosa* infection by active immunization have not been successful. An earlier study showed no benefit of polyvalent *Pseudomonas* vaccine and predisposed some patients to more severe pulmonary disease with infection.[103] A more recent study with a conjugate vaccine capable of inducing high affinity, opsonic anti-lipopolysaccharide (LPs) antibodies found protection in only a subgroup of patients.[104] A *P. aeruginosa* flagella vaccine capable of inducing high long-lasting antibody titer systematically and in respiratory secretions was being studied in a multi-center European trial in 400 CF patients.[105] However, a result of this trial has not been published to date.

## 4.6 Adjunctive Therapy for Pulmonary Exacerbation

Defective mucociliary transport and retention of mucus predispose to bacterial overgrowth, which triggers repeated cycles of infection and airway inflammation. Attempts to restore airway surface liquid in CF and improve airway clearance may decrease exacerbations from infections and improve or preserve lung function and prolonged survival. Previous studies of inhalation of hypertonic saline showed increased mucociliary transport and encouraging short-term results, but were limited by small sample sizes.[106] Hence, routine use for treatment of CF patients was not recommended until further proof of benefit. Since topical application of saline to the epithelium of the airway would likely be short-lived, prolonged effect was not expected. However, two recent studies have supported the use of this simple and relatively inexpensive therapy. Donaldson et al.[107] studied 24 CF patients with inhaled hypertonic saline (5 ml of 7% sodium chloride) four times daily. There was a sustained increase of mucus clearance at 8 h and 24 h over baseline and improved lung function as measured by FEV and FVC compared to baseline. In the other study the long-term benefit of inhaled hypertonic saline was reported in a controlled, double-blind trial.[108] CF patients 6 years or older with stable disease were randomized to inhale 4 ml of either 7% hypertonic saline ($N = 83$) or 0.9% (control) saline ($N = 81$) twice daily for 48 weeks. A bronchodilator was given before each dose as hypertonic saline can cause acute transient airflow obstruction. The hypertonic-saline group had significant improvement in lung function compared to controls (higher FVC by 82 ml) and $FEV_1$ (by 64 ml) $p = 0.03$, during the 48-week period. Moreover the hypertonic-saline resulted in 56% fewer pulmonary exacerbation ($p = 0.02$), and 76% higher number of patients without exacerbations ($p = 0.03$).[108] Some issues and limitations to these studies have been raised by the accompanying editorial.[109] In the controlled therapeutic trial[108] the decrease in pulmonary exacerbation was largely confined to the first 3 months of treatment, associated by a decrease in compliance by patients over time. Also, inhaled tobramycin was only received by less than 15% of the participants, despite the fact that about 80% were chronically infected with *P. aeruginosa* (much less than the standard practice in the United States). However, this raises the issue that hypertonic saline inhalation could result in a use of less chronic tobramycin therapy, which may result in lower-resistant organisms. The mechanism of the therapeutic benefit was not elucidated by these studies, as the improvement of mucus clearance could have resulted from increased surface liquid or from increased induction of cough or both.[109]

The only other proven therapy for increasing mucus clearance in CF patients is recombinant human DNAse (rh DNAse) licensed by the Food and Drug Administration (FDA) as Pulmozyme, for chronic maintenance therapy for CF patients.[25] The purified rh DNAse digests polymeric extracellular DNA and reduces sputum viscosity and improves airway mucus clearance. In a phase III trial of Pulmozyme 2.5 mg nebulized once daily resulted in 6% improvement in FEV, and a 22% reduction in pulmonary exacerbations in CF patients older than 5 years.[110] The main side-effects were transient laryngitis and hoarseness. A 2-year randomized trial in CF children with mild lung disease showed only modest improvement in FEV (~3%) and FEF (~8%), but 34% reduction in pulmonary exacerbations.[111] In a review of 14 trails assessing inhaled rh DNAse, 11 were placebo-controlled and two were compared with hypertonic saline.[112] There was evidence that inhaled rh DNAse improve lung function significantly in CF patients at 1, 2, 6 months, and 2 years, but a nonsignificant difference at 3 years.[112] The reduction in exacerbations at 2 years was nonsignificant. A previous crossover trial showed that hypertonic saline was inferior to rh DNAse in improving lung function at 3 months but did not assess pulmonary exacerbation for outcome.[113] In the recent controlled trial with hypertonic saline noted before[108] the beneficial effects seen were independent of concurrent use of rh DNAse, thus hypertonic saline would be an inexpensive adjunctive therapy rather than replacement for rh DNAse (which is more expensive). Another osmotic agent, mannitol, which can be administered as a dry powder by metered-dose inhaler, thus more convenient, is also being evaluated.[109]

## *4.6.1 Anti-inflammatory Therapy*

Pulmonary complications in CF are thought to be related to recurrent inflammatory response to infections, with chronically activated neutrophils and cytokines causing loss of lung function and premature death. Anti-inflammatory treatment strategies have resulted in some success. Systemic steroids and possibly ibuprofen have been shown to decrease the rate of respiratory decline in patients with CF but adverse effects and tolerability have limited their usefulness.[114] There is no evidence of clinical efficacy in CF of inhaled steroids, unless there is underlying asthma or bronchial hyperresponsiveness.[25]

In the most recent review of nonsteroidal anti-inflammatory drugs in CF to prevent pulmonary deterioration, five controlled trials were identified.[115] There was some evidence to suggest that nonsteroidal anti-inflammatory drugs may prevent pulmonary deterioration in subjects with mild lung disease due to CF, but their routine use was not recommended. As previously mentioned part of the benefit seen with chronic use of macrolides in CF patients may be due to an anti-inflammatory action. Pilot studies on other anti-inflammatory therapies that are being evaluated in CF patients include simvastatin, N-acetylcysteine supplementation, and oral glutathione.[81]

Simvastatin, a HMG-CoA reductase inhibitor and other "statins" used to lower cholesterol blood levels are also considered as anti-inflammatory agents. Simvastatin can also block a protein that may contribute to the low concentration of nitric oxide (NO) in the CF lung. NO has antibacterial and anti-inflammatory properties and is an important component of the host defence. Volunteers will receive simvastatin for 1 month and the levels of inflammatory markers from nasal cells, lung mucus, and blood, as well as NO in their exhaled breath measured before and after treatment.[81]

It is postulated that the lung changes in CF patients from repeated infection and inflammation is partly related to release of oxidants from neutrophils. The human body normally controls inflammation by production of substances (antioxidants) that reduce or counteract the effects of these oxidants. Imbalance of these factors, such as deficiency in the antioxidant glutathione may contribute to the lung disease in CF. N-acetylcysteine can replenish glutathione levels, and a phase I study has shown that it appropriately can produce an anti-inflammatory effect.[81] A phase II study to assess clinical effectiveness of oral N-acetylcysteine is currently ongoing. Another study is to provide an oral formulation of glutathione that is buffered, microencapsulated, and enteric-coated to enable more efficient absorption. Glutathione levels and various inflammatory markers are being measured in plasma and sputum, and lung function is monitered.[81]

## 4.7 Future Directions

The ultimate cure for CF would be to correct the basic genetic defect that causes the disease. In vitro studies demonstrated that introduction of CFTR complementary DNA into affected cells could correct the chloride channel defect.[116] Gene therapy remains in an evolving, developmental stage in CF, while some initial human studies with adenovirus associated vectors have been encouraging several barriers remain including efficient delivery and long-term expression of the CFTR transgene in the airway. CF gene therapy has made milestones along the way. While the treatment can restore CFTR function in cultured cells and animal models, the optimal vector or delivery method for CF gene therapy has yet to be found.[25] Advances have been made in viral vector design (using viruses deleted of their harmful potential) and nonviral approaches to gene therapy.

## 4.7 Future Directions

Protienomics is a cutting edge tool to identify proteins important to the functioning of CFTR in the airway (including the CFTR protein itself). Sets of protein involved in shaping, moving CFTR to the proper place in the cell and critical to the function are under investigation. Approximately 15 proteins were identified in 2004 and are under evaluation for therapy and as biomarkers to assess activity and response to treatment.[117]

Other approaches to treatment would be to block the adhesion of bacteria to the airway epithelium early in children with CF to prevent chronic colonization and infection with *P. aeruginosa*, *S. aureus*, and *B. cepacia*. Dextrans (neutral polymers of glucose) have been shown in vitro to block adherence of *P. aeruginosa* and *B. cepacia* to respiratory epithelial cells.[118,119] Aerolized dextran has also been shown to protect mice from *P. aeruginosa* pneumonia.[120] In vitro dextran can decrease the viscosity of sputum from CF patients, thus may improve mucus clearance,[121] and it is also easy to produce and is inexpensive. Thus, large randomized, controlled trials in CF subjects are warranted with inhaled dextran. Endogenous cationic antimicrobial peptides produced by epithelial cells and neutrophils is part of the innate immunity against the early infection, and have broad antibacterial activity in respiratory secretion against gram-positive and gram-negative pathogens (including *P. aeruginosa*).[122] Although there is no evidence of deficiency of these peptides in CF, it has been postulated that the raised ionic content of the airway surface fluid may inactivate these salt-sensitive peptides or the slow mucociliary clearance may allow bacterial pathogens to overwhelm these molecules' antibactericidal activity.[123] To date there is no evidence of cross-resistance to these peptides and available antimicrobials, thus direct application to the bronchial mucosa in higher concentrations may be an attractive form of therapy for even multi-resistant bacteria. A phase I trial of a Protegrin-derived peptides, 1B-367 (Intra Biotics Pharmaceuticals Inc, Palo Alto, CA), has shown good tolerance and safety profile in CF adults by inhalation, but further clinical trials are needed to prove efficacy.[124] The cost of production of these antimicrobial peptides may prohibit commercial development, and pathogenic bacteria such as *P. aeruginosa* can acquire mechanisms to evade killing by these peptides, such as employing proteases to digest the peptides or modifying the anionic surface charge on their surface lipopolysaccharide.[125]

As previously mentioned new macrolides (ie azithromycin) may be beneficial in CF by improving clearance of *P. aeruginosa* alginate biofilms (thus reducing severity of lung pathology) by blockage of quorum sensing, and increased sensitivity to hydrogen peroxide and the complement system.[126] Other potentially useful novel therapy to prevent pseudomonas biofilm formation include human host defense peptide LL-37 (decreases attachment of bacterial cells, stimulating twitching motility, influence two major quorum sensing system (Las and Rh1), leading to down regulation of genes essential for biofilm development).[127] Utilization of maggot excretions/secretions products are of potential therapeutic benefit as they are effective against biofilms of *S. aureus* and *P. aeruginosa*.[128]

Further antimicrobial trials are needed to define the optimum therapy to eradicate *P. aeruginosa* in the early colonization stage; also proper randomized multicenter trials are needed to prove the benefit of combination versus single agents; to define optimum duration of therapy that provide maximum benefit and limiting toxicity and development of resistance.

# References

1. Lehtzin, N., John, M., Irizarry, R., Merlo, C., Diette, G., Boyle, M., (2006), Outcomes of adults with cystic fibrosis infected with antibiotic-resistant *Pseudomonas aeruginosa*. Respiration 73:27–33.
2. Boucher, R., (2005), Cystic fibrosis, in: Harrison's Principles of Internal Medicine, 16th Edition, Kasper, D.C., Braunwald, E., Fauci, A.S., Hauser, S.L., Longo, D.L., Jameson, J. L., (eds), McGraw-Hill, New York, pp. 1543–1546.
3. Brennan, A.L., Geddes, D.M., (2002), Cystic fibrosis. Curr. Opin. Infect. Dis. 15:175–182.
4. Fredericksen, B., Koch, C., Hoiby, N., (1997), Antibiotic treatment of initial colonization with *Pseudomonas aeruginosa* postpones chronic infection and prevents deterioration of pulmonary function in cystic fibrosis. Pediatr. Pulmonol. 23:330–335.
5. Starner, T.D., McCray, P.B., Jr. (2005), Pathogenesis of early lung disease in cystic fibrosis: A window of opportunity to eradicate bacteria. Ann. Intern. Med. 14:816–822.
6. Li, Z., Kosork, M.R., Farrell, P.M., Laxova, A., West, S.E.H., Green, C.G., Collins, J., Rock, M.J., Splaingord, M.L., (2005), Longitudinal development of mucoid *Pseudomonas aeruginosa* infection and lung disease progression in children with cystic fibrosis. JAMA 293: 581–588.
7. Goldman, M.J., Anderson, G.M., Stolzenberg, E.D., Kari, U.P., Zasloff, M., Wilson, J.M., (1997), Human beta-defensins is a salt-sensitive antibiotic in lung that is inactivated in cystic fibrosis. Cell 88:553–560.
8. Smith, J.J., Travis, S.M., Greenberg, E.P., Welsh, M.J., (1996), Cystic fibrosis airway epithelia fail to kill bacteria because of abnormal airway surface fluid. Cell 85:229–236.
9. Matsui, H., Grubb, B.R., Torran, R., Randell, S.H., Gatzy, J.T., Davis, C.W., Boucher, R.C., (1998), Evidence for periciliary liquid layer depletion, not abnormal ion composition, in the pathogenesis of cystic fibrosis airways disease. Cell 95:1005–1015.
10. Poschet, J.F., Boucher, J.C., Tatterson, L., Skidmore, J., VanDyke, R.W., Deretic, V., (2001), Molecular basis for defective glycosylation and *Pseudomonas* pathogenesis in cystic fibrosis lung. Proc. Natl. Acad. Sci USA 98:13972–13977.
11. Bryan, R., Kube, D., Perez, A., Davis, P., Prince, A., (1998), Overproduction of the CFTR, R domain leads to increased levels of asialoGMI, and increased *Pseudomonas aeruginosa* binding by epithelial cells. Am. J. Respir. Cell Mol. Biol. 19:269–277.
12. De Bentzmann, S., Roger, P., Dupuit, F., Bajolet-Laudinat, O., Fuchey, C., Plotkowski, M.C., Puchelle, E., (1996), Asialo-GMI is a receptor for *Pseudomonas aeruginosa* adherence to regenerating respiratory epithelial cells. Am. J. Respir. Cell Mol. Biol. 64:1582–1588.
13. Schroeder, T.H., Reiniger, N., Meluleni, G., Grout, M., Colemon, F.T., Pier, G.B., (2001), Transgenic cystic fibrosis mice exhibit reduced early clearance of *Pseudomonas aeruginosa* from the respiratory tract. J. Immunol. 166:7410–7418.
14. Meng, O., Springall, D.R., Bishop, A.E., (1998), Lack of inducible nitric oxide synthase in bronchial epithelium: a possible mechanism of susceptibility to infection in cystic fibrosis. J. Pathol. 164:323–331.
15. Sturgess, J., Imrie, J., (1982), Quantitative evaluation of the development of tracheal submucosal glands in infants with cystic fibrosis and control infants. Am. J. Pathol. 106:303–311.
16. Inglis, S.K., Wilson, S.M., (2005), Cystic fibrosis and airway submucosal glands. Pediatr. Pulmon. 40:279–284.
17. Aichele, D., Schnare, M., Saake, M., Rollinghoff, M., Gessner, A., (2006), Expression and antimicrobial function of bactericidal permeability increasing protein in cystic fibrosis patients. Infect. Immun. 74:4708–4714.

18. Miller, M.B., Gilligan, P.H., (2003), Laboratory aspects of management of chronic pulmonary infections in patients with cystic fibrosis. J. Clin. Microbiol. 41:4009–4015.
19. Cystic Fibrosis Foundation, (2002), Patient registry 2001 annual report. Cystic Fibrosis Foundation, Washington, DC.
20. Jarry, T.M., Cheung, A.L., (2006), *Staphylococcus aureus* escapes more efficiently from the phagosome of a cystic fibrosis bronchial epithelial cell line than from it's normal counterpart. Infect. Immun. 74:2565–2577.
21. Lyczak, J.B., Cannon, C.C., Pier, G.B., (2002), Lung infections associated with cystic fibrosis. Clin. Microbiol. Rev. 15:194–222.
22. Thomas, S.R., Ray, A., Hodson, M.E., Pitt, T.L., (2000), Increased sputum amino-acid concentration and auxotrophy of *Pseudomonas aeruginosa* in severe cystic fibrosis lung disease. Thorax 55:795–797.
23. Costerton, W., Veeh, R., Shirtliff, M., Paomore, M., Post, C., Ehrlich, G., (2003), The application of biofilm science to the study and control of chronic bacterial infections. J. Clin. Invest. 112:1466–1477.
24. Hoiby, N., (2002), Understanding bacterial biofilms in patients with cystic fibrosis: Current and innovative approaches to potential therapies. J. Cystic Fibrosis. 1:249–254.
25. Gibson, R.L., Burns, J.L., Ramsey, B.W., (2003), Pathophysiology and management of pulmonary infections in cystic fibrosis. Am. J. Respir. Crit. Care Med. 168:918–951.
26. Oliver, A., Canton, R., Campo, P., Baquero, F., Blazquez, J., (2000), High frequency of hypermutable *Pseudomonas aeruginosa* in cystic fibrosis lung infection. Science 288: 1251–1254.
27. Soong, G., Muir, A., Gomez, M.I., Waks, J., Reddy, B., Planet, P., Singh, P.K., Kanoko, Y., Wolfgang, M.C., Hsiao, Y.S., Tony, L., Prince, A., (2006), Bacterial neuramidases faciliatates mucosal infection by participating in biofilm production. J. Clin. Invest. 116:2297–2305.
28. Van Alst, N.E., Picardo, K.F., Iglewski, B.H., Haidaris, C.G., (2007) Nitrate sensing and metabolism modulate motility, biofilm formation, and virulence in *Pseudomonas aeruginosa*. Infect. Immun. 75:3780–3790.
29. MacEachran, D.P., YE, S., Bomberger, J.M., Hogan, D.A., Swiatecka-Urban, A., Stanton, B. A., O'Toole, G.A., (2007), The *Pseudomonas aeruginosa* secreted protein PA2934 decreases apical membrane expression of the Cystic Fibrosis Trans-membrane Conductance Regulator. Infect. Immune 75:3902–3912.
30. Isles, A., Maclusky, I., Corey, M., Gold, R., Prober, C., Flemig, P., Levison, H., (1984), *Pseudomonas cepacia* infection in cystic fibrosis: an emerging problem. J. Pediatr. 104: 206–210.
31. Heath, D.G., Hohreker, K., Carriker, C., Smith, K., Routh, J., LiPuma, J.J., Aris, R.M., Weber, D., Gilligan, P.H., (2002), Six-year molecular analysis of *Burkholderia cepacia* complex isolates among cystic fibrosis patients at a referral center for lung transplantation. J. Clin. Microbiol. 40:1188–1193.
32. Chen, J.S., Witzmann, K.A., Spilker, T., Fink, R.J., LiPuma, J.J., (2001), Endemicity and inter-city spread of *Burkholderia cepacia* genomovar III in cystic fibrosis. J. Pediatr. 139: 643–641.
33. Chaparro, C., Maurer, J., Gutierrez, C., Krajden, M., Chan, C., Winton, T., Keshavjce, S., Scavuzzo, M., Tullis, E., Hutcheon, M., Kesten, S.E., (2001), Infection with *Burkholderia cepacia* complex isolates among cystic fibrosis: outcome following lung transplantation. Am. Rev. Respir. Crit. Care Med. 163:43–48.
34. Aris, R.M., Routh, J.C., LiPuma, J.J., Heath, D.G., Gilligan, P.H., (2001), Lung transplantation for cystic fibrosis patients with *Burkholderia cepacia* complex. Survival linked to genomovar type. Am. J. Respir. Crit. Care Med. 164:2102–2106.
35. Henry, D., Campbell, M., Mc Gimpsey, C., Clarke, A., Louden, L., Burns, J.L., Roe, M.H., Vandamme, P, Speert, D., (1999), Comparison of isolation media for recovery of *Burkholderia cepacia* complex from respiratory secretions of patients with *cystic fibrosis*. J. Clin. Microbiol. 37:1004–1007.

36. Sun, L., Jiang, R.Z., Stainbach, S., Holmes, A., Campanelli, C., Forstner, J., Sajjan, U., Tan, Y., Riley, M., Goldstein, R., (1995), The emergence of a highly transmissible lineage of Cbl+ *Pseudomonas (Burkholderia) cepacia* causing CF centre epidemics in North America and Britain. Nat. Med. 7:626–627.
37. Graff, G.R., Burns, J.L., (2002), Factor affecting the incidence of *Stentotrophomonas maltophilia* isolation in cystic fibrosis. Chest 121:1754–1760.
38. Saiman, L., Chen, Y., Tabibi, S., San Gibriel, R., Zhou, J., Lui, Z., Lai, L., Whittier., S., (2001), Identification and antimicrobial susceptibility of *Alcaligenes xylosoxidans* isolated from patients with cystic fibrosis. J. Clin. Microbiol. 39:3942–3945.
39. Goss, C.H., Otto, K.L., AiKen, M.L., Rubenfeld, G.D., (2002), Detecting *Stentotrophomonas maltophilia* does not reduce survival of patients with cystic fibrosis. Am. J. Respir. Crit Care Med. 166:356–361.
40. Tan, K.K., Conway, S.P., Brownlee, K.G., Etherington, C., Peckham, G., (2002), Alcaligenes infection in cystic fibrosis. Pediatr. Pulmonol. 34:101–104.
41. McMenamin, J.D., Zaccone, T.M., Coenye, T., Vandamme, P., LiPuma, (2000), Misidentification of *Burkholderia cepacia* in US cystic fibrosis treatment centers: an analysis of 1,051 recent sputum isolates. Chest 177:1661–1665.
42. Krzewinski, J.W., Nguyen: C.D., Foster, J.M., Burns, J.L., (2001), Use of random amplified polymorphic DNA PCR to examine epidemiology of *Stentotrophomonas maltophilia* and *Achromobactor (Alcaligenes) xylosoxidans* from patients with cystic fibrosis. J. Clin. Microbiol. 39:3597–3602.
43. Kilby, J.M., Gilligan, P.H., Yankaskas, J.R., Highsmith. W.E. Jr., Edwards, L.J., Knowles, M. R., (1992), Nontuberculous mycobacteria in adult patients with cystic fibrosis. Chest 102: 70–75.
44. Oliver, K.N., Weber, D.J., Wallace, R.J. Jr., Faiz, A.R., Lee, J.H., Zhang, Y., Brown-Elliot, B. A., Handler, A., Wilson, R.W., Schechter, M.S., Edwards, L.J., Chakraborti, S., Knowles, M. R., (2003), Nontuberculous mycobacteria I: multicenter prevalence study in cystic fibrosis. Am. J. Respir. Crit. Care Med. 167:828–834.
45. Sermet-Gaudelus, I., Le Bourgeois, M., Pierre-Audigier, C., Offredo, C., Guillemot, D., Halley, S., Akoua-Koffi, C., Vincent, V., Sivadon-Tardy, V., Ferroni, A., Berche, P., Scheinmann, P., Lenoir, G., Gaillard, J.-L., (2003), *Mycobacterium* abscessus and children with cystic fibrosis. Emerg. Infect. Dis. 9:1587–1591.
46. Pierre-Audigier, V., Ferroni, A., Sermet – Gaudelius, I., Le Bourgeois, M., Offredo, C., Vu-Tien, H., Fauroux, B., Mariani, P., Munck, A., Binger, E., Guillemot, D., Quesne, G., Vincent, V., Berche, P., Gaillard, J.L., (2005), Age-related prevalence and distribution of nontuberculous mycobacterial species among patients with cystic fibrosis. J. Clin. Microbiol. 43: 3467–3470.
47. Olivier, K.N., Weber, D.J., Lee, J.H., Handler, A., Tuder, G, Molina, P.L., Tomashefski, J., Knowles, M.R., (2003), Nontuberculous mycobacteria: II. Nested-cohort study of impact on cystic fibrosis lung disease. Am. J. Respir. Crit. Care Med. 167:833–840.
48. Ferroni, A., Vu-Thien, H., Lanotte, P., Le Bourgeois, M., Sermet-Gaudelus, I., Fauroux, B., Marchand, S., Varaigne, F., Berche, P., Gaillard, J.L., Offredo, C., (2006), Value of Chorhexidine decontamination method for recovery of nontuberculous mycobacteria from sputum samples of patients with cystic fibrosis. J. Clin. Microbiol. 44:2237–2239.
49. Bakore, N., Rickerts, V., Bargon, J., Just-Nubbling, G., (2003), Prevalance of *Aspergillus fumigatus* and other fungal species in the sputum of adult patients with cystic fibrosis. Mycoses 46:19–23.
50. Stevens, D.A., Moss, R.B., Kurup, V.P., Knutsen, A.P., Greenberger, P., Judson, M.A, Denning, D.W., Crameri, R., Brody, A.S., Light, M., Skove, M., Maish, W., Mastella, G., and Participants in the Cystic Fibrosis Foundation Consensus Conference, (2003), Allergic bronchopulmonary aspergillosis in cystic fibrosis state of the art: Cystic Fibrosis Foundation Consensus Conference. Clin. Infect. Dis. 37(Suppl. 3):S225–S264.

# References

51. Taccetti, G., Procopio, E., Morianelti, C., Campama, S., (2000), Allergic bronchopulmonary aspergillosis in Italian cystic fibrosis patients: prevalence and percentage of positive tests in the employed diagnostic criteria. Eur. J. Epidemiol. 16:837–842.
52. Mastella, G., Rainisio, M., Harmes, H.K., Hodson, M., Koch, C., Navarro, J., Strandvik, B., McKenzie, S.G., (2001), Epidemiologic Registry of Cystic Fibrosis: allergic bronchopulmonary aspergillosis in cystic fibrosis, a European epidemiologic study. Eur. Respir. J. 16: 464–471.
53. Cimon, B., Carrere, J., Vinatier, J.F., Chazalette, J.P., Chabasse, D., Bouchara, J.P., (2001), Clinical significance of *Scedosporium apiospermum* in patients with cystic fibrosis. Eur. J. Clin. Microbiol Infect. Dis. 19:53–56.
54. Diemert, D., Kunimoto, D., Sard, C., Rennie, R., (2001), Sputum isolation of *Wangiella dematitidis* in patients with cystic fibrosis. Scand. J. Infect. Dis. 33:777–779.
55. Cimon, B., Carrere, J., Chazalette, J.P., Vinatier, J.F., Chabasse, D., Bouchara, J.P., (1999), Chronic airway colonization by *Penicillium emesonii* in a patient with cystic fibrosis. Med. Mycol. 37:291–293.
56. Prober, C.G., (1991), The impact of respiratory viral infections in patients with cystic fibrosis. Clin. Rev. Allergy 9:87–102.
57. Hiatt, P.W., Grace, S.C., Kozinetz, C.A., Raboudi, S.H., Treece, D.G., Taber, L.H., Piedra, P. A., (1999), Effects of viral lower respiratory tract infection on lung function in infants with cystic fibrosis. Pediatr. 103:619–626.
58. Thomassen, M.J., Demko, C.A., Doershuk, C., (1987), Cystic Fibrosis: a review of pulmonary infections and interventions. Pediatr. Pulmonol. 3:334–351.
59. Ratjen. F., Comes, G., Paul, K., Posselt, H.G., Wagner, T.O., Harmes, K., (2001), German Board of the European Registry for Cystic Fibrosis (ERCF): effect of continuous antistaphylococcal therapy on the rate of *P. aeruginosa* acquisition in patients with cystic fibrosis. Pediatr. Pulmonol. 31:13–16.
60. Stutman, H.R., Lieberman, J.M., Nussbaum, E., Marks, M.I., (2002), Antibiotic prophylaxis in infants and children with cystic fibrosis: a randomized controlled trial. J. Pediatr. 140: 299–305.
61. Valerius, N.H., Koch, C., Hoiby, N., (1991), Prevention of chronic *Pseudomonas aeruginosa* colonization in cystic fibrosis by early treatment. Lancet 338:725–726.
62. Burns, J.L., Gibson, R.L., McNamara, S., Yim, D., Emerson, J., Rosenfeld, M., Hiatt, P., McCoy, K., Castile, R., Smith, A.L., Ramsey, B.W., (2001), Longitudinal assessment of *Pseudomonas aeruginosa* in young children with cystic fibrosis. J. Infect. Dis. 183:444–452.
63. Munck, A., Bonacorsi, S., Mariani-Kurkdijian, P., Lebourgeois, M., Gérardin, M., Brahimi, N., Navarro, J., Bingen, E., (2001), Genotype characterization of *Pseudomonas aeruginosa* strains recovered from patients with cystic fibrosis after initial and subsequent colonization. Pediatr. Pulmonol. 32:288–292.
64. Gibson, R.L., Emerson, J., McNamara, S., Burns, J.L., Rosenfeld, M., Yunker, A., Hamblett, N., Accurso, F., Dovey, M., Hiatt, P., Korstan, M.W., Moss, R., Retsch-Bogert, G, Wagener, J., Waltz, D., Wilmott, R., Zeitlin, P.I., Ramsey, B,: Cystic Fibrosis Therapeutic Development Network Study Group, (2003), Significant microbiological effect of inhaled tobramycin in young children with cystic fibrosis. Am. J. Respir. Crit. Care Med. 167:841–849.
65. Frederiksen, H.K., Norregaard, L., Gotzche, P.C., Pressler, T., Koch, C., Hoiby, N., (1999), Changing epidemiology of *Pseudomonas aeruginosa* infection in Danish cystic fibrosis patients (1974–1995). Pediatr Pulmonol. 28:159–166.
66. Johansen, H.K., Norregaard, L., Gotzche, P.C., Presster, T., Koch, C., Hoiby, N., (2004), Antibody response to *Pseudomonas aeruginosa* in cystic fibrosis patients: a marker of therapeutic success? A 30year cohort study of survival in Danish CF patients after onset of chronic *P. aeruginosa* lung infection. Pediatr. Pumonol. 37:427–432.
67. Hoiby, N., Frederiksen, B., Pressler, T., (2005), Eradication of early *Pseudomonas aeruginosa* infection. J. Cyst. Fibrosis. 4 (Suppl. 2):49–54.

68. Armstrong, D.S., Grimwood, K., Carlin, J.B., Carzino, R., Gutierrez, J.P., Hull, J., Olinsky, A., Phelan, E.M., Robertson, C.F., Phelan, P.D., (1997), Lower airway inflammation in infants and young children with cystic fibrosis. Am. J. Respir. Crit. Care. 156:1197–11204.
69. Chiron-Corporation. Chiron Announces Launch of ELITE Trial. Accessed at http: 11phx. corporate-ir/phoenix:zhtml?C=105850&p=irol-news Article & ID=552967&highlight=on18October2005.
70. Early *Pseudomonas* Infection Control (EPIC) Trial. National Heart, Lung and Blood Institute (NHLBI). Accessed at www.clinicaltrials.gov./ct/gui/show/NCT00097773.
71. Illowite, J.S., Gorvoy, J.D., Smaldowe, G.C., (1987), Quantitative deposition of aerolized gentamicin in cystic fibrosis. Am. Rev. Respir. Dis. 136:1445–1449.
72. Geller, D.E., Pitlick, W.H., Nardella, P.A., Tracewell, W.G., Ramsey, B.W., (2002), Pharmacokinetics and bioavailability of aerosolized tobramycin in cystic fibrosis. Chest 122: 219–226.
73. Ramsey, B.W., Pepe, M.S., Quan, J.M., Otto, K.L., Montgomery, A.B., Williams-Warren, J., Vansiljev, K.M., Borowitz, D., Bowman, C.M., Marshall, B.C., Marshall, S., Smith, A.L., (1999), Intermittent administration of inhaled tobramycin in patients with cystic fibrosis. Cystic Fibrosis Inhaled Tobramycin Study Group. N. Engl. J. Med. 340:23–30.
74. Moss, R.B., (2001), Administration of aerolized antibiotic in cystic fibrosis patients. Chest 120(Suppl. 3):107S–113S.
75. Cystic Fibrosis Foundation Patient Registry, (2002), 2001 Annual Data Report to the Center Directors. Cystic Fibrosis Foundation, Bethesda, MD.
76. Cystic Fibrosis Foundation Patient Registry, (2005), 2004 Annual Data Report to the Center Directors. Cystic Fibrosis Foundation, Bethesda, MD.
77. Littlewood, J.M., Mitter, M.G., Ghoneim, A.T., Ramsden, C.H., (1985), Nebulized colomycin for early *Pseudomonas* colonization in cystic fibrosis. Lancet 1:865.
78. Hodson, M.E., Gallagher, C.G., Govan, J.R., (2002), A randomized trial of nebulized tobramycin or colistin in cystic fibrosis. Eur. Respir. J. 20:658–664.
79. Cunningham, S., Prasad, A., Collyer, L., Carr, S., Lynn, I.B., Wallis, C., (2001), Bronchoconstriction following nebulized colistin in cystic fibrosis. Arch. Dis. Child. 84:432–433.
80. Fernandez, J.D., Santiago, R.T., Matacon, M.P., Mayo, R.C., Sańchez, G.T., (1994), Inhaled aztreonam therapy in patients with cystic fibrosis colonized with *Pseudomonas aeruginosa*. An. Esp. Pediatr. 40:185–188.
81. Cystic Fibrosis Foundation Clinical Trials & Studies, (2006), Anti-Infection therapies. Cystic Fibrosis Foundation, Besthesda, MD, http://www.cff.org/research/clinical-trials/ongoing-trials/anti-infection/#IV_VS/Inhaled-Antibiotics.
82. Reed, M.D., Stern, R.C., Myers, C.M., Yamashita, T.S., Blumer, J.L., (1988), Lack of unique ciprofloxacin pharmacokinetic characteristics in patients with cystic fibrosis. J. Clin. Pharmacol. 28:691–699.
83. Ball, P., (1990), Emergent resistance to ciprofloxacin amongst *Pseudomonas aeruginosa* and *Staphylococcus aureus*: clinical significance and therapeutic approaches. J. Antimicrob. Chemother 26(Suppl. F):165–179.
84. Chysky, V., Kapila, K., Hullman, R., Arcieri, G., Schacht, P., Echols, R., (1991), Safety of ciprofloxacin in children: worldwide clinical experience based on compassionate use: emphasis on joint evaluation. Infections 19:289–296.
85. Jaffe, A., Bush, A., (2001), Antiinflammatory effects of macrolides in lung disease. Pediatr. Pulmonol. 31:464–473.
86. Tateda, K., Ishii, Y., Matsumoto, T., Furuya, N., Nagasluma, M., Matsunaga, T., Ohno, A., Miyazaki, S., Yomaguchi, K., (1996), Direct evidence for antipseudomonal activity of macrolides: exposure-dependent bactericidal activity and inhibition of protein synthesis by erythromycin, clarithromycin, and azithromycin. Antimicrob. Agents Chemother. 40: 2271–2275.
87. Wozniak, D.J., Keyser, R., (2004), Effects of subinhibitory concentration of macrolide antibiotics on *Pseudomonas aeruginosa*. Chest 125(Suppl. 2):62S–69S.

# References

88. Labro, M.T., (1998), Antiinflammatory effects of macrolides: a new therapeutic potential? J. Antimicrob. Chemother. 41:37–46.
89. Equi, A., Balfour-Lynn, I.M., Bush, A., Rosenthal, M., (2002), Long term azithromycin in children with cystic fibrosis: a randomized, placebo-controlled crossover trial. Lancet 360:978–984.
90. Wolter, J., Seeney, S, Bell, S., Bowler, S., Masel, P., McCormach, J., (2002), Effect of long term treatment with azithromycin on disease parameters in cystic fibrosis: a randomized trial. Thorax 57:212–216.
91. Saiman, L., Marshall, B.C., Mayer-Hamblatt, N., Burns, J.L., Quittner, A.L., Cibene, D.A., Coquillette, S., Fieberg, A.Y., Accurso, F.J., Campbell, P.W.3rd, (2003), The Macrolide Study Group: a multicenter, randomized, placebo controlled, double-blind trial of azithromycin in patients with cystic fibrosis chronically infected with *Pseudomonas aeruginosa*. JAMA 290:1749–1756.
92. Elphick, H.E., Tan, A., (2006), Single versus combination therapy for people with cystic fibrosis. Cochrane Database of Systematic Reviews; accessed at: 00075320–100000000–01458.
93. Aaron, S.D., Vandemheen, K.L., Ferris, W., Fergusson, D., Tullis, E., Haase, D., Berthiaume, Y., Brown, N., Wilcox, P., Yizghatlion, V., Bye, P., Bell, S., Chan, F., Rose, B., Jeanneret, A., Stephenson, A., Noseworthy, M., Freitag, A., Paterson, N., Doucette, S., Harbour, C., Ruel, M., MacDonald, N., (2005), Combination antibiotic susceptibility testing to treat exacerbation of cystic fibrosis associated with multiresistant bacteria: a randomized, double-blind controlled trial. Lancet 366:463–471.
94. Etherington, C., Hall, M., Conway, S., Peckham, D., Denton, M., (2008), Clinical impact of reducing routine susceptibility testing in chronic *Pseudomonas aeruginosa* infections in cystic fibrosis. J. Antimicrob. Chemother. 61:425–427.
95. Lechtzin, N., John, M., Irizarry, R., Merlo, C., Diette, G.B., Boyle, M.P., (2006), Outcomes of adults with cystic fibrosis infected with antibiotic-resistant *Pseudomonas aeruginosa*. Respiration 73:27–33.
96. Burkhardt, O., Lehmann, C., Madabushi, R., Kumar, V., Derendorf, H., Welte, T., (2006), Once-daily tobramycin in cystic fibrosis: better for clinical outcome than thrice daily but more resistance development. J. Antimicrob. Chemother. 58:822–829.
97. Lewin, C., Doherty, C., Gowan, J., (1993), Invitro activities of meropenem, PD127391, PD131628, ceftazidime, chloramphenical, co-trimoxazole, and ciprofloxacin against *Pseudomonas cepacia*. Antimicrob. Agents. Chemother. 37:123–125.
98. Burns, J., Saiman, L., (1999), *Burkholderia cepacia* infection in cystic fibrosis. Pediatr. Infect. Dis. J. 18:123–125.
99. Vartivarian, S., Anaissie, E., Bodey, G., Spingg, H., Rolston, K., (1994), A changing pattern of susceptibility of *Xanthomonas maltophilia* to antimicrobial agents; implications for therapy. Antimicrob. Agents Chemother. 38:624–627.
100. Saiman, L., Chen, Y., Tabibi, S., San Gabriel, P., Zhou, J., Liu, Z., Lai, L., Whittier, S., (2001), Identification and antimicrobial susceptibility of *Alcaligenes xylosoxidans* isolated from patients with cystic fibrosis. J. Clin. Microbiol 39:3942–3945.
101. Maiz-Carro, L., Navas-Elorza, E., (2002), Nontubercilous mycobacterial pulmonary infection in patients with cystic fibrosis. Am. J. Resp. Med. 1:107–117.
102. Petrini, B, (2006), *Mycobacterium abscessus*: an emerging-rapid-growing potential pathogen. APMIS 114:319–328.
103. Langford, D.T., Hiller, J., (1984), Prospective, controlled study of a polyvalent *Pseudomonas* vaccine in cystic fibrosis: three year results. Arch. Dis. Child 59:1131–1134.
104. Lang, A.B., Schaad, U.B., Rudeberg, A., Wedgwood, J., Que J.U., Furer, E., Cryz, S.J., Jr., (1995), Effect of high-affinity anti-*Pseudomonas aeruginosa* lypopolysaccharide antibodies

induced by immunization on the rate of *Pseudomonas aeruginosa* infection in patients with cystic fibrosis. J. Pediatr. 127:711–717.
105. Doring G, Dorner, F., (1997), A multicenter vaccine trial using the *Pseudomonas aeruginosa* flagella vaccine immunization in patients with cystic fibrosis. Behring Inst. Mitteilungen 98:338–344.
106. Wark, P.A.B., McDonald, V., Jones, A.P., (2006), Nebulized hypertonic saline for cystic fibrosis. Cochrane Database of Systematic Review. Access: 00075320–100000000–00452.
107. Donaldson, S.H., Bennett, W.D., Zeman, K.L., Knowles, M.R., Tarran, R., Boucher, R.C., (2006), Mucus clearance and lung function in cystic fibrosis with hypertonic saline. N. Engl. J. Med. 354:241–250.
108. Elkins, M.R., Robinson, M., Rose, B.R., Harbour, C., Moriarty, C.P., Marks, G.B., Belousova, E.G., Xuan, W., Bye, P.T.P, for the National Hypertonic Saline in Cystic Fibrosis (NHSCF) Study Group, (2006), A controlled trial of long-term inhaled hypertonic saline in patients with cystic fibrosis N. Engl. J. Med. 354:229–240.
109. Ratjen, F., (2006), Restoring airway surface liquid in cystic fibrosis. (Editorial), N. Engl. J. Med. 354:291–293.
110. Fuchs H.J., Borowitz, D.S., Christiansen, D.H., Morris, E.M., Nash, M.L., Ramsey, B.W., Rosenstein, B.J., Smith, A.L., Wohl, M.E., (1994), The Pulmozyme Study Group: Effect of aerolized recombinant human DNASE on exacerbations of respiratory symptoms and pulmonary function in patients with cystic fibrosis. N. Engl. J. Med. 331:637–642.
111. Quan, J.M., Tiddens, H.A., Sy, J.P., McKenzie, S.G., Montgomery, M.D., Robinson, P.J., Wohl, M.E., Konstan, M.-W., (2001), The Pulmozyme Early Intervention Trial Study Group: a two year randomized, placebo-controlled trail of dornase alfa in young patients with cystic fibrosis with mild lung function abnormalities. J. Pediatr. 139:813–820.
112. Jones, A.P., Wallis, C.E., Kearney, C.E., Kearney, C.E., (2006), Recombinant human deoxyribonuclease for cystic fibrosis. Cochrane Database of Systematic Reviews. Access no: 00075320–100000000–00909.
113. Suri, R., Metcalf, C., Lees, B., Grieve, R., Flather, M., Normand, C., Thompson, S., Bush, A., Wallis, C., (2001), Comparison of hypertonic saline and alternate-day or daily recombinant human deoxy-ribonuclease in children with cystic fibrosis: a randomized trial. Lancet 358:1316–1321.
114. Korstan, M.W., Davis, P.B., (2002), Pharmacological approaches for discovery and development of new anti-inflammatory agents for the treatment of cystic fibrosis. Adv. Drug Deliv. Rev. 54:1409–1423.
115. Lands, L.C., Desateux, C., Crighton, A., (2006), Oral non-steroidal anti-inflammatory drug therapy for cystic fibrosis. Cochrane Database Systematic Reviews. Access no: 00075320–100000000–003494.
116. Rich, D.P., Anderson, M.P., Gregory, R.J., Chery, S.H., Paul, S., Jefferson, D.M., McCann, J. D., Klirger, K.W., Smith, A.E., Welsh, M.J., (1990), Expression of cystic fibrosis transmembrane conductance regulator corrects defective chloride channel regulation in cystic fibrosis airway epithelial cells. Nature 347:358–363.
117. Cystic Fibrisis Foundation, (2004), Annual Report: Research. Cystic Fibrosis Foundation, Bethesda, MD access: no:http://www.cff.org/uploadedfiles/publications/files/2004AnnualReportFinal.pdf.
118. Borghouthi, S., Guerdoud, L.M., Speert, D.P., (1996), Inhibition by dextran of *Pseudomonas aeruginosa* adherence to epithelial cells: Am. J. Respir. Crit. Care Med. 154:1788–1793.
119. Chiu, C.H., Wong, S., Hancock, R.E., Speert, D.P., (2001), Adherence of *Burkholderia cepacia* to respiratory tract epithelial cells and inhibition with dextrans. Microbiol. 147:2651–2658.
120. Bryan, R., Feldman, M., Jawetz, S.C., Rajan, S., DiMargo Tang, H.B., Scheffler, L., Speert, D.P., Prince, A., (1999), The effects of aerolized dextran in a mouse model of *Pseudomonas aeruginosa* pulmonary infection. J. Infect. Dis. 179:1449–1458.

# References

121. Feng, W., Garrett, H., Speert, D.P., King, M., (1998), Improved clearability of cystic fibrosis sputum with dextran treatment in vitro. Am. J. Respir. Care Med. 184:29–32.
122. Cole, A.M., Liao, H., Stuchlik, O., Tilan, J., Pohl, J., Ganz, T., (2002), Cationic polypeptide are required for antibacterial activity of human airway fluid. J. Immunol. 169:6985–6991.
123. Goldman, M.J., Anderson, G.M., Stolzenberg, E.D., Kari, U.P., Zasloff, M., Wilson, J.M., (1997), Human beta-defensin-1 is a salt-sensitive antibiotic that is inactivated in cystic fibrosis. Cell 88:553–560.
124. Ramsey, B, Rodman, D., Redman, R., Haeslsen, M., Johnson, C., Hamblett, N., Fugii, C., Loury, D., (2001), Phase I safety and tolerability study of ascending multiple doses of aerolized isegaran HCL solution (1B-367) in adults with cystic fibrosis. Pediatr. Pulmonol. 32:A263.
125. Ganz, T., (2001), Fatal attraction evaded: how pathogenic bacteria resist cationic polypeptides. J. Exp. Med. 193:F31–F34.
126. Hoffman, N., Lee, B., Rasmussen, T.B., Song, Z., Johansen, H.K., Givskow, M., Hoiby, N., (2007), Azithromycin block quorum sensing and alginate polymer formation and increases sensitivity to serum and stationary-growth-phase killing of *Pseudomonas aeruginosa* and attenuates chronic *P. aeruginosa lung* infection in CFTR(-/-) mice. Antimicrob. Agents Chemother. 51:3677–3687.
127. Overhage, J., Campisano, A., Bains, M., Torfs, ECW, Rehm, BHA, Hancock, REW, (2008), Human host defense peptide LL-37 prevents bacterial biofilm formation. Infect. Immun. 76:4176–4182.
128. van der Plas, M.J., Jukema, G.N., Wai, S.W., Dogterom-Ballering, H.C., Lagendijk, E.L., van Gulpen, C., van Dissel, J.T., Bloemberg, G.V., Nibbesring, P.H., (2008), Maggot excretions/secretions are differentially effective against biofilms of *Staphylococcus aureus* and *Pseudomonas aeruginosa*. J. Antimicrob. Chemother. 61:117–122.

# Chapter 5
# Re-Emergence of Childhood Respiratory Infections in Adults (RSV & Pertussis)

## A: Respiratory Syncytial Virus infection in Adults

## 5.1 Introduction

Respiratory syncytial virus (RSV) is a major cause of lower respiratory tract illness in young children, responsible for significant yearly morbidity and life-threatening infections in the first 2 years of life. It is a major cause of outbreaks of tracheobronchitis, bronchiolitis, and pneumonia in young children in the winter and spring. Nearly 100% of children worldwide will be infected with RSV by 3 years of age and 95% will have antibodies by 2 years.[1] However, immunity is incomplete and short lived and recurrent infection is common. Although the attack rates are most common in infants, between 38% and 47% of older children and adults in families acquire RSV infection after exposure[2] Although RSV infection in adults has been recognized for decades its importance has been overlooked until more recently.

## 5.2 Microbiology and Pathogenesis

RSV is an enveloped single strand, negative-sense RNA virus of the Paramyxoviridae family. It belongs to the fourth genus of the Pneumoviridae subfamily. Within this genus are the pneumonia virus of mice, bovine RSV, ovine RSV, caprine RSV, and turkey rhinotracheitis virus. RSV isolates can be divided into two major groups, A & B and into subtypes within each group.[3] The antigenic relatedness of the two strain groups is about 25%.[4] In outbreaks of RSV, strains of both groups can circulate simultaneously, but the relative proportion of the strains can vary.[5,6]

The infectivity and pathogenicity of the virus are associated with two glycosylated surface proteins, the F and G proteins.[1] The F protein is structurally similar to the fusion protein of the paramyxoviruses with two disulfide-linked fragments (F1 and F2). The fusion (F) protein initiates viral penetration by fusing viral and cellular membranes, promoting viral spread and fusion of infected to adjacent uninfected cells to form the characteristic syncytia. The co-expression of three surface glycoproteins F, G, and SH is necessary for efficient fusion. The G protein appears to mediate attachment of the virus to the host cells. The incubation period of RSV infection ranges from 2 to 8 days and the virus is inoculated through the nose or eyes, and less commonly the mouth. The infection is usually confined to the respiratory tract from the upper airway to the entire lower respiratory tract. The characteristic feature of RSV infection is development of bronchitis and bronchiolitis with edema of the mucosa of the respiratory tract associated with narrowing of the airway and obstruction from mucus secretion and sloughed epithelium. The result is airway obstruction with wheezing, areas of hyperinflation, and segments of atelectasis. Lymphocytic peribronchial infiltration and edema of the bronchiolar walls, and interstitial mononuclear infiltration with areas of edema and necrosis can be seen in the lung alveoli (respiratory pneumonia) on histology.

The exact pathogenesis of RSV infection is unclear and may represent immunologic mechanisms, as most infants with severe disease have circulating maternally derived antibodies at the time. Furthermore, previous trials of a formalin-inactivated RSV vaccine found immunized infants were not protected from disease and some developed exaggerated illness with severe lower respiratory tract disease.[7] However, several studies have demonstrated that high levels of maternal antibodies correlate with lower rates of infections and less severe disease.[1,8] Moreover, the trials of hyperimmune RSV globulin in young children showed high antibody levels protected against more severe disease.[9,10] Studies in B-cell depleted mice indicate that antibodies protect against severe illness and reinfections but are not required for clearance of primary RSV infections.[11]

RSV infection in children induce virus specific IgE homocytotropic antibodies in the respiratory tract, with mast cell stimulation and increased concentration of histamine and inflammatory mediators, including increased levels of leukotrienes and eosinophil cationic protein.[12,13] This cascade of events leads to enhanced inflammation and edema to the lower bronchi/bronchioles resulting in bronchospasm and wheezing. There is good evidence from clinical studies in children and experimental models with RSV that early respiratory infections may contribute to early sensitizations to other antigens in a child genetically prone to develop asthma.[13]

### 5.2.1 *Immunity*

Primary RSV infection induces IgM response in 5–10 days, with lower levels less than 6 months old, persisting for 1–3 months, and occasionally for a year.[14] RSV-specific IgG antibody appears soon after IgM response and reaches maximum levels 20–30 days after onset of symptoms (mainly IgG1 and IgG3 subclasses). Younger infants often have lower antibody response and a year after primary infection IgG levels decline to very low levels,[13] but a booster effect is noted within 5–7 days after reinfection.[15] Free anti-RSV IgA appears within 2–5 days after infection in the respiratory tract and peak titers are present between 8 and 13 days, and serum IgA appears several days later than IgM and IgG responses.

Infection with RSV also induces specific cell-mediated immune responses, including lymphocyte transformation, cytotoxic T-cell enhancement, and antibody-dependent cellular cytotoxic responses.[16] The fact that children and adults with impairment of cellular immunity, as well as experimentally immunosuppressed animals, demonstrate more severe disease and protracted viral shedding, indicate that cell-mediated immunity is important for recovery.[1,17] This could also explain increased prevalence and severe disease in the elderly with waning cell-mediated immunity. In the last decade there has been increased interest in the role of cell-mediated immune responses in the mechanism of immunopathology in the respiratory tract. Th1 and Th2 types of CD4 cells, as well as CD8 cells have been implicated in the immunopathogenesis of RSV and influenza virus infections.[16,17] A balance between the expression of different pro-inflammatory cytokines, chemokines, and the evolvement of Th1 versus Th2 or CD4 versus CD8 responses in RSV infection, may determine the pathology, and degree of protection against respiratory disease.[18]

## 5.2.2 Epidemiology

In young, healthy adults RSV infection is not considered as a cause of respiratory infection, and the importance and manifestations in this population has been little studied. RSV occurs in yearly outbreaks and is highly contagious and repeated infections occur throughout life. In most cases these recurrent infections involve the upper respiratory tract and do not receive a specific diagnosis or differentiated from the "common cold."

A prospective study of 2,960 healthy adults (18–60 years of age) during 1975–1995, was carried out in Rochester (New York) to determine the prevalence and manifestations of RSV infections.[19] Of these subjects, 211 (7%) acquired RSV infection, 199 (94%) were medical personnel or students, and 12 were family members of households with children. The infections were symptomatic in 84% of subjects, with upper respiratory tract symptoms only in 74% and included lower respiratory tract symptoms in 26%. Fever developed in 40% of the subjects and lower respiratory tract signs were present in 26%. Compared to influenza, RSV infections were associated with significantly more nasal congestion, ear, and sinus involvement, and productive cough but less frequent fever and headaches.[19] The mean duration of RSV illness (9.5 days) was significantly longer than that of influenza (6.8 days), but absenteeism from work was greater with influenza (66%) compared to RSV infections (38%).

In another epidemiology study of RSV infection in adults in France, RSV was identified in 20 (11.7%) of 170 influenza-like illness, 13 (4.8%) of 270 cases of non-severe lower respiratory tract illnesses in the community.[20] RSV was the cause of 11 (6.3%) of 164 cases of acute bronchitis, and in 51 acute pneumonias hospitalized with respiratory distress syndrome a virus was identified in 17 (33.3%) with influenza A in 6 and RSV in 3 (5.5%). All the hospitalized RSV-infected patients were older people with chronic pulmonary or cardiac disease.[20]

Surveillance data on emergency hospital admissions among residents of Greater London collected from 1994 to 2001 were reported for the association with RSV and influenza infections.[21] The rate of hospitalization attributable to RSV infection in children aged <1 year was 5 per 1,000 infants per year. The association in people > 65 years old was much lower with an attributable rate of hospitalization of 0.7 per 1,000 population, with influenza being 1.1 per 1,000 population in the same age group.[21] Another recent study evaluated the effect of RSV infections and influenza A in community-dwelling elderly persons and high-risk adults (21 years of age or older with chronic pulmonary disease, congestive heart failure) prospectively over two winters.[22] RSV infection was identified in 102 (8.8%) of 1,148 prospective cohorts and 142 (10.2%) of 1,388 hospitalized patients, and influenza A in 44 patients in the prospective cohorts and 154 hospitalized patients. RSV infection accounted for 10.6% of hospitalization for pneumonia, 11.4% for chronic obstructive pulmonary disease exacerbation, 5.4% for congestive heart failure, and 7.2% for asthma.[22] In the hospitalized cohort, RSV infection and influenza A resulted in similar lengths of stay, rates of use of intensive care (15% and 12%, respectively), and mortality (8% and 7%, respectively).

These studies strongly indicate then RSV is a significant pathogen in the elderly, particularly with coexisting cardiac and pulmonary diseases. However, the exact mechanism of worsening pulmonary function is not clear. Whether it is due primarily to the virus itself or viral–bacterial interaction, with simultaneous or sequential infections is unclear.[23] Future studies will need to analyze for simultaneous viral and bacterial infection.

Nosocomial infection with RSV with outbreaks each year are frequent in pediatric hospitals but also has been recognized in the adult wards or hospitals. Transmission of the virus appears to occur through the staff becoming infected or possibly by the spread of contaminated secretions from infected patients to other patients by the staff.[1] During outbreaks almost 50% of the hospital personnel have acquired RSV infection and visitors sometimes are important in the spread of infection.[1] Elderly institutionalized populations are at particular risk for RSV infection and may result in severe disease, including pneumonia in 5–50% of the cases with respiratory failure and mortality rate of up to 20%.[1]

#### 5.2.2.1 Immunosuppressed Subjects

RSV has been reported to cause severe lung disease in lung transplant[24] and bone marrow transplant recipients,[25] in isolated case reports or case series. Immunocompromised patients who develop pneumonia and subsequent respiratory failure requiring mechanical ventilation have a mortality rate approaching 100%. A prospective study to assess RSV infections after stem cell transplantation (SCT) from

37 European centers was recently reported.[26] The frequency of documented respiratory virus infection was 3.5% among 819 allogeneic and 0.4% among 1,154 autologous SCT patients. The deaths of five (10.6%) allogeneic SCT patients were directly attributed to respiratory virus infection (three RSV; two influenza A). Lymphocytopenia was a significant risk factor for lower respiratory tract RSV infection. The overall mortality in RSV infection was 30.4% and the direct RSV-associated mortality was 17.4%. For influenza A virus infection the corresponding percentages were 23.0% and 15.3%.[26]

In another report from a single center in Britain between 1997 and 2001, 35 episodes of respiratory virus infection were noted in 25 of 83 allogeneic SCT recipients.[27] Parainfluenza virus was the commonest isolate (45.7%) followed by RSV (37%). More than half of the episodes of respiratory virus infection progressed to the lower respiratory tract, but the mortality was low (8%), possibly due to early initiation of antiviral therapy and reduced-intensity conditioning (chemotherapy).[27] A more recent study from a hematology unit in Switzerland (a university referral center for adults) between 2002 and 2007, identified 34 adult immunosuppressed patients with RSV infection.[28] Most of the patients (22 or 65%) had upper respiratory tract infection and 12 (35%) developed lower respiratory infection, 5 of whom required intensive care, and the RSV-attributable mortality was 18% (6 patients). The major risk factors for lower respiratory infection and RSV-attributable mortality was severe immunodeficiency and pre-engraftment. RSV-specific reverse-transcriptase-polymerase chain reaction (RT-PCR) from nasal aspirate or bronchoalveolar lavage was the most rapid and sensitive technique for diagnosis (100% sensitivity), antigen testing (only 40% positive), and viral culture (57% positive after 2–4 days) were less reliable.[28]

## 5.2.3 Management in Adults

The traditional methods of viral culture and serology for confirming the diagnosis of RSV infections are inadequate and time dependent, and thus not useful in the management of patients.

Molecular diagnostics of the respiratory secretions for detecting the virus such as RT-PCR or by direct immunofluorescence staining with monoclonal antibodies are more accurate and provide rapid results.[29] Treatment of RSV infection in the elderly is largely supportive. In infants with lower respiratory tract RSV infection requiring hospitalization, aerolized ribavirin is the only approved specific theory. Ribavirin is a broad-spectrum synthetic antiviral nucleoside that has shown some marginal benefit in infants. The effectiveness of aerolized ribavirin monotherapy in immunocompromised adults is controversial, and reports of effectiveness are conflicting and limited to small case series.[30,31] The most common therapies for RSV infection in immunocompromized patients are aerolized ribavirin and immunoglobulin products. Animal experiments and some uncontrolled studies suggest that the combination of ribavirin and RSV-hyperimmune globulin are more beneficial than monotherapy for immunosuppressed patients.[32–34] However, other studies have not confirmed these findings of improved response with combined therapy versus monotherapy or supportive care.[26,30,35] In most reports ten patients with severe immunodeficiency and lower respiratory tract RSV infection received a combination of oral ribavirin and intravenous immunoglobulin (IVIG, 0.5 g/kg every other day), and seven patients also received palivizumab, with a survival rate of only 50%.[28] Despite the limitations of available data some groups continue to recommend combinations of ribavirin and intravenous polyclonal immunoglobulin for immunosuppressed patients with RSV pneumonia.[36] An important factor in the management of RSV infections in the immunosuppressed is initiation of early therapy, as mortality increases with delay in treatment.[30,34,37]

## 5.2.4 Prevention

The key for effective prevention and control of RSV infection is an effective vaccine, which has eluded investigators and pharmaceutical companies so far. This will be a daunting task for developing an effective vaccine that will provide immunity even greater than natural infection. It is likely, however, that failure of natural infection to provide protection against RSV infection is probably related to the rapid decline in antibodies. The presence of secretory neutralizing antibodies appear to protect against upper respiratory tract infection, and serum-neutralizing antibodies protect against lower respiratory tract RSV infection, and cell-mediated responses appear to terminate infection.[38] Clinical trials with passive immunizations support the feasibility of developing an effective vaccine,[23] but repeated booster doses will likely be required to maintain adequate neutralizing antibodies. Although the World Health Organization has designated RSV as a high-priority pathogen for vaccine development, vaccine-developing companies have declining interest.[39]

Preventative strategies include good infection control practice in both acute and chronic health care facilities to limit nosocomial transmission. RSV may be spread by close or direct contact and by droplet secretions from an infected person. Standard universal precautions with hand washing between patients should be followed by medical personnel. Respiratory isolation with contact precautions with gloves and gowns are recommended. However, most cases of RSV infection will not be recognized early enough on adult wards for these measures to be effective. For prevention of household transmission it has been recommended to include educating parents and family about hand washing, cleaning environmental surfaces, isolating infants and children with infection, and avoiding crowded places such as day-care centers.[40] However, the value of these measures have not been proven or may not be practical. It is reasonable, however, that family members (adults or children) should not have close contacts with the elderly, debilitated, or immunosuppressed subjects for any symptoms of respiratory tract infections, as presentations of RSV infection can be indistinguishable from the "common cold."

Palivizumab, a humanized monoclonal IgG antibody specific for RSV (F glucoprotein) inhibits fusion of the virus to the respiratory epithelium and this neutralizes the virus and prevents establishment of infection. It has been approved and is the standard for the prevention of RSV infection in high-risk infants; however it is untested or unproven for the elderly and immunosuppressed adults. A Phase I study in adult recipients of SCT has recently shown that palivizumab is safe and well tolerated.[41]

### 5.2.5 Future Directions

The main emphasis for future research should be to find and develop an effective vaccine for infants and adults. Recombination technology can be used to create live attenuated RSV vaccines that contain a combination of attenuating vaccines. In a recent study of two live attenuated recombinantly derived RSV candidates, rA2cp 248/404/Delta SH and rAcp248/404/1030 Delta SH, were found to be highly attenuated in adults and RSV-seropositive children, and were well tolerated and immunogenic in RSV-seronegative children.[42] Additional studies are needed to determine whether the vaccines can induce protective immunity against wild type RSV. Another recombinant RSV subunit vaccine (BBG2Na) was previously shown to be well tolerated and highly immunogenic in RSV-seropositive young adults.[43] A further Phase II clinical trial with this vaccine was reported to induce protective antibodies in subjects over 60 years of age; and passive transfer of serum from these subjects protected SCID mouse lungs against RSV challenge.[44]

There is also a need for more efficacious RSV antiviral agents as the current treatment is not very effective. A greater understanding of the viral fusion process and the RSV genomics may lead to development of better agents than ribavirin such as $2'-5'$ oligoadenylate antisense (2–5 A – Antisense) compound.[45]

To prove the value of ribavirin alone or with RSV-hyperimmune globulin in the immunosuppressed patients will be a daunting task. A recent attempt by NIAID collaborative group to determine the value of early administration of ribavirin in hematopoietic cell transplant recipients with upper respiratory infection failed to recruit sufficient number of subjects after 5 years.[46] Future design should involve an international collaborative effort to obtain adequate sample size.

## References for A

1. Hall, C.B., McCarthy, C.A., (2000), Respiratory Syncytial Virus, in: Principles and Practice of Infectious Diseases, 5th Edition, Mandell, G.L., Bennett, J.E., Dolin, R., (eds). Churchill Livingstone, Philadelphia, pp. 1782–1801.
2. Hall, C.B., Geiman, J.M., Biggar, R., Kotok, D.I., Hogan, P.M., Douglas, G.R. Jr., (1976), Respiratory syncytial virus infection within families. N. Engl. J. Med. 294:414–419.

3. Mufson, M.A., Orvell, C., Rafnar, B., Norrby, E., (1985) Two distinct subtypes of human respiratory syncytial virus. J. Gen. Virol 66: 2111–2124.
4. Walsh, E.E., Brandriss, M.W., Schlesinger, J.J., (1987), Immunological differences between the envelope glycoproteins of two strains of human respiratory syncytial virus. J. Gen. Virol. 68: 2169–2176.
5. Hendry, R.M., Talis, A.L., Godfrey, E., Anderson, L.J., Fernie, B.F., McIntosh, K., (1986), Concurrent circulation of antigenically distinct strains of respiratory syncytial virus during community outbreaks. J. Infect. Dis. 153: 291–297.
6. Hall, C.B., Walsh, E.E., Schnabel, K.C., Long, C.E., McConnochie, K.M., Hildreth, S.W., Anderson, L.J., (1990), Occurrence of groups A and B of respiratory syncytial virus over 15 years; associated epidemiological and clinical characteristics in hospitalized and ambulatory children. J. Infect. Dis. 162: 1283–1290.
7. Kim, H.W., Canchola, J.G., Brandt, C.D., Pyles, G., Chanock, R.M., Jensen, K., Parrott, R.H., (1969), Respiratory syncytial virus disease in infants despite prior administration of antigenic inactivated vaccine. Am. J. Epidemiol. 89: 422–434.
8. Lamprecht, C.L., Krause, H.E., Mufson, M.A., (1976), Role of maternal antibody in pneumonia and bronchiolitis due to respiratory syncytial virus. J. Infect. Dis. 134: 211–217.
9. Groothuis, J.R., Simoes, E., Levin, M.J., Hall, C.B., Long, C.E., Rodriguez, W.J., Arrobio, J., Meissner, H.C., Fulton, D.R., Wellive, B.C., Tristram, D.A., Siber, G.R., Prince, G.A., VanRaden, M., Hemming, V.A., for The Respiratory Syncytial Virus Immunoglobulin Study Group, (1993), Prophylactic administration of respiratory syncytial virus immune globulin to high-risk infants and young children. The RSVIG Study Group, N. Engl. J. Med. 329:1524–1530.
10. The Prevent Study Group, (1977), Reduction of respiratory syncytial virus hospitalization among premature infants and infants with bronchopulmonary dysplasia using respiratory syncytial virus immune globulin prophylaxis. Pediatrics 99: 93–99.
11. Graham, B.S., Bunton, L.A., Rowland, J., Wright, P.F., Karzon, D.T., (1991), Respiratory syncytial virus infection in anti -µ treated mice. J. Virol. 65: 4936–4942.
12. Welliver, R.C., Wong, D.T., Sun, M., Middleton, E,J.R., Vaugh, R.S., Ogra, P.L., (1981), The development of respiratory syncytial virus-specific IgE and the release of histamine in nasopharyngeal secretions after infections; N. Engl, J.Med. 305: 841–846.
13. Ogra, P.L., (2004), Respiratory syncytial virus: The virus, the disease and the immune response. Pediatr. Resp. Rev. 5 (Suppl A): S119–S126.
14. Ruuskanen, O., Ogra, P.L., (1993), Respiratory syncytial virus. Curr. Probl. Pediatr. 23: 50–79.
15. Welliver, R.C., Kaul, T.N., Putnam, T.I., Sun, M., Riddlesberger, K., Ogra, P.L., (1980), The antibody responses to primary and secondary infection with respiratory syncytial virus: Kinetics of class-specific responses. J. Pediatr. 96: 808–813.
16. Kimpen, J.L., Simoes, E.A.F., (2001), Respiratory syncytial virus and reactive airway disease. Am.J. Respir. Crit. Care Med. 163: S1–S6.
17. Englund, J.A., Sullivan, C.J., Jordan, M.C., Dehner, L.P., Vercelloti, G.M., Balfour, H.H. Jr., (1988), Respiratory syncytial virus infection in immunocompromised adults. Ann. Intern. Med. 109: 203–208.
18. Umetsu, D.T., Dekmyff, R.H., (1997), Th1 and Th2 $CD_4$ + cells in the pathogenesis of allergic diseases. Proc. Soc. Exp. Biol. Med. 215: 11–20.
19. Hall, C.B., Long, L.E., Schnabel, K.C., (2001), Respiratory syncytial virus infections in previously healthy working adults. Clin. Infect. Dis. 33: 792–796.
20. Freymuth, F., Vabret, A., Gouarin, S., Pettijean, J., Charlonneu, P., Lehoux, P., Galateau-Salle, F., Tremolieres, F., Canette, M.F., Maynaud, C., Mosnier, A., Burnouf, L., (2004), Epidemiology and diagnosis of respiratory syncytial virus in adults. Revu Malad. Respir. 21: 35–42.
21. Mangtani, P., Hajat, S., Kovats, S., Wilkinson, P., Armstrong, B., (2006). The association of respiratory syncytial virus infection and influenza with emergency admissions for respiratory disease in London: An analysis of routine surveillance data. Clin. Infect. Dis. 42: 640–646.

22. Falsey, A.R., Hennessey, P.A., Formica, M., Cox, C., Walsh, E.E., (2005), Respiratory syncytial virus infection in elderly and high-risk adults. N. Engl. J. Med. 352: 1749–1759.
23. Sethi. S., Murphy, T.F., (2005), RSV infection - not for kids only (Editorial) N. Engl. J. Med. 352: 1810–1812.
24. Flynn, J.D., Akers, W.S., Jones, N., Stevkovic, N., Waid, T., Mullett, T., Jaharia, S., (2004), Treatment of syncytial virus pneumonia in a lung transplant recipient: case report and review of the literature. Pharmacotherapy; 24: 932–938.
25. Khushaloni, N.I., Bakri, F.G., Wentling, D., Brown, K., Mohr, A., Anderson, B., Keesler, C., Ball, D., Bernstein, Z.P., Bernstein, S.H., Czuczman., M.S., Segal, B.H., McCarthy, P.L. Jr., (2001), Respiratory syncytial virus infection in the late bone marrow transplant period; report of three cases and review. Bone Marrow Trans. 27: 1071–1073.
26. Ljungman, P., Ward, K.N., Crooks, B.N., Parker, A., Martino, R., Shaw, P.J., Birch, L., Brune, M., DeLa Camara, R., Dekker, A., Pauksen, K., Russell, N., Schwarer, A.P., Cordonnier, C., (2001), Respiratory virus infections after stem cell transplantation: a prospective study from the Infectious Diseases Working Party of the European Group for Blood and Marrow Transplantation. Bone Marrow Trans. 28: 479–484.
27. Chakrabarti, S., Avivi, I., Mackinnon, S., Ward, K., Kottaridis, P.D., Osman, H., Waldmann, H., Hale, G., Fegan, C.D., Yong, K., Goldstone, A.H., Linch, D.C., Milligan, D.W., (2002), Respiratory virus infections in transplant recipients after reduced – intensity conditioning with Campath - 1H: high incidence but low mortality. Brit. J. Haematol. 119: 1125–1132.
28. Khanna, N., Widmer, A.F., Decker, M., Steffen, I., Halter, J., Heim, D., Weisser, M., Gratwohl, A., Fluckiger, U., Hirsch, H., (2008), Respiratory syncytial virus infection in patients with hematological disease; single-center study and review of the literature. Clin. Infect. Dis. 46: 402–412.
29. Rovida, F., Percivalle, E., Zavattoni, M., Torsellini, M., Sarasini, A., Companini, G., Paolucci, S., Baldanti, F., Revello, M.G., Gerna, G., (2005), Monoclonal antibodies versus reverse transcription - PCR for detection of respiratory viruses in a patient population with respiratory tract infections admitted to hospital. J. Med. Viral, 75: 336–347.
30. Anaissie, E.J., Mahfuoz, T.H., Aslam, T., Pouli, A., DesiKan, R., Fassas, A., Barlogie, B., (2004), The natural history of respiratory syncytial virus infection in cancer and transplant patients: implications for management, Blood 103: 1611–1617.
31. Englund, J.A., Piedra, P.A., Whimbey, E., (1997), Prevention and treatment of respiratory syncytial virus and parainfluenza viruses in immunocompromised patients, Am. J. Med. 102: 61–70.
32. Ottolini, M.G., Porter, D.D., Hemming, V.G., Zimmerman, M.N., Schwab, N.M., Prince, G. A., (1999), Effectiveness of RSV hyperimmune globulin prophylaxis and therapy of respiratory syncytial virus in an immunosuppressed animal model. Bone Marrow Trans. 24: 41–45.
33. DeVincenzo, J.P., Hirsch, R.L., Fuentes, R.J., Top, F.H., Jr. (2002), Respiratory syncytial virus immune globulin treatment of lower respiratory tract infection in pediatric patients undergoing bone marrow transplantation: a compassionate use experience. Bone Marrow Trans. 25: 161 165.
34. Zamora, M.R., Hodges, T., Nicholls, M.R., Astor, T.L., Marquesen, J., Weill, D., (2004), Impact of respiratory syncytial virus pneumonia following lung transplantation: a case controlled study. J. Heart Lung Trans. 23(Suppl 2): S43–S441.
35. Nichols, W.G., Gooley, T., Boeckh, M., (2001), Community- acquired respiratory syncytial virus and parainfluenza virus infections after hematopoietic stem cell transplantation: the Fred Hutchinson Cancer Research Centre experience. Biol. Blood Marrow Trans. 7:115–117.
36. Swedish Consensus Group, (2001), Management of infections caused by respiratory syncytial virus. Scand. J. Infect. Dis. 33: 323–328.
37. Ljungman P., (2002), Prevention and treatment of viral infections in stem cell transplant recipients. Br. J. Haematol. 118: 44–57.
38. Polack, F.P., Kamon, R.A., (2004), The future of respiratory syncytial virus vaccine development. Pediatr. Infect. Dis. J. 23(Suppl): S65–S73.

39. Maggon, K., Barik, S., (2004), New drugs and treatment for respiratory virus. Rev. Med. Virol. 14: 149–168.
40. Jafri, H.S., (2003), Treatment of respiratory syncytial virus: antiviral therapies. Pediatr. Infect. Dis. J. 22: 589–583.
41. Boeckh, M., Berrey, M.M., Bowden, R.A., Crawford, S.W., Balsley, J., Corey, L., (2001), Phase I evaluation of the respiratory syncytial virus-specific monodoral antibody palivizumab in recipients of hematopoietic stem cell transplantation. J. Infect. Dis. 184: 350–354.
42. Kamon, R.A., Wright, P.F., Belshe, R.B., Thumar, B., Casey, R., Newman, F., Polack, F.P., Randolph, V.B., Dently, A., Hackell, T., Gruber, W., Murphy, B.R., Collins, P.L., (2005), Identification of a recombinant live attenuated respiratory syncytial virus vaccine candidate that is highly attenuated in infants. J. Infect. Dis. 191: 1093–1104.
43. Power, U.F., Nguyen, T.N., Rietveld, E., de Swart, R.L., Groen, J., Osterhaus, A.D., deGroot, R., Corvaia, N., Beck, A., Bouveret-Le-Cam, N., Bonnefoy, J.Y., (2001), Safety and immunogenicity of a novel recombinant subunit respiratory syncytial virus vaccine (BBG2Na) in healthy young adults. J. Infect. Dis. 184: 1456–1460.
44. Plotnicky-Gilquin, H., Cyblat-Chanal, D., Goetsch, L., Lacheny, C., Libon, C., Champion, T., Beck, A., Pasche, H., Nguyen, T.N., Bonnefoy, J.Y., Bouveret-Le-Cam, N., Corvaia, N., (2002), Passive transfer of serum antibodies induced by BBG2Na, a subunit vaccine, in the elderly protects SCID mouse lungs against respiratory syncytial virus challenge. Virology 303: 130–137.
45. Torrence, P.F., Powell, L.D., (2002), The quest for an efficacious antiviral for respiratory syncytial virus. Antiviral Chem. Chemother. 13: 325–344.
46. Boeckh, M., Englund, J., Li, Y., Miller, C., Cross, A., Fernandez, H., Kuypers, J., Kim, H., Gnann, J., Whitley, R., NIAD Collaborative Antiviral Study Group, (2007), Randomized controlled multicenter trial of aerolized ribavirin for respiratory syncytial virus upper respiratory tract infection in hematopoietic cell transplant recipients. Clin. Infect. Dis. 44: 235–249.

# Chapter 5B
# Re-Emergence of Childhood Respiratory Infections in Adults (RSV & Pertussis)

## B: Pertussis in Adults

## 5.3 Introduction

Pertussis (whooping cough) remains an uncontrolled infectious disease despite the institution of universal vaccination in children since the early 1940s. In fact in many developed countries in North America and Europe pertussis has been increasing since 1980. In the United States the number of annually reported cases has increased sixfold since 1980, with 11,647 cases reported in 2003, despite vaccination compliance of more than 80% of young children.[1] Pertussis whole-cell vaccine was introduced in Canada in 1943, and the incidence of whooping cough declined by 90% over the subsequent 40 years.[2] However, it has increased again in the early 1990s and has remained high since then. The incidence of whooping cough has also increased in recent years in Norway, especially in older children and adults, and in 2004 it was 168 cases per 100,000 of the population.[3] The reported incidence rates probably underestimate the true burden of the disease because of incomplete reporting and lack of recognition of the illness.[4,5]

Young children with pertussis are more easily diagnosed because of presentations with whooping cough, paroxysmal cough episodes followed by an audible inspiratory whoop and sometimes vomiting. Although most children have a persistent but benign illness, serious sequale may occur in infants such as pneumonia, seizures, encephalopathy, and death. Infants can also present with cough and apneic episodes. Immunized infants, older children, adolescents, and adults do not exhibit whooping cough but may have prolonged cough for several weeks.

**Table 5.1** Species of *Bordettella* genus (Compiled from data obtained from Loeffelholz,[6] Preston,[8] and Preston et al.[34])

|    | Species | Host range | Diseases |
| --- | --- | --- | --- |
| 1. | *B. pertussis* | Humans | Whooping cough |
| 2. | *B. parapertussis* | Humans | Mild whooping cough |
|    |                    | Sheep  |                     |
| 3. | *B. bronchiseptica* | Mammals | Kennel cough (dogs) |
|    |                     |         | Rhinitis (swine)    |
| 4. | *B. avium* | Birds | Rhinotracheitis |
| 5. | *B. trematum* | Humans? | Wound infection, otitis media |
| 6. | *B. holmseii* | Humans? | Septicemia |
| 7. | *B. hinzii* | Humans, domestic fowl | Asymptomatic |
| 8. | *B. petrii* | Environment | Not known |

## 5.3.1 Microbiology and Pathogenesis

*Bordetella pertussis*, a small encapsulated gram-negative coccobacillus, is the cause of whooping cough. There are eight members of the *Bordetella* genus (Table 5.1), and three of the species cause respiratory tract infection in mammals, *B. pertussis*, *B. parapertussis*, and *B. bronchiseptica*. *B. parapertussis* can cause a mild pertussis-like syndrome but clinical illness occurs only in 3–4% of infected persons, compared to 75% in pertussis.[6] *B. bronchiseptica* is rarely isolated from the respiratory tract of humans, mainly after close contact with animals (rabbits, cats, guinea pigs) or in immunosuppressed subjects. These three bordetellae share numerous bacterial components involved in pathogenesis which are similar. The bacterial factors important to the disease process have been characterized (Table 5.2).[7,8] These virulence factors include toxins (pertussis toxin, tracheal cytotoxin, adenylate cyclase), adhesion factors (filamentous hemagglutinin, pertactin, fimbriae), and others.

Humans are the only natural hosts of *B. pertussis* and infection is acquired from infected droplets. The organism has a strong tropism for the ciliated respiratory mucosa, the only site of infection. Attachment and colonization of the respiratory epithelium is followed by proliferation on the surface, ciliostasis, damage to the respiratory epithelium, and induction of inflammatory mediators and mucus into the respiratory tract. Damage to the respiratory epithelium and impairment of normal ciliated mucosal function are the primary outcome of *Bordetella* infection.

Genomic studies suggest that the three respiratory *Bordetella* species recently evolved from a common ancestor with a largely identical core genome.[8] Only 11 genes in *B. pertussis* have been found to be species specific (genes found only in that species and not in the other bordetellae). It was initially thought that pertussis toxin was responsible for much of the pathology in whooping cough, but the fact that *B. parapertussis* does not express the toxin yet causes a similar illness, is against a major role of this toxin. The only difference in clinical profile between the diseases produced by the two bacteria that may be ascribed to pertussis toxin

**Table 5.2** Bacterial components in pathogenesis of disease (Compiled from data obtained from Cotter & Miller,[7] and Preston[8])

| Bacterial components | Function | Acellular vaccine component |
| --- | --- | --- |
| Filamentous hemagglutinin | Moderates adherence (adhesin) | Yes |
| Pertactin | Adhesin | Yes |
| Fimbriae | Adhesin | Yes |
| Pertussis toxin | Catalyze ADP Ribosylation of host G-Proteins. Role in disease unclear | Yes (Inactivated) |
| Adenylate cyclase | Cytotoxin, antiinflammatory effects | No |
| Type III secretion system | Alters host immune function. Important in chronic Infection? | No |
| Dermonecrotic toxin | Adhesin | No |
| Lipopolysaccharide | Proinflammatory activity, resist host defence | No |
| Tracheal cytotoxin | Cytotoxin. Damage respiratory epithelium | No |
| Br KAB system | Resistance to serum-medicated killing | No |
| Bug AS system | Regulator of expressions of most Bordetellae virulence factors | No |

expression is increased lymphocytosis observed in *B. pertussis* infection.[9] *B. parapertussis* besides producing a milder illness only accounts for 5% of the pertussis syndrome or whooping cough.

The recently determined genome of *B. pertussis* makes it possible to apply functional genomics, such as transcriptomics and systemic knock-out mutagenesis. The expression of most *B. pertussis* virulence genes is controlled by the two component system Bvg A/S.[10] The functional genomics approach has uncovered two strongly Bvg A/S activated genes, named hot A and hot B (for "homology of toxin"), the products showing high-sequence similarities to pertussins toxin subunit.[10]

## 5.3.2 *Immunity*

Both infection and vaccine-induced immunity to *B. pertussis* wane in adolescence, thus the population is vulnerable to reinfection and a source of infection to susceptible infants.[8] The reason for the short-lived immunity is unknown. Maternal antibodies do not confer protection to babies, probably because the level is too low. By 4 months of age most infants had no measurable antibody to pertussis toxin or filamentous hemagglutinin.[11]

Infection with *B. pertussis* elicits both IgG and IgA antibody responses to pertussis toxin, filamentous hemagglutinin (FHA), pertactin (PRN), and fimbriae types 2 and 3 (FLM).[12] Primary immunization of children results in IgG antibody response but not IgA response to the same antigens (if present in the vaccine). Surveys of IgA antibody are used as a marker of past infection rather than previous immunization; however, IgA antibody is relatively short lived. In a recent study of the prevalence of antibody to four *B. pertussis* antigens obtained from 1,793 adolescents and adults, only 20% demonstrated IgG antibody to pertussis toxin >6 EU/ml.[13] In contrast 68%, 59%, and 39% had concentrations of IgG >8 EU/ml to FHA, PRN, and FLM, respectively. Some investigators have concluded from analysis of previous data that anti-pertussis toxin protect against typical pertussis, anti-PRN and anti-FLM correlate with protection against typical and mild pertussis while anti-FHA levels showed no correlation to protection.[14] In a recent study from Finland 303 adolescents who were previously immunized 5 years earlier with booster pertussis immunization, or only diphtheria/tetanus booster, had a measurement of cellular and humoral immunity to pertussis toxin, FHA, and PRN.[15] Cell-mediated immunity levels to all three antigens persisted above the prebooster levels measured 5 years earlier. IgG antibodies to the three pertussis vaccine antigen decline overtime, but with the exception of pertussis toxin antibodies, were still higher than the prevaccination levels. The results indicate that the interval between acellular pertussis booster immunization might be extended beyond 5 years.

Although antibodies to some *B. pertussis* antigen seem more strongly linked to protection than others, little is known of the role of cell-mediated immunity.[16] It appears that cell-medicated immunity is essential for recovery from natural infection and in long-term protective immunity.[17] Both naturally acquired and vaccine-induced immunity decline over time but boosting from natural subclinical infection does occur.[16] It has been estimated that the duration of immunity post-infection ranged from 7 to 20 years and post-vaccination from 4 to 12 years.[18] The duration of protection after vaccination varies, however, with vaccine type, age at first vaccination, schedule, and level of exposure. In general whole-cell tends to have higher short- and long-term potency similar to that of one or two component acellular vaccines, but efficacy similar to three or five component acellular vaccines.[16]

## 5.3.3 Epidemiology

It is estimated that there are 20–40 million cases of whooping cough annually worldwide, 90% of which occur in developing countries, with about 200,000 to 300,000 fatalities each year. In the past decade there have been numerous reports of increased pertussis in the immunized population, especially in adolescents and adults. However, the burden of disease or prevalence in adults is difficult to determine. In populations where children are routinely immunized, adolescents and adults are the main source of infection for infants. Reported cases of pertussis only represent a fraction of the infections in the population, because of under-reporting, failure to recognize cases by physicians due to lack of awareness, and

## 5.3 Introduction

low index of suspicion.[19] Insensitive or poorly performed laboratory tests, or lack of availability, also contributes to confirmation and reporting of B. pertussis infection. Unlike most respiratory tract infections in which the incubation period is short and duration of illness brief (1–2 weeks), pertussis can have incubation period of days to weeks (6–21 days) and symptoms of persistent cough for prolonged periods ("cough of 100 days").[1] The organism can be recovered from patients only during the first 3–4 weeks of illness and is difficult to isolate in the previously immunized subjects. Studies of prolonged cough illnesses in adults and adolescents indicate that between 12% and 32% are the result of B. pertussis.[20] Serological surveys of adults using IgA antibody suggest that infections in the United States and Germany (where pertussis has been endemic) are of similar frequency. In recent years, almost one half of the reported cases of pertussis were in persons >10 years of age, with the greatest increase between 10 and 19 years of age. It has been estimated that about 1 or 2 in 1,000 adolescents and adults develop pertussis each year, and >12% of persons with acute cough illness of at least 1–2 weeks duration have evidence of pertussis infection.[21] Several studies have suggested that mothers, in particular, are a significant source of infection for infants.[22] Adolescents, grand parents, and health care workers can also play a role. Most adolescents acquire the infection from schoolmates and friends, whereas the main source for adults are children and work colleagues.[22]

In recent years outbreaks of pertussis have been reported in several states of the United States, some of which involved health care workers. In New York State in 1998 and 1999, more than 600 cases of pertussis were confirmed by a single private laboratory.[23] In Texas in 2005, more than 2,000 cases of pertussis were reported and nine patients died, eight of them infants.[24] In 2003, more than 1,900 cases of pertussis were reported in Wisconsin, mainly among adults and adolescents.[25] In Lebanon, New Hampshire more than 4,500 hospital employees were vaccinated with the acellular pertussis vaccine in response to cases of pertussis among health care workers in the spring of 2006.[24] Pertussis has seasonal annual peaks and a 2–5 yearly epidemic cycles. These epidemic cycles continue despite vaccination but widespread vaccination result in increase in interepidemic period and mean age of infection.[16]

After the introduction of whole-cell pertussis vaccine in North America in the 1940s, whooping cough incidence drastically declined and reached the lowest level in the 1980s. There was frequent local and systemic reactions to the vaccine, mostly mild in nature (fever, irritability, erythema, swelling or tenderness at the injection site), but occasionally more severe reactions would occur (febrile seizures, hypotonic-hyporesponsive episodes). In the 1990s a less reactogenic acellular vaccine replaced the whole-cell vaccine and rates of adverse reaction declined, but since then the incidence of pertussis has continued to increase in the United States and Canada. Rises in Canada have been linked to use of a poorly effective vaccine[26] and in the Netherlands partly to the emergence of non-vaccine variants.[27]

The shift in epidemiology of pertussis is likely multifactorial.[24] Immunity after vaccination is short lived, after whole-cell pertussis vaccination there is decrease in immunity after 3–5 years, with no protective immunity by 10–12 years. The acellular pertussis vaccine-induced immunity also appears to decline in a similar time span,[24] in view of the increase in outbreaks, since the widespread use of this vaccine suggest less protective immune response than with the whole-cell vaccine. However, the apparent increase may be partly attributed to increased recognition and reporting of pertussis in adolescents and adults. The immunity after natural pertussis is not sustained or lifelong, and apparent control of infection in the community may be related to continued circulation of the bacteria with subclinical and mild infection with subsequent immune boosting.[24] False positive test results because of contamination in the laboratory (particularly problematic with in-house PCR) may result in pseudo-outbreaks and apparent increase in pertussis reporting. For instance, the "outbreak" in New York State in 1998 to 1999 was the result of positive PCR from a single laboratory and did not correlate with pertussis-like clinical illness.[23]

### *5.3.4 Diagnosis and Management*

The average incubation period of pertussis is 6–10 days, and begins with a catarrhal phase for 1–2 weeks, during which patients are most contagious and indistinguishable from mild viral upper respiratory tract infection. The cough increases in severity as the catarrhal stage progresses. The subsequent paroxysmal phase, which lasts 3–6 weeks, is characterized by spells of coughing with the characteristic whooping, vomiting, cyanosis, and apnea in children. The symptoms gradually decrease in severity in the convalescent phase, which can last up to several months. Adolescents and adults usually experience a milder form of the three typical stages of pertussis (without the whooping, cyanosis, and apnea), but can present with protracted cough.[28] Most (80%) of adolescents and adults with pertussis have a cough lasting >21 days, and many (27%) are still coughing at 90 days after onset. Immunized children also may present with only coughing lasting a medium of 3 weeks, and only 6% of vaccinated children had the classic whoop.[29]

The laboratory methods of diagnosis of pertussis includes collection of posterior nasopharyngeal secretion for culture on selective media or polymerase chain reaction (PCR) methods for rapid diagnosis or serological methods using acute and convalescent sera for > fourfold rise in titers. The sensitivity of cultures is greatest in the early phase of infection and the positive predictive value approaches 100% in severe cases of unvaccinated children and infants during the first 2 weeks.[29] The sensitivity of cultures decreases with duration of illness, previous antibiotic therapy, and vaccination. The sensitivity of culture can be as low as 15–45% when symptoms are less than 3 weeks, falling to 0% by 3 weeks and after.[16] Serology is not useful for early diagnosis and more valuable for epidemiological or prevalence surveys. PCR methods are most reliable for early rapid diagnosis even when the organism is no longer culturable. In a recent French study of 217 adults with persistent cough, 70 had confirmed laboratory diagnosis by any of three methods, culture was only positive in one case compared to 36 by PCR.[30] However, the sensitivity of PCR decreases with the duration of symptoms, varies on the primers used, and false positive results can occur from cross contamination, especially in an inexperienced laboratory. A commercial test approved by the US FDA is not yet available, thus results might vary from laboratory to laboratory. Use of the insertion sequence IS 481 target for PCR can result in false positives produced by *B. bronchoseptica* and *B. holmessii*, which possess similar sequences.[30]

Diagnosis by means of serological testing may be difficult in vaccinated or adult patients. Only humoral responses to pertussis toxin have been shown to be consistent among vaccinated and unvaccinated patients.[28] However, the antibody response to pertussis toxin is variable in magnitude and duration between individuals. Although a single serum IgG antipertussis toxin antibody level above 100–125 EU/ml has been considered a reasonable threshold for diagnosis,[32] the usefulness of this late in the clinical course of the disease is of limited value.

Treatment with antibiotics for pertussis can limit the severity of illness and eradicate the bacteria only if started in the catarrhal phase. Treatment can be initiated with a macrolide, for 5 days (azithromycin) to 7 days (erythromycin and clarithromycin) with about equal efficacy for proven pertussis in the first 1–2 weeks of illness. Erythromycin is less tolerated and compliance-poor but newer macrolides are more expensive. For intolerance or rare macrolide allergies or resistance, trimethoprim-sulfamethoxazole can be used.[28] Starting antimicrobials after 7 days of symptoms is likely not effective in clinical outcome. The management of adolescents and adults with prolonged persistent cough is mainly supportive and symptomatic. Although various modalities to suppress paroxysmal cough has been used such corticosteroids, salbutamol, antihistamines and even pertussis-specific immunoglobulin there is no proof of their efficacy.[33] However, the most effective nonspecific antitussive therapy are opioids (codiene) and dextromethorphan, which act centrally on the brainstem but also have a placebo affect.[34]

### 5.3.5 *Prevention*

The mainstay of control of pertussis in children and adults is vaccination and revaccination. Although routine vaccination of infants and children for pertussis has been standard practice for many years in developed countries, pertussis is on the rise again. Whole-cell vaccines of killed organisms were introduced in the 1940s and are highly effective, but associated with frequent local and systemic reactions. A s-component acellular pertussis vaccine became available in the 1990s, and has largely replaced the whole-cell vaccine in the United States and other countries, because of the lower incidence of adverse reaction. This acellular vaccine may also be more effective than the whole-cell vaccine, three doses prevented 85% of cases over a 2-year period versus <60% for the whole cell vaccine (5 doses) in Canada.[2]

Since the immunity wanes after vaccination or infection in early life, repeated vaccinations in adolescence or adulthood had been proposed. In a large multicenter, randomized, double-blind trial of an acellular vaccine in adolescents and adults, 2,781 healthy subjects were monitored for 2.5 years for illness with cough for more than 5 days.[35] Each illness was evaluated with use of a nasopharyngeal aspirate for culture and PCR, and acute and convalescent serology for *B. pertussis*. On the basis of case definition for pertussis the incidence of pertussis in controls ranged from 370 to 450 cases per 1,000,000 person-years, and vaccine efficacy was 92% (95% confidence interval, 32–99%).[35]

In a recent cost-effective analysis the benefits of seven independent strategies for revaccination (booster) of adolescents and adults, in the form of diphtheria-tetanus-acellular pertussis (dtap) was undertaken.[36] Of these strategies, the most economical was revaccination of adolescents 10–19 years of age, which would prevent 0.7–1.8 million cases and save $0.6–1.6 billion over a decade. Routine adult booster vaccination every decade, although justified by the analysis, was more expensive and would be difficult to implement.[36] A few countries, Australia, Canada, Austria, Germany, and France, and recently the United States have now recommended routine booster doses of dtap in adolescents, and some for adults (the United States, Australia, Austria); and it is expected that other developed nations will soon adopt this policy. Vaccination should be considered to protect staff and indirectly their families and contacts for occupational exposures such as obstetric, midwifery, pediatric, laboratory, and child care workers.[37]

Prophylaxis after exposure to known cases (secondary prevention) should be considered for unvaccinated infants and high-risk adults, in health care and in household settings. The US Center for Disease Control and Prevention (CDC) recommends the macrolides (same as treatment) over 14 days for prevention of health-care-associated pneumonia.[38] Patients are considered noncontagious after 5 days of antimicrobial therapy, or 21 days after onset of cough. Antimicrobial prophylaxis is more effective if initiated within 21 days (preferably 14 days) of onset of paroxysmal cough in the index case.[39]

## *5.3.6 Future Directions*

Basic science research is still needed to evaluate the exact cause of the prolonged severe cough in pertussis, as the mechanism remains unclear. It is still not elucidated whether patients are contagious during the paroxysmal coughing phase, as nasopharyngeal cultures are usually negative after 3 weeks of illness.

Clinical trials in pregnant women are needed to determine the value of acellular vaccine in preventing infection in infants. Maternal antibodies to *B. pertussis* are usually low but can be actively transported in cord blood. Active immunization of newborns with acellular pertussis vaccines is underway in the United States. Further clinical trials are needed in adults on booster vaccination every 10 years to determine duration of immunity, program costs, compliance and non-medical costs associated with pertussis.[36]

There has been an increasing trend in developed countries for grandparents to act as surrogate parents or assist in caring for infants, and thus be a source of infection to nonimmunized infants. Previous studies indicate that the elderly are also susceptible to symptomatic pertussis, and in one study of 100 adults over 66 years of age for 3 years, the rate of pertussis infection was 19.7/100 person-years.[40] Thus, consideration should be given for booster immunization of the elderly, and studies should be performed to assess their immune response to the acellular pertussis vaccine.

An alternative strategy to prevent pertussis in the population besides booster vaccination is to develop new, more effective vaccines that will provide lifelong immunity to *B. pertussis*. However, this may be a daunting task as natural infection does not result in lifelong immunity. Moreover, there is no enthusiasm for this approach by vaccine-producing pharmaceutical companies. Genome sequence information may be helpful in identifying bacterial components that are highly conserved among species that could be used as cross-protective antigens.[8,41]

However, in the meantime as a prelude to universal adult vaccination it has been recommended by the Global Pertussis Initiative (an expert scientific forum) that immediate universal adolescent vaccination should be instituted in countries in which it is economically feasible.[42] Expanded vaccination should include adding booster doses to existing childhood schedules (preschool or adolescent) and booster doses for specific adult subgroups with the highest risk of transmission of *B. pertussis* to infants (i.e., new parents, other contacts of new born, and health care workers).[42]

Since 90% of the global burden of pertussis and the associated mortality are borne by developing nations, without the resources to institute universal childhood vaccination programs for many infectious diseases, it should be the goal of richer developed nations to assist the World Health Organization in implementing universal vaccination with dtap for all children.

# References

1. Hewlett, E.L., Edwards, K.M., (2005), Pertussis – not just for kids. N. Engl. J. Med. 352: 1215–1222.
2. Galonis, E., King, A.S. Varughese, P., Halperin, S.A., (2006), Changing epidemiology and emerging risk groups for pertussis. C M A J 174: 451–452.
3. Dudman, S.G., Troseid, M., Jonassen, T.O., Steinbak, K.M., (2006), Whooping cough – an increasing problem in Norway. Tidss Krift fur Den Norske Laegeforening; 126: 305–308.
4. Deeks, S., DeSemes, G., Boulianne, N., Duval, B., Rochette, L., Dery, P., Halperin, S., (1999), Failure of physicians to consider the diagnosis of pertussis in children. Clin. Infect. Dis. 28: 840–846.
5. Crowcroft, N.S., Stein, C., Duclos, P., Birmingham, M., (2003), How best to estimate the global burden of pertussis? Lancet Infect. Dis. 3: 413–418.
6. Loeffelholz, M.J., (2003), Bordetella, in Manual of Clinical Microbiology, 8th Edition; Murray, P.R., Baron, E.J., Jorgensen, J.H., Pfaltler. M.A., Yorken, R.H., A S M Press, Washington DC, pp. 780–788.

7. Cotter, P.A., Miller, J.F., (2001), Bordetella, in: Principles of bacterial pathogenesis, Groisman, E.A. (Ed) Academic Press, San Diego, CA, pp. 619–674.
8. Preston, A., (2005), *Bordetella pertussis*: the intersection of genomics and pathobiology. C M A J 173: 55–62.
9. Heininger, U., Stehr, K., Schmitt-Grohe, S., Lerenz, C., Rost, R., Christenson, P.D., Uberal, M., Cherry, J.D., (1994), Clinical characteristics of illness caused by *Bordetella parapertussis* compared with illness caused by *Bordetella pertussis*. Pediatr. Infect. Dis. J. 13: 306–309.
10. Locht, C., Antoine, R., Raze, d., Mielcarek, N., Hot, D., Lemoine, Y., Mascart, F., (2004), *Bordetella pertussis* from functional genomics to intranasal vaccination. Int. J. Med. Microbiol. 293: 583–588.
11. Edwards, K.M., (2003). Pertussis an important target for maternal immunization. Vaccine 21: 3483–3486.
12. Stehr, K., Cherry, J.D., Heininger, U., Schmitt-Grohe, S., Uberall, M., Laussucq, S., Eckhardt, T., Meyer, M., Engelhardt, R., Christensen, P., (1998), A comparative efficay trial in Germany in infants who received either the Lederle/Takeda acellular pertussis component DTA (DtaP) vaccine, the Lederle whole- cell component DT P vaccine or DT vaccine. Pediatrics 101: 1–11.
13. Cherry, J.D., Chang, S.J., Klein, D., Lee, M., Barenkamp, S., Bernstein, D., Edelman, R., Decker, M.D., Greenberg, D.P., Keitel, W., Treanor, J., Ward, J.I., (2004), Prevalence of antibody to *Bordetella pertussis* antigens in serum specimens obtained from 1793 adolescents and adults. Clin. Infect. Dis. 39: 1715–1718.
14. Olin, P., Hallander, H.O., Gustafsson, L., Reizenstein, E., Storsacter, J., (2001), How to make sense of pertussis immunogenicity data. Clin. Infect. Dis. 33 (Suppl.4): S288–S291.
15. Edelman, K., He, Q., Mäkinen, J., Sahlberg, A., Haanperä, M., Schuermna, L., Wolter, J., Mertsola, J., (2007), Immunity to pertussis 5 years after booster immunization during adolescence. Clin Infect. Dis. 44: 1271–1277.
16. Crowcroft, N.S., Pebody, R.C., (2006), Recent developments in pertussis. Lancet 367: 1926–1936.
17. Mills, KH, (2001), Immunity to *Bordetella pertussis*. Microbes. Infect. 3: 655–677.
18. Wendelboe, AM., van Rie, A, Salmaso, S, Englund, JA (2005), Duration of immunity against pertussis after natural infection or vaccination. Pediatr. Infect. Dis. 24: s58–s61.
19. Cherry, J.D., Grimprel, E., Guiso, N., Heininger, U., Mentsola, J., (2005), Defining pertussis epidemiology: Clinical, microbiologic and serologic perspectives. Pediatr. Infect. Dis. J. 24 (Suppl 5): S25–S34.
20. Cherry, J.D., (1999). Epidemiological, clinical and laboratory aspects of pertussis in adults. Clin. Infect. Dis. 28(Suppl 2): S112–S117.
21. Orenstein, W.A., (1999), Pertussis in adults: Epidemiology, signs, symptoms and implications for vaccination. Clin. Infect. Dis. 28 (Suppl 2): S147–S150.
22. Schellekens, J., von Konig, C.H., Gardner, P., (2005), Pertussis sources of infection and routes of transmission in the vaccination era. Pediatr. Infect. Dis. J. 24 (Suppl. 5): S19–S24.
23. Lievano, F.A., Reynolds, M.A., Waring, A.L., Ackelsberg, J., Bisgard, K.M., Sanden, G.N., Guris, D., Golaz, A., Bopp, D.J., Limberger, R.J., Smith, P.F., (2002), Issues associated with and recommendation for using PCR to detect outbreaks of pertussis. J. Clin. Microbiol 40: 2801–2805.
24. Halperin, S.A., (2007), The control of pertuiss – 2007 and beyond. N. Engl. J. Med. 356: 110–113.
25. Advisory Committee on Immunization Practices (ACIP), (2006), Preventing tetanus, diphtheria, and pertussis among adolescents: use of tetanus toxoid, reduced diphtheria toxoid and acellular pertussis vaccines: recommendations of the Advisory Committee on Immunization Practices (ACIP). MMWR Recommen. Rep. 55 (RR-3): 1–34.
26. Ntezayabo, B., De Serres, G., Duval, B., (2003), Pertussis resurgence in Canada largely caused by a cohort effect. Pediatr. Infect. Dis. 22: 22–27.

27. Mastrantonio, P., Spigagha, P., van Oirschot, H., van der Heide, H.G., Heuvelman, K., Stefanelli, P., Mooi, F.R., (1999), Antigenic variants in *Bordetalla pertussis* strains isolated from vaccinated and unvaccinated children. Microbiology; 145: 2069–2075.
28. Tozzi, A.E., Celentano, L.P., Ciofi degli Atti, M.L., Salmaso, S., (2005), Diagnosis and management of pertussis. C M A J : 172: 509–515.
29. Yaari, E., Yafe-Zimerman, Y., Schwartz, S.B., Slater, P.E., Schvartzman, P., Andoren, N., Branski, D., Kerem, E., (1999), Clinical manifestation of *Bordetella pertussis* infection in immunized children and young adults. Chest:115: 1254–1258.
30. Kosters, K., Riffelmann, M., Wirsing vonKonig, C.H., (2001), Evaluation of a real-time PCR assay for detection of *Bordetella pertussis* and *B. parapertussis* in clinical samples. . J. Med. Microbiol. 50: 436–440.
31. Gilberg, S., Njamkepo, E., Schlumberger, M., Guiso, N, (2002), Evidence of *Bordetella pertussis* infection in adults presenting with persistent cough in a French area with very high whole-cell vaccine coverage. J. Infect. Dis. 186: 415–418.
32. Wirsing von Konig, C.H., Halperin, S., Rifflemann, M., Guiso, N., (2002), Pertussis of adults and infants. Lancet Infect. Dis. 2: 744–750.
33. Pillay, V., Swingler, G., (2003), Symptomatic treatment of the cough in whooping cough. Cochrane Database Syst. Rev. (4): CD 003257.
34. Widdecombe, J., Shankar, K., (2004), Acute cough in the elderly: aetiology, diagnosis and therapy. Drugs Aging 31: 243–258.
35. Ward, J.I., Cherry I.D., Chang, S.J., Partridge, S., Lee, H., Treanor, J., Greenberg, D.P., Keitel, W., Borenkamp, S., Bernstein, D.I., Edelman, R., Edwards, K., APERT Study Group, (2005) Efficacy of an acellular pertussis vaccine among adolescents and adults. N. Engl. J. Med. 353: 1615–1617.
36. Purdy, K.W., Hoy, J.W., Botterman, M.F., Ward, I.F., (2004), Evaluation of strategies for use of acellular pertussis vaccine in adolescents and adults. A cost - benefit analysis. . Clin. Infect. Dis. 39: 20–28.
37. Ward, A., Caro, J., Bassinet, L., Housset, B., O'Brien, J.A., Guiso, N., (2005), Health and economic consequences of an outbreak of pertussis among healthcare workers in a hospital in France. Infect. Control. Hosp. Epidemiol. 26: 288–292.
38. Tablan, O.C., Andersen, J, Besser-May, T., Bridges, C., Hayjeh, R., CDC: Healthcare Infection Control Practices Advisory Committee, (2004), Guidelines for preventing healthcare associated pneumonia, 2003: recommendations of CDC and the HealthCare Infection Control Practices Advisory Committee. M M W R: 53 (RR-3) 1–36.
39. Dodhin, H., Crowcroft, N.S., Bramley, J.C., Miller, E., (2002), U.K. Guidelines for use of erythomycin chemoproplylaxis in persons exposed to pertussis. J. Public Helath Med. 24: 200–206.
40. Hodder, S.L., Cherry, J.D., Montimer, E.A. Jr., Ford, A.B., Gombein, J., Papp, K., (2002) Antibody responses to *Bordetella pertussis* antigens and clinical correlations in elderly community residents. Clin. Infect. Dis. 31: 7–14.
41. Preston, A., Parkhill, J., Maskell, D.J., (2004), The Bordettellae: lessons from genomics. Nat. Rev. Microbiol. 2: 379–390.
42. Forsyth, K.D., Campins-Marti, Caro, J., Cherry, J.D., Greenberg, D., Guiso, N., Heininger, U., Schellekens, J., Tan, T., Wirzing von Konig, C.H., Plotkin S., for the Global Pertussis Initiative, (2004), New pertussis vaccination strategies beyond infancy: Recommendation by the Global Pertussis Initiative. Clin. Infect. Dis. 39: 1802–1809.

# Section C
# New Concepts and Trends

# Chapter 6
# New Concepts and Emerging Issues in Sepsis

## 6.1 Introduction

Severe sepsis and septic shock are manifestations of the host's immune uncontrolled response to infection. The term sepsis is a poorly defined, but commonly used term in the medical literature, and it is derived from the Greek word "Sépsis" meaning decay. Sepsis is best defined as a life-threatening condition or complex caused by overwhelming inflammatory response to infection associated with dysregulation of the body's immune mechanism. Sepsis is the leading cause of death in critically ill patients in most intensive care units (ICUs). It has been estimated that in the United States sepsis develops in 750,000 people annually, and more then 210,000 of those die[1,2]! Infants and children in >42,000 cases of severe sepsis occur annually in the United States and millions worldwide.[2] The incidence of septicemia and sepsis have been increasing in the past 3 decades in many countries because of several factors, including longer lifespan with a greater population of the elderly; treatment with immunosuppressives with a greater number of subjects with organ transplantations and cancers; use of invasive and novel treatment with prosthesis, long-term or permanent catheters; and the expanding acquired immunodeficiency syndrome (AIDS) epidemic. In national hospital discharge surveys in the United States, the incidence of septicemia had increased from 73.6 per 100,000 patients in 1979 to 175.9 per 100,000 patients in 1987.[3] Surveys in the United States and Europe have estimated that severe sepsis accounts for 2–11% of all admission to hospital or ICUs.[1] Observational studies indicate that 30–50% of the cases are admitted through the emergency department, rather than developing in hospitals.[4,5] The incidence of sepsis appears to continue to increase by 8.7% annually (with an adjusted rate of increase of nearly 300% from 1979 to 2000),[6] but may be greater in the United States (US) with an incidence of 240–300 per 100,000 populations, compared to some European countries (Austria, Germany) with rates of 54–116 per 100,000 population.[7]

Despite progress in our understanding of the pathophysiology of sepsis, the mortality rate is still high (in those with severe sepsis and septic shock). Although the mortality rate overall has fallen in the United States from 27.8% to 17.9% in septic patients over 2 decades, the mortality rate was 30% in those with any organ failure and 70% in those with multiple organ failure.[6] Patients with infections and severe sepsis require prolonged stay in ICU and hospital, resulting in increase health care costs. Estimates of direct costs per sepsis patient in the United States are about $50,000 whereas European costs are lower, $26,450–33,350.[7] Thus a crude estimate of the direct annual cost of severe sepsis in the United States is about $17.0 billion.[1]

## 6.2 Definitions

Sepsis, severe sepsis, and septic shock represent progressive stages of the same disease. The transition from sepsis to septic shock can occur in a few hours, but most occurs during the first 24 h of hospitalization. Since 1992 an expert panel from the American College of Chest Physicians and the Society of Critical Care Medicine produced a consensus statement on definition of sepsis and the stages (see table[8]). A systemic inflammatory response syndrome (SIRS) was defined as a systemic inflammatory reaction, regardless of their etiology (infectious or noninfectious). Sepsis was, therefore, defined as SIRS resulting from a documented infection; severe sepsis as sepsis with organ dysfunction or hypoperfusion; and septic shock as presence of sepsis with refractory hypotension. The above criteria have recently been updated, dismissing the SIRS criteria and proposing prediction/insult/response/organ dysfunction (PIRO) criteria.[9] The application of the definitions for epidemiological and clinical reporting can be problematic but does provide a framework for classification of patients. However, it is likely that the official health statistics will still underestimate the true incidence.

## 6.3 Immune Response

Sepsis or septic shock syndrome need not be associated with documented bacteremia, but should be accompanied by the pathophysiological changes of SIRS with a site or source of infection. Gram-negative bacteria were the predominant causes of sepsis in the 1960s up until the 1980s but gram-positive bacterial infections have now accounted for more than half the cases in the past 2 decades. Fungal infections such as systemic candidiasis are an increasing cause of sepsis in the ICU and immunosuppressed patients. Among the organisms causing sepsis in 2000 in the United States, gram-positive bacteria accounted for 52.1% of cases, gram-negative bacteria for 37.6%, polymicrobial infections for 4.7%, anaerobes for 1%, and fungi 4.6%.[6]

The first line of defense against invading microorganisms is the innate immune system, which then triggers the adaptive component organized around specialized cells, T-cells and B-cells. There are a limited number of receptors involved in innate immune recognition (in the hundreds) which would not be able to recognize every possible foreign antigen. Thus, the innate immune system by evolution has adapted

## 6.3 Immune Response

to focus on highly conserved structures present in large groups of microorganisms.[10] These structures are named pathogens-associated molecular patterns: i.e., bacterial lipopolysaccharide (LPS), peptoglycan, lipoteichoic acid (plasma membrane of gram-positive bacteria), mannan (cell wall of fungi), bacterial DNA, double-stranded RNA (viral), and glucans. The pathogens-associated molecular patterns are produced only by the microorganisms and not by the hosts, and are invariant structures shared by the entire classes of pathogens. The innate immune system evolve to recognize them by pattern-recognition receptors, which are expressed on many effector cells, such as the macrophages, dendritic cells, and B-cells professional antigen-presenting cells. For example, the LPS present on all gram-negative bacteria can be detected by the pattern-recognition receptor of the host to virtually any gram-negative bacterial infections.[10] Once the pathogen-recognition receptor binds to the pathogen-associated molecular pattern, it activates the effecter cells immediately without delaying after proliferation, thus initiating a rapid host defense.

The pattern recognition receptors can be divided into three classes: secreted, endocytic, and signalling.[10] The secreted pattern-recognition molecules (e.g., mannose-binding lectin) functions as opsonins by binding to microbial cell wall and triggers the complement system and phagocytosis. The mannose-binding lectin (MBL) is an acute phase reactant synthesized by the liver that binds carbohydrates on gram-positive and gram-negative bacteria and yeast, as well as some viruses and parasites.[11] MBL-associated serine proteases are activated by microbial ligands binding to MBL with direct activation of the complement pathway, independent of adaptive immune response.

Endocytic pattern-recognition receptors occur on the surface of phagocytes, and mediate the uptake and delivery of the invaders into lysosomes for destruction. Pathogen-derived peptides are present and form a complex with the major histocompatibility – complex (MHC) molecules on the surface of macrophages. The macrophage mannose receptor, (member of the mannose-lectin family) is an endocytic pattern-recognition receptor that recognizes carbohydrates in a large number of microorganisms and mediates their phagocytosis by macrophages.[12] The macrophage scavenger receptor is another endocytic pattern-recognition receptor that binds to bacterial cell wall and enhances phagocytosis and clearance from the circulation.[13] Other recently identified pattern-recognition receptors with relevance to innate immunity include nucleotide-binding and oligomerization-domain proteins, and caspase-recruitment domain helicase.[14]

Signaling receptors include the family of toll receptors that have a major role in the induction of immune and inflammatory responses by mediating the intracellular signaling of microbial products. These toll-like receptors (TLRs) recognize pathogen-associated molecule patterns and activate signal-transduction pathways that induce inflammatory cytokines and costimulatory molecules, essential to the adaptive immune response.[10] TLR4 and TLR2 function as receptors of the innate immune system and activate the transcription nuclear factor (NF-$_\kappa$B) signaling pathway. TLR4 is essential for the recognition of LPS and interacts with LPS-binding protein and another protein, MD-2, to interact with CD14, a receptor on macrophages and B-cells to form a complex. Thus, for any one microbe, there are a variety of molecules that can activate many different pattern-recognition receptors. The binding of pathogen-associated molecules with pattern-recognition receptor activate several signaling intracellular pathways, resulting in activation of transcription factors (NF-κB, AP-1, FOS, JUN) that control immune response genes (including interferon regulatory factor families) for the release of numerous effector molecules and proinflammatory cytokines. Cytokines are essential for orchestrating the innate and adaptive immune defenses to invading pathogens. The adaptive immune system responds to a pathogen only after recognition by the innate immune system. T-cells antigen receptors recognize ligand (peptide) bound to MHC class II molecules on the surface of antigen-presenting cells. T-cells require signals from the peptide-MHC molecule complex plus a costimulatory signal (CD80 and CD86 molecules) on the surface of antigen-presenting cells to be activated. After activation helper T-cells control activation of cytotoxic T-cells, B-cells, and macrophages (adaptive immune responses).[10]

## 6.4 Pathogenesis

Although bacterial infections are by far the most common causes of sepsis and septic-like syndrome, this clinical complex can be seen with severe disseminated fungal infections (about 5%) and even rarely with viral illnesses, such as severe acute respiratory syndrome (SARS), avian influenza and hemorrhagic viral infections (dengue, Lassa fever, etc.). Whereas gram-negative bacteria initiate the sepsis syndrome mainly by LPS interacting with LPS-binding protein and CD14 via TLR4 (coreceptor for LPS), gram-positive bacteria (*Staphylococci* and *Streptococci*) can initiate the mechanism of SIRS by the components of their cell wall (peptoglycin, lipoprotein, lipoteichoic acid, and phenol soluble modulin) by binding to TLR2.[15] There is also recent evidence that although pneumococcal lipoteichoic acid induces profound inflammatory response and activation of the coagulation pathway through TLR2-dependent route, it is likely amplified by endogenous TLR4 ligands.[16] Gram-positive bacteria can also cause severe sepsis or septic shock by producing exotoxins that act as superantigens, as in staphylococcal or streptococcal toxic shock syndrome and streptococcal necrotizing fasciitis. Superantigens are not processed for clonotypic presentation by antigen presenting cells. Superantigens are a group of powerful antigens that bind directly to MHC class II molecules of antigen-presenting cells and to Vβ chain of T-cell receptors, outside of the normal T-cell receptor site, and are able to react with multiple T-cell receptor molecules.[15] Thus, activating a large number of T-cells nonspecifically (>fivefold than conventional antigens) to produce massive amounts of proinflammatory cytokines.

Macrophages and neutrophils contain the inflammasome, a complex of proteins involved in the innate defense mechanism.[17] At least two types of inflammasome exist, composed mainly of the "NALP" family of proteins, NALP1 inflammasome and NALP3 (the central component of the cryopyrin inflammasome). Stimulation of the cryoprin inflammasome by pathogenic bacteria results in activation of

## 6.4 Pathogenesis

caspase I, which in turn activates interleukin-1β (1L-1β) through cleavage of pro-1L-1β. This proinflammatory cytokine (secreted by macrophages) triggers another cascade of molecular events (including -TNFα) that result in inflammation.[17] Cryopyrin-deficient macrophages do not respond efficiently to gram-positive bacteria (i.e., *S. aureus* or *Listeria monocytogenes*) but can recognize gram-negative bacteria (which require other inflammasome components).[18]

Nuclear factor (NF)-κB is involved in regulating the transcription of many of the immunomodulatory mediators involved in sepsis and associated organs dysfunction or failure. Signaling pathways stimulated by bacterial products (LPS, lipoteichoic acid, etc.) or cytokine receptors, including those for TNF-α, 1L-1 via TLRs, enhance nuclear activation of NF-κB and transcription of genes encoding expression of cytokines, chemokines, adhesion molecules, apoptotic factors, and other mediators of inflammation and coagulation (Table 6.2).[19] Since NF-κB plays a central role in sepsis modulation of this factor may have therapeutic implications, and suppression in animal models of sepsis decrease acute inflammation and organ dysfunction.[20] Activation of caspase-8 (a cysteine protease required for monocyte differentiation into macrophages) may have therapeutic implications, as it prevents sustained NF-κB activation by down-regulation through cleavage of a kinase receptor-interacting protein1 (RIP1).[21]

Interferon – γ (IFN-γ) plays a major role in immune-modulation after immune stimulation of T-lymphocytes by infectious agents. IFN-γ is essential for killing intracellular organisms by enhancing the synthesis of inducible nitric oxide (NO). However, the role of IFN-γ in immune defense against gram-negative bacterial infection is inconsistent. Interleukin – 18 (IL-18), an IFN-γ inducing factor, essential for IFN-γ production appears to play an important role in sepsis.[22] In mice neutralization of IL-18 protects against endotoxin and ischemia-induced liver damage. Thus, IL-18 blockade may be a therapeutic target to neutralize the pathologic consequences of sepsis via IFN-γ mechanisms.[22]

Monocytes and macrophages are effector cells of the innate immunity which are central in the recognition and elimination of invading pathogens. Molecules and cytokines secreted by macrophages orchestrate the innate and adaptive host immune response. An important cytokine released in large amounts by monocytes and macrophages on exposure to bacterial products is macrophage inhibitory factor (MIF). MIF acts by regulating the expression of TLR4-LPS complex, which are important in the innate immune responses to endotoxin and gram-negative bacterial sepsis.[23] Immunoneutralization of MIF protects mice against lethal endotoxemia, gram-positive toxic syndrome and experimental bacterial peritonitis.[15] High blood levels of MIF in children and adults with gram-negative sepsis is associated with parameters of disease severity (shock, disseminated intravascular coagulopathy [DIC], lactic acidosis, etc.), dysregulated pituitary-adrenal function, and early mortality.[24] Excessive production of this potent proinflammatory cytokine appears to play an important role on the sepsis syndrome and associated mortality, and inhibitory agents may help to treat severe sepsis.

High mobility group proteins superfamily, particularly high mobility group box-1 (HMGB1), a DNA-binding protein regulating gene transcription and stabilizing nucleosome formation has been shown to be a late mediator of inflammation and sepsis,[25] HMGB1 is released by activated macrophages, induces the delayed release of other proinflammatory mediators (TNF-α, IL-1α, 1L-1β, IL-1 receptor agonist, 1L-6, 1L-8, and macrophage inflammatory protein [MIP]), and thus mediates lethality when overexpressed. Administration of anti-HMGB1 antibodies protects against lethal endotoxemia, even after peak activity of circulating TNF.[26] Delayed treatment with anti-HMGB1 prevents lung pathology independent of pulmonary levels of TNF, 1L-1β, and MIP-2,[27] indicating that HMGB1 is an independent mediator of endotoxin-induced inflammation.

A recently discovered receptor of the immunoglobulin superfamily, TREM-1 (triggering receptor expressed on myeloid cells), activates neutrophils and monocytes/macrophages by signaling through the adaptor protein DAP12.[28] TREM-1 amplifies TLR-initiated responses after microbial invasion and enhances secretion of proinflammatory chemokines and cytokines to bacterial and fungal infections. In animal models of acute sepsis blockade of TREM-1 signaling with TREM-1-IgG fusion protein reduces hyperinflammatory responses and death.[29]

Neutrophils play a pivotal role in the defense against bacterial and some fungal infections (i.e., invasive candidiasis). However, overwhelming activation of neutrophils can result in tissue damage. Elimination or neutralization of pathogenic bacteria by neutrophils is accomplished by their large stockpile of proteolytic enzymes and rapid production of reactive oxygen radicals to degrade internalized invaders.[30] Local accumulation of neutrophils in the microvasculature, and release of lytic factors and proinflammatory cytokines extracellularly from tissue-infiltrating neutrophils can result in local damage. During sepsis the homeostatic environment in the microculation is compromised partly by formation of leukocytic aggregates, endothelial hyperactivity, fibrin deposition, and tissue exudates that predispose to microvascular occlusion and impairment of tissue oxygenation.[31] Large numbers of neutrophils accumulate in organs developing failure in sepsis, and widespread recruitment and sequestration probably contribute to subsequent organ dysfunction.[30] Experimental interventions that deplete or antagonize the activity of neutrophils ameliorate organ dysfunction.[32] The fact that neutrophil-mediated lung injury (acute respiratory distress syndrome [ARDS]) occurs in patients with neutropenia, indicate that organ dysfunction can be initiated by a few neutrophils sequestered in the microvasculature. A distinct subpopulation of neutrophils with characteristic secretary profiles may account for the organ dysfunction. In animal models of sepsis, immature neutrophils preferentially accumulate in the pulmonary microvasculature, and activation with release of proteolytic enzymes (defensins) induces tissue damage.[33,34]

## 6.4.1 *Hemodynamics*

Sepsis classically produces a vasodilatory shock with low systemic vascular resistance, normal or increased cardiac output, hypovolemia due to arterial and venous vasodilatations, and leakage of plasma into the extravascular space, tachycardia (a hyper-dynamic shock syndrome), and ultimately hypotension and hypoperfusion (if uncorrected) in 90% of patients.[35] Although sepsis is the most frequent cause of vasodilatory shock, other causes include carbon monoxide intoxication, nitrogen intoxication, prolonged and severe hypotension of any cause (hemorrhage and cardiogenic shock, severe heart failure with mechanical assist devise, prolonged cardiopulmonary bypass), and other conditions such as lactic acidosis due to drug intoxication, certain mitochondrial disease, cyanide poisoning, and cardiac arrest with pulseless electrical activity (anaphylaxis, liver failure and glucocorticoid deficiency are sometimes listed as causes of vasodilatory shock, but the data is inconclusive[36]). The basic mechanism responsible for vasodilatory shock is failure of the vascular smooth muscle to contract. This is in contrast to the usual cases of acute hemorrhage or acute cardiogenic shock, or severe dehydration where profound vasoconstriction in the venous and arteriolar circulation is a compensatory mechanism via the neuroendocrine response. In the late stages of septic shock profound vasoconstriction and increased peripheral vascular resistance can occur.

## 6.4.2 Mechanisms

In all form of vasodilatory shock the plasma vasodilators such as atrial natriuretic peptide and nitric oxide concentrations are markedly elevated and the potassium ($K_{ATP}$) channels or neurohormonal system is activated.[36] Atrial natriuretic peptide and nitric oxide activate a kinase that interact with myosin phosphatase, dephosphorylate myosin and prevents muscle contraction. Moreover, nitric oxide, atrial natriuretic peptide, calcitonin gene-related peptide, and adenosine (all greatly increased in septic shock) activate the $K_{ATP}$ channels, allowing efflux of potassium and thus hyperpolarization of the plasma membrane and preventing entry of calcium into the cells, thus, inhibiting catecholamine or angiotensin II-induced vasoconstriction. Activation of the $K_{ATP}$ channels in arterioles is a critical mechanism in the hypotension and vasodilation characteristic of septic shock. $K_{ATP}$ channels are further activated by increased intracellular concentration of hydrogen ion and lactate,[36] consequences of hypoperfusion and tissue anoxia accompanying shock.

Activation of the sympathetic nervous system and the rennin-angiotensin-aldosterone axis, the nonosmotic release of vasopressin, and an increase in cardiac output (secondary to decreased cardiac afterload) are compensatory mechanisms of the body to maintain arterial circulation in patients with severe sepsis and septic shock, but may lead to acute renal failure.[37] Arginine vasopressin initially increases in septic shock (200–300 pg/ml) and after an hour the plasma levels fall ($^\wedge$30 pg/ml), as the neurohypophysial stores are depleted.[38] This may play a role in septic shock as arginine vasopressin decreases the synthesis of nitric oxide and inactivate the $K_{ATP}$ channels, thus attenuating the arterial vasodilatation and pressor resistance during sepsis.[37]

Thus, vasodilatation and hypotension is due to the failure of the smooth muscle to constrict. However, the pathophysiology of sepsis leading to vasodilatation is very complex. Molecules expressed by microbial pathogens interact with plasma

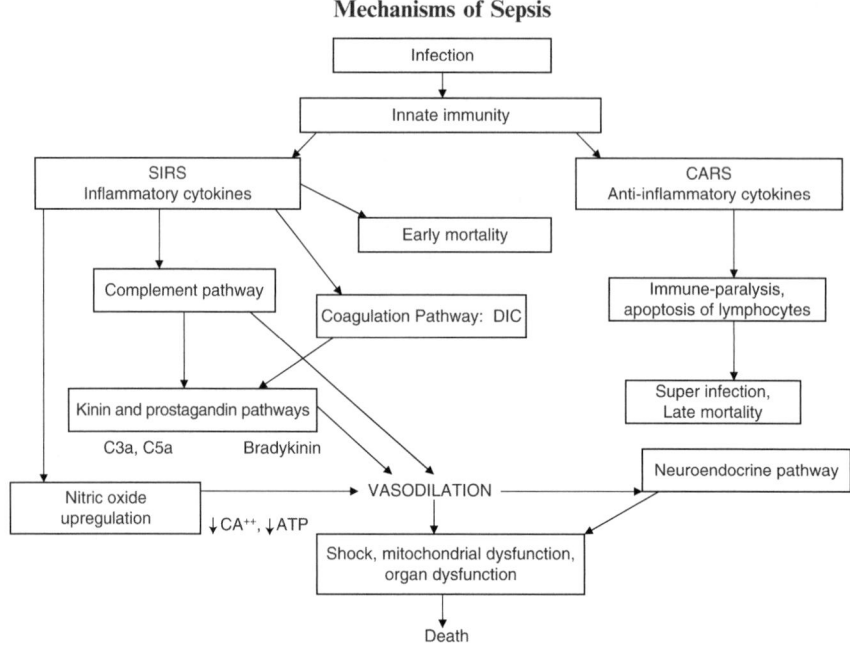

**Fig. 6.1** Mechanisms of sepsis

mediators, monocytes or macrophages, endothelial cells, neutrophils, and platelets to activate the inflammatory cytokine cascade, the complement system, arachidonic acid and the prostaglandin pathway, the coagulation and kinin cascade, the endorphin system, and finally the nitric oxide pathway (see Fig. 6.1). These mediators stimulate widespread vasodilatation, increase vascular permeability, with microvascular dysfunction, acute renal failure, acute respiratory distress syndrome, hepatic failure, and disseminated intravascular coagulation (DIC).

Although the general paradigm is that sepsis is a manifestation of an uncontrolled inflammatory response, the failure of anti-inflammatory agents in randomized clinical trials have raised doubts about this concept.[39] A clear picture of the pathogenesis of sepsis has been evolving over the past decade, and a new paradigm appears to focus on a dysregulated immune response, with an imbalance between proinflammatory and anti-inflammatory cytokines. Moreover the initial stages of sepsis is characterized by hyper-inflammation with excessive proinflammatory cytokines (SIRS) followed by a phase of – compensatory anti-inflammatory response (CARS), with anergy and immunodepression (Fig. 6.1).[40]

Activated CD4 T-cells are programmed to secrete cytokines of two distinct and antagonistic profiles (proinflammatory and anti-inflammatory).[40] The proinflammatory (TH1) response include secretion and induction of tumor-necrosis factor (TNF)-α, interferon-γ, and interleukin (1L)-1 and 2. The anti-inflammatory (TH-2) response results in secretion of 1L-4, 1L-10, and 1L-12. Some studies have shown that 1L-10 is increased in sepsis and that the level predicts mortality[41,42] and

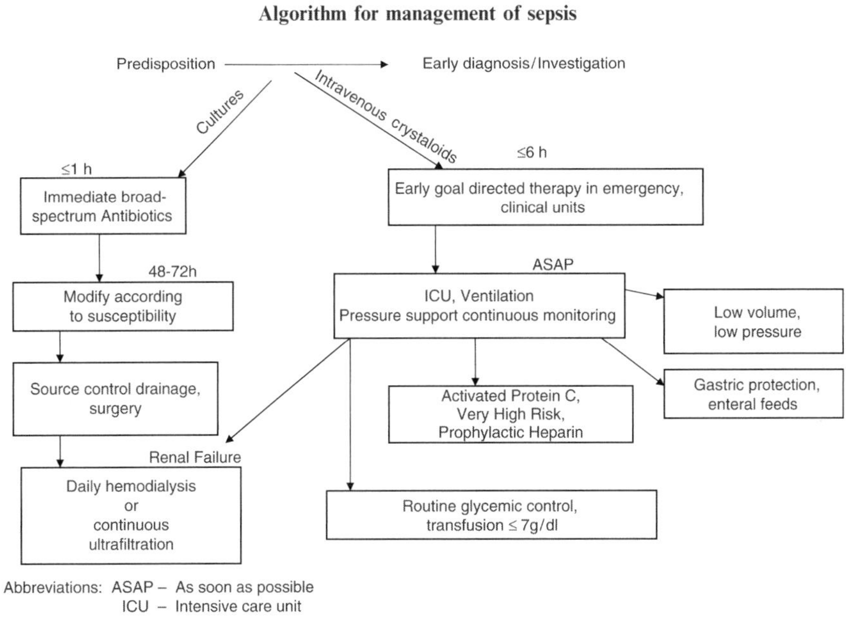

## Algorithm for management of sepsis

**Fig. 6.2** Algorithm for management of sepsis

that reversal of TH2 response improves survival among septic patients.[40] The anti-inflammatory cytokines can inhibit the synthesis of proinflammatory cytokines and exert several direct opposing effects on different cell types. Thus, 1L-10 represents an important autoregulatory mechanism that controls the inflammatory response and toxicity of these mediators.

### 6.4.3 Apoptosis of Immune Cells

Sepsis results in the dysregulation of normal apoptosis which may account for immunosuppression associated with severe sepsis, and in part the excessive inflammatory response. Recent studies of patients dying of sepsis have found profound, progressive apoptosis-induced loss of cells of the adaptive immune system.[43–45] There are markedly decreased levels of B cells, CD4 T-cells, and follicular dendritic cells, but no significant loss of CD8 T-cells, natural killer cells, or macrophages in severe sepsis. Depletion or loss of these lymphocytes can cause decreased antibody production, macrophage activation, and impaired antigen presentation. In one study of 19 patients with sepsis 15 (78.9%) had severe lymphopenia with absolute lymphocyte count of $500 \pm 270/mm^3$ (normal being above $1,200/mm^3$).[43] Bacterial lipoproteins also can initiate apoptosis of monocyte cells and epithelial cells through TLR-2, providing a molecular link between microbial products, apoptosis and the host defense mechanism. The type of cell death may determine the immune response. Apoptotic cells increase anergy or anti-inflammatory cytokines that impair the response to pathogens, whereas necrotic cells cause immune stimulation and enhance antimicrobial defence.[46,47] The mechanism of lymphocyte apoptosis in sepsis is not completely understood but may be related to stress-induced endogenous release of glucocortecoids[48] and bacteria have evolved molecules that deregulate caspases to induce apoptosis.[46]

Neutrophils play a major role in the host's response to invading pathogens and are essential for their eradication. However, neutrophils through release of oxidants and proteases are believed to be responsible for injury to organs with inflammatory conditions, including sepsis. Excessive neutrophil activation and sequestration in the lungs may play a role in the acute respiratory distress syndrome (ARDS), commonly present with severe sepsis. Neutrophils are recruited to the site of infections and normally die within 6–8 h after their release into the circulation. Inflammation is terminated and controlled in part, by the apoptosis of neutrophils. There is recent evidence that apoptosis is delayed in neutrophils from patients with sepsis.[49] This may result in failure to down-regulate proinflammatory cells, leading to prolongation of inflammation.[50] Failure of the regulatory pathway of apoptosis can prolong survival of neutrophils, resulting in death by necrosis with up-regulation of inflammation. The mechanism of delayed apoptosis involves activation of NF-κB, via caspase-1 and generation of 1L-1.[51] Pre-B cells colony enhancing factor (PBEF) a growth factor for B cells (produced by activated lymphocytes), and up-regulated by LPS stimulation, appears to inhibit apoptosis of neutrophils.[52]

Thus it is clear that there is deregulation of apoptosis in sepsis which appears to play a role in the pathogenesis. Enhanced apoptosis of organ tissues may contribute to increased intestinal permeability (gastrointestinal epithelial cells exhibit external apoptotic cell death) and organ failure. Large numbers of lymphocytes and gastrointestinal epithelial cells die by apoptosis during sepsis.[53] While failure to initiate apoptosis process in neutrophils may prolong and enhance the inflammatory reaction, enhanced lymphocytic apoptosis may result in immunosuppression.

### 6.4.4 Immunoparalysis

It has become evident over the past decade that the early mortality of fulminant sepsis is associated with excessive systemic inflammation mediated by various proinflammatory cytokines. After this initial phase (few days), counter-regulatory pathways activation with excessive anti-inflammatory cytokines and increased apoptosis of lympocytes is associated with immunodepression or "immunoparalysis," which probably contribute to late mortality from secondary nosocomial infections.[54] Sepsis is thus associated with reduced responsiveness of immune cells to release proinflammatory cytokines at a later stage. There is diminished responsiveness of circulating monocytes, granulocytes, and lymphocytes. It has been proposed that the hyporesponsiveness of immune cells is confined to circulating blood cells, and not to local-tissue immune cells which remain responsive to bacterial antigen.[55]

The mechanism of secondary immune paralysis in sepsis is not fully understood, but may involve the anti-inflammatory cytokines 1L-10 and transforming growth factor-β (TGFβ). In an animal model of sepsis depression of splenocyte immune responses was mediated by 1L-6 and TGFβ[56] and plasma from septic patients greatly depress normal monocyte secretion of TNF-γ through functional deactivation by 1L-10.[57] Since immunoparalysis could contribute to the late mortality of the septic syndrome, strategies to restore immune function in septic patients are being investigated. Biologics that may reverse monocyte deactivation in vitro and animals, thus of potential therapeutic benefit in sepsis, include interferon-γ (INF-γ) and granulocyte-macrophage colony-stimulating factor (GM-CSF).[55] In a small pilot study of nine patients with sepsis and immunoparalysis (defined as <30% HLA-DR-positive monocytes), daily subcutaneous injection of INF-γ for 3 days restored TNF-production capacity of monocytes and eight patients survived.[58] Thus, further clinical trials with IFN-γ in late sepsis is warranted.

The type of cell death also determines the immunologic function of surviving immune cells.[40] Apoptotic cells induce anergy or anti-inflammatory cytokines that impair host response to pathogens, and necrotic cells cause immune stimulation and increase host immune defence.[59] Thus, in late sepsis immunodepression is a result of quantitative depletion of circulating lymphocytes and monocytes, as well as functional impairment of the remaining mononuclear cells.

Although clinical and animal experiments support the concept of early deaths in sepsis being related to hyper-inflammation and late mortality being associated with excessive anti-inflammatory cytokines, this is likely an oversimplification of a complex process. Thus, a simple plasma measurement of cytokines may not be adequate to define the status of immune response during sepsis as suggested.[60] Two recent studies in a murine model of sepsis with monitoring of plasma cytokines during the evolution of the syndrome have been reported from the same laboratry.[61,62] In the early phase there was simultaneous increase in proinflammatory (1L-6, TNF, 1L-1β, M1P-1 and -2, exotoxin) and anti-inflammatory (TNF-soluble receptors, 1L-10, 1L-1 receptor antagonist) cytokines in early deaths (day 1–5).[61] Both pro- or anti-inflammatory cytokines were reliable in predicting mortality up to 48 h. During the later phase of sepsis, some mice die with evidence of immunosuppression (increased bacterial growth and low 1L-6), while others die with immunostimulation (high 1L-6 and bacterial growth) none of the surviving mice after day 4 exhibited increased 1L-6.[62] This complex response does not support the use of proinflammatory cytokine measurement for classifying the inflammatory status during sepsis.

## 6.4.5 Tissue Oxygenation

While microvascular blood flow redistribution undoubtedly occurs in sepsis, investigators have shown increased tissue oxygen tension in the organs of animals and patients with sepsis.[63,64] Thus, suggesting that the predominant defect might be in cellular oxygen use (tissue dysoxia) rather than in oxygen delivery. Studies on skeletal muscles biopsies of critically ill patients with sepsis have found that ATP concentration was significantly lower in patients who subsequently died than survivors and controls.[65] There was an association of nitric oxide overproduction, antioxidant depletion, mitochondrial dysfunction, and decreased ATP concentrations that relate to organ failure and eventual outcome. Therefore, bioenergetics failure appears to be a pathophysiological mechanism underlying multiorgan dysfunction in sepsis.[62]

## 6.4.6 Coagulation

Dysfunction of the blood coagulation cascade and fibrinolysis are common in patients with sepsis but clinically overt DIC is uncommon. However, septic shock is nearly always associated with some degree of DIC, with microvascular thrombosis, consumption of platelets and coagulation of proteins, and stimulation of the fibrinolytic system, with increased risk of hemorrhage.[66] Hemostatic abnormalities and endothelial changes are some of the earliest manifestations of a wide spectrum of infections. Changes in the fibrinolytic system are seen soon after a single infusion of endotoxin with many of the abnormalities seen in early clinical sepsis.[67] Rapid release of tissue plasminogen activator ($\tau$-PA) was followed by an early increase in plasminogen activation, reaching a maximum by 2–3 h and decreased by 3–5 h. The decrease in fibrinolytic activity was due partly to appearance of plasminogen-activator inhibitor (PAI)-1 activity at 3–5 h. Sepsis can activate the coagulation pathway at multiple sites, via activation of chemical mediators on the endothelium and monocytes, and through activation of the proinflammatory cascade. Endotoxin and other toxins can directly activate the extrinsic pathway by up-regulation of tissue factor (TF) and factor VII leading to thrombin and clot formation. TF activation is considered the primary initiator of coagulation in sepsis.[68] In addition, sepsis activates the contact system (intrinsic pathway) through induction of TNF-$\alpha$ and interleukins via activation of Hageman factor (XII), to factor XIa, which acts as trigger of the intrinsic coagulation pathway. Activated factor XII (a) also hydrolyses pre-kallikrein to the proteolytic kallikrein which cleaves kininogen to release bradykinin (a potent vasodepressor), which is thought to contribute to hypotension in early sepsis.[69]

General activation of the coagulation depletes the natural antithrombotic factors, protein C, antithrombin, and TF pathway inhibitor. Protein C is converted to activated protein C (APC) by thrombin binding to thrombomodulin on endothelium surface, and counter prothrombotic state, and exhibit anti-inflammatory properties by decreasing proinflammatory cytokines and neutrophil rolling on endothelium. Protein C and protein S inhibit endotoxin-induced production of TNF, 1L-1$\beta$, and 1L-6 by monocytes in vitro and in vivo, activated protein C reduce TNF secretion in endotoxemic rats.[55] Activated protein C controls coagulation by proteolytically inactivating factors Va and VIIa. In sepsis conversion of protein C to the activated form is impaired by increased consumption of its cofactor protein S. Several processes during sepsis and inflammation have been associated with the reductions in endothelial-cell thrombomodulin and endothelial protein C receptor. These include down-regulation of transcription genes encoding these factors in response to cytokines and sepsis,[70] and enzymatic cleavage of protein C activation complex.[71] Thus, disruption of the activated protein C complex in sepsis is an early event that leads to widespread thrombosis and DIC, and may play a role in perpetuation of an uncontrolled inflammatory response. In severe sepsis the activities, besides activated protein C, of TF pathway inhibitor, antithrombin, and fibrinolysis are impaired, resulting in a procoagulant state.

Plasminogen activator inhibitor type I (PAI-1), a major inhibitor of the fibrinolytic system, has been implicated in the pathogenesis of sepsis. High circulating levels of PAI-1 are predictive of poor outcome in septic patients,[72] and polymorphism in the gene encoding PAI-1 influences the development of septic shock in patients with meningococcal sepsis.[73] However, experiments in gene knockout mice found that PAI-1 is essential for host defense against severe gram-negative pneumonia. Mice with deletion of PAI-1 had increased bacterial overgrowth and lethality, whereas, mice with transgenic overexpression of PAI-1 protected the animals against *Klebsiella* pneumonia, by promoting neutrophil recruitment to the pulmonary compartment.[74]

### 6.4.7 Complement System

The complement-activation pathways play integral roles in the immune defense against invading pathogens, and are therefore important in the pathogenesis of the sepsis syndrome. All the three major pathways and other neutrophil/macrophage-associated pathway can be activated in sepsis.[75] Activation of the classical pathway occurs after contact with IgG- and IgM-immune complexes and C-reactive protein, with interaction of the subunits of C 1 (qr and s). The lectin pathway involves interaction of MBL and mannose residue on bacterial surfaces, resulting in activations of MBL-associated serine protease complex. Both the classical and lectin pathways converge resulting in cleavage of C4 and C2, and generation of C3 convertase (C4b–C2a).[75] The alternative pathway is stimulated by bacterial LPS, interacting with C3b, factors B and D to subsequently generate C3 convertise. At this stage the three main pathways converge, resulting in generation of C3a fragment which is an anaphylatoxin that causes vasodilation and increased vascular permability.[75] The C3b fragment is an opsonic factor which combines with C3 convertase to form C5 convertase, which cleaves C5 into C5a and C5b. C5a is also an anaphylotoxin, whereas C5b interacts with C6, C7, C8, and C9 to form the membrane attack complex (C5b–C9). Another associated pathway involves cleavage of C5 by proteases from neutrophils and macrophages to generate C5a and other fragments.[75]

C5a enhances the innate immune response by interacting with a receptor (C5aR) on neutrophils, macrophages, and endothelial cells that leads to induction of localized, contained inflammation. Phagocytic cells (neutrophils and macrophages) ability to engulf and kill bacteria by release of granule enzyme and generation of superoxide anion is enhanced by contact with C5a.[76,77] C5a also induces chemotactic response of neutrophils and confer resistance to apoptosis.[78]

Although low and locally regulated concentrations of C5a have positive priming effects on neutrophils and macrophages, excessive generation of C5a, as occurs during sepsis, can have deleterious systemic effects.[75] Generation of large amounts of C3a and C5a in animals can cause circulatory failure, hypotension, and diffuse capillary leakage.[79] Relatively high levels (10–100 nM) of C5a in plasma can impair neutrophil function, stimulate macrophages and endothelial cells to produce excessive amounts of proinflammatory mediators, and generate prothrombotic activity that can lead to DIC.[75] Furthermore, increased levels of C5a can also induce activation of caspase 3 leading to apoptosis of thymocytes and probably lymphocytes.[80] In experimental animal models of sepsis blockade of C5a or C5aR (by specific antibody against C5a or C5aR antagonist) greatly improve survival in rodents from 20% to 70%.[81]

## 6.4.8 ARDS in Sepsis

Pulmonary dysfunction is very common in severe sepsis and almost 85% of these patients will require ventilatory support, typically for 7–14 days. Overall, sepsis is associated with the highest risk of progression to acute lung injury or ARDS ($\wedge$ 40%).[82] Although some of the deaths are attributable to ARDS the majority are due to sepsis itself and multiorgan failure. This illness has an early acute phase in all patients with ARDS, and a smaller variable fraction have a late (chronic) phase secondary to pulmonary fibrosis (rare in sepsis-induced ARDS). The acute early phase is characterized by the influx of protein-rich edema fluid into the airspace, due to increased permeability of the alveolar-capillary barrier.[82]

Although histologic studies and animal models implicate the sequestration and activation of neutrophils (releasing protease and oxygen radicals) as the main pathogenic mechanism in the acute lung injury, there is still some controversy. Patients with profound neutropenia and sepsis can also develop ARDS and some animal models of ARDS are neutrophils independent.[82] Furthermore, in clinical trials of severe infection patients receiving granulocyte colony-stimulating factor (G-CSF) did not have increased risk of ARDS, despite very high peripheral circulating neutrophils (40,000–70,000/mm$^3$).[83,84]

ARDS is an inflammatory disease with endothelial and epithelial injury, loss of epithelial integrity, increases alveolar-capillary permeability and development of hyaline membranes. It is very likely that there are multiple factors and pathways involved in the pathogenesis. Undoubtedly local and systemic hyperproduction of proinflammatory cytokines (or the imbalance of proinflammatory and anti-inflammatory cytokines) and disturbances of coagulation are important, leading to platelet-fibrin thrombi in small pulmonary vessels. Other factors that may contribute to ARDS include overdistension of alveoli from mechanical ventilation and disturbance in the production and function of surfactant.[82] Despite the undisputed role of inflammation in the development of ARDS, anti-inflammatory agents such as corticosteroids have not been beneficial in the early acute or later stage of the disease.[85,86]

The three main pathogenic processes of ARDS: unchecked inflammation, interstitial/alveolar protein accumulation, and destruction of pulmonary epithelial cells can be controlled by the up-regulation of the host's heat shock protein (HSP)-70.[86] Thus, the consequences of ARDS from severe sepsis may be due to a dysregulation or impaired expression in lungs of HSP-70. Administration of adenovirus vector containing HSP-70 cDNA driven by a cytomegalovirus (CMV) promoter in septic rats reduced pathological changes of ARDS and improved outcome by 50%.[87] The surprising aspect of this study is the improvement in mortality from amelioration of the ARDS, as patients with sepsis rarely die from ARDS but succumb to multiple organ dysfunction syndrome,[88] or recurrent sepsis. This suggests that the lung itself represents a motor of systemic inflammation that contributes significantly to the overall SIRS.[88] Another possibility is that generation of HSP-70 in the lungs produces a systemic protective effect on extra-pulmonary organ failure.

## 6.5 Management in Sepsis

Improvement in survival of patients with sepsis has been realized in recent years by a combination of factors: rapid institution of resuscitative measures and broad-spectrum antibiotics in the Emergency Department, and a multidisciplinary approach, are largely responsible for evident improved outcome. Consensus guidelines have been published by an international, multiorganization, multidisciplinary body – the "Surviving Sepsis Campaign" in 2004,[89] in an attempt to reduce the dismal morbidity and mortality from severe sepsis. The guidelines cover more than 50 aspects of care in the septic patient. The approach to antibiotic therapy was based on expert opinion and common sense rather than on controlled randomized trials.[90] The main body of these guidelines has focused on resuscitation and management "bundles" (core issues).

## 6.6 Early Goal-Directed Therapy

Early resuscitative measures before admission to the ICU in the Emergency Department or on the clinical units, is a key component of management of severe sepsis (to correct hypotension and lactic acidosis). An elevated serum lactate concentration can provide clues of tissue hypoperfusion even before overt hypotension. Management during the first 6 h of sepsis is the cornerstone of "early goal-directed therapy."

Previously, two large randomized controlled trials had shown that supranormal hemodynamic goals (maintaining high cardiac output and high oxygen delivery) at various stages of sepsis had no survival benefit.[91,92] A criticism of these earlier studies is that goal-directed hemodynamic optimization was started too late, usually when patients arrive in the ICUs. Moreover, besides initiating earlier goal-directed therapy within the "golden period" of opportunity the aims should be to attain more normal hemodynamic optimization, rather than supranormal parameters. Furthermore, reliance on early hemodynamic assessment on physical findings, vital signs, central venous pressure, and urinary output may fail to detect persistent tissue hypoxia.[93,94] A more definitive early resuscitation strategy to achieve a balance between systemic oxygen delivery and oxygen demand, using a goal-orientated manipulation of cardiac preload, afterload, and contractility has been proposed and tested. Resuscitation end points used in a previous trial of early-goal-directed therapy by Rivers et al.,[95] include normalization of mixed venous oxygen saturation (central venous oxygen saturation $\geq 70\%$ by continuous monitoring), arterial lactate concentration, base deficit, and pH. Crystalloids in 500 ml bolus was given every 30 min to achieve a central venous pressure of 8–12 mmHg; and vasopressors given to maintain a mean arterial pressure of 65–90 mmHg; and urine output maintained $\geq 0.5$ ml/kg/h (similar parameters as standard are). Transfusion of blood was used to maintain a hematocrit of $\geq 30\%$ (equivalent to hemoglobin 10 g/dl).

In the randomized trial by Rivers et al.,[95] 263 patients with severe sepsis and septic shock were enrolled, with 130 assigned early-goal-directed therapy and 133 to standard therapy. During the first 72 h, the patients assigned to early-goal directed therapy had significantly higher mean central venous oxygen saturation (70.4% vs 65.3%), a lower lactate concentration (3.0 vs 3.9 mmol/l), a lower base deficit (2.0 vs 5.1 mmol/l), and a higher pH (7.4 vs 7.36). In-hospital mortality was lower in the early goal-directed therapy (46.5% vs 30.5%, $p = 0.009$); 28-day mortality (49.2% vs 33.3%, $p = 0.01$); and 60-day mortality (56.9% vs 44.3%, $p = 0.03$) were also significantly lower.[95] However, multiorgan failure between the groups was not significantly different (21.8% vs 16.2%, $p = 0.27$). Although early-goal-directed therapy is considered standard for severe sepsis and septic shock at present, this approach is based on a relatively small number of patients from a single randomized, control trial. Moreover, in a national survey of 100 emergency departments in the US, multiple barriers to time-sensitive resuscitation of septic patients existed in more than half the respondents (due to shortage of nursing staff and central venous pressure monitoring availability).[96] In another survey in England, of the 78 emergency departments responding as of March 2006, only 18.5% initiated early goal-directed-therapy and a further 10% were about to initiate the protocol.[97]

## 6.7 Antimicrobial Therapy in Severe Sepsis

There is no specific antibiotic regimen of choice for sepsis or septic shock, nor randomized comparative trials to address this issue. Choice of antibiotics should be chosen according to likely microorganisms responsible for each individual setting. For instance, community-acquired versus hospital-acquired; site or source of

## 6.7 Antimicrobial Therapy in Severe Sepsis

infection – i.e. pneumonia, urinary tract, intraabdominal, or intravascular catheter. In general, community-acquired infections are usually more susceptible to standard antibiotics except in those on previous antibiotics, prolonged urethral, or intravascular catheters with multiple healthcare unit exposure. It is important to take into consideration the local epidemiology of the types of microorganisms causing sepsis, and the resistance pattern in each individual hospital, ICU, city, or region before selecting appropriate empiric therapy.

Although international and mulitcenter studies provide useful insight on the microbial patterns and level of antimicrobial resistance there is tremendous variation at the national and local level.[98] This is exemplified by the wide geographic variation in the incidence of community-acquired MRSA infection between cities and countries. Even in hospitals that are geographically close different spectra of microorganisms and different patterns of antibiotic resistance may exist in ICUs, due to differences in case loads and antibiotic practices.[99]

Current guidelines recommend rapid institution of broad-spectrum antibiotics to cover the most likely pathogen in the given clinical scenario. There is reasonably good data to indicate that prompt administration of appropriate antibiotics is important in modifying the outcome in severe sepsis (based largely on review of observational literature reports).[100] The effect of initial antimicrobial choice and results of microbial cultures in 904 patients with conformed severe sepsis or early septic shock was analyzed from a prospective multicenter trial of an immunomodulating agent.[101] The 28-day mortality was 24% (168/693) for patients adequately treated, versus 39% (82/211) for those receiving inappropriate antimicrobial therapy ($p < 0.001$). A more recent prospective (nonrandomized) study assessed the benefit of appropriate empiric antibiotic therapy in 920 patients with documented sepsis from three medical centers in Israel, Italy, and Germany.[102] In this study the mortality rate were 20.1% (64/319) and 11.8% (68/576) for patients receiving inappropriate empiric therapy and appropriate therapy, respectively ($p = 0.001$). Presumably, patients receiving initial inappropriate therapy would be switched to susceptibility-directed therapy, results of which are usually available after 2–4 days. Similar results were reported from a randomized, controlled sepsis (MONARS) trial subgroup analysis of 2,634 patients (as part of the monoclonal anti-TNF trial.[103] Mortality rate among adequately treated patient was 33% versus 43% in those initially inadequately treated ($p < 0.001$). These three prospective studies indicate that rapid institution of appropriate antibiotics results in improved outcome (38–41% improvement), but delaying appropriate therapy for 2–3 days (pending culture and susceptibility) still result in a 60–80% survival in patients with sepsis. Recent reports, however suggests that, outcome with delayed appropriate antibiotic treatment for bacteremias may be organism dependent. In a cohort of 215 patients with *S. aureus* bacteremia from Taiwan (30 with community-acquired MRSA) there was no significant difference in 30-day mortality between methicillin-sensitive *S. aureus* or MRSA infection, even though most patients (83%) with MRSA bacteremia did not receive initial appropriate therapy within the first 48 h.[104] On the other extreme, outcomes of *Pseudomonas aeruginosa* bacteremia with relatively reduced susceptibility to piperacillin-tazbactam is markedly reduced compared to those infected with highly susceptible strains treated with the same agent.[105] In this retrospective cohort the 30-day mortality rate was 85.7% (6/7) in patients treated with piperacillin-tazobactam with MIC 32–64 mg/l (considered susceptible by the Clinical Laboratory Standards Institute, ≤64 mg/l), but only 30% in those whose organisms were more susceptible (≤16 mg/l) treated with the same antibiotic ($N =$ 10).[104] This small study suggest that the resistance breakpoint for piperacillin-tazobactam should be reduced to >16 mg/l, more in line with the British Society of Antimicrobial Chemotherapy guidelines.[105] Perhaps the most convincing data on relationship between delay in the initiation of effective antimicrobial therapy and mortality was recently reported from a large retrospective cohort of septic chock in adults.[106] In a multicenter study 2,731 patients with septic shock were evaluated, 77.9% of whom had documented infection, and the mortality rate of the entire cohort was 56.2% (higher than recent reports). The median time for initiation of effective antibiotic after identification of recurrent/persistent hypotension was 6 h. In multivariate analysis (including APACHE II score), time to initiation of effective antimicrobial therapy was the single strongest predictor of outcome.[106] Administration of an effective antibiotic within the 1st hour of documented hypotension was associated with a survival rate of 79.9%. Each hour of delay in antimicrobial administration over the ensuing 6 h was associated with an average decrease in survival of 7.6%. In this large cohort collected between 1989 and 2004, only 50% of septic shock patients received effective antibiotic therapy within 6 h of documented hypotension. Although the major limitation of this important study is the retrospective design and, thus, the accuracy of the timing of therapy in relationship to documented shock, current guidelines is to initiate antibiotic therapy immediately after onset of shock or before in suspected severe sepsis. The implications of this study would be more compelling and robust if the data were collected prospectively.

It has been generally recommended to reassess and modify antimicrobial therapy after 2–3 days according to microbiological results and susceptibility, and to step down to a narrow spectrum, less toxic and less expensive agent to reduce resistance, toxicity, and cost. There is no evidence that this strategy is detrimental to the patients' well being. Empirical antifungal therapy should not be used on a routine basis for severe sepsis or septic shock, but may be considered for selected patients with high risk for invasive candidiasis and for high clinical suspicion.[100] Besides specific treatment directed at likely pathogens, source control or eradication is important to control the infection by drainage of abscesses or infected fluid collections and debridement of necrotic tissue. Although this approach is highly logical the evidence to support these recommendations are based on observational data and thus lower tier.[107]

## 6.8 Activated Protein C

Recombinant human activated protein C (drotrecogin alpha) is an anti-inflammatory, antithrombotic, profibrinolytic treatment for specific pathophysiologic derangements in severe sepsis. Experimented studies in sepsis models indicate that activated protein C (APC) has direct anti-inflammatory effect at a cellular level. In a sepsis microcirculation model APC effectively reduced leucocyte rolling and leucocyte firm adhesion in systemic endotoxemia, but the action was unlikely to be related or caused by thrombin inhibition-associated anticoaguatory mechanism.[108] Recombinant APC was approved by the US Food and Drug Administration (FDA) for treatment of patients with severe sepsis, based on the 19.4% reduction in the relative risk of death (absolute risk reduction of 6.1%) found in the PROWESS study.[109] In a post hoc analysis performed by the FDA, the benefit of APC was restricted to the more severely ill patients (APACHE II score of 25 or more or with $\geq 2$ organ dysfunction). A subsequent randomized trial (ADDRESS) showed no significant benefit of APC in patients with severe sepsis and low risk of death.[110] The cost of APC per therapeutic course was $6800(US) in 2002, and an economic evaluation estimated that it was cost-effective to treat severely septic patients with an APACHE II score of $\geq 25$ ($24,484 per life-year gained[111]). Although APC can result in excessive bleeding sepsis results in a procoagulant state which may predispose to thromboembolic and ischemic conditions. Hence heparin thromboprophylaxis is still required. In a recent multicenter randomized, blinded, control trial with all patients receiving APC, 493 were given subcutaneous enoxaparin prophylaxis and 990 were given placebo.[112] Patients receiving heparin prophylaxis had no greater risk of bleeding but had lower risk of ischemic stroke (71% relative risk reduction) lower venous thromboembolism (1.2% absolute risk reduction) and lower mortality (3.6% absolute risk reduction), not statistically significant.[112]

## 6.9 Corticosteroids in Severe Sepsis

Controversy on the value of corticosteroids for the management of severe sepsis (septic shock) has existed for several decades. The pendulum of consensus for using corticosteroids in severe sepsis has swing back and forth over this time. Previous trials have shown that early, short course (48 h) of high-dose corticosteroids did not improve the outcome in severe sepsis.[113] Renewed interest in lower-dose corticosteroids for stress-induced relative adrenal insufficiency (secondary to severe sepsis) has been in vogue for the past 5 years. This was based on initially two (of five) small randomized, controlled trials showing that relatively low-dose hydrocortisone decreased the need for vasopressor support for septic patients.[114,115] An adequately powered study by Annare et al.[116] ($N = 300$) subsequently showed that hydrocortisone plus fludrocortisone for 7 days significantly improved survival in septic shock syndrome in patients with inadequate response to 250 μg corticotrophin-stimulation test.[116] However, the concept of relative adrenal insufficiency in sepsis and the criteria for this diagnosis has been controversial. Furthermore, total serum corticosal does not reflect the unbound free cortisol (the physiologically active form), and critically ill patients with hypoalbuminemia commonly have high free serum cortisol but low total cortisol levels after corticotrophin-stimulation.[117]

In a more recent larger multicenter, randomized, double-blind trial of 499 patients with septic shock, hydrocortisone (50 mg every 6 h for 5 days) did not improve survival or reversal of shock.[118] Of the total cohort 233 (46.7%) did not respond to corticotrophin (125 in the hydrocortisone group and 108 in the placebo group). At 28 days, there was no difference in survival between the two study groups with "relative adrenal insufficiency" (mortality rate 39.2% vs 36.1%).[118] Thus this somewhat larger study did not support use of low-dose corticosteroids or routine corticotrophin testing in severe sepsis. However, the sample size is too small to even show a relative reduction of 15–20% in mortality from a baseline of 35%, which would require a trial of at least 2,600 patients.[119] Whether such a large daunting trial should be undertaken is open for debate. At present corticosteroids and corticotrophin test should not be routinely used in the management of severe sepsis or septic shock.

## 6.10 Intensive Insulin Therapy

Intensive insulin therapy to maintain strict glycemic control (even in non-diabetics) have been advocated for the management of severe sepsis.[89] This was based on a study by Van den Berghe et al.[120] involving critically ill surgical patients, which showed that strict euglycemia (4.4–6.1 mmol/l or 80–10 mg/dl) resulted in lower in-hospital mortality from 10.9% to 7.2%, mainly by reducing deaths from multiple organ failure in septic patients. In this study of 1,548 patients over 12 months intensive insulin therapy reduced mortality exclusively in the long-stay cohort (10.6% mortality vs 20.2%, $p = 0.005$). The strict glycemic control in this trial not only reduced overall in-hospital mortality by 34%, but also bloodstream infections by 46%, severe acute renal failure requiring dialysis by 41%, reduction in median number of blood transfusions by 50%, and critical illness polyneuropathy by 44%.[120] The mechanisms by which intensive insulin therapy could achieve such remarkable results were not clear, unless hyperglycemia or insulin resistance play a major role in the pathophysiology of these complications.

A recent trial confined to patients with severe sepsis ($N = 537$) did not confirm the extraordinary benefit with intensive insulin therapy.[121] At 28 days there was no significant difference between conventional and intensive insulin therapy in mortality or organ failure, but significantly higher rate of severe hypoglycemia (17.0% vs 4.1%, $p < 0.001$). This study also assessed the value of colloid (10% pentastarch, a low molecular-weight hydroxyethyl starch) compared to crystalloid (modified Ringer's lactate) for fluid resuscitation. The colloid used in this study appeared to be harmful, with greater risk of renal impairment at recommended doses, and impairment of long-term survival at high doses.[121] Thus, neither intensive insulin therapy nor colloid should be used in the management of severe sepsis and septic shock.

## 6.11 Vasopressin and Vasopressors

Persistent hypotension after infusion of crystalloids in septic shock is generally treated with vasopressors such as dopamine, dobutamine, adrenaline, noradrenaline, and vasopressin (as recommended by guidelines). It is unclear if there is a vasopressor of choice for the treatment of septic shock or for the treatment of shock in general. In a systematic review of eight randomized controlled trials (RCT) comparing various vasopressors, there was inadequate evidence to determine superiority of any one vasopressor to other agents in the treatment of states of shock.[122] In contradiction a recent recommendation, supposedly on the basis of an evidence-based review, maintain that norepinephrine or dopamine is the vasopressor of choice in the treatment of septic shock.[123] Norepinephrine may be combined with dobutamine when cardiac output is being measured. Epinephrine, phenylephrine, and vasopressin were not recommended as first-line agents in the treatment of septic shock. Vasopressin may be considered for salvage therapy, and low-dose dopamine was not recommended for the purpose of renal protection. Dobutamine was recommended as the agent of choice to increase cardiac output to physiological levels.[123]

Vasopressin is an endogenously released stress hormone that is important in shock, and there is a deficiency of vasopressin in patients with septic shock.[124] Low-dose vasopressin is widely used in septic shock based largely on observational studies,[125] and on the postulate that vasopressin administration can restore vascular tone and blood pressure, thus reducing the need for the use of catecholamines. In a recent multicenter, randomized, double-blind trial of 778 patients with septic shock low-dose vasopressin (0.01–0.03 u/minute) or norepinephrine (5–15 µg/minute) in addition to open-label vasopressors were compared.[126] There was no significant difference in the 28-day mortality rate (35.4% and 39.3%, $p = 0.26$) or 90-day mortality (43.9% and 49.6%, respectively; $p = 0.11$. In patients with less severe shock the mortality rate was lower in the vasopressin group than in the norepinephrine group at 28 days (26.5% vs 35.7%, $p = 0.05$), but no difference was noted in those with severe septic shock.[126] The statistical difference in the subgroup with less severe shock should be considered as hypothesis-generating concept to be confirmed by larger trials in subjects with less severe septic shock.

## 6.12 Blood Products in Sepsis

Anemia is common in critically ill patients, especially in those with severe sepsis. This may be due to a combination of factors including hemolysis from DIC, poor utilization of iron in the reticuloendothelial system secondary to inflammatory mediators, bleeding tendency from stress ulceration of the stomach and thrombocytopenia, as well as decreased generation of erythropoietin from decreased expression of the erythropoietin gene and protein mediated by TNF-$\alpha$ and 1L-1$\beta$.[127] The indications for blood transfusion in the critically ill patients are somewhat controversial, as there is evidence that blood transfusion can be immunosuppressive. Furthermore some studies suggest that liberal blood transfusion in these critically ill patients may worsen the outcome. Rivers et al.[95] as part of the 6 h early goal-directed-therapy recommended a hemacrit of 30% (corresponding to hemoglobin value of about 10 g/dl), as threshold for blood transfusion. However, a previously randomized controlled, multicenter study on transfusion requirements in critically ill patients with hemoglobin <9 g/dl, compared liberal transfusion with hemoglobin <10 g/dl to restrictive transfusion below hemoglobin 7.0 g/dl to maintain up to 9 g/dl.[128] The overall 30-day mortality was similar between the two groups. The mortality rate during hospitalization was significantly lower in the restrictive-strategy groups (5.7% vs 13.0%, $p = 0.02$), as well as in subgroups with less acute illness, and under 55 years of age.[128] Restrictive use of blood transfusion was thus least as effective and possible better to liberal red-cell transfusion, except for patients with acute myocardial infarction and unstable angina. This latter study however, was not specially addressing anemia in severe sepsis. Although Rivers et al.[95] noted marked decrease in mortality when transfusion was provided early (within 6 h) of severe sepsis, this was not the primary intervention of the study.

More recently a large multicenter, observational study was conducted in 198 European ICUs to assess the effect of blood transfusion and mortality in a cohort of 3,147 critically ill patients, 1,040 (33.0%) received a blood transfusion.[129] Although there was a direct relationship between number of blood transfusions and the mortality rate, after multivariate analysis and adjustment for confounding variables, blood transfusion itself was not significantly associated with a worse outcome.[129]

A systemic review of use of blood products in sepsis in 2004[130] concluded that blood transfusion should be targeted to maintain hemoglobin at 7.0–9.0 g/dl; that erythropoietin is not recommended for sepsis associated anemia; fresh-frozen plasma should be given for documented deficiency of coagulation factors in the presence of active bleeding or before surgical procedures. Although erythropoietin decreases transfusion requirements there is no evidence of improved survival in a RCT in patients with severe sepsis or critical illness.[130] High-dose antithrombin-III is also not recommended based on a large RCT which failed to show improved survival in patients with severe sepsis.[131] However, reanalysis of the data in patients with high risk of death (30–60%, showed lower mortality in the antithrombin-III group versus placebo at day-90 ($p = 0.04$).[132] Thus more studies are needed to confirm this effect in sicker patients, similar to the observation with activated protein C.

## 6.13 Ventilation and Other Adjunctive Therapy

Mechanical ventilation is a critical component of the management strategy in severe sepsis and acute lung injury or ARDS is a common complication. Lung protection strategy (use of relatively low tidal volumes) is an important component of the overall ventilation management. There is evidence from RCTs that small tidal volume ventilation decreases mortality in patients with ARDS,[133] and is beneficial in acute lung injury in septic patients.[134] In a review on mechanical ventilation in sepsis-induced lung injury it was also recommended that a minimum amount of positive end-expiratory pressure should be maintained to prevent lung collapse.[135] Prone positioning should be considered in those with severe ARDS, but the role of high-frequency oscillatory ventilation and airway pressure release ventilation in ARDS was uncertain.[135] Unfortunately the ideal fluid management strategy in ARDS is unknown.

Acute renal failure occurs in approximately 19% of patients with moderate sepsis, 23% with severe sepsis, and 51% with septic shock.[136,137] The combination of acute renal failure and sepsis is associated with a higher mortality (up to 70%) than sepsis without renal failure (35–45% mortality).[37] The mechanism for renal failure in sepsis is probably multifactorial. Early in sepsis as arterial vasodilatation occurs, it results in renal sympathetic and angiotensin activities leading to renal vasoconstriction with sodium and water retention.[37] Renal perfusion is then further compromised by systemic hypotension, intravascular hypovolemia, diffuse coagulapathy (DIC) with subsequent acute tubular necrosis. Patients with sepsis and acute renal failure are hypercatabolic and studies suggest that increased duration and frequency of dialysis can improve survival. A recent study showed that daily hemodialysis as compared to alternate-day hemodialysis was associated with less systemic inflammatory response of sepsis (22% vs 46%, $p < 0.01$), lower mortality (28% vs 46%, $p < 0.01$) and a shorter duration of acute renal failure/mean $\pm$ SD, $9 \pm 2$ vs $16 \pm 6$ days, $p = 0.001$).[138]

Continuous renal replacement therapy by veno-venous hemofiltration is becoming more popular for the management of acute renal failure in sepsis. However, there is no definite proof of its superiority over hemodialysis.[37] There is evidence, however, that in patients with sepsis-related acute renal failure, better survival was achieved with aggressive ultrafiltration rate of 45 ml/kg/h than with a rate of 35 ml/kg/h.[139]

## 6.14 Immunotherapies for Sepsis

Polyvalent intravenous immunoglobulins (IVIG) modulate the expression and function of FC receptors, activation of complement and cytokine networks, production of idiotype antibodies, and activation, differentiation, and effector functions of T and B cells[140]; thus, could be beneficial in severe sepsis. However, small RCT of an adjunctive IVIG in bacterial sepsis has shown conflicting results. Two recent systematic reviews and meta-analysis of the value of IVIG in sepsis have arrived at different conclusions. In a review by Paldal and Gotzche,[141] the meta-analysis of all trials showed a relative risk of death with IVIG of 0.77 (95% CF, 0.68–0.88). High-quality trials, however, showed no significant survival benefit, whereas other less stringent trials showed a relative risk of death of 0.61 (95% CI, 0.5–0.73). Since high-quality trials failed to demonstrate a reduction in mortality, IVIG was not recommended for treatment of sepsis[141]. A more recent review and meta-analysis analyzed 20 RCT (*n* = 2,621) and found an overall survived benefit with IVIG (risk ratio 0.74 (95% CI, 0.62–0.89)). The benefit was greatest for those with severe sepsis or septic shock (risk ratio 0.64, CI 0.52–0.79), receiving a total dose of $\geq 1$ g/kg for >2 days.[142] A large randomized trial of IVIG was recommended by the authors. However, a sensitivity analysis on high-quality trials found no evidence that IVIG was beneficial in severe sepsis,[143] similar to Rildal and Gotzche[141] results.

In a recent multicenter, relatively large RCT (*n* = 653) of (score defined severity) septic patients there was no significant reduction of mortality with IVIG vs placebo at 7 or 28 days (39.3% vs 37.3%, respectively).[144] Although exploratory finding revealed a 3-day shortening of mechanical ventilation in the surviving patients, IVIG did not improve the 4-day pulmonary function, and had no effect on plasma levels of IL-6 and TNF-receptors I and II.[144] Thus, IVIG at the dose used 10.9 g/kg total dose) does not appear beneficial in severe sepsis.

Granulocyte-colony-stimulating factor (G-CSF) besides its role on granulopoiesis enhances many functions of mature granulocytes such as chemotaxis, phagocytosis, and microbicidal and oxidative activity. G-CSF seems to combine its proinflammatory effects on several granulocyte function but with anti-inflammatory effects on mononuclear cells.[54] G-CSF exerts its anti-inflammatory effects on monocytes by lowering the release of proinflammatory cytokines and increasing the release of anti-inflammatory mediators. There have a few small RCTs of G-CSF in non-neutropenic patients with sepsis. In one of the larger RCT of hospitalized patients with multilobar pneumonia (*n* = 480), there was no survival benefit with G-CSF but a trend to reduced mortality was noted in patients with pneumococcal bacteremia.[83] In a small RCT of 44 preterm neonates with clinical diagnosis of early-onset sepsis, G-CSF did not affect mortality but reduced the incidence of secondary nosocomial infections.[84] The clinical benefit of future immunotherapy should be defined by large multicenter RCT utilizing INF-γ and GM-CSF as these drugs might correct the immunoparalysis seen in late severe sepsis.

## 6.15 Genetics and Sepsis

Wide variability exists in the susceptibility to and outcome from sepsis even within similar cohorts matched for age and comorbid illnesses. Some of this variability may be due to genetic variation (polymorphisms) in genes encoding components of the innate immune response. Although experimental models have provided insight on the effects of these genetic polymorphisms in sepsis, there are disparate results observed in many studies of polymorphisms and sepsis outcome in humans.[145] Polymorphisms in genes encoding proteins involved in the recognition of bacterial pathogens (TLR-4, CD14, MBL, Fc(gamma) RIIIa) and the response to bacterial pathogens (TNF-α, IL-1α and β, IL-1R agonist, IL-6, IL-10, HSPs, ACE-1, and PAI-1) could all potentially influence the manifestation and outcome of sepsis. In a review of clinical studies on two candidate genes, TNF-α and $TLR_4$, studies examining the relationships between single nucleotide polymorphisms (SNPs) and sepsis risk and outcome have found, inconsistencies in the literature.[146] The main limitations relate to the translation of experimental observations into reproducible genotype–phenotype associations. The reasons for these deficiencies are mainly due to insufficient sample size because of the complexities and multifactorial nature of the predisposing and prognostic variables as well as the background genetic heterogeneity.[146]

The complexity of genetic predisposition to sepsis is compounded by the many interacting pathways involved in the sepsis syndrome. Not only genetic variations in genes encoding the innate immune response and the inflammatory cascade that need to be considered, but also polymorphisms of genes regulating the coagulation and fibrinolytic systems, and ARDS need to be included. For instance, deletion polymorphism, within the promoter region of the plasminogen-activator inhibitor-1 gene leads to impaired fibrinolysis and influences the severity and outcome of meningococcal disease and susceptibility to severe sepsis.[147] Also factor V Leiden mutation (associated with thrombotic events) can exacerbate purpura fulminans in meningococcal sepsis, but can provide survival advantage in severe sepsis.[147]

Another genetic factor that could be useful as a predictor of clinical outcome for patients with sepsis is the HLA-DR antigen expression on monocytes which reflects the individual's immune status.[148] Reports suggest that long-term sharp declines in HLA-DR antigen expression on monocytes corresponds to the level of immunoparalysis and reflects a poor outcome.

In the future it is predicted that therapeutic trials and actual treatment regimens for patients with sepsis are likely to be designed to target specific genotypes and associated cellular responses, to maximize clinical response and patient safety.[149] However, we are many years away from achieving this goal of individualized targeted treatment. To confirm the predictive value of multiple allelic variants and risk for severe sepsis will require large population based studies of thousands of subjects; and to assess prognostic outcome will need several hundreds of septic patients in trials.

## 6.16 Future Directions

Although our understanding of the pathogenesis of the sepsis syndrome has increased remarkably in the past 2 years, the advances in new therapeutics have been disappointing. In the past 2 decades numerous promising immunomodulatory agents have been tested in clinical trials (see Table 6.1) but only one has proven but limited value (activated proteins C). There are several biological agents which appears very promising in experimental models that need to be tested in large clinical trials (see Table 6.2). However, it is unclear and somewhat dubious that any of these agents will be of proven clinical value to be used in the future for the management of severe sepsis. Even if one or more of these biologics prove to be effective in RCT, it would take several years for approval for marketing and they would likely be very expensive with limited indications for specific subgroups.

**Table 6.1** Immunomodulatory agents tested in sepsis in clinical trials (Data compiled from [55, 118, 144, 152, 153, 154])

| Anti-inflammatory agents | Comments |
| --- | --- |
| • Glucocorticoid (high and low dose) | No proven benefit |
| • TNFα antibodies | Mixed results |
| • Recombinant Type I & II soluble (TNFα) receptors | No survival benefit |
| • Recombinant 1L-1Ra | No survival benefit |
| • Platelet activity factor antagonist | No survival benefit |
| • Bradykinin inhibitor | No survival benefit |
| • Ibuprofen | No survival benefit |
| *Anti-Endotoxin compounds* | |
| • Endotoxin antiserum | No survival benefit |
| • Endotoxin monoclonal antibody | No survival benefit |
| • Recombinant bactericidal/permeability-increasing protein | Improved morbidity but not survival; further studies needed |
| *Immunostimulatory agents* | |
| • Granulocyte colony-stimulating factor (G-CSF) | No benefit in larger trials |
| • Macrophage-granulocyte-CSF | Needs larger trials |
| • Intravenous immunoglobulin | No proven benefit |
| *Anticoagulation agents* | |
| • Activated Protein C | Some improved survival in poor risk |
| • Antithrombin III | Overall no survival benefit, potential benefit in poor risk |
| • Tissue factor pathway inhibitor | No improvement |

Drugs currently approved for other medical conditions have been proposed as novel therapies for the sepsis syndrome and are inexpensive. These include the statins (HMG-CoA reductase inhibitors), which alter the lipid metabolism and also have anti-inflammatory activity, and have proven benefits in many diseases involving vascular inflammation and injury. Recent animal experiments suggest that the statins may reduce morbidity and mortality in sepsis, when administered before the insult.[150] The pleiotropic effects of statins as anti-inflammatory and immunomodulatory agents lend support to the potential for these agents as new therapy for prevention or treatment of severe sepsis. However, many therapeutic interventions, shown effective in animal experiments when administered before onset of sepsis, are not effective in the clinical settings of sepsis syndrome. Although large well-designed randomized, blinded trials should be undertaken with statins for sepsis, it would best be tested in critically ill (high risk) patients even before the onset of sepsis (similar to trials of prophylactic heparin).

**Table 6.2** Potential new therapies for sepsis (Compiled from data obtained from [23, 24, 26, 58, 81, 155–159])

| Agent | Comments |
|---|---|
| • Interferon-gamma | Restore monocyte function, counter late immune paralysis |
| • 1C14 ($CD_{14}$ monoclonal antibody) | Suppresses inflammatory response to endotoxin |
| • C5a antibodies | Restores neutrophils function |
| • CD40-receptor monoclonal antibodies | Decreases lymphocyte apoptosis |
| • Anti-HMGB1 antibodies | Inhibit systemic inflammation |
| • Anti-macrophage migration inhibitory factor (MIF) antibodies | Suppresses inflammatory reaction |
| • Ethyl pyruvate | Anti-inflammatory effect |
| • ClinHibitor (CIINH) | Interacts with endotoxin to modify inflammation |
| • Antioxidants | Counter-free radicals (i.e., reactive oxygen and nitrogen species) |

HMGB1 = high mobility group box-1

Another group of agents, thiazolidinediones, now in use for diabetes mellitus may also have therapeutic benefit in the septic patients.[151] Peroxisome proliferator-activator receptor-gamma (PPARγ) is a member of the nuclear receptor superfamily and a ligand-activated transcription factor with pleiotropic effects on lipid metabolism, inflammation, and cell proliferation. The thiazolidinediones (pioglitazone, rosiglitazone, troglitazone, and ciglitazone) are synthetic PPARγ agonists used mainly as insulin-sensitizing drugs. There are several in vitro and in vivo studies that have demonstrated that these agents may be useful in sepsis and inflamation.[151] Thus large clinical trials are warranted in critically ill patients with high risk of sepsis, early or before the event, with these agents.

It should not be surprising that any one biologic agent acting on a single pathway in the complex multisystem pathway process of sepsis should fail (i.e., anti-TNF antibodies). Although excessive production of a molecule (proinflammatory cytokine) may be harmful, blockage will often be harmful as well as these substances serve a useful purpose. Hence we should consider the sepsis syndrome in a different perspective, liken to a polyendocrine acute disorder (without the luxury of time), where we need to achieve a "normal balance" of inflammatory and anti-inflammatory and immune mediators. The distance in the future seems to be far (many years from now), when we can simply do a blood test to determine which mediator(s) need suppression and which needs replacement.

A promising approach for treatment of severe sepsis is a combination of immunomodulatory agents, thymosin α1 (a naturally occurring thymic peptide to augment T cell function) combined with ulinastatin (a Kunitz-type protease inhibitor found in urine) that can control a series of proinflammatory mediators and cytokines.[160] In a preliminary prospective randomized trial of 120 patients with sepsis caused by carbapenem resistant intra-abdominal infection, 60 patients received the combination study agents and the others placebo. Although there was only a trend in improved survival (due to small sample size) on day 28, there was significantly greater survival in the immunomodulatory group vs control at 60 and 90 days ($p = 0.033$).[160] Moreover, the treated study group had significantly shorter duration of mechanical ventilation and ICI stay ($p < 0.001$), and a lower incidence of shock compared to control group ($p = 0.026$). Another intriguing approach would be to combine immunomodulators with anticholinergic agents to block α 7 cholinergic receptors, as there is evidence in a murine model of intra-abdominal sepsis that deficiency of α 7 receptor is associated strongly with increased clearance of coliform bacteria and reduced dissemination.[161] The α 7 cholinergic receptors are key to anti-inflammatory cell signaling induced by acetylcholine and the cholinergic anti-inflammatory pathway.

## 6.17 Conclusion

Sepsis syndrome still carries a high mortality in high-risk patients with organ(s) dysfunction. The pathogenic mechanism is extremely complex and involves several interacting pathways and networks. The end result is dysregulation of the inflammatory and immunomodulatory systems. A new sepsis classification known as "PIRO" has been proposed. PIRO stands for predisposition, infection, response, and organ dysfunction.[162] It is hoped that this system will facilitate better understanding and improved therapeutic interventions for sepsis, but this is doubtful. The evidence suggests that early recognition and early intervention (immediate appropriate antibiotics and early-goal-directed therapy) are most important in affecting outcome. A recent national educational effort to promote bundles of care (a resuscitator tasks to begin immediately and be accomplished within 6 h; and a management bundle – four tasks completed within 24 h), for severe sepsis and septic shock in Spain was associated with improved guideline compliance and lower hospital mortality.[163] However, compliance rates were still low and the improvement in the resuscitation bundle lapsed by 1 year.

## References

1. Angus, D.C., Linde-Zwirble, W.T., Lidicker, J., Clermont, G., Carcillo, J., Pinsky, M.R., (2001), Epidemiology of severe sepsis in the United States: analysis of incidence, outcome, and associated costs of care. Crit. Care Med. 29: 1303–1310.
2. Murphy, S.L., (2000), Deaths: final statistics for 1998. National vital statistics report. Vol. 48., No 11. National Center for Helath Statistics: Hyattsville, MD (DHHS publication no. (PH5) 2000-11200-0487).
3. Center for Disease Control, (1990), Increase in national hospital discharge survey rates for septicemia – United States, 1979–1987. JAMA 269: 937–938.
4. Rivers, E.P., Nguyen, H.B., Huang, D.T., Donnino, M.W., (2002), Critical care and emergency medicine. Curr. Opin. Crit. Care 8: 600–606.

# References

5. McIntyre, L.A., Herbert, P.C., Cook, D.J., Magder, S., Dhingra, V., Bell, D.R., (2003), Are delays in the recognition and initial management of patients with severe sepsis associated with hospital mortality? Crit. Care Med. 31 (12 Suppl.): A75.
6. Martin, G.S., Mannino, D.M., Eaton, S., Moss, M., (2003), The epidemiology of sepsis in the United States from 1979 through 2000. NEJM 348: 1546–1654.
7. Burchardi, H., Schneider, H., (2004), Economic aspects of severe sepsis. A review of intensive care unit costs, cost of illness and cost effectiveness of therapy. Pharmacoeconomics 22: 793–813.
8. Bone, R.C., Balk, R.A., Cerra, F.B., Dellinger, R.P., Fein, A.M., Krans, W.A., Schein, R.M., Sibba Ld, W.J., (1992), Definition for sepsis and organ failure and guidelines for the use of innovative therapies in sepsis. The ACCP/SCCM consensus conference committee, American College of Chest Physicians/Society of Critical Care Medicine. Chest 101: 1656–1662.
9. Levy, M.M., Fink, M.P., Marshall, J.C., Abraham, E., Angus, D., Cook, D., Cohen, J., Opal, S. M., Vincent, J.L., Ramsey, G., International Sepsis Definition Conference, (2003), 2001 SCCM/ESICM/ACCP/ATS/SIS International Sepsis Definition Conference. Int. Care Med. 29: 530–538.
10. Medzhitov, R., Janeway, C. Jr., (2000), Innate Immunity (Advances in Immunology). N. Engl. J. Med 343: 338–344.
11. Epstein, J., Eichbaum, Q., Sheriff, S., Ezckowitz, R.A., (1996), The collectins in innate immunity. Curr. Opin. Immunol. 8: 29–35.
12. Fraser, I.P., Koziel, H., Ezekowitz, R.A., (1998), The serum mannose-binding protein and the macrophage mannose receptor are pattern recognition molecules that link innate and adaptive immunity. Semin. Immunol. 10: 363–372.
13. Thomas, C.A., Li, Y., Kodama, T., Suzuki, H., Silverstein, S.C., EL Khoury, J., (2000), Protection from lethal gram-positive infection by macrophage scavenger receptor-dependent phagocytosis. J. Exp. Med. 191: 147–156.
14. Mizgerd, J.P., (2008), (Mechanisms of disease) Acute lower respiratory tract infection. NEJM 358: 716–727.
15. Bochud, P.Y., Calandra, T., (2003), Pathogenesis of sepsis. New concepts and implications for future treatment. BMJ 326: 262–264.
16. Dessing, M.C., Schoiuten, M., Draing, C., Levi, M., von Aulock, S., van der Poll, T., (2008), Role played by toll-like receptors 2 and 4 in lipoteichoic acid-induced lung inflammation and coagulation. J. Infect. Dis. 197: 245–252.
17. Drenth, J.P.H., van der Meer, J.W.M., (2006), The inflammasome a linebacker of innate defence. N. Engl. J. Med. 355: 730–732.
18. Mariathasan, S., Weiss, D.S., Newton, K., McBride, J., O'Rourke, K., Roose-Girma, M., Lee, W.P., Weinrauch,Y., Monack, D.M., Dixit, V.M., (2006), Cryopyrin activates inflammasome in response to toxins and ATP. Nature 440: 228–232.
19. Abraham, E., (2003), Nuclear factor-κB and its role in sepsis associated organ failure. J. Infect. Dis. 187(Suppl. 2): s364–s369.
20. Liu, S.F., Ye, X., Malik, A.B., (1997), In vivo inhibition of nuclear factor-κB activation prevents inducible nitric oxide synthase expression and systemic hypotension in a rat model of septic shock. J. Immunol. 159: 3976–3983.
21. Rebe, C., Cathelin, S., Launay, S., Filomenko, Prévotat, L., L'OLlivier, C., Gyan, E., Michaeu, O., Grant, S., Dupart-Kupperschmitt, A., Fontenay, M., Solary, E., (2007), Caspase-8 prevents sustained activation of NF-κB in monocytes undergoing macrophage differentiation. Blood 109: 1442–1450.
22. Dinarello, C.A., Fantuzzi, G., (2003), Interleukin-18 and host defence against infection. J. Infect. Dis. 187(Suppl 2): s370–s380.
23. Calendra, T., Froidevaux, C., Martin, C., Roger, T., (2003), Macrophage migration inhibitory factor and host immune defenses against bacterial sepsis. J. Infect. Dis. 187(Suppl 2): s385–s390.

24. Emonts, M., Sweep, F.C.G.J., Grebenchtchikov, N., Geurts-Moespot, Knaup, M., Chonson, A. L., Erard, V., Renner, P., Hermans, P.W.M., Hazelzet, J.A., Calandra, T., (2007), Association between high levels of blood macrophage migration inhibitory factor, inappropriate adrenal response, and early death in patients with severe sepsis. Clin. Infect. Dis. 44: 1321–1328.
25. Wang, H., Yang, H., Czura, C.J., Sama, A.E., Tracey, K.J., (2001), HMGB1 as a late mediator of lethal systemic inflammation. Am. J. Respir. Crit. Care Med. 164: 1768–1773.
26. Czura, C.J., Yang, H., Tracey, K.J., (2003), High mobility group box-1 as a therapeutic target downstream of tumor necrosis factor. J. Infect. Dis. 187(Suppl 2): s391–s396.
27. Abraham, E., Arcaroli, J., Carmody, A., Wang, H., Tracey, K.J., (2000) HMG-1 as a mediator of acute lung inflammation. J. Immunol. 165: 2950–2954.
28. Colonna, M., Facchetta, F., (2003) TREM-1 (triggering receptor expressed on myeloid cells): a new player in acute inflammatory response. J. Infect. Dis. 187(Suppl 2): s397–s401.
29. Bouchon, A., Facchetti, F., Weigand, MA, Colonna, M, (2001) TREM-1 amplifies inflammation and is a crucial mediator of septic shock. Nature 410: 1103–1107.
30. Brown, K.A., Brain, S.P., Pearson, J.D., Edgeworth, J.D., Lewis, S.M., Treacher, D.F., (2006), Neutrophils in development of multiple organ failure in sepsis. Lancet 368: 157–168.
31. Astiz, M.E., DeGent, G.E., Lin, R.Y., Rackow, E.C., (1996), Microvascular function and rheologic changes in hyperdynamic sepsis. Crit. Care Med. 23: 265–271.
32. Sato, T., Shinzawa, H., Abe, Y, Takahashi, T., Arai, S., Sendo, F., (1993), Inhibition of *Corynebacterium parvum*-primed and lipopolysaccharide-induced hepatic necrosis in rats by selective depletion of neutrophils using monoclonal antibody, J. Leukoc. Biol. 53: 144–150.
33. Van eden, S.F., Kitigawa, Y., Klut, M.E., Lawrence, E., Hogg, J.C., (1997), Polymorphonuclear leucocytes released from the bone marrow preferentially sequester in lung microvessels. Microcirc. 4: 369–380.
34. Zhang, H., Porro, G., Orzech, N., Muller, B., Liu, M., Slutsky, A.S., (2001), Neutrophil defensins mediate acute inflammatory response and lung dysfunction in dose-related fashion. Am .J. Physiol. Lung Cell Mol. Physiol. 80: 947–954.
35. Parrillo, J.E., (1993) Pathogenetic mechanisms of septic shock. N. Engl. J. Med. 328: 1471–1477.
36. Landry, D.W., Oliver, J.A., (2004), The pathogenesis of vasodilatory shock. N. Engl. J. Med 345: 588–595.
37. Schrier, R.W., Wang, W., (2004), Acute renal failure and sepsis. N. Engl. J. Med. 351: 159–169.
38. Landry, D.W., Levin, H.R., Gallant, G.M., Ashton, R.C. Jr., Seo, S., D'Alessandro, D., Oz, M. C., Oliver, J.A., (1997) Vasopressin deficiency contributes to the vasodilation of septic shock. Circulation 95: 1122–1125.
39. Zeni, F., Freeman, B.F., Natanson, C, (1997), Antiinflammatory therapies to treat sepsis and septic shock: a reassessment. Crit. Care. Med. 25: 1095–1000.
40. Hotchkiss, R.S, Karl, I.E., (2003), The pathophysiology and treatment of sepsis. NEJM 348: 138–150.
41. Opal, S.M., DePalo, V.A., (2000), Anti-inflammatory cytokines. Chest 117: 1162–1172.
42. Gogos, C.A., Drosou, E., Bassaris, H.P., Skoutelis, A., (2000), Pro-versus anti-inflammatory cytokine profile in patients with severe sepsis: a marker for prognosis and future therapeutic options. J. Infect. Dis. 181: 176–180.
43. Hotchkiss, R.S., Swanson, P.E., Freeman, B.D., Tinsley, K.W., Cobb, J.P., Matuschak, G.M., Buchman, T.G., Karl, I.E., (1999), Apoptotic cell death in patients with sepsis, shock and multiple organ dysfunction. Crit. Care Med. 27: 1230–1251.
44. Hotchkiss, R.S., Tinsley, K.W., Swanson P.E., Schmieg, R.E. Jr., Hui, J.J., Chang, K.C., Osborne, D.F., Freeman, B.D., Cobb, J.P., Buchman, T.G., Karl, I.E. (2001), Sepsis-induced apoptosis causes profound depletion of B and $CD_4+$ T Lymphocytes in humans. J. Immunol. 166: 6952–6963.

# References

45. Hotchkiss, R.S., Tinsley, K.W., Swanson, P.E., Grayson, M.H., Osborne, D.F., Wagner, T.H., Cobb, J.P., Coppersmith, C., Karl, I.E., (2002), Depletion of dendritic cells but not macrophages in patients with sepsis. J. Immunol. 168: 2493–2450.
46. Aliprantis, A.O., Yang, R.-B., Mark, M.R., Suggett, S., Devaux, B., Radolf, J.D., Klimpel, G. R., Godowski, P., Zychlinsky, A., (1999), Cell activation and apoptosis by bacterial lipoproteins through toll-like receptor-2. Science 285: 736–739.
47. Voll, R.E., Herrmann, M., Roth, E.A., Stach, C., Kalden, J.R., Girkontaite, I., (1997), Immunosuppressive effects of apoptotic cells. Nature 390: 350–351.
48. Ayala, A., Herdon, C.D., Lehman, D.L., Demaso, C.M., Ayala, C.A., Chaudry, I.H., (1995), The induction of accelerated thymic programmed cell death during polymicrobial sepsis: control by corticosteroids but not tumour necrosis factor. Shock 3: 259–267.
49. Taneja, R., Parodo, J., Jia, S.H., Kapus, A., Rotstein, O., Marshall, J.C., (2004), Delayed neutrophil apoptosis in sepsis is associated with maintenance of mitochondrial transmembrane potential and reduced caspase-9 activity, Crit. Care Med. 32: 1460–1469.
50. Mahidara, R., Billiar, T.R., (2000), Apoptosis in sepsis. Crit. Care Med. 28 (Suppl): N105–113.
51. Watson, G., Rotstein, O.D., Parodo, J., Bitar, R., Marshall, J.C., (1998), The 1L-1 converting enzyme (caspase-1) inhibits apoptosis of inflammatory neutophils through activation of 1L-1. J. Immunol. 161: 957–962.
52. Jia, S.H., Li, Y., Parodo, J., Kapus, A., Fan, L., Rotstein, O.D., (2004), Pre-B cell colony-stimulating factor inhibits neutrophil apoptosis in experimental inflammation and clinical sepsis. J. Clin. Invest. 113: 1318–1327.
53. Hotchkiss, R.S., Schmieg, R.E., Swanson, P.E., Freeman, B.D., Tinsley, K.W., Cobb, J.P., Karl, I.E., Buchman, T.G., (2000), Rapid onset of intestinal epithelial and lymphocyte apoptotic cell death in patients with trauma and shock. Crit. Care Med. 28: 3207–3217.
54. Volk, H.D., Reinke, P., Docke, W.D., (2000) Clinical aspects from systemic inflammation to "immunoparalysis". Chem. Immunol. 74: 162–177.
55. Van der Poll, T., (2001), Immunotherapy of sepsis. Lancet Infect. Dis. 1: 165–174.
56. Ayald, A., Knotts, J.B., Ertel, W., Perrin, M.M., Morrison, M.H., Chaudry, I.H., (1993), Role of interleukin 6 and transforming growth factor-beta in the induction of depressed splenocyte responses following sepsis. Arch. Surg. 128: 89–94.
57. Brandtzaeg, P., Osnes, L., Ovstebo, R., Joo, G.B., Westwik, A.B., Kierulf, P., (1996), Net inflammatory capacity of human septic shock plasma evaluated by a monocyte-based target cell assay: identification of interleukin-10 as a major functional deactivator of human monocytes. J. Exp. Med. 184: 51–60.
58. Döcke, W.D., Randow, F., Syrbe, U., Krausch, D., Asadullah, K., Reinke, P., Volk, H.D., Kox, W., (1997), Monocyte deactivation in septic patients: restoration by IFN-γ treatment. Nat. Med. 3: 678–681.
59. Kalden, J.R., Girkontaite, I., (1997), Immunosuppressive effects of apoptotic cells. Nature 390: 350–351.
60. Mokart, D., Merlin, M., Santinnini, A., Brun, J.P., Delpero, J.R., Houvenaeghel, G., Moutardier, V., Blache, J.L., (2005), Procalcitocin, interleukin 6 and systemic inflammatory response syndrome (SIRS): early markers of postoperative sepsis after major surgery. Br. J. Anaesh. 94: 767–773.
61. Osuchowski, M.F., Welch, K., Siddiqui, J., Remick, D.G., (2006), Circulatory cytokine/inhibitor profiles reshape the understanding of the SIRS/CARS continuum in sepsis and predict mortality. J. Immunology 177: 1967–1974.
62. Xiao, H., Siddiqui Remick, D.G., (2006), Mechanisms of mortality in early and late sepsis, Infect. Immun. 74: 5227–5235.
63. Rosser, D.M., Stidwill, R.P., Jacobson, D., Singer, M., (1995), Oxygen tension in the bladder epithelium increases in both high and low output endotoxemic sepsis. J. Appl. Physiol. 79: 1878–1882.

64. Boekstegers, P., Weidenhofer, S., Pilz, G., Werdan, K., (1991), Peripheral oxygen availability within skeletal muscle in sepsis and septic shock: comparison of limited infection and cardiogenic shock. Infection 19: 317–323.
65. Brealey, D., Brand, M., Hargreaves, I., Heales, S., Land, J., Smolenski, R., Davies, N.A., Cooper, C.E., Singer, M., (2002), Association between mitochondrial dysfunction and severity and outcome of septic shock. Lancet 360: 219–223.
66. Veruloet, M.G., Thijs, L.G., Hack, C.E., (1998), Derangements of coagulation and fibrinolysis in critically ill patients with sepsis and septic shock. Semin. Thromb. Hemost. 24: 33–44.
67. Suffredini, A.F., Harpel, P.C., Parrillo, J.E., (1989), Promotion and subsequent inhibition of plasminogen activation after administration of intravenous endotoxin to normal subjects. N. Engl. J. Med 320: 1165–1172.
68. Esmon, C.T., (2005), The interactions between inflammation and coagulation. Br. J. Haematol. 131: 417–430.
69. Mason, J.W., Colman, R.W., (1971), The role of Hageman factor is disseminated intravascular coagulation induced by septicemia, neoplasia or liver disease. Thromb. Diath. Haemorrh. 26: 325–331.
70. Moore, K.L., Andreoli, S.P., Esmon, N.L., Esmon, C.T., Bang, Nu., (1987), Endotoxin enhances tissue factor and suppresses thrombomodulin expression of human vascular endothelium in vitro. J. Clin. Invest. 79: 124–130.
71. Esmon, C.T., Xu, J., Gu, J.M., Qu, D., Laszik, Z., Ferrall, G., Steams-Kurosawa, D.J., Kurosawa, S., Taylor, F.B., Esmon, N.L., (1999), Endothelial protein receptor. Thromb. Haemostat. 82: 251–258.
72. Raaphorst, J., Johan Groenveld, A.B., Bossick, A.W., Erik Hack, C., (2001), Early inhibition of activated fibrinolysis predicts microbial infection, shock and mortality in febrile medical patients. Thromb. Haemostat. 86: 543–549.
73. Hermans, P.W., Hazelzet, J.A., (2005), Plasminogen activator inhibitor type I gene polymorphism and sepsis. Clin. Infect. Dis; 41(Suppl. 7): s453–s458.
74. Renckens, R., Roelofs, J.T.H., Bonta, P.I., Florquin, S., de Vries, C.J.M., Levi, M., Carmeliet, P., van't Veer, C., van der Poll, T., (2007), Plasminogen activator inhibitor type I is protective during severe gram-negative pneumonia. Blood 109: 1593–1601.
75. Ward, P., (2004), The dark side of C5A in sepsis. Nature Rev. Immunol. 4: 133–142.
76. Goldstein, I.M., Weissmann, G., (1974), Generation of C5 – derived lysosomal enzyme releasing activity (C5A) by lysates of leucocyte lysosomes. J. Immunol. 113: 1583–1588.
77. Mollnes, T.E., Brekke, O.L., Fung, M., Fure, H., Christianseu, D., Bergseth, G., Videm, V., Lappegard, K.T., Köhl, J., Lambris, J.D., (2002), Essential role of the C5A receptor in *E.coli*-induced oxidative burst and phagocytosis revealed by a novel lepirudin-based human whole blood model of inflammation. Blood 100: 1869–1877.
78. Perianayagam, M.C., Balakrishnan, V.S., King, A.J., Pereira, B.J., Jaber, B.L., (2002), C5a delays apoptosis of human neutrophils by a phosphatidylinositol 3-kinase-signaling pathway, Kidney Internat. 61: 456–463.
79. Younger, J.G., Sasaki, N., Delgado, J., Ko, A.C., Ngheim, T., Waite, M.D., Till, G.O., Ward, P.A., (2001), Systemic and lung physiological changes in rats after intravascular activation of complement, J. Appl. Physiol. 90: 2289–2295.
80. Riedermann, N.C., Guo, R.F., Laudes, I.J., Keller, K., Sarma, V.J., Padgaonkar, V., Zetoune, F.S., Ward, P., (2002), C5a receptor and thymocyte apoptosis in sepsis. FASEB J. 16: 887–888.
81. Czermak, B.J., Sarma, V., Pierson, C.L., Warner, R.L., Huber-Lang, M., Bless, N.M., Schmal, H., Fried, H.P., Ward, P.A., (1999), Protective effects of C5a blockade in sepsis. Nature Med. 5: 788–792.
82. Ware, L.B., Matthay, M.A., (2000), The acute respiratory distress syndrome. N. Engl. J. Med 342: 1334–1349.
83. Nelson, S., Heyder, A.M., Stone, J., Bergeron, M.G., Daugherty, S., Peterson, G., Fotheringham, N., Welch, W., Milwee, S., Root, R., for the Multilobar Pneumonia Study Group, (2000),

A randomized controlled trial of filgrastin for the treatment of hospitalized patients with multilobar pneumonia. J. Infect: Dis. 181: 970–973.
84. Miura, E., Procianoy, R.S., Bittar, C., Miura, C.S., Miura, M.S., Mello, C., Christensen, R.D., (2001), A randomized, doubled-masked placebo-controlled trial of recombinant granulocyte colony-stimulating factor administration to preterm, infants with the clinical diagnosis of early-onset sepsis. Pediatrics 107: 30–35.
85. Bernard, G.R., Luce, J.L., Sprung, C.L., Rinaldo, J.E., Tate, R.M., Sibbald, W.J., Kariman, K., Higgins, S., Bradley, R., Metz C.A., (1989), High-dose cortiosteroids in patients with the adult respiratory distress syndrome. N. Engl. J. Med. 317: 1565–1570.
86. The National Heart, Lung, and Blood Institute Acute Respiratory Distress Syndrome (ARDS) Clinical Trials Network, (2006), Efficacy and safety of corticosteroid for persistent acute respiratory distress syndrome. N. Engl. J. Med 354: 1671–1684.
87. Weiss, Y.G., Maloyan, A., Tazelaar, J., Raj, N., Deutschman, C.S., (2002), Adenoviral transfer of HSP-70 into pulmonary epithium ameliorates experimental acute respiratory distress syndrome. J. Clin. Invest. 110: 801–806.
88. Slutsky, A.S., (2002). Hot new therapy for sepsis and the acute respiratory distress syndrome. J. Clin. Invest. 110: 737–739.
89. Dellinger, R.P., Carlet, J.M., Masur, H., GerLach, H., Calandra, H., Cohen, J., Gea-Banacloche, J., Keh, D., Marchall, J.C., Parker, M.M., Ramsay, G., Zimmerman, J.C., Vincent, J.L., Levy, M.M., for the Surviving Sepsis Campaign Management Guidelines Committee, (2004) Surviving Sepsis Campaign guidelines for management of severe sepsis and septic shock. Crit. Care Med. 32: 858–873.
90. Poulton, B., (2006), Advances in management if sepsis: the randomized controlled trials behind the surviving sepsis campaign recommendations. Internat. J. Antimicrob. Agents 27: 97–101.
91. Gattinoni, L., Brazzi, L., Pelosi, P., Latini, R., Tognoni, G., Pesenti, A., Fumagelli, R., for the $SVO_2$ Collaborative Group, (1995) A trial of goal-orientated hemodynamic therapy in critically ill patients. N. Engl. J. Med. 333: 1025–1032.
92. Hayes, M.A., Timmins, A.C., Yau, E.H., Pallazo, M., Hinds, C.J., Watson, D., (1994), Elevations of systemic oxygen delivery in the treatment of critically ill patients. N. Engl. J. Med 330: 1717–1722.
93. Rady, M.Y., Rivers, E.P., Nowak, R.M., (1996), Resuscitation of the critically ill in the ED: responses of blood pressure, heart rate, shock index, central venous oxygen saturation, and lactate, Am. J. Emerg. Med. 14: 218–225.
94. Cortez, A., Zito, J., Lucas, C.E., Gerrick, S.J., (1977), Mechanism of inappropriate polyuria in septic patients. Arch. Surg. 112: 471–476.
95. Rivers, E., Nguyen, B., Havstad, S., Ressler, J., Muzzin, A., Knoblich, B., Peterson, E., Tomlanovich, M., for the Early Goal-Directed Therapy Collaborative Group, (2001), Early goal-directed therapy in the treatment of severe sepsis and septic shock. N. Engl. J. Med. 345: 1368–1377.
96. Corlbom, D.J., Rubenfeld, G.D., (2007), Barriers to implementing protocol-based sepsis resuscitation in the emergency department-results of a national survey. Crit. Care Med. 35: 2525–2532.
97. Sivayohan, N., (2007), Management of severe sepsis and septic shock in the emergency department: a survey of current practice in emergency departments in England. Emer. Med. J. 24: 422.
98. Llewelyn, M.J., Cohen, J., (2007), Tracking the microbes in sepsis: advancements in treatment bring challenges for microbial epidemiology. Clin. Infect. Dis. 44: 1343–1348.
99. Rello, J., Sa-Borges, M., Correa, H., Leal, S.R., Barraibar, J. (1999) Variations in etiology of ventilator – associated pneumonia across four treatment sites: implications for antimicrobial prescribing practices. Am. J. Respir. Crit. Care Med. 160: 608–613.

100. Bochud, P.-Y., Bonten, M., Marchetti, O., Calandra, T., (2004), Antimicrobial therapy for patients with severe sepsis and septic shock: an evidence-based review. Crit. Care Med. 32 (Suppl): s495–s511.
101. Harbarth, S., Garbino, J., Pugin, J., Romand, J.A., Lew, D., Pittet, D., (2003), Inappropriate initial antimicrobial therapy and its effect on survival in a clinical trial of immunomodulating therapy for severe sepsis. Am. J. Med. 115: 529–535.
102. Fraser, A., Paul, M., Almanasreh, N., Tacconelli, E., Frank, U., Cauda, R., Borok, S., Cohen, M., Andereassen, S., Nielson, A.D., Leibovici, L.: Treat Study Group, (2006), Benefit of appropriate empirical antibiotic treatment: thirty-day mortality and duration of hospital stay. Am. J. Med. 119: 970–976.
103. MacArthur, R.D., Miller, M., Albertson, T., Panacek, E., Johnson, D., Teoh, L., Barchuk, W., (2004), Adequacy of early empiric antibiotic treatment and survival in severe sepsis: experience from the MONARCS trial. Clin. Infect. Dis. 38: 284–288.
104. Wang, J.-L., Chen, S.-Y., Wang, J.-T., Wu, G.H.-M., Chiang, W.-C., Hsueh, P.-R., Chen, Y.-C., Chang, S.-C., (2008), Comparison of both clinical features and mortality risk associated with bacteremia due to community-acquired methicillin-resistant *Staphylococcus aureus* and methicillin-susceptible *S. aureus*. Clin. Infect. Dis. 46: 799–806.
105. Tam, V.H., Gamez, E.A., Weston, J.S., Gerard, L.N., LaRocco, M.T., Caeiro, J.P., Gentry, L.O., Garey, K.W., (2008), Outcomes of bacteremia due *Pseudomonas aeruginosa* with reduced susceptibility to piperacillin-tazobactam: implications on the appropriateness of the resistance breakpoint. Clin. Infect. Dis. 46: 862–867.
106. Kumar, A., Roberts, D., Wood, K.E., Light, B., Parrillo, J.E., Sharma, S., Suppes, R., Feinstein, D., Zanotti, S., Taiberg, L., Gurka, D., Kumar, A., Cheang, M., (2006), Duration of hypotension before initiation of effective antimicrobial therapy is the critical determinant of survival in human septic shock. Crit. Care. Med. 34: 1589–1596.
107. Marshall, J.C., Maier, R.V., Jimenez, M., Dellinger, E.P., (2004), Source control in management of severe sepsis and septic shock: an evidence-based review. Crit. Care. Med. 32: s513–s526.
108. Hoffman, J.N., Vollmar, B., Laschke, M.W., Fertmann, J.M., Jauch, K.-W., Menger, M.D., (2005), Microcirculatory alterations in ischemia-reperfusion injury and sepsis: effects of activated protein C and thrombin inhibition. Crit. Care: 9(Suppl 4): s33–s37.
109. Bernard, G.R., Vincent, J.-L., Laterre, P.-F., La Rosa, S.P., Dhainaut, J.-F., Lopez-Rodriguez, Steingrub, J.S., Garber, G.E., Helterbrand, J.D., Ely, E.W., Fisher, C.J. Jr., for the Recombinant Human Activated Protein C Worldwide Evaluation in Severe Sepsis (PROWESS) Study Group, (2001), Efficacy and safety of recombinant human activated protein C for severe sepsis. N. Engl. J. Med. 344: 699–709.
110. Abraham, E., Laterre, P.F., Garg, R., Levy, H., Talwar, D., Trzaskoma, B.L., Francois, B., Guy, J.S., Brückman, M., Reu-neto, A., Rossaint, R., Perrotin, D., Sablotzki, A., Arkins, N., Utterback, B.G., Macias, W.C., for the Administration of Drotreogin Alfa (Activated) in Early Stage Severe Sepsis (ADDRESS) Study Group, (2005), Drotreogin alfa (activated) for adults with severe sepsis and a low risk of death. N. Engl. J. Med. 353: 1332–1341.
111. Manns, B.J., Lee, H., Doig, C.J., Johnson, D., Donaldson, C., (2002), An economic evaluation of activated protein C treatment for severe sepsis. N. Engl. J. Med. 347: 993–1000.
112. Levi, M., Levy, M., Williams, D.I., Artigas, A., Antonelli, M., Wyncoll, D., James, J., Booth, F.V., Wang, D., Sundin, D.P., Macias, W.L., Xigris and Prophylactic Heparin Evaluation in Severe Sepsis (XPRESS) Study Group (2007), Heparin prophylaxis did not increase mortality and was beneficial in adults with sepsis receiving drotrecogin alfa. Am. J. Respir. Crit. Care. Med. 176: 483–490.
113. Sprung, C.L., Caralis, P.V., Marcial, E.H., Pierce, M., Gelbard, M.A., Long, W.M., Duncan, R.C., Tendler, M.D., Karpf, M., (1984), The effects of high-dose corticosteroids in patients with septic shock: a prospective controlled study. N. Engl. J. Med. 311: 1137–1143.
114. Briegel, J., Forst, H., Haller, M., Schelling, G., Kilger, E., Kuprat, G., Hemmer, B., Hummel, T., Lenhart, A., Heyduck, M., Stoll, L., Peter, K., (1999), Stress doses of hydrocortisone

reverses hyperdynamic septic shock: a prospective, randomized, double-blind, single-center study. Crit. Care Med. 27: 723–732.
115. Annane, D., Bellissant, E., Bollaert, P.E., Briegel, J., Keh, D., Kupfer, Y., (2004), Corticosteroids for severe sepsis and septic shock: a systematic review and meta-analysis. BMJ 329: 480 (online).
116. Annane, D., Sébille, V., Charpentier, C., Bollaert, P.E., Francois, B., Korach, J.M., Capellier, G., Cohen, Y., Azoulay, E., Troché, G., Chaumet-Riffaut, P., Bellissant, E., (2002), Effect of treatment with low doses of hydrocortisone on mortality in patient with septic shock. JAMA 288: 862–871.
117. Hamrahian, A.H., Oseni, T.S., Arafah, B.M., (2004), Measurements of serum free cortisol in critically ill patients. N. Engl. J. Med. 350: 1829–1638.
118. Sprung, C.L., Annane, D., Keh, D., Moreno, R., Singer, M., Freivogel, K., Weiss, Y.G., Benbenishty, J., Kalenka, A., Forst, H., Laterre, P.-F., Reinhart, K., Cuthbertson, B.H., Payen, D., Briegel, J., for the Corticus Study Group (2008), Hydrocortisone therapy for the patients with septic shock. N. Engl. J. Med. 358: 111–124.
119. Finfer, S., (2008), Corticosteroids in septic shock (Editorial). N. Engl. J. Med. 358: 188–190.
120. Van den Berghe, G., Wouters, P., Weekers, F., Verwaest, C., Bruyninckx, F., Schetz, M., Vlasselaers, D., Ferdinande, P., Lauwers, P., Bouillion, R., (2001), Intensive insulin therapy in critically ill patients. N. Engl. J. Med. 345: 1359–1367.
121. Brunkhorst, F.M., Engel, C., Blous, F., Meier-Hellmann, A., Regaller, M., Weiler, N., Moerer, O., Gruendling, M., Oppert, M., Grond, S., Olthoff, D., Jaschinski, U., John, S., Rossaint, R., Welte, T., Schaefer, M., Kern, P., Kuhnt, E., Kiehntopf, M., Hartog, C., Natanson, C., Loeffler, M., Reinhart, K., for the German Competence Network Sepsis (Sepnet), (2008), Intensive insulin therapy and pentastarch resuscitation in severe sepsis. N. Engl. J. Med. 358: 125–139.
122. Mullner, M., Urbanek, B., Havel, C., Losert, H., Waechter, F., Gamper, G., (2004), Vasopressors for shock. [Review]. Cochrane Database Syst. Rev. CD003709.
123. Beale, R.J., Hollenberg, S.M., Vincent, J.L., Parrillo, J.E., (2004), Vasopressors and inotropic support in septic shock: an evidence-based review. Crit. Care. Med. 32(Suppl 11): s455–s465.
124. Russell, J.A., (2007), Vasopressin in septic shock. Crit. Care Med. 35(Suppl): s609–s615.
125. Luckner, G., Dunser, M.W., Jochberger, S., Mayr, V.D., Wenzel, V., Ulmer, H., Schmid, S., Knotzer, H., Pajk, W., Hasibeder, W., Mayr, A.J., Frieseneker, B., (2005), Arginine vasopressor in 316 patients with advanced vasodilatory shock. Crit. Care Med. 33: 2659–2566.
126. Russell, J.A., Walley, K.R., Singer, J., Gordon, A.C., Hebert, P.C., Cooper, J., Holmes, C.L., Mehta, S., Grnaton, J.T., Storms, M.M., Cook, D.J., Presnail, J.J., Ayers, D., for the VASST Investigators, (2008), Vasopressin versus norepinephrine infusion in patients with septic shock. N. Engl. J. Med. 358: 877–887.
127. Jelkmann, W., (1998), Proinflammatory cytokines lowering erythropoietin production. J. Interferon Cytokine Res. 18: 555–559.
128. Hebert, P.C., Wells, Blajchman, M.A., Marshall, J., Martin, C., Pagliarello, G., Tweeddale, M., Schweitzer, I., Yetisir, E., (1999), A multicenter, randomized, controlled trial of transfusion requirements in critical care. Transfusion Requirements in Critical Care Investigators, Canadian Critical Care Trials Group. N. Engl. J. Med. 340: 409–417.
129. Vincet, J.L., Sakr, Y., Sprung, C., Harboe, S., Damas, P., Sepsis Occurrence in Acutely Ill Patients (SOAP) Investigators, (2008), Are blood transfusion associated with a greater mortality rates? Results of the Sepsis Occurrence in Acutely Ill Patients Study. Anesthesiology 108: 31–39.
130. Corwin, H.L., Gettinger, A., Rodriguez, R.M., Pearl, R.G., Gubler, K.D., Enny, C., Colton, T., Corwin, M.J., (1999), Efficacy of recombinant human erythropoietin in the critically ill patient: a randomized, double-blind, placebo-controlled trial. Crit. Care Med. 27: 2346–2350.

131. Warren, B.L., Eid, A., Singer, P., Pillay, S.S., Carl, P., Novak, I., Chalupa, P., Atherstone, A., Pénzes, I., Kübler, A., Knaubs, Keinecke, H.O., Heinrichs, H., Schindel, F., Juers, M., Bone, R.C., Opal, S.M., Kybersept Trial Study Group, (2001), Caring for the critically ill patient; High dose antithrombin III in severe sepsis: a randomized controlled trial. JAMA 286: 1869–1878.
132. Wiedermann, C.J., Hoffman, J.N., Juers, M., Ostermann, H., Kienast, J., Briegel, J., Strauss, R., Keinecke, H.O., Warren, B.C., Opal, S.M.; Kybersept Investigators, (2006), High-dose antithrombin III in the treatment of severe sepsis in patients with a high risk of death: efficacy and safety. Crit. Care Med. 34: 285–292.
133. The Acute Respiratory Distress Syndrome Network, (2000), Ventilation with lower tidal volumes as compared with traditional tidal volumes for acute lung injury and the acute respiratory distress syndrome. N. Engl. J. Med. 342: 1301–1308.
134. Eisner, M.D., Thompson, T., Hudson, L.D., Luce, J.M., Hayden, D., Schoenfeld, D., Matthay, M.A.; Acute Respiratory Distress Syndrome Network, (2001), Efficacy of low tidal volume ventilation in patients with different clinical risk factors for acute lung injury and the acute respiratory distress syndrome. Am. J. Respir. Crit. Care Med. 164: 231–236.
135. Sevransky, J.E., Levy, M.M., Marini, J.J., (2004), Mechanical ventilation in sepsis-induced acute lung injury/acute respiratory distress syndrome: an evidence-based review. Crit. Care Med. 32 (Suppl 11): s548–s583.
136. Riedemann, N.C., Guo, R.F., Ward, P.A., (2003), The enigma of sepsis. J. Clin. Invest. 112: 460–467.
137. Rangel-Frausto, M.S., Pittet, D., Costigan, M., Hwang, T., Davis, C.S., Wenzel, R.P., (1995), The natural history of the systemic inflammatory response syndrome (SIRS): a prospective study. JAMA 273: 117–123.
138. Schiffl, H., Lang, S.M., Fischer, R., (2002), Daily hemodialysis and the outcome of acute renal failure. N. Engl. J. Med. 346: 305–310.
139. Ronco, C., Belloma, R., Homel, P., Brendolan, A., Dan, M., Piccinni, P., La Greca, G., (2000), Effects of different doses in continuous veno-venous hemofiltration on outcomes of acute renal failure: a prospective randomized trial. Lancet 356: 26–30.
140. Kazatchkine, M.D., Kaveri, S.V., (2001), Immunomodulation of autoimmune and inflammatory diseases with intravenous immune globulin. N. Engl. J Med. 345: 747–755.
141. Pildal, J., Gotzche, P.C., (2004), Polyclonal immunoglobulin for treatment of bacterial sepsis: a systematic review. Clin. Infect. Dis. 39: 38–46.
142. Turgeon, A.F., Hutton, B., Ferguson, D.A., McIntyre, L., Tinmouth, A.A., Cameron, D.W., Hebert, P.C., (2007), Meta-analysis: intravenous immunoglobulin in critically ill adult patients with sepsis. Ann. Intern Med. 146: 193–203.
143. Alejandria, M.M., Lancing, M.A., Dans, L.F., Mantaring, J.B., (2002), Intravenous immunoglobulin for treating sepsis and septic shock. Cochrane Database Syst. Rev 1: CD001090.
144. Werdan, K., Pilz, G., Bujdoso, O., Fraunberger, P., Neeser, G., Schmieder, R.E., Viell, B., Marget, W., Seewald, M., Walger, P., Stuttmann, R., Speichermann, N., Peckelsen, C., Kurowski, V., Osterhues, H.H., Verner, L., Neumann, R., Muller-Werdan, U., Score-based Immunoglobulin Therapy of Sepsis (SBITS) Study Group, (2007), Score-based immunoglobulin G therapy of patients with sepsis: the SBITS study. Crit. Care Med. 35: 2693–2701.
145. Dahmer, M.K., Randolph, A., Vitali, S., Quasney, M.W., (2005), Genetic polymorphisms in sepsis (review). Pediatr. Crit. Care Med. 6 (3 Suppl): s61–s73.
146. Imahara, S.D., O'Keefe, G.E., (2004), Genetic determinants of the inflammatory response. (Review). Curr. Opin. Crit. Care 10: 318–324.
147. Texereau, J., Pene, F., Chiche, J.D., Rousseau, C., Mira, J.P., (2004), Importance of hemostatic gene polymorphisms for susceptibility to and outcome of severe sepsis. Crit. Care Med. 32(Suppl 5): s313–s319.
148. Yoshida, S., (2004), Monocyte HLA-DR expression as predictors of clinical outcome for patients with sepsis. Japan. J. Clin. Med. 62: 2281–2284.

149. Arcaroli, J., Fessler, M.B., Abraham, E., (2005), Genetic polymorphisms and sepsis. Shock 24: 300–312.
150. Terblanche, M., Almog, Y., Rosenson, R.S., Smith, T.S., Hackman, D.G., (2006), Statins: panacea for sepsis? Lancet Infect. Dis. 6:242–248.
151. Zingarelli, B., Cook, J.A., (2005), Peroxisome proliferators-activated receptor-gamma is a new therapeutic target in sepsis and inflammation. Shock 23: 393–399.
152. Marshall, J.C., (2000), Clinical trials of mediator-directed therapy in sepsis: what have we learned? Inten. Care Med. 26: 575–583.
153. Polderman, K.H., Girbes, A.R.J., (2004), Drug intervention trials in sepsis: divergent results. Lancet 363: 1721–1723.
154. Levin, M., Quint, P.A., Goldstein, B., Barton, P., Bradley, J.S., Shenie, S.D., Yeh, T., Kim, S. S., Cafaro, D.P., Scannon, P.J., Giroir, B.P., and the rBPI$_{21}$ Meningococcal Sepsis Study Group, (2000), Recombinant bactericidal/permeability-increasing protein (rBPI$_{21}$) as adjunctive treatment for children with severe meningococccal sepsis: a randomized trial. Lancet: 356: 961–967.
155. Axtelle, T., Pribble, J., (2003), An overview of clinical studies in healthy subjects and patients with severe sepsis with IC14, a CD14-specific chimeric monoclonal antibody. J. Endoxin. Res. 9: 385–389.
156. Schwulst, S.J., Grayson, M.H., Di Pasco, P.J., Davis, C.G., Brahmbhatt, T.S., Ferguson, T. A., Holchkiss, R.S., (2006), Agonistic monoclonal antibody against CD40 receptor decreases lymphocyte apoptosis and improves survival in sepsis. J. Immunol. 177: 557–565.
157. Fink, M.P., (2004), Ethyl pyruvate: a novel treatment for sepsis and shock. Minerva Anestesiol. 70: 365–371.
158. Liu, D., Cai, S., Gu, X., Scafidi, J., Wu, X., Davis, A.E. 3rd, (2003), C1 inhibitor prevents endotoxin shock via a direct interaction with lipopolysaccharide. J. Immunol. 171: 2594–2601.
159. Victor, V.M., Rocha, M., Esplugues, J.V., De La Fuente, M., (2005), Role of free radicals in sepsis: antioxidant therapy. Curr. Pharmaceut. Design. 11: 3141–3158.
160. Zhang, Y., Chen, H, Li, Y., Zheng, S., Chen, Y., Li, L., Zhou, L., Xie, H., Praseedom, R.K., (2008), Thymosin α1 and ulinastatin-based immunomodulatory strategy for sepsis arising from intra-abdominal infection due to carbapenem-resistant bacteria. J. Infect. Dis. 198: 723–730.
161. Giebelen, IAJ, Le Moine, A., van den Pangaart, P.S., Sadis, C., Goldman, M., Florquin, S., van der Poll, T., (2008), Deficiency of α 7 cholinergic receptors facilitates bacterial clearance in *Escherichia coli* peritonitis. J. Infect. Dis. 198: 750–757.
162. Opal, S.M., (2005), Concept of PIRO as a new conceptual framework to understand sepsis. Pediatr. Crit. Med. 6 (Suppl 3): s55–s60.
163. Ferrer, R., Antigas, A., Levy, M.M., Blanco, J., González-Diaz, G., Garnacho-Montero, J., Ibáñez, J., Palencia, E., Quintana, M., de la Torre-Prados, M.V.; for the Edusepsis Study Group, (2008), Improvement in process of care and outcome after a multicenter severe sepsis educational program in Spain. JAMA 299: 2294–2303.

# Chapter 7
# Febrile Neutropenia: Management Issues

## 7.1 Introduction

Neutrophils (granulocytes) are vital components of the effector mechanisms of the host defense. They represent part of the first-line defense against invading microbes (particularly bacteria and fungi), and are essential as part of the innate immune response. Neutrophils circulate as quiescent cells, and their main functions as phagocytic and bactericidal defenders are performed in tissues where microbial invasion occurs. The neutrophil microbicidal defense mechanisms for microbial killing can be either oxidative or non-oxidative. The principal oxidative killing of microbes is via the myeloperoxidase (MPO) – hydrogen peroxide ($H_2O_2$) pathway. The microbicidal products generated by the MPO – $H_2O_2$ pathway include hypochlorous acid, chlorination products, tyrosine radicals, and nitrogen intermediates.[1]

The neutrophils also produce a host of antimicrobial substances used to fight invading pathogens. These include (1) bacterial permeability-increasing (BPI) protein, which binds to lipopolysaccharide (LPS), with antimicrobial activity against gram-negative bacteria; (2) defensins, small amphipathic pore-forming antibacterial cationic peptides with broad antibacterial spectrum; (3) serine proteases (elastase, cathepsin G) with direct antibacterial activity, besides enzymatic function; (4) lysozyme which cleave peptoglycan-polymers of bacterial cell wall (i.e. gram-positive bacteria); (5) lactoferrin, iron chelator to sequester iron (essential for bacterial growth), but also the proteolytic fragments have direct bactericidal activity; (6) B2 integrins to mediate cellular adhesions and regulate phagocytosis; (7) cathelicidin protein (hcap-18), binds endotoxin, and has antibacterial activity against gram-positive bacteria as well.

The hosts' normal response to bacterial infection usually involves increase in the neutrophil count as a result of proinflammatory cytokine and granulocyte-colony-stimulating factor (GCSF) up regulation. Neutropenia (granulocytopenia) is normally defined as two standard deviations below the mean of the population studied.

## 7.2 Pathogenesis

The definition of neutropenia is age related, in children under 10 years of age, neutropenia is <1.5 granulocytes X $10^3/\mu L$ ($< 1.5 \times 10^9/L$); in older children and adults neutropenia is defined as <1.8 granulocytes × $10^3/\mu L$ (or $<1.8 \times 10^9/L$)[2]. The mechanisms of neutropenia are by several means: (1) hypoplastic neutropoiesis (as with myelotoxic agents); (2) ineffective neutropoiesis (resulting from enhanced apoptosis of late precursors); (3) increased removal or utilization of circulating neutrophils (acute bacterial infections, autoimmune neutropenia, hypersplenism); (4) shifts of cells from the circulation to the marginal pool (endotoxinemia, exposure to dialysis membrane); (5) combination of the above factors.[2] Neutropenia can be acquired or congenital (cyclical neutropenia); and can be from disorders of intrinsic abnormalities of hematopoietic progenitor cells, or from extrinsic factors, such as tumor infiltration, fibrosis, or irradiation. Drug-induced neutropenia now account for the commonest cause of severe neutropenia, 3–12 cases per million population.[2] The two mechanisms of drug-induced neutropenias are (a) dose-related toxicity from interference with protein synthesis and cell replication (nonselective), e.g. myelotoxic chemopeutic agents; (b) dose-unrelated idiosyncratic, allergic, or immunologic mechanisms (i.e., phenothiazines, chloramphenicol, sulfonamides, etc.).[2] Cancer chemotherapeutic agents are the commonest cause of severe neutropenia because of high proliferative activity of neutrophil precursors in bone marrow and short half-life of granulocytes in blood. The neutrophil count reaches its nadir (lowest value) at approximately 10–14 days from initiation of the cytotoxic therapy cycle. Chemotherapeutic regimens for lymphomas and for solid tumors tend to induce periods of severe neutropenia less than 7 days, whereas regimens for acute myeloid leukemia and bone marrow transplant produce profound neutropenia usually lasting more than 10–14 days. Marrow recovery does not usually occur in the latter circumstances until the 4th week after initiating therapy. However, G-CSF may accelerate the recovery period.

The risk of infection is inversely related to the severity of neutropenia, see Table 7.1. However, risk and severity of infection also depends on the duration and cause of neutropenia. Severe acute neutropenia ($<0.5 \times 10^3/\mu L$) that occurs over hours or days (i.e., post-chemotherapy) results in greater risk of severe infection than severe chronic neutropenia (present for months or years).[2] Similarly, for the same degree of neutropenia disorders of production that affect early hematopoietic precursor cells (aplastic anemia, post-chemotherapy, severe congenital neutropenia) leads to greater susceptibility to infection than conditions with adequate marrow precursors (Felty syndrome, rheumatoid arthritis, autoimmune neutropenia).[2] Moreover, risk of infection is greater when the granulocytes are falling than when they are in recovery for similar counts. There is also more serious and increased risk of infection when neutropenia accompanied by monocytopenia, lymphocytopenia, or hypogammaglobulinemia than with isolated neutropenia. Other risk factors for infection that are commonly present in patients with malignancy receiving myelotoxic chemotherapy, include breaks in the integrity of the mucous membranes and skin, impaired vascular supply to tissues, and poor nutritional status of the hosts. Cytotoxic agents such as the antimetabolites and the alkylating agents can damage the epithelial cells of the oral cavity and gastrointestinal mucosa. The time of maximal gut epithelial damage coincides with the time of neutrophil nadir and greatest opportunity for microbial invasion. Endogenous microbial flora colonizing the oral mucosa or gut epithelium are often responsible for causing infection and fever.

Recent introduction of novel agents to treat malignancy such as monoclonal antibodies directed against cell receptors on B and T cells precursors used for treatment of lymphoma and acute leukemia, have added new problems and may increase the risk for infection, especially systemic fungal infections.[3] Some genetic factors are being identified that may affect the risk of infection in neutropenic cancer patients. Genetically determined deficiency of mannose-binding lectin (MBL), an important component of the innate immune system might influence the duration of fever during neutropenic episodes.[4] In a recent study the duration of fever for patients with MBL deficiency was twice that for patients in the control group (20.5 vs 10.0 days, $p = 0.014$) with febrile neutropenia.[4]

## 7.3 Febrile Neutropenia Definition

Febrile neutropenia is usually defined as the presence of a single oral temperature of >38.3°C (101° F) or a temperature of >38.0°C (100.4°F) for >1 h, with a neutrophil count <500 cells/mm$^3$ (0.5 × 10$^3$/µL); or a count <1,000 cells/mm$^3$ (1.0 × 10$^3$/µL), with a predicted decrease <500 cells/mm.[3,5] The incidence of febrile neutropenic events varies with the patient population and the type of cytotoxic therapy. Eighty to 100% of patients undergoing remission-induction therapy for acute leukemia or patients receiving conditioning therapy for bone marrow transplantation experience febrile episodes during neutropenia.[6] In contrast the rates are much lower for neutropenia associated with chemotherapy for lymphoma (approximately 25%).

At least one-half of neutropenic patients who become febrile have an established or occult infection, and at least 20% of patients with neutrophil count <100 cells/mm$^3$ (0.1 × 10$^3$/µL) have bacteremia.[5] However, febrile episodes occurring during neutropenia may not represent infection. Noninfectious causes of fever include

Table 7.1 Neutrophil count and risk of infection

| Neutropenic score | Absolute granulocytes (× 10$^3$/µL) | Infection |
| --- | --- | --- |
| Mild | 1.0–1.8 | No increase |
| Moderate | 0.5–1.0 | Slight increase |
| Severe | 0.5–0.1 | Substantial increase |
| Critical | <0.1 | Life threatening, extreme increase |

drugs, blood products, underlying cancer, thrombophlebitis, hematomas, and possible absorption of bacterial products from the gut because of damaged epithelium.

In recent years the mortality and treatment of febrile neutropenia has greatly improved, but the mortality rate not only varies with underlying disease, co-morbid factors, age, severity and duration of neutropenia, type and source of infection, but between countries. The overall mortality rate from documented cases of bacteremia decreased from 21% in 1978 to 7% in 1994 in Europe.[7] The 30-day mortality rate from any cause for patients with gram-negative or gram-positive bacteremia are now as low as 10% and 6%, respectively.[8] These dramatic improvements are likely from multiple factors, but rapid treatment with empirical, broad-spectrum antibacterial therapy using very active antimicrobial agents after development of fever has played a pivotal role. Although similar trends are found in many centers of Europe and North America; a recent report of hospitals across the United States involving 2,340 patients with underlying malignancy and nosocomial bacteremia was not confirmatory.[9] A high mortality rate was associated with gram-positive bacteria including coagulase – negative staphylococci (33.4%), methicillin – susceptible *Staphylococcus aureus* (22.8%), and methicillin-resistant *S. aureus* (MRSA) (17.7%).[9] The discrepancies between these reports are difficult to reconcile, but the European data might have the bias of being derived from clinical trials of empiric antibiotic therapy, in which patients are selected or excluded based on specific criteria. The experience at a large cancer center in the United States (M.D. Anderson Cancer Center) underscore the fact that bacteremia accounts for only 35% of proven infections among patients with hematologic malignancies and 20% of infection among patients with solid tumors.[10] Infection occurring at other sites (e.g., pneumonia) or polymicrobial infections had higher mortality rates.[10] It should be noted, however, that the majority of patients presenting with febrile neutropenia do not have bacteremia, pneumonia nor any clinically identifiable site of infection (except oral mucositis) and their prognosis is very good. The most important prognostic factors are usually rate of recovery of the granulocyte count, and response of the underlying cancer to chemotherapy.

## 7.4 Microbiology and Etiology

Previous studies in the 1990s of over 1,700 episodes of febrile neutropenia had found nearly 60% was associated with infections and 43% was unexplained.[11] However, in some studies the group with fever of unknown origin (FUO) can be as high as 60% of febrile neutropenia. In the European Organization for Research and Treatment of Cancer (EORTC) trial[11] 29% of patients had microbiological confirmed bacterial infection (25% with bacteremia), 29% clinically defined infectious, and 3.5% confirmed viral, fungal, or mixed infection. The most common sites of clinically defined infection are usually oral mucositis, intravascular catheter, pneumonia, perianal cellulitis, and neutropenic enterocolitis predominantly in children with acute leukemia, but can occur in adults with prolonged neutropenia.

## 7.4 Microbiology and Etiology

In the past several decades the etiology of bacteremia in febrile neutropenic patients has undergone significant changes. Gram negative bacteria, especially *Escherichia coli* and *Pseudomonas aeruginosa*, were the dominant organisms in the 1960–1970s. The predominant pathogens shifted during the 1980s (internationally), until presently from gram-negative to gram-positive pathogens.[12,13] The reason for the changing microbiology is likely multi-factorial, and these include increased use of prolonged intravascular catheters, prophylaxis with oral quinolones and changes in chemotherapy that leads to greater mucosal damage. The most common infective agents worldwide in febrile neutropenic hosts are coagulase-negative staphylococci (CNS), *S. aureus* (including MRSA), viridans streptococci, enterococci, and gram-negative bacteria. However, there are a few recent reports of resurgence of gram-negative bacteria in neutropenic patients, after prophylaxis.[14,15] In one of these studies from Spain, *E. Coli* was the most common pathogen isolated from blood among febrile neutropenic cancer patients.[16] *P. aeruginosa* infection may also be more prevalent in warmer climates, as it accounted for 27% of pathogens isolated from febrile neutropenic patients in an Indian hospital.[17] In a large 1,000 bed tertiary care hospital in Japan gram-negative organisms were more prevalent during 1985–1996, but gram-positive bacteria became the predominant isolates since 1997 in neutropenic patients.[18] However, *Pseudomonas* species and *Candida* species each accounted for 11.6% of the blood isolates, and MRSA was recovered in about 14%.[18] Polymicrobial infections account for ~15% of infections in the cancer immunocompromised patients, and polymicrobial bacteremia in large trials of neutropenic patients varies from 5% to 32% of those with bacteremia.[19]

### 7.4.1 Initial Antibiotic Therapy

Empiric broad-spectrum antibiotics are always started for febrile neutropenic patients because of the risk of rapid spread of bacterial infection. Prior to the mid-1990s broad-spectrum parenteral agents, singly or in combination, were routinely used to treat febrile neutropenic patients. The greatest advance in the approach to management of febrile neutropenia, in the past decade, has been the advent and general acceptance of oral antibiotics, as initial therapy for low-risk neutropenic patients. The landmark randomized, controlled studies from Pakistan in 1992 and 1995[20,21] confirmed the efficacy of oral antibiotic therapy given to inpatients or outpatients with febrile neutropenia. Since then progress has been made in the development and validation of rules that attempt to predict a low risk (<10%) of severe infection or complication in cancer patients with febrile neutropenia.[22]

Oral out-patient management of selected patients with febrile neutropenia is now widely accepted and recent critical reviews and meta-analyses have endorsed this therapeutic approach.[23–25] Factors associated with a lower risk of complication and a favorable outcome in febrile neutropenia are shown in Table 7.2.[5] A recent international collaborative study of 1,139 febrile neutropenic patients with cancer established and validated a scoring system to identify low-risk patients.[26] A risk

**Table 7.2** Low-risk factors in febrile neutropenia

- Age <60 years
- Cancer in partial or complete remission
- Temperature <39°C
- Mild to moderate symptoms
- Absolute neutrophil count ≥100 cells/mm$^3$
- Absolute monocyte count ≥100 cells/mm
- Evidence of bone marrow recovery
- Duration of neutropenia <7 days
- Resolution of neutropenia expected <10 days
- Normal chest radiograph
- Near normal hepatic and renal function tests
- No neurological or mental changes
- No comorbidity complications: hypoxia, vomiting, diarrhea, shock, dehydration
- No intravenous catheter-site infection

index of ≥21 indicated that the patient is at a low risk (<10%) for developing serious medical complications during the course of febrile neutropenia, and would be suitable for oral out-patient antibiotics (Table 7.3). A risk-index score of ≥21 identified low-risk patients with a positive predictive value of 91%, specificity of 68%, sensitivity of 71%, and negative predictive values of 91%.[22–26] In the multinational study[26] there were only two deaths among low-risk patients, although global misclassification occurred in 30% of the predictive model.[22] The database did not include infants and children but recently Klassent et al.[27] prospectively derived and validated a clinical presentation guideline for pediatric oncology patients with febrile neutropenia. Children with no comorbities, with a normal radiograph and an initial absolute monocyte count >100 cells/mm$^3$ are at the lowest risk for significant bacterial infections.

Although, the initial study in Pakistan[20] used oral ofloxacin the subsequent international validated study[26] used a combination of oral ciprofloxacin and amoxicillin – clavinate for low-risk patients. The risk-index score of >21 in the latter study predicted a <5% risk for severe complication. In an ongoing evaluation of this scoring system the success rate in the out-patient management with oral therapy is about 96%.[28] Theoretically, based on the microbiological spectrum a suitable oral agent would be moxifloxacin which should provide similar coverage as the ciprofloxacin/amoxicillin–clavilanate, and could be an alternative in penicillin allergic subjects. In the most recent Cochrane review of oral versus intravenous antibiotics for febrile neutropenia, 15 trials were analyzed and the mortality and treatment failures were similar between the two modes of therapy; also quinolones alone or combined with another antibiotic were used with comparable results.[29]

## 7.4 Microbiology and Etiology

**Table 7.3** Scoring for febrile neutropenia (Based on data from Klatersky et al.[25])

| Characteristics | Score |
|---|---|
| Outpatient presentation | 3 |
| Age <60 years | 2 |
| Extent of illness: | |
| No or mild symptoms | 5 |
| Moderate symptoms | 3 |
| No hypotension | 5 |
| No dehydration | 3 |
| No chronic obstructive lung disease | 4 |
| Solid tumor or no previous invasive fungal disease | 4 |

A score of >20 is predictive of a low risk.

### 7.4.2 High-Risk Patients

Febrile neutropenic patients with a risk-index score <21 should be considered high risk and be admitted to hospital for intravenous antibiotic therapy. Evaluation of all febrile neutropenic patients, irrespective of score, should include thorough physical examination, especially to identify signs of mucositis, intravenous site inflammation, perianal cellulites, and pneumonia; routine complete blood counts, creatinine, liver enzymes and 2–3 sets of blood cultures (obtained from peripheral vein and any intravascular catheter); chest radiograph and urine culture and urine analysis.

In a prospective multicenter survey in progress,[28] among 663 patients with febrile neutropenia serious complications have occurred in 40% of the high-risk patients and only 13% of the low-risk patients. Mortality rates have been 15% for high-risk subjects and only 1% for the low-risk groups. With respect to prognosis and clinical presentation, fever of unknown origin (usually benign course) has been more frequent in the low-risk than high-risk patients (49% vs 35%). Whereas in the sub-population with bacteremia gram-negative organisms (usually associated with higher mortality), have been more common among high-risk than among low-risk patients (59% vs 31%).[28] However, the opposite has been seen with gram-positive bacteria (reflecting the low virulence, indolent course of CNS, diphtheroids, and viridans streptococci) with 62% vs 38%, in low-risk and high-risk patients, respectively. In the subgroups of patients with bacteremia, complications and mortality were much higher in the high-risk (68% and 28%) than the low-risk patients (24% and 2%).[28]

Empiric broad-spectrum antibiotics to cover gram-positive and gram-negative bacteria are recommended; however, there is no specific agent or combination of choice. Most centers rely on a single broad-spectrum newer beta-lactam agent (such as cefepime, ceftazidime, pipercillin–tazobactam, or imipenem), and others use a combination of aminoglycoside or quinolone (ciprofloxacin) with a beta-lactam agent. Choice of antibiotic should be selected depending on the local antimicrobial resistance pattern in that center, allergy history of the subject, and renal function. Several randomized, controlled studies have compared the response to a single broad-spectrum agent to a combination of agents (usually with an aminoglycoside) in febrile neutropenia. In a recent systematic review and meta-analysis of this topic (47 trials with 7,807 patients), it was concluded that broad-spectrum monotherapy with a beta-lactam was just as effective as combination with an aminoglycoside.[29] A similar conclusion was also reached by a previous meta-analysis.[30]

Although a large randomized study of 543 febrile neutropenic patients showed similar response between a beta-lactam–ciprofloxacin combination compared to a beta-lactam-tobramycin combination,[31] a recent meta-analysis of eight randomized, controlled studies suggested that ciprofloxacin–beta-lactam combination may be somewhat more effective and safer than aminoglycoside–beta-lactam combination.[32] Although there is no proof that combination therapy is better than monotherapy, concerns have been raised about reliance on a broad-spectrum beta-lactam monotherapy, in view of the increasing recognition worldwide of multi-resistant strains to these agents, including extended spectrum beta-lactamase (ESBL) producing gram-negative bacteria. Moreover, gram-positive bacteria which have superseded gram-negative bacilli as the commonest cause of bacteremia are frequently resistant to these agents (i.e. MRSA, MRSE (methicillin-resistant *Staphylococcus epidermidis*, and J.K. diphtheroids). However, empiric addition of vancomycin is not indicated unless mandated by microbiological susceptibility data. In a recent review and meta-analysis of randomized, controlled trials comparing one antibiotic regimen versus the same regimen with a glycopeptide, there was no difference in mortality and response.[33] Thus vancomycin or other glycopeptide should be deferred until the documentation of resistant gram-positive bacteremia, or highly suspicious of MRSA sepsis.

Patients with gram-negative bacteremia are often treated with a combination of antibiotics to broaden the spectrum, to reduce risk of emergence of resistant strains, and to exploit synergism between beta-lactam drugs and aminoglycoside. Although, many randomized, controlled trials and even meta-analysis of monotherapy versus combination therapy showed no difference in outcome in febrile neutropenic patients, the total numbers with gram-negative bacteremia may be too small to avoid a type II error. Earlier observation studies before the advent of highly active beta-lactam agents had shown reduced mortality in *P. aeruginosa* bacteremia with combination therapy.[34] In a more recent prospective observational study of monotherapy versus beta-lactam -aminoglycoside combinations for gram-negative bacteremia, only for neutropenic patients was there a greater benefit with combination therapy (odd ratio [OR], 0.2: 95% confidence interval [CI], 0.05–0.7).[35] For neutropenic patients the mortality rates were 30% (8 of 27) and 7% (4 of 54), for monotherapy versus combination, respectively. However, in a recent meta-analysis of 17 studies addressing this issue (not restricted to neutropenic subjects) combination antimicrobial therapy for gram-negative bacteremia was found not to be superior over monotherapy, but the data suggest that *P. aeruginosa* bacteremias, especially in neutropenic subject may do better with combination of anti-pseudomonas beta-lactam with an aminoglycoside (i.e., tobramycin) or ciprofloxacin.[36,37]

## 7.4.3 Choice of Monotherapy

Although, early empirical broad-spectrum antibiotic has now become established treatment for febrile neutropenia, several beta-lactams are considered acceptable for monotherapy. Numerous clinical trials have compared various beta-lactam therapy and no one agent is clearly superior. However, carbapenems (imipenem–cilistatin and meropenem), piperacillin-tazobactam, and cefepime have advantages over ceftazidime monotherapy because of broader spectrum of activity against gram-positive bacteria and oral flora (prominent causes of febrile neutropenia). Although most comparative studies with ceftazidime versus other monotherapy show similar outcomes in febrile neutropenia, the need for modification or adding gram-positive antibacterial agent is usually significantly higher in the ceftazidime groups. In a relatively large multicentre, randomized controlled study of 411 cancer patients with febrile neutropenia although the differences between groups of patients treated with ceftazidime or meropenem were not statistically significant for clinically defined or microbiologically defined infections, there was some evidence of ceftazidime inferiority.[38] For instance, the rate of clinical response was significantly higher with meropenem for all episodes (54% vs 44%), fever of unknown origin (62% vs 46%), critically neutropenic (<100 cells/μL) patients (55% vs 43%), and bone marrow transplant patients (73% vs 27%).[38] In a recent preliminary data meta-analysis (12 trials of 3,306 patients) ceftazidime was found to be inferior to carbapenems for treatment of febrile neutropenic patients (OR 0.75, $p = 0.001$).[39]

Cefepime (a fourth-generation cephalosporin) has been recommended for monotherapy in febrile neutropenia because of high in vitro activity against most gram-negative and gram-positive bacteria.[5] Moreover, several studies had shown, similar response to other broad-spectrum monotherapy or combination therapy.[40–42] However, in a recent review and meta-analysis of randomized, controlled trials on monotherapy in febrile neutropenia, cefepime was found to be associated with higher all-cause mortality at 30 days than other beta-lactams (relative risk [RR] 1.44, 95 CI 1.06–1.94) in 3,123 participants.[43]

The IDSA guideline in 2002[5] for management of febrile neutropenia did not list any beta-lactam-beta-lactamase inhibitor for monotherapy. However, over the past several years there have been accumulating data on the efficacy of piperacillin/tazobactam as monotherapy for febrile neutropenia. A recent review of Paul et al.[43] listed six trials that assessed piperacillin/tazobactam comparing it with imipenem and meropenem (one trial each) and with cefepime (four trials). Treatment response was similar between piperacillin/tazobactam and with cefepime or carbapenems. A more recent large randomized, controlled study of 528 patients with febrile neutropenia, found similar response between cefepime and piperacillin/tazobactam.[42] In another recent study of febrile neutropenia in patients with acute leukemia or autologous peripheral blood stem cell transplantation piperacillin/tazobactam was comparable to ceftazidime in efficacy.[44] Piperacillin/tazobactam has also been found to be more effective than ceftriaxone plus gentamicin in febrile neutropenic patients with hematological malignancies.[45] Moreover, combination with amikacin was no more effective than with monotherapy with piperacillin/tazobactam.[46] Recent experience of the EORTC group in 763 eligible patients with fever and neutropenia receiving piperacillin/tazobactam as monotherapy has confirmed its value and role in management of febrile neutropenia.[47]

Carbapenems are listed as initial empiric monotherapy for febrile neutropenia by several practice guidelines, including IDSA, NCCN (National Comprehensive Cancer Network), IHOI Infectious Diseases Working party of the German Society of Hematology and Oncology), SEQ (Chemotherapy Society of Spain).[48] Reviews and recent meta-analysis of empiric antibiotic monotherapy for febrile neutropenia have concluded that carbapenems are associated with fewer treatment modifications than other comparators.[43] However, adverse events were significantly more frequent with carbapenems, specifically pseudomembranous colitis (RR 1.94, 95% CI 1.24–3.04).[43] Furthermore, carbapenems daily acquisition costs are higher than piperacillin/tazobactam. For instance in Canada the daily cost of piperacillin/tazobactam (4.5 g 8 hourly) is $64.50, imipenem/cilastatin (500 mg 6 hourly) is $97.52, and meropenem (1 g 8 hourly) is $146.10.

## 7.5 Duration of Therapy

The median time for defervescence for febrile neutropenia after starting monotherapy or combination therapy is 5–7 days in high-risk patients, and 2 days for low-risk subjects.[49,50] Antibiotic regimen may be changed if a causative microbe is identified, according to susceptibility results, but broad-spectrum coverage should be maintained. It has been recommended that antibiotic treatment should be continued for a minimum of 7 days and the patient is free of symptoms and signs.[5] Therapy can be stopped if the neutrophil count has increased to >500 cells/mm$^3$ for 2 consecutive days, and the patient has been afebrile for 48 h in those without documented infection. Although many hematologists prefer to continue antibiotics in those persistently severely neutropenic (<500 cells/mm$^3$) and afebrile for several days, there is no support for this practice in prospective studies. Therapy can be discontinued in persistently neutropenic patients if the patient has been afebrile (preferably >4 days), provided close monitoring continues and signs of infection (if any) have resolved.[51] Patients with persistent severe neutropenia should be treated for at least 2 weeks. However, this is an area which requires further study as guidelines are based on opinions of authorities rather than hard evidence.

In cases of persistent fever despite resolution of neutropenia and no clinical or imaging evidence of infection, all antibiotics should be discontinued and assessed for possible drug fever. Persistent fever may be secondary to underlying disease (i.e., lymphoma), blood products, and occasionally chronic hepatosplenic candidiasis. A clue to this latter diagnosis is increased alkaline phosphatase with or without mild increase in transaminases, and target lesions visible on liver ultrasound or computerized tomography. Rarely other systemic mycosis or viral infection (i.e., cytomegalovirus infection in bone marrow transplants) may account for persistent fever despite resolution of severe neutropenia.

Persistent fever while on broad-spectrum antibiotics for >3–5 days, in the presence of continued severe neutropenia, requires clinical and therapeutic reassessment. The presence of a central intravenous catheter infection or resistant bacterial infection need to be excluded; and the presence of *Clostridia difficile* colitis or drug reaction should be eliminated. Once these possibilities have been ruled out in the reassessment then addition empirical antifungal agents should be considered (especially after 5 days antibiotic therapy). Initial improvement with antibiotic therapy, then subsequent development of fever while still neutropenic can be due to secondary infections. In a recent review of 1,720 patients with their first episode of febrile neutropenia, 836 responded to initial antibiotic therapy but a secondary infection developed in 129 (15%) patients, after a median of 10 days.[52] Thirty-percent of these patients had clinically documented infection (oropharynx and respiratory tract in the majority, followed by skin and soft tissue, gastrointestinal tract, and intravenous device insertion site). Of the 40 patients with microbiologically documented infections there were recovery of gram-positive bacteria in 50% of isolates, gram-negative bacteria in 8%, fungi in 4.2%, and viruses in 9% (herpes simplex and cytomegalovirus).[52]

## 7.6 Empiric Antifungal Therapy

It has become standard practice in most oncology centers to start empiric antifungal therapy for persistent febrile neutropenic patients after 5 days of broad-spectrum antibiotics, with no detectable source or cause of the persistent fever evident. Earlier studies in the 1980s[53,54] found that up to one third of febrile neutropenic patients who fail to respond to 1 week of broad-spectrum antibiotics have systemic fungal infections. The addition of amphotericin B to the broad-spectrum antibiotics became therapy of choice to treat *Candida* or *Aspergillus* species, the most commonly recovered fungi. In some cases antifungal therapy may be withheld if the patient is clinically stable and the neutrophil count is rising. In these cases stopping the antibiotics may be considered to exclude drug fever, particularly if the granulocyte count has risen above 200–300 cells/μL.

Performing other investigations to confirm a systemic fungal infection may be implemented. These include imaging studies such as computerized tomography (CT) of the sinuses, thorax, and the abdomen. Newly developed blood tests to detect *Candida* and *Aspergillus* antigens for rapid, early diagnosis are used by some centers in research settings but are not of established value or commercialized for routine use. The difficulty in making a firm diagnosis of invasive fungal disease is the driving force for empiric antifungal therapy.

In the initial study by Pizzo et al.,[53] after 7 days of antibiotic therapy patients randomized to receive addition of amphotericin B had decreased rate of fungal infection from 31% to 6%. The EORTC trial[54] also confirmed fewer documented invasive fungal infections and fewer fungal-related deaths in the amphotericin treated group versus controls. Comparative trials with more expensive lipid formulations of amphotericin B have found similar success rates compared to the deoxycholate preparation, but fewer side effects.[55,56]

*Candida* species is the most common fungal pathogen in neutropenic patients and is recognized most frequently during the 2nd or 3rd week of neutropenia. Previous studies have shown that the mean interval for development of *Candida sepsis* is 9–11 days after onset of granulocytopenia.[57,58] Aspergillus infection is infrequent during the first 2 weeks of neutropenia but have an increasing incidence over the course of time. Other emerging but less frequent fungal pathogens include *Fusarium* and *Trichosporon* species. Reviews of the experience of large oncology centers in the 1970s–1990s found that *Candida albicans* and *C. tropicalis* were the most frequent *Candida* species causing disseminated infection in neutropenic subjects. Hence, fluconazole which has poor activity against *Aspergillus* species and less frequent *Candida species* (i.e., *C. krusei* and some strains of *C. glabrata*) has been used for low-risk patients in the first 2 weeks of persistent febrile neutropenia. Fluconazole is less toxic than amphotericin B, less expensive than the lipid compounds and available in parenteral and oral preparations, thus would be a suitable alternative if found to be just as effective. Two previous prospective studies in the late 1990s demonstrated that fluconazole was an acceptable alternative to amphotericin B for empirical antifungal therapy at institutions with low drug-resistant *Candida* species or mold infection.[59,60] Empirical fluconazole therapy has not been recommended for patients receiving fluconazole as prophylaxis, or have evidence of pulmonary or sinus infection. However, more recent studies from Europe have found that non-*albicans Candida* spp. accounted for 168 (65%) of 257 candidemic isolates in hematological malignancies.[61] Thus fluconazole may be inappropriate for empiric therapy in febrile neutropenia because of limited spectrum.[62]

Itraconazole, available orally and parenterally (in some countries) has a broader spectrum of activity than fluconazole against non-*albicans Candida* species and *Aspergillus* species. However, the capsule formulation has variable and unpredictable bioavailability and the oral solution is preferable for oral therapy as the intestinal absorption is better and more predictable. In one randomized, controlled study of 384 neutropenic cancer patients, itraconazole (initial 48 h intravenously) and amphotericin B were equivalent in efficacy as empirical therapy, but there was less toxicity with itraconazole.[63] Voriconazole, a new triazole, broad-spectrum antifungal agent available orally and parenterally, with activity against fluconazole-resistant *Candida* species, *Aspergillus* species, and several emerging moulds (*Fusarium* spp. and *Scedosporium* spp) is another alternative to amphotericin B for empiric treatment of febrile neutropenia. In a randomized international study of 837 patients with persistent febrile neutropenia, 415 were assigned to voriconazole and 422 to liposomal amphotericin B.[64] The overall success of treatment was similar but there were fewer documented breakthrough fungal infections in patients treated with voriconazole than in those treated with liposomal amphotericin B (1.9% vs 5%, $p = 0.02$).[64] However, significantly more patients stopped voriconazole due to persistent fever and voriconazole is not approved by the FDA for empirical treatment of febrile neutropenia as it did not meet non-inferior criteria.

Caspofungin, an echinocandin agent available for parenteral use only, has activity against *Candida* species (but *Candida parapsilosis* may respond less readily to treatment)[62] and *Aspergillus* species. Caspofungin was compared to liposomal amphotericin B in a randomized, controlled trial involving over 1,000 neutropenic patients, and was found to be just as effective and better tolerated.[65]

To date alternatives to amphotericin B have shown less toxicity but no clear improvement in efficacy, but at much higher acquisition costs. Recent studies have highlighted problematic issues in trial design and interpretation: inclusion criteria and definition of success are main controversial issues. The criteria in the various randomized studies as to onset of starting antifungal therapy after initiating antibiotic therapy varied from 3 days to greater than 5 days. Most patients receiving empiric antifungal therapy do not need these agents, as only a minority of the persistent febrile episodes are caused by occult invasive fungal infection.[66]

Another controversial issue is the definition of successful therapy in these trials.[67,68] The primary end point of all these trials was a composite criterion of clinical success based with defervescence as a major component of this end point. However, there are numerous causes of fever in these cancer patients including underlying disease and the medications (especially amphotericin B). In fact, the main objective of empiric antifungal therapy is to treat occult invasive fungal infection, or prevent them from breaking through or occurring. Hence, it could be argued that although voriconazole failed the primary objective set forth by the trial design, it achieved the main clinical objective of reduced numbers of invasive fungal infections.[68] Future research in this area should focus on identifying patients of greatest need for antifungal therapy, or patient risk groups stratification for developing invasive candidiasis or aspergillosis, and use or development of new diagnostic techniques for identifying patients at an early stage of infection.[67]

## 7.7 Prevention

### 7.7.1 *Prophylactic Antibiotics*

Attempts to reduce the risk of bacterial infection with severe neutropenia after cancer chemotherapy with prophylactic antimicrobials has been used and studied over the past 2 decades. However, controversy still persists on the overall value and role of antibiotic prophylaxis in this setting. Several earlier studies showed that oral trimethoprim–sulfamethoxazole (TMP–SMZ) reduced the incidence of gram-negative bacterial infection in randomized, controlled trials of patients with severe granulocytopenia.[68–70] However, this soon led to emergence of TMP–SMZ resistance in colonizing coliform bacteria and infections caused by multi-resistant microorganisms in centers using this prophylaxis.[71,72]

Recent studies using fluoroquinolone prophylaxis compared to placebo have shown decreased rates of fever and infection,[73,74] but were not adequately powered for effects on mortality. However, in a recent meta-analysis of antibiotic prophylaxis with fluoroquinolones in afebrile neutropenic patients ($N = 10,274$) in 100 randomized, controlled trials, prophylaxis reduced all-cause mortality and infection-related mortality but did not increase fungal infection.[75] The absolute risk reductions found in this review are small, 4% for all-cause mortality and 4% for infection-related mortality. Moreover, the overall mortality for neutropenia cancer patients with documented bacteremia is only about 7%.[76] Most of the studies included in the analysis were not specifically designed to measure emergence of fluoroquinolone-resistant bacteria, thus pooling of their results was insufficient to provide a firm answer. The potential for emergence, amplification, and dissemination of antibiotic-resistant organisms is a major issue with prophylaxis. There is already a worldwide increase of fluoroquinolone-resistant bacteria, not only in cancer centers[77] but in the community populations.[78] Once these resistant clones become established, they are difficult to control. Based on past experiences it is very likely that centers that use antibiotic prophylaxis in neutropenic patients will eventually experience multi-resistant gram-negative bacteria infections induced by these agents. This will compromise future use of febrile neutropenic oral quinolone therapy for the low-risk patients. Moreover, there are disadvantages of increased adverse effects and increased risk of *Clostridium difficile* colitis. For these and other reasons current guidelines do not recommend routine antibiotic prophylaxis for neutropenic subjects.[5,79]

## 7.7.2 Colony-Stimulating Factors

Colony-stimulating factors (CSF) mainly granulocyte – CSF (GCSF) and less commonly granulocyte – macrophage CSF (GMCSF), have been used as supplemental therapy in many cancer centers for management of febrile neutropenia. Clinical trials have reported conflicting results on the value of CSFs on the improvement of outcomes in patients with febrile neutropenia. In a recent meta-analysis of randomized controlled trials comparing CSFs plus antibiotics versus antibiotics alone for treatment of febrile neutropenia 13 studies met the inclusion criteria.[80] The overall mortality was not influenced by the use of CSF but a marginally significant reduction of infection related mortality was found ($p = 0.05$). However, patients with CSFs had shorter length of hospitalization ($p = 0.0006$) and shorter time to neutrophil recovery ($p = <0.00001$).[80] Thus, adding CSFs also reduces the duration of antibiotic therapy and decreases hospital costs in patients with high-risk febrile neutropenia.[81,82]

CSFs have also been used prophylactically to decrease febrile neutropenia after chemotherapy in various types of cancers. In a systematic review of CSFs to prevent infection and febrile neutropenia in patients undergoing chemotherapy for malignant lymphoma, these agents reduced the relative risk (RR) for severe neutropenia (RR 0.67), febrile neutropenia (RR 0.74), and infection (RR 0.74).[83] However, surprisingly CSFs did not reduce the number of patients requiring intravenous antibiotics nor reduced the infection related mortality, or improved complete tumor response. In children with acute lymphoblastic leukemia (ALL), the use of CSF significantly reduced febrile neutropenic episodes ($p = 0.003$), length of hospitalization ($p = 0.03$), and number of infectious episodes ($p = 0.002$).[84] However, there was no evidence for a shortened duration of neutropenia nor fewer treatment days, and insufficient data to assess the benefit on survival. In another meta-analysis of prophylaxis CSFs after chemotherapy in children with cancer these agents were associated with a 20% reduction in febrile neutropenia and shorter duration of hospitalization (by almost 2 days), but there was no reduction of infection-related mortality.[85] In conclusion, CSFs are of most value for treatment of high-risk patients with severe febrile neutropenia and are cost-effective but do not improve survival.

### 7.7.3 Antifungal Prophylaxis

The incidence of fungal infections has been increasing over the past 2 decades, associated with a greater number of older subjects receiving cancer chemotherapy and organ transplantations. Since invasive fungal infections are difficult to diagnose and treat effectively in the presence of severe neutropenia, antifungal prophylaxis is a consideration in some settings. Fluconazole has been shown to reduce the prevalence of both superficial and systemic fungal infections in bone marrow transplant recipients.[86–88] A meta-analysis of 16 randomized, controlled trials showed that fluconazole reduced the incidence of both superficial and invasive fungal infections in centers in which the incidence of systemic fungal infections exceeds 15%.[89] However, fluconazole has limited activity against *C. krusei* and *C. glabrata* and increased frequency of infection with these strains have been reported in some institutions using prophylaxis with fluconazole.[90] Prophylactic fluconazole 400 mg/day has been used for 75 days following bone marrow transplantation at the Fred Hutchinson Cancer Research Center (Seattle) and 655 patients were enrolled in a study protocol between 1994 and 1997.[91] *C. albicans* was the most frequent colonizing species before fluconazole exposure, but after initiation of fluconazole prophylaxis 53% of colonized patients carried non-*albicans* strains (predominantly, *C. glabrata* and *C. krusei*). Thirty of 651 (4.7%) patients developed candidemia after bone marrow transplantation – the most common species were *C. glabrata* ($N = 14$ or 47%), *C. parapsilosis* ($N = 7$ or 23%), *C. krusei* ($N = 6$ or 20%), *C. albicans* ($N = 2$ or 6.6%). The blood isolates of *C. albicans* were highly resistant to fluconazole (MIC > 64 µL/mL). However, overall the use of prolonged prophylaxis with fluconazole resulted in a low incidence of candidemia and attributable mortality from azole-resistant strains.[91]

Itraconazole oral solution or capsules have been studied in two relatively large randomized, controlled trials for prophylaxis in neutropenic patients with malignancies (including bone marrow recipients).[92,93] The frequency of systemic fungal infections due to *Candida* species were reduced in both, and one trial showed a decrease in candidiasis-related mortality.[94] In a recent multicenter trial of 140 patients undergoing allogeneic hematopoietic stem-cell transplantation, itraconazole was compared to fluconazole for long-term prophylaxis (100 days).[95] Both agents were administered intravenously initially for 2 days followed by oral formulations (itraconazole oral solution was used). Proven invasive fungal infection occurred in 9% of itraconazole recipients versus 25% of fluconazole recipients within 180 days of transplantation, $p = 0.001$. Although the overall mortality rate was similar between the groups, fewer fungal infection related deaths were present in the itraconazole group (9% vs 18%). Itraconazole is more effective than fluconazole for long-term prophylaxis after stem-cell transplantation but gastrointestinal side effects were greater with itraconazole.[95] A recent meta-analysis of five randomized, controlled trials on this topic concluded that itraconazole is more effective in preventing fungal infections in neutropenic patients, but more adverse events may limit its use.[96] In a multicenter randomized trial of high-risk patients with severe prolonged neutropenia, posaconazole ($N = 304$) was compared to oral fluconazole ($N = 240$) or itraconazole ($N = 58$) and found to be superior than the standard azoles in preventing invasive fungal infections (2% vs 8%, $p = 0.003$), and in reducing overall mortality within 100 days after randomization (16% vs 22%, $p = 0.035$).[97] Posaconazole is a new triazole with broader spectrum against yeast and molds, including some zygomycetes and fusarium. Significantly fewer patients receiving posaconazole had invasive aspergillosis (1% vs 7%, $P < 0.001$).[97]

A novel approach to antifungal prophylaxis (mainly to prevent invasive aspergillosis) in patients with prolonged neutropenia is the administration of aerolized amphotericin B. In a recent randomized, placebo-controlled trial of 271 cancer neutropenic patients aerolized liposomal amphoterium B or placebo inhalation twice a week, until neutrophils counts >300 cells/mm$^3$, was administered.[98] Both intent-to-treat and on-treatment analyses demonstrated statistical significant protection against invasive pulmonary aspergillosis in the treated group (OR 0.26 and 0.14, $p = 0.005$ and 0.007, respectively). Main side effects noted was increased coughing with liposomal anphotericin B. This should be a safe, relatively inexpensive means of antifungal prophylaxis. Larger, multicenter trials should be performed with amphotericin B deoxycholate, which theoretically should be just as effective and safe, and would be more cost-effective.

## 7.8 Future Directions

The management of febrile neutropenia has improved greatly in recent years, and the declining trends in mortality are a reflection of successful early adaptation of empirical anti-infective therapy. However, as new cancer treatments are introduced and as microorganisms evolve under selective pressure of antimicrobial agents, we can predict increasing outbreaks of multi-resistant and unusual opportunistic pathogens for the future. Monoclonal antibodies directed against cell receptors on B and T cell precursors used to treat lymphoma and acute leukemia, which may predispose to greater risk of fungal infection, tuberculosis, viral infections, and other intracellular pathogens.[3] In the last decade there has been great progress in the understanding of the molecular pathogenesis of many malignancies, as well as to their genetic determinants, thus scientists and pharmaceuticals are already developing novel antineoplastic agents that will have more specificity against cancer cells and hence, hopefully less toxicity on hematopoietic cells (i.e., granulocytes) and epithelial mucosal cells. There is, however, no stockpile of new promising anti-infectives in development to combat multi-resistant organisms. This area of drug development is seen by many pharmaceuticals as an investment with diminishing returns or profit. Thus collaborative efforts with governments' financial support may be needed for stimulating interest in this area. Widespread use of antibiotic or antifungal prophylaxis will eventually result in selection of resistant microorganisms,[99] and compromise the therapeutic value of our effective armamentarium. Other means of preventing infection in neutropenic subjects are urgently needed. So far routine use of granulocyte-colony-stimulating factors prophylactically does not appear to be the answer. Exploration of novel non-pharmacological products for prophylactic benefit is needed. Bacterial translocation via the intestinal mucosa is a possible mechanism of fever and bacteremia in severe neutropenia. A small pilot project has been recently reported on the safety and dose of a probiotic strain of *Enterococcus faecium* M-74, which may inhibit bowel colonization by pathogenic microorganisms by lactic acid production.[100]

Identification of genetic factors (such as MBL deficiency) that can predispose to extremely high incidence of infection with neutropenia, could be used in the future for selective use of CSFs or antibiotic prophylaxis.

Future research should also concentrate on more sensitive and specific non-invasive tests in accurately diagnosing fungal infections in the neutropenic subjects. This would allow early prompt directed antifungal therapy, rather than treating many patients with prolonged fever without fungal infections with potentially toxic and expensive antifungal agents. Although, newer techniques such as PCR for detecting fungal antigens appear promising, there is still a way to go before they become standard diagnostic tools.[101] Although the risk of invasive aspergillosis in hematopoietic stem transplant correlates with the degree of immunosuppression and exposure to fungal spores, other factors are likely important as only 5 to 10% of transplanted patients develop these infections.[102] Thus these high risk groups should be particularly targeted for aspergillosis prophylaxis, such as subjects with toll-like receptor (TLR) – 1 and TLR6 polymorphisms,[102] and recipients of allogeneic hematopoetic-cell transplants from donors with TLR4 polymorphism, especially S4 haplotype.[103]

# References

1. Borregaard, N., Boxer, L.A., (2006), Disorders of neutrophil function, in: Williams Hematology, 7th Edition; Lichtman, M.A., Beutler, E., Kipps, T.J., Seligsohn, U., Kaushansky, K., Prchal, J.T., (eds); McGraw-Hill Medical, New York, pp. 921–957.

2. Dale, D.C., (2006), Neutropenia and neutrophilia, in: Williams Hematology, 7th Edition; Licktman, M.A., Beutler, E., Kipps, T.J., Seligsohn, U., Kaushansky, K., Prchal, J.T. (eds); McGraw-Hill Medical, New York, pp. 907–919.
3. Marty, F.M., Lee, S.J., Fahey, M.M., Alyea, E.P., Soiffer, R.J., Antin, J.H., Baden, L.R., (2003), Infliximab use in patients with severe graft-versus-host disease and other emerging risk factors of non-Candida invasive fungal infections in allogeneic hematopoietic stem cell transplant recipients: a cohort study. Blood 102: 2768–2776.
4. Neth, O., Hann, I., Turner, M.W., Klein, N.J., (2001), Deficiency of mannose-binding lectin and burden of infection in children with malignancy: a prospective study. Lancet 358: 614–618.
5. Hughes, W.T., Armstrong, D., Bodey, G.P., Bow, E.J., Brown, A.E., Calondra, T., Feld, R., Pizzo, P.A., Rolston, K.V.I., Shenep, J.L., Young, L.S., (2002) 2002 Guidelines for the use of antimicrobial agents in neutropenic patients with cancer. Clin. Infect. Dis. 34: 730–751.
6. Van der Anwera, P., Gerain, J., (1993), Use of quinolones in the prophylaxis and treatment of granulocytopenic immunocompromised cancer patients. Drugs 45(Suppl 3): 81–90.
7. Viscoli, C., EORTC International Antimicrobial Therapy Group, (2002), Management of infection in cancer patients: studies of the EORTC (International Antimicrobial Therapy Group (IATG). Eur. J. Cancer 38(Suppl 4): S82–S87.
8. Viscoli, C., Castagnola, E., (1998), Planned progressive antimicrobial therapy in neutropenic patients. Br. J. Hematol. 102: 879–888.
9. Wisplinghoff, H., Seifert, H., Werzel, R.P., Edmond, M.P., (2003), Current trends in the epidemiology of noscomial blood stream infections in patients with hematological malignancies and solid neoplasms in hospitals in the United States. Clin. Infect. Dis. 36: 1103–1110.
10. Yadegarynia, D., Turrand, J., Raad, I., Rolston, K., (2003), Current spectrum of bacterial infections in patients with cancer. Clin. Infect. Dis. 7(Suppl): S1144–S1145.
11. The International Antimicrobial Therapy Cooperative Group of the European Organization for Research and Treatment of Cancer (1993), Efficacy and toxicity of single doses of amikacin and ceftriaxone versus multiple daily doses of amikacin and ceftazidime for infection in patients with cancer and granulocytopenia. Ann. Intern. Med. 119: 584–593.
12. Zinner, S.H., (1999), Changing epidemiology of infections in patients with neutropenia and cancer: emphasis on gram-positive and resistant bacteria. Clin. Infect. Dis. 29: 490–494.
13. Ramphal, R., (2004), Changes in the etiology of bacteremia in febrile neutropenic patients and the susceptibilities of the currently isolated pathogens. Clin. Infect. Dis. 39(Suppl I): S25–S31.
14. Catorratala, J., Fernandez Sevilla, A., Tubau, F., Callis, M., Gudiol, F., (1995), Emergence of quinolone-resistant *Escherichia coli* bacteremia in neutropenic patients with cancer who have received prophylactic norflxacin. Clin. Infect. Dis. 20: 557–560.
15. Haupt, R., Rumanengo, M., Fears, T., Viscoli C., Castagnola, E., (2001), Incidence of septicemias and invasive mycoses in children undergoing treatment for solid tumors: a 12 year experience at a single Italian institution. Eur. J. Cancer, 37: 2413–2419.
16. Gaytan-Martinez, J., Mateos-Garcia, E., Sanchez-Cortes, Gonzalez-Llaven, J., Casanova-Cardiel, L.J., Fuentes-Allen, J.L., (2002), Microbiological findings in febrile neutropenia. Arch. Med. Res. 31: 388–392.
17. Raje, N.S., Rao, S.R., Iyer, R.S., Kelkar, R.S., Pai, S.K., Nair, C.N., Kurkure, R.A., Magrath, I. T., Advani, S.H., (1994), Infection analysis in acute lymphoblastic leukemia: a report of 499 consecutive episodes in India. Pediatr. Hematol. Oncol. 3: 271–280.
18. Kanamaru, A., Tatsumi, Y., (2004), Microbiological data for patients with febrile neutropenia. Clin. Infect. Dis. 39(Suppl. I) S7–S10.
19. Rolston, VI, Bodey, GP, Safdar, A, (2007), Polymicrobial infection in patients with cancer: an under appreciated and underreported entity. Clin. Infect. Dis. 45: 225–233.
20. Malik, A., Abbas, Z., Karim, M., (1992), Randomized comparison of oral ofloxacin alone with combination of parenteral antibiotics in neutropenic febrile patients. Lancet 339: 1092–1096.

21. Malik, I.A., Khan, W.A., Karim, M., Aziz, Z., Khan, M.A. (1995), Feasibility of outpatient management of fever in cancer patients with low-risk neutropenia: results of a prospective randomized trial. Am. J. Med. 98: 224–231.
22. Kern, W.V., (2006), Risk assessment and treatment of low-risk patients with febrile neutropenia. Clin. Infect. Dis. 42: 533–540.
23. Klastersky, J., (2004), Management of fever in neutropenic patients with different risks of complications. Clin. Infect. Dis. 39(Suppl 1): S32–S37.
24. Vidal, L., Paul, M., Ben-Dor, I., Soares-Weiser, K., Leibovici, L., (2004), Oral versus intravenous antibiotic treatment for febrile neutropenia in cancer patients: a systemic review and meta-analysis of randomized trials. J. Antimicrob. Chemother: 54: 29–37.
25. Sipsas, N.V., Bodey, G.P., Kontoyiannis, D. P., (2005), Perspectives for the management of febrile neutropenic patients with cancer in the 21st century. Cancer 103: 1103–1113.
26. Klatersky. J., Paesmans, M., Rubenstein, E.B., Boyer, M., Elting, L., Feld, R., Gallagher, J., Herrstedt, J., Rapoport, B., Rolston, K., Talcott, J; for the Study Section of Multinational Association for Supportive Care in Cancer, (2000), The Multinational Association for Supportive Care in Cancer risk index: a multinational scoring system for identifying low-risk febrile neutropenic cancer patients. J. Clin. Oncol. 18: 3038–3051.
27. Klassen, R.J., Goodman, R., Pham, B.A., Doyle, J.J., (2000), "Low-risk" prediction rule for pediatric oncology patients presenting with fever and neutropenia. J. Clin. Oncol. 18: 1012–1019.
28. Vidal, L., Paul, M., Ben- Dor, I., Pokroy, E., Soares-Weiser, K., Leibovic L., (2006), Oral versus intravenous antibiotic treatment for febrile neutropenia in cancer patients. Cochrane Database Syst. Rev. 3: Access no.00075320–100000000–03018.
29. Paul, M., Soares-Weiser, K., Leibovici., L., (2003), Beta-lactam monotherapy versus beta-lactam-aminoglycoside combination therapy for fever with neutropenia: a systematic review and meta-analysis. B.M.J 326: 1111.
30. Furno, P., Bucaneve, G., Del Favero, A., (2002), Monotherapy or aminoglycoside- containing combinations for empirical antibiotic treatment of febrile neutropenic patients: a meta-analysis. Lancet Infect. Dis. 2: 231–242.
31. Peacock, J.E., Herrington, D.A., Wade, J.C., Lazarus, H.M., Reed, M.D., Sinclair, J.W., Havestock, D.C., Kowalsky, S.F., Hurd, D.D., Cushing, D.A., Harman, C.P., Donowitz, G. R., (2002), Ciprofloxacin plus piperacillin compared with tobramycin plus piperacillin as empirical therapy in febrile neutropenic patients. A randomized, double-blind trial. Ann. Intern. Med. 137: 77–87.
32. Bliziotis, I.A., Michalopoulos, A., Kasiakou, S.K., Samonis, G., Christodoulou, C., Chrysanthopoulou, S., Falagas, M.E., (2005) Ciprofloxacin vs an aminoglycoside in combination with a beta-lactam for the treatment of febrile neutropenia: a meta-analysis of randomized controlled trials. Mayo Clin, Proc. 80: 1146–1156.
33. Paul, M., Borok, S., Fraser, A., Vidal, L., Cohen, M., Leibovici, L., (2005), Additional anti-Gram-positive antibiotic treatment for febrile neutropenic cancer patients. Cochrane Database Syst. Rev. (3): CD 003914.
34. Hilf, M., Yu, K.L., Sharp, J., Zuravleff, J.J., Korvick, J.A., Muder, R.R., (1989), Antibiotic therapy for *Pseudomonas aeruginosa* bacteremia: outcome correlations in a prospective study of 200 patients. Am. J. Med. 83: 119–123.
35. Leibovici, L., Paul, M., Poznanski, O., Drucker, M., Samra, S., Konigsberger, H., Pitlik, S.D., (1997), Monotherapy versus β-lactam-aminoglycoside combination treatment for gram-negative bacteremia: a prospective observational study. Antimicrob. Agents Chemother. 41: 1127–1133.
36. Safdar, N., Handelsman, J. Maki, D.G., (2004), Does combination antimicrobial therapy reduce mortality in Gram-negative bacteremia? A meta-analysis. Lancet Infect. Dis. 4: 519–527.
37. Chow, J.W., Yu, V.L., (1999), Combination antibiotic therapy versus monotherapy for gram-negative bacteremia: a commentary. Int. J. Antimicrob. Agents 11: 7–12.

38. Feld, R., DePauw, B., Berman, S., Keating, A., Ho, W., (2000), Meropenem versus ceftazidime in the treatment of cancer patients with febrile neutropenia: a randomized, double blind trial. J. Clin. Oncol 18: 3690–3698.
39. Glasmacher, A., von Lilienfeld., Toal, M., Schulte, S., Hahn, C., Schmidt-Wolf, Prentice, A., (2005), An evidence-based evaluation of important aspects of empirical antibiotic therapy in febrile neutropenic patients. Clin. Microbiol. Infect. 11(Suppl 5): 17–23.
40. Cherif, H., Bjorkholm M., Engervall, P., Johansson, P., Ljungmar, P., Hast, R., Kalin, M., (2004), A prospective, randomized study comparing cefepime and imipenem-cilastatin in the empirical treatment of febrile neutropenia in patients treated for haematological malignancies. Scand. J. Infect. Dis. 36: 593–600.
41. Tamura, K., Imajo, K., Akiyama, N., Susuki, K., Urabe, A., Ohyashiki, K., Tanimoto, M., Masaoka, T., Japan Febrile Neutropenic Study Group, (2004), Randomized trial of cefepime monotherapy or cefepime in combination with amikacin as empirical therapy for febrile neutropenia Clin. Infect. Dis. 39(Suppl 1): S15–S24.
42. Bow, E.J., Rotstein, C., Noskin, G.A., Laverdiere, M., Schwarer, A.P., Segal, B.H., Seymour, J.F. Szer, J., (2006), A randomized, open-label, multicenter comparative study of the efficacy and safety of piperacillin-tazobactam and cefepime for the empirical treatment of febrile neutropenic episodes in patients with hematologic malignancies. Clin. Infect. Dis. 43: 447–459.
43. Paul, M., Yahav, D., Fraser, A., Leibovici, I., (2006), Empirical antibiotic monotherapy for febrile neutropenia: systematic review and meta-analysis of randomized controlled trials. J. Antimicrob. Chemother. 57: 176–189.
44. Harter, C., Schulze, B., Goldschmidt, H., Benner, A., Geiss, H.K., Hoppe-Tichy, T., Ho, A.D., Egerer, G., (2006), Piperacillin/tazobactam vs ceftazidime in the treatment of neutropenic fever in patients with acute leukemia or following autologous peripheral blood stem cell transplantation: a prospective randomized trial. Bone Marrow Transpl. 37: 373–379.
45. Gorschluter, M., Hahn, C., Fixson, A., Mey, U., Ziske, C., Molitor, E., Horre, R., Sauerbruch, T., Marklein, G., Schmidt-Wolf, I.G., Glasmacher, A., (2003), Piperacillin/tazobactam is more effective than ceftriaxone plus gentamicin in febrile neutropenic patients with hematological malignancies: a randomized comparison. Support Care Cancer: 11: 362–370.
46. Del Favero, A., Menichetti, F., Martino, P., Bucaneve, G., Micozzi, A., Gentile, G., Furno, P., Russo, D., (2001), A multicenter, double-blind, placebo-controlled trial comparing piperacillin/tazobactam with and without amikacin as empiric therapy for febrile neutropenia. Clin. Infect. Dis. 33: 1295–1301.
47. Viscoli, C., Cometta, A., Kern, W.V., Bock, R., Paesmans, M., Crokaert. F., Glauser, M.P., Calandra, T., (2006), Piperacillin/tazobactam monotherapy in high-risk febrile and neutropenic cancer patients. Clin. Microbiol. Infect. 12: 212–216.
48. Glasmacher, A., von Lilienfeld-Toal, M., Schulte, S., Hahn, C., Schmidt-Wolf, I.G.H., Prentice, C., (2005), An evidence based evaluation of important aspects of empirical antibiotic therapy in febrile neutropenic patients. Clin, Microbiol. Infect. 11(Suppl 5): 17–23.
49. Elting, L.S., Rubenstein, E.B., Rolston, K., Cantor, S., Martin, G.G., Kurtin, D., Rodriguez, S., Lam, T., Kanesan, K., Bodey, G., (2000), Time to clinical response and outcome of antibiotic therapy of febrile neutropenia with implications for quality and cost of care. J. Clin. Oncol. 18: 3699–3706.
50. Freifeld, A., Marchigiani, D., Walsh, T., Chanock, S., Lewis, L., Hiemenz, J., Hiemenz S., Hicks, J.E., Gill, V., Steinberg, S.M., Pizzo, P.A., (1999), A double-blind comparison of empirical oral and intravenous antibiotic therapy for low-risk febrile patients with neutropenia during cancer chemotherapy. N. Engl. J. Med. 341: 305–311.
51. Rolston, K.V.I., (2004), The Infectious Diseases Society of America 2002 Guidelines for the use of antimicrobial agents in patients with cancer and neutropenia: salient features and comments. Clin. Infect. Dis. 39(Suppl 1): S46–S48.
52. Akova, M., Paesmans, M., Calandra, T., Viscoli, C., for the International Antimicrobial Therapy Group of the European Organization for Research and Treatment of Cancer

# References

(2005), A European Organization for Research and Treatment of Cancer-International Antimicrobial Therapy Group study of secondary infections in febrile, neutropenic patients with cancer. Clin. Infect. Dis. 40: 239–245.

53. Pizzo, P.A., Robichaud, K.J., Gill, F.A., Witebsky, F.G., (1982), Empiric antibiotic and antifungal therapy for cancer patients with prolonged fever and granulocytopenia. Am. J. Med. 72: 101–111.

54. E O R T C International Antimicrobial Therapy Cooperative Project Group, (1989), Empiric antifungal therapy in febrile granulocytopenic patients. Am. J. Med. 86: 668–672.

55. Walsh, J.T., Finberg, R.W., Arndt, C., Hiemenz, J., Schwartz C., Bodensteiner, D., Pappas, P., Seibel, N., Greenberg, R.N., Dummer, S., Schuster, M., Holcenberg, J.S. for the National Institute of Allergy and Infectious Diseases Mycoses Study Group (1999) Liposomal amphotericin B empirical therapy in patients with persistent fever and neutropenia, National Institute of Allergy and Infectious Diseases Mycoses Study Group. N. Engl. Med. 340: 764–771.

56. Wingard, J.R., White, M.H., Anaissie, E., Raffalli, J., Goodman, J. Arrieta, A., and the L-Amph./ABLC Collaborative Study Group, (2000), A randomized, double-blind comparative trial evaluating the safety of liposomal amphotericin B versus amphotericin lipid complex in the empirical treatment of febrile neutropenia. Clin. Infect. Dis. 31: 1155–1163.

57. Saral, R., (1991), Candida and aspergillus infections in immunocompromized patients: An overview. Rev. Infect. Dis. 13: 487–492.

58. Horn, R., Wong, B., Kiehn, T.E., Armstrong, D., (1985), Fungemia in a cancer hospital: changing frequency, earlier onset and results of therapy. Rev. Infect. Dis. 7: 646–655.

59. Viscoli, C., Castagnola C., VanLint, M.T., Moroni, C., Gararenta, A., Rossi, M.R., Fanci, R., Menichetti, F., Casselli, D., Giacchino, M., Congiu, M., (1996), Fluconazole versus Amphotericin B as empirical antifungal therapy of unexplained fever in granulocytopenic cancer patients. Eur. J. Cancer 32A: 814–820.

60. Winston, D. J., Hathorn, J. W., Schuster, M.G., Schiller, G. J., Territo, M.C., (2002), A multicenter randomized trial of fluconozole versus amphotericin B for empiric antifungal therapy of febrile neutropenic patients with cancer. Am. J. Med. 108: 282–289.

61. Tortorano, A.M., Peman, J., Bernhardt, H., Klingspor, L., Kibbler, C.C., Faure, O., Biraghi, E., Canton, E., Zimmermann, K., Seaton,S., Grillot, R., the ECMM Working Group on Candidaemia, (2004), Epidemiology of candidaemia in Europe: Results of 28 – month European Confederation of Medical Mycology (ECMM) hospital- based surveillance study. Eur. J. Clin. Micriobial Infect. Dis. 23: 317–322.

62. Pappas, P. G., Rex, J.H., Sobel, J., Filler, S.G., Dismukes, W.E., Walsh, T.J., Edwards, J.E., (2004), Guidelines for treatment of candidiasis. Clin. Infect. Dis. 38: 161–189.

63. Boogaerts, M., Winston, D.J., Bow, E.J., Garber, G., Reboli, A.C., Schwarer, A.P., Novitzky, N., Boehome, A., Chwetzoff, E., De Beule, K., and the Intraconazole Neutropenic Study Group, (2001), Intravenous and oral itraconazole versus intravenous amphotericin B deoxycholate as empirical antifungal therapy for persistent fever in neutropenic patients with cancer who are receiving broad-spectrum antibacterial therapy. Ann. Intern. Med. 135: 412–422.

64. Walsh, T.J., Pappas, P., Winston, D.J., Lazarus, H.M., Petersen, F., Raffalli, J., Yanovich, S., Stiff, P., Greenberg, R., Danowitz, G., Schuster, M., Reboli, A., Wingard, J. Arndt, C., Reinhardt, J. Hadley, S., Finberg, R., Laverdierre, M., Perfect, J., Garber, G., Fioritoni, G., Anaissie, E., Lee, J. National Institute of Allergy and Infectious Diseases Mycoses Study Group, (2002), Vorionazole compared with liposomal amphotericin B for empirical antifungal therapy in patients with neutropenia and persistent fever. N. Engl. J. Med. 346: 225–234.

65. Walsh, T.J., Teppler, H., Donowitz, G.R., Maertens, J.A., Baden, L.R., Dmoszynska, A., Cornely, O.A., Bourque, M.R., Lupinacci, R.J., Sable, C.A., dePauw, B.E., (2004), Caspofungin versus liposomal amphotericin B for empirical antifungal therapy in patients with persistent fever and neutropenia. N. Engl. J. Med. 351: 1391–1402.

66. Winegard, J.R., (2004), Empirical antifungal therapy in treating febrile neutropenic patients. Clin. Infect. Dis. 39(Suppl): S38–S43.

67. Martino R., Viscoli, C., (2005), Empirical antifungal therapy in patients with neutropenia and persistent or recurrent fever of unknown origin. Brit. J. Haematol. 132: 138–154.
68. Sobel, J.D., (2006), Design of Clinical trials of empiric antifungal therapy in patients with persistent febrile neutropenia: considerations and critiques. Pharmacotherapy: 26 (Suppl): 47S–54S.
69. Gurwith, M.J., Brunton, J.L., Lank, B.A., Harding, G.K.M., Ronald, A.R., (1979), A prospective controlled investigation of prophylactic trimethoprim/sulfamethoxazole in hospitalized granulocytopenic patients. Am. J. Med. 66: 248–256.
70. Wade, J.C., Schimpff, S.C., Hargadon, M.T., Fortner, C.L., Young, V.M., Wiernik, P.H., (1981), A comparison of trimethoprim-sulfamethoxazole plus nystatin with gentamicin plus nystatin in the prevention of infections in acute leukemia. N. Engl. J. Med. 304: 1057–1062.
71. Dekker, A.W., Rozenberg-Arska, M., Sixma, J.J. Verhoef, J., (1981), Prevention of infection by trimethoprim-sulfamethoxazole plus amphotericin B in patients with acute nonlymphocytic leukemia. Ann. Intern. Med. 95: 555–5591.
72. Wilson, J.M., Guiney, D.G., (1982), Failure of oral trimethoprim-sulfamethoxazole prophylaxis in acute leukemia. Isolation of resistant plasmids from strains of Enterobacteriaceae are causing bacteremia. N. Engl. J. Med. 306: 16–20.
73. Murray, B.E., Rensimer, E.R., Du Port, H.L., (1982), Emergence of high level trimethoprim, resistance in fecal *Escherichia coli* during oral administration of trimethoprim–or trimethoprim-sulfamethoxazole, N. Engl. J. Med. 306: 130–135.
74. Bucaneve, G., Micozzi, A., Menichetti, F., Martino, P., Dionisi, M.S., Martirelli G., Allione, B., D'Antonio, D., Buelli, M., Nosari, A.M., Cilloni, D., Zuffa, E., Cantaffa, R., Specchia, G., Amadori, S., Fabbiano, F., Deliliers, G.L., Lauria, F., Foa, R., Del Favero, A., for the Gruppo Italiano Malattié Ematologiche dell □ Adulto (GIMEMA) Infection Program, (2005), Levofloxacin to prevent bacterial infection in patients with cancer and neutropenia. N. Engl. J. Med. 353: 977–987.
75. Cullen, M., Steven, N., Billingham, L., Gaunt, C., Hastings, M., Simmonds, P., Stuart, N., Rea, D., Bower, M., Fernando, I., Huddart, R., Gollins, S., Phil, D., Stanley, A., for the Simple Investigation in Neutropenic Individuals of the Frequency of Infection after chemotherapy + / − Antibiotic in a Number of Tumours (SIGNIFICANT) Trial Group, (2005), Antibacterial prophylaxis after chemotherapy for solid tumors and lymphomas. N. Engl J. Med. 353: 988–998.
76. Gafter-Gvilli, A., Fraser, A., Paul, M., Leibovici, L., (2005), Meta-Analysis: Antibiotic prophylaxis reduces mortality in neutropenic patients. Ann. Intern. Med. 142: 979–995.
77. Viscoli, C., Varnier, O., Machetti, M., (2005), Infections in patients with febrile neutropenia; epidemiology, microbiology and risk stratification. Clin. Infect. Dis. (Suppl.4): S240–S245.
78. Kern, W.V., Andriof, E., Oethinger, M., Kern, P., Hacker, J., Morre, R., (1994) Emergence of fluoroquinolone-resistant *Escherichia coli* at a cancer center. Antimicrobial Agents Chemother. 38: 681–687.
79. Hooper, D.C., (2001), Emerging mechanisms of flouroquinolone resistance. Emerg. Infect. Dis. 7: 337–341.
80. Sullivan, K.M., Dykewicz, C.A., Longworth, D.L., Boeckh, M., Baden, C.R., Rubin, R.H., Sepkowitz, K.A., Centers for Disease Control and Prevention; Infectious Diseases Society of America, American Society for Blood and Marrow Transplantation Practice Guidelines and beyond, (2001), Preventing opportunistic infections after hematopoietic stem cell transplantation: the Centers for Disease Control and Prevention, Infectious Diseases Society of America, and American Society for Blood and Marrow Transplantation Practice Guidelines and beyond. Hematology (Am. Soc. Hematol. Educ. Program): 392–421.
81. Clark, O.A., Lyman, G.H., Castro, A.A., Clark, L.G., Djulbegovic, B., (2005), Colony–stimulating factors for chemotherapy − induced febrile neutropenia: a meta-analysis of randomized controlled trials. J. Clin. Oncol. 23: 4198–4214.
82. Garcia-Carbonero, R., Mayordomo, J.I., Tornamira, M.V., Lopez − Brea, M., Rueda, A., Guillem. V., Arcediano, A., Yubero, A., Ribera, F., Gomez, C., Tres, A., Perez-Garcia, J.L.,

Lumbreras, C., Hornedo, J., Cortes-Funes, H., Poz-Ares, L., (2001) Granulocyte colony-stimulating factor in treatment of high-risk febrile neutropenia: a multicenter randomized trial. J. National Cancer Inst. 93: 31–38.
83. Lyman, G., H., Kuderer, N.M., (2004), The economics of the colony – stimulating factors in the prevention and treatment of febrile neutropenia. Crit. Rev. Oncol. Hematol. 50: 129–146.
84. Bohlius, R., Reiser, M., Schwarzer G., Engert, A., (2004), Granulopoiesis-stimulating factors to prevent adverse effects in the treatment of malignant lymphoma. Cochrane Database Syst. Rev., C.D 003189: PMID: 14974009.
85. Sasse, E.C., Sasse, A.d., Brandalise, S., Clark, O.A., Richards, S., (2005) Colony stimulating factors for prevention of myelosuppressive therapy induced febrile neutropenia in children with acute lymphoblastic leukemia. Cochrane Database Syst. Rev. CD004139.
86. Sung, L., Nathan, P.C., Lange, B., Beyene, J., Buchanan, G.R., (2004), Prophylactic granulocyte colony stimulating factor and granulocyte-macrophage colony-stimulating factor decreases febrile neutropenia after chemotherapy in children with cancer: a meta-analysis of randomized trials. J. Clin. Oncol. 22: 3350–3356.
87. Goodman, J.L., Winston, D.J., Greenfield, A., Chandrasekar, P.N., Fox, B., Kaizer, H., Shadduck, R.K., Shea, T.C., Stiff, P., Friedman, D.J., (1992), A controlled trial of fluconazole to prevent fungal infections in patients undergoing bone marrow transplantation: a prospective, randomized, double-blind study. N. Engl. J. Med. 326: 845–851.
88. Slavin, M.A., Osborne, B., Adams, R., Levenstein, M.J., Schoch, H.G., Feldman, A.R. Myers, J.D., Bowden, R.A., (1995), Efficacy and safety of fluconazole prophylaxis for fungal infections after marrow-transplantation – a prospective, randomized, double-blind study. J. Infect. Dis. 171: 1545–1552.
89. Ellis, M.E., Clink, H., Ernst, P., Halim, M.A., Padmos, A., Spence, D., Kalin, M., Hussain Qadri, S.M., Burnie, J., Greer, W., (1994) Controlled study of fluconazole in the prevention of fungal infections in neutropenic patients with haematological malignancies and bone marrow transplant recipients. Eur. J. Clin Microbiol. Infect. Dis. 13: 3–11.
90. Kanda, Y., Yamamoto, R., Chizuka, A., Hamaki T., Suguro, M., Arai, C., Matsuyama, T., Takezako, N., Miwa, A., Kern, W., Kami, M., Akiyama, H., Hirai, H., Togawa, A. (2000) Prophylactic action of oral fluconazole against fungal infection in neutropenic patients: a meta-analysis of 16 randomized, controlled trials, Cancer: 89 1611–1625.
91. Wingard, J.R., Mertz, M.G., Rinaldi, M.G., Johnson, T.R., Karp, J.E., Saral, R., (1991), Increases in *Candida krusei* infection among patients with bone marrow transplantation and neutropenia treated prophylactically with fluconazole. N. Engl. J. Med. 325: 1274–1277.
92. Marr, K.A., Saidel, K., White, T.C., Bowden, R.A., (2000), Candidemia in allogeneic blood and marrow transplant recipients: Evolution of risk factors after the adoption of prophylactic fluconazole. J. Infect. Dis. 181: 309–316.
93. Menichetti, F., Del Favero, A., Martino, P., Bucaneve, G., Micozzi, A., Girmenia, C., Barbabietola, G., Pagano, L., Leoni, P., Specchia, G., Caiozzo, A., Raimondi, R., Mandelli, F., and the GIMEMA Infection Program, (1994), Itraconazole oral solution as prophylaxis for fungal infection in neutropenic patients with hematologic malignancies: a randomized, placebo – controlled, double-blind, multicenter trial. Clin. Infect. Dis. 28: 250–255.
94. Nucci, M., Biasoli, I., Akiti, T., Silveira, F., Solza, C., Barreiros, G., Spector, N., Derossi, A., Pulcheri, W., (2000), A double-blind, randomized, placebo-controlled trial of itraconazole, capsules as antifungal prophylaxis for neutropenic patients. Clin. Infect. Dis. 30: 300–305.
95. Winston, D.J., Maziarz, R.T., Chandrasekar, P.H., Lazarus, H.M., Goldman, M., Blumer, J.L. Leitz, G. J., Territo, M.C., (2003), Intravenous and oral itraconazole versus intravenous and oral fluconazole for long-term antifungal prophylaxis in allogeneic hemotopoietic stem-cell transplant recipients. Ann. Intern. Med. 138: 705–713.
96. Vardakas, K.A., Michalopoulos, A., Falagas, M.E., (2005), Fluconazole versus itraconazole for antifungal prophylaxis in neutropenic patients with hematological malignancies: a meta-analysis of randomized-controlled trials. Brit. J. Haematol. 131: 22–28.

97. Cornely, O.A., Maertens, J., Winston, D. J., Perfect, J., Ullmann, A.J., Helfgott, D., Walsh, T.J., Holowiecki, J., Stockelberg, D., Goh, Y.T., Petrini, M., Hardalo, C., Suresh, R., Angulo-Gonzalez, D., (2007) Posoconazole vs fluconazole or itraconazole prophylaxis in patients with neutropenia. N. Engl. J. Med. 356: 348–359.
98. Rijnders, B.J., Cornelissen, J.J., Slobbe, L., Becker, M.J., Doorduijn, J.K., Hop, W.C., Ruijgrok, E.J., Löwenberg, B., Vulto, A., Lugtenburg, P.J., de Marie, S., (2008), Aerolized amphotericin B for the prevention of invasive pulmonary aspergillosis during prolonged neutropenia: a randomized, placebo-controlled trial. Clin. Infect. Dis. 46: 1401–1408.
99. Imbof, A., Arunmozhi Balajee, A., Fredricks, D.N., Englund, J.A., Marr, K.A., (2004), Breakthrough fungal infections in stem cell transplant recipients receiving voriconazole. Clin. Infect. Dis. 39: 743–746.
100. Mego, M., Ebringer, L., Drgona, L., Mordiak, J., Trupl, J., Greksak, R., Nemova, I., Oravcova, E., Zajac, V., Koza, I., (2005), Prevention of febrile neutropenia in cancer patients by probiotic strain *Enterococcus faecium* M-74. Pilot study phase I. Neoplasma; 52: 159–164.
101. Donnelly, J.P., (2006), Polymerase chain reaction for diagnosing invasive aspergillosis: getting closer but still a ways to go. Clin. Infect. Dis. 42: 487–489.
102. Pamer EG., 2008, TLR polymorphisms and the risk of invasive fungal infections (Editorial). N. Engl. J. Med. 359: 1836–1838.
103. Bochud, P.Y., Chien, J.W., Marr, K.A., Leisenring, W.M., Upton, A., Janer, M., Rodrigues, S. D., Li, S., Hansen, J.A., Zhao, L.P., Aderem, A., Boeckh, (2008), Toll-like receptor 4 polymorphism and aspergillosis in stem-cell transplantation. N. Engl. J. Med. 359: 1766–1777.

# Chapter 8
# Emerging Issues and Trends in *Clostridium difficile* Colitis

## 8.1 Introduction

*Clostridium difficile*-associated diarrhea (CDAD) is a major cause of nosocomial and antibiotic-associated diarrhea, and it is the commonest recognized cause of pseudomembranous colitis. Despite the recognition of this pathogen since 1978 as the major cause of antibiotic-associated diarrhea, availability of treatment, and recognized infection control measures, CDAD has remained a persistent problem in most hospitals. Moreover, since 2002 renewed interest in this infection has been stimulated by epidemic outbreaks in hospitals in Canada, United States, United Kingdom, and the Netherlands secondary to a hypervirulent strain of *C. difficile*, associated with high recurrence and increased severity.

Although, a large body of literature exists on the pathogenesis, epidemiology, diagnostic methods, and management of CDAD, we still have no effective prevention and no optimal therapy for recurrences. The disease, is mostly a nuisance to healthy, young subjects, complicating antibiotic therapy, but can be a fatal disease in the elderly and high-risk population. It should be noted that despite our inability to conquer and prevent CDAD, there has been no new treatment on the market for this condition in the past 25 years.

## 8.2 Microbiology

*C. difficile* is the most important and clinically relevant identified species of the genus *Clostridium*, which consists of over 150 species of aerotolerant but anaerobic spore-forming gram-positive rods. The organism has been isolated from diverse natural habitats including soil, hay, sand, dung from various large mammals (cows, donkeys horses) and the feces of smaller animals (pigs, dogs, cats, rodents) and humans.[1] Investigation has found that *C. difficile* can survive in nature and indoor for at least 4 years in inoculated equine feces.[2] *C. difficile* is carried asymptomatically as a normal colonic flora in up to 50% of healthy neonates, but the carriage decreases in children older than 2 years to about 3% in healthy adult carriers.[3] In a recent longitudinal study of 139 healthy adults (cultured at 3-monthly intervals) 18 (12.9%) were found to carry C. difficile at some time, 10 (55.6%) once, 3 (16.7%) twice, 2 (11.1%) thrice, and 3 (16.7%) all four times over 9 months.[4] Although, C. difficile colonization is transient in most subjects, there are healthy adults that are persistently colonized and these individuals have higher concentrations of enterococci in their feces.[4] In another large study from Japan 1,234 healthy individuals were cultured for fecal carriage of C. difficile and 94 (7.6%) were carriers (range from 4.2% to 15.3% in different groups).[5] Repeat cultures at 5–7 months after initial culture in 38 carriers reveal persistence in 12 (32%). However, six (50%) of these individuals had a new strain on repeat culture.[5] These results suggest that intestinal carriage may play a role as a reservoir for community-acquired CDAD, but cross-transmission of C. difficile among family members occurred infrequently.[5]

Recent investigations of the C. difficile genome have revealed that presence of a cluster of 17 genes, 11 of which encode proteins with similar two-domain structures (probably surface-anchored proteins).[6] Two of these genes have been proven to encode proteins involved in cell adherence: slpa encodes the precursor of two proteins of the S-layer (p 36 and p 47), and Cwp66 encodes the Cwp66 adhesin.[6] Cwp84 gene encodes a putative surface-associated cysteine protease, which may have a role in the physiopathology of C. difficile infection. Multilocus sequence analysis of virulence-associated genes in C. difficile isolated from various origins has defined some associated functions and polymorphisms.[7] Colonization-factor-encoding genes includes Cwp66, Cwp64, fbp66, flic (flagellarcap protein), flid, groEL (heat shock protein), and slpa; a pathogenicity locus (Paloc) that includes toxin A and B genes (tcdA and tcdB), positive regulator gene (tcdD), a negative-regulator gene (tcdC), and a gene of uncertain function (tcdE)[8]; and a binary toxin gene (CDT), that encodes actin-specific ADP-ribosyltransferase.[9] Recent analysis indicates that a large proportion (11%) of the C. difficile genome consists of mobile genetic elements, mainly in the form of conjugative transposons.[10] These mobile elements involve an extensive array of genes that control antimicrobial resistance, virulence, host interaction, and production of surface proteins.[10]

For epidemiological investigations of outbreaks, methods used for typing included pulsed-field gel electrophoresis (PFGE), serotyping by Western immuno-blotting, PCR ribotyping, PCR-restriction fragment length polymorphism (RFLP), multilocus variable-number tandem-repeat (MLVTR) analysis, and restriction-endonuclease analysis (REA). Large clostridial toxin (A and B) production is highly correlated with REA typing designations.[11]

## 8.3 Pathogenesis

The primary initiating event in CDAD is disruption of the gut normal protection barrier provided by the intestinal flora, during treatment with antibiotics and occasionally by antineoplastic agents. The mechanism of protection by the normal

## 8.3 Pathogenesis

indigenous biomass of enteric bacteria, $\geq 10^{12}$ bacteria per gram of feces, is poorly understood. Ingestion of toxigenic strains of *C. difficile* by fecal-oral transmission allows for colonization and multiplication of the vegetative form throughout the colon, facilitated by a reduced microbial ecosystem. The infective dose (ID) or $ID_{50}$ (inoculation to produce infection in 50% of subjects) of *C. difficile* has not been elucidated. Although the vegetative form is normally destroyed by gastric acid, the spores are acid resistant and vegetate in the small bowel.

Studies in mice indicate that the concentration of bacterial metabolic products (both volatile and nonvolatile), which can be influenced by antibiotics and fermentable fiber in the diet, play a role in eliminating or harboring *C. difficile* and affect the $ID_{50}$.[12] Although, attachment of the organism to the intestinal mucosa is not considered essential to produce disease, indirect evidence suggest otherwise. Molecular characterization of the flic gene encoding flagellar cap protein showed that this protein is very well conserved, and this high degree of conservation suggests that is has a very specific function in attachment to cell or mucus receptors.[13] Furthermore, in vitro *C. difficile* adhere to tissue culture cells, augmented by GroEL heat shock protein[14] and inhibited by colostrum and xylitol.[15]

Although both toxigenic and non-toxigenic strains of *C. difficile* can colonize the intestines, only the toxin-producing isolates can produce disease. The 19.6 kb pathogenicity locus (PaLoc) that includes the genes for toxins A and B are always present in toxigenic isolates and absent from non-toxigenic isolates, but strains with defective PaLoc with variable gene expression still can cause disease.[8] Variations in toxin A and B genes have been described, and more recently polymorphism in the negative-regulator toxin-gene (tcdC) have been found and these variants may affect toxin production differently.[16]

Initially it was thought that both toxins A and B (A+/B+) were necessary to produce disease by *C. difficile* and that toxin-variant strains (A−/B+) with deletion of the toxin A gene or encoding a nonfunctional toxin A were nonpathogenic. These variations in the pathogenicity locus of the toxin gene were classified into 15 toxinotypes by using molecular techniques.[17] However, these variant toxin strains (A−/B+) have been documented to produce diarrhea[18] and nosocomial outbreak of CDAD in hostpitals,[19] and fatal pseudomembranous colitis.[20] The prevalence of these toxin A variant strains of *C. difficile* is not well established, but nosocomial outbreaks have been described in Canada,[19] the Netherlands,[21] and Japan.[22] In a study from France these *C. difficile* variant strains were detected in 2.7% of 334 patients with CDAD,[23] and in 11% of 159 strains isolated in Poland.[24] During a nosocomial outbreak in a hospital in Japan the toxin A variant strain accounted for 30 of 77 ($\approx$39%) of *C. difficile* isolates causing disease over a year.[22] There were no differences in clinical presentation, severity of disease and usual risk factors between infection caused by the usual isolates (A+/B+) and variant strains (A−/B+) of *C. difficile*.[22] In the animal model, hamsters infected with A+/B+ strains of *C. difficile* showed higher colonization and mortality rate (100%) compared to A−/B+ variant strains (30% mortality).[18]

A feature of these A−/B+ isolates is the deletion of a large region within the portion of toxin A gene encoding the binding portion of the toxin.[25] Nearly all strains of *C. difficile* producing disease have been found to be toxin B positive. However, there is one report of a patient with recurrent CDAD where the original isolates contained toxins A and B, but reinfection was caused by toxin B mutant with decrease in vancomycin susceptability.[26]

Toxigenic isolates of *C. difficile* produce and release toxins as the cells grow and lyse. Although toxin A (308 kDa) is considered primarily an enterotoxin that induces positive fluid secretion in the rabbit ligated ideal loop model, there is also evidence that is has cytotoxic properties. Toxin B is a 270 kDa cytotoxin that induces cytopathogenic effects in numerous tissues culture cell lines. Both toxins interfere with the actin cytoskeletons of intestinal epithelial cells, rendering the cells nonfunctional. They act intracellularly by monoglucosylation of the Rhd proteins, a subfamily of small guanosine triphosphatase (GTPase) that regulate actin cytoskeleton and various signal transduction processes.[27] Disassembly of the actin cytoskeleton can then lead to disruption of the intestinal epithelium and excessive fluid leakage. Recent evidence indicate that toxin A requires a substance P receptor to initiate disease, as mice genetically deficient in the neurokinin-1 receptor are protected from epithelia cell damage induced by toxin A.[28] Furthermore, a human colonocyte-binding protein for toxin A has just been described as glycoprotein 96 (gp96), a member of the heat shock protein family expressed on apical membranes and in the cytoplasm of colonocyte.[29] Thus, gp96 serves as a plasma membrane-binding protein to enhance entry of toxin A and allowing cellular signaling events. A similar cell receptor for toxin B has yet to be identified.

Both toxins A and B are potent stimulators of the inflammatory cascade, as evidence by massive infiltration of neutrophils, macrophages, and lymphocytes in the intestinal (colonic) mucosa.[30] In animals there is receptor-mediated endocytosis of the toxins, followed by endosomal acidification, a necessary step for conversion of the toxin to its active form in the cytosol.[31] The toxins are potent stimulators of the pro-inflammatory cytokines (tumour necrosis factor-$\alpha$, interleukin (IL)-1, IL-6, and IL8, and the prostaglandin pathway.[27,30] Prostaglandins produced through cyclooxygenase (COX)-2 expression are involved in the mediation of the secretion of electrolytes and water and the inflammatory response induced by toxin A.[32] Interferon-gamma (IFN-$\gamma$) appears to be important in the toxin A-induced gene expression of the pro-inflammatory cytokines. In gene knockout mice with IFN-$\gamma$ deficiency or pretreatment with neutralizing anti-IFN-$\gamma$ antibodies of wild-type mice prevented toxin A-induced enteritis.[33] There is also evidence that toxin A activates the three main mitogen-activated protein (MAP) kinases, which mediates intestinal inflammation and monocyte necrosis,[34] and there is also increased apoptosis of monocytes via increased caspase-3 activity.[35]

### *8.3.1 Binary Toxin and New Hypervirulent Strains*

Although the role of toxins A and B are well established in the pathogenesis of CDAD, a third toxin, binary toxin CDT found in some *C. difficile* strains, is of questionable importance in producing disease. Binary toxin CDT is unrelated to

## 8.3 Pathogenesis

tcdA and tcdB but instead is related to the group of clostridial binary toxins with two unlinked molecules, both of which are necessary for toxic activity. CDTa is the enzymatic component, and CDTb is the receptor-binding component.[36] This toxin is an ADP-ribosyltransferase and, similar to toxins A and B, acts by disruption of the epithelial actin cystoskeleton.[37] It is very likely that this was the substance, originally described in 1982, that inhibited bowel motility in the rabbit model, distinct from tcdA and tcdB.[38]

*C. difficile* strains carrying the binary toxin CDT genes are found in <10% of most surveys.[39-41] Most binary toxin CDT-positive strains of *C. difficile* also produce toxins A and B. However, strains that produce the binary toxin CDT but neither of the large clostridial toxins (A and B) have been described.[35,42] Binary toxin-positive strains accounted for 2% (8 of 402) of *C. difficile* isolates that do not produce toxins A and B.[42] Moreover, two of the eight strains that were CDT-positive (A−/B−) were isolated from symptomatic patients (but causality could not be proved).[42] A hospital outbreak of CDAD in Pittsburg over a year recently found that 65.3% of 49 *C. difficile* isolates carried the binary toxin genes, and their presence was associated with more severe disease.[43] In Paris a case control cohort analysis of 26 cases of CDAD due to binary toxin-producing stains were compared with 52 controls (CDAD due to binary toxin-negative strains).[44] Diarrhea was more often community acquired, a cause of hospitalization, more frequently associated with abdominal pain and with liquid stools in cases with binary toxin than controls.[44]

Recent reports in the United States indicate that the rate and severity of CDAD are increasing and may be associated with a toxin-gene variant strain of *C. difficile*, highly resistant to fluoroquinolones.[45] The Center for Disease Control and Prevention (CDC) collected 187 *C. difficile* isolates from six states between 2000 and 2003, and compared them to results of more than 6,000 isolates obtained before 2001.[44] This report outlines the emergence of an epidemic strain REA group B1/PFGE Type NAPI in eight health care facilities over the previous 5 years. This strain was noted for the presence of the binary toxin CDT and deletion of the negative-regulator gene tcdC. Clindamycin resistance was the same between two groups (79%) but all the current strains and none of the historic B1/NAP isolates were resistant to gatifloxacin and moxifloxacin.[45]

Experimental study using four binary toxin CDT-positive only (A- B- CDT$^+$) *C. difficile* strains, demonstrated that the binary toxin CDT required exogenous tripsinization to produce marked fluid assimilation in the rabbit ideal loop model.[46] However, challenge of clindamycin-treated hamsters with these strains resulted in colonization but not diarrhea or death.[46] Hence binary toxin CDT my play an adjunctive role with the presence of toxins A and B in the pathogenesis of CDAD but by itself is not very pathogenic. The epidemic of hypervirulent *C. difficile* infections with severe disease has been spreading across North America with large outbreaks in Quebec, Canada,[47] and to the Netherlands.[48] These outbreaks are primarily related to the *C. difficile* ribotype 027, toxinotype III, which appears to produce more severe disease because of hyper-production of toxins A and B.[49]

This feature of these strains of *C. difficile* appears to be related to the deletion of tcdC gene, which is an 18-base pair sequence in the PaLoc responsible for down-regulation of toxin production.[45,49] These hypervirulent strains produce 16 and 23 times higher concentrations of toxin A and B in vitro then other isolates of *C. difficile*.

## 8.4 Clinical Aspects

The spectrum of disease produced by toxigenic strains of *C. difficile* is quite variable, from asymptomatic infection or mild diarrhea to florid disease resulting in toxic megacolon, colectomy, and death. Besides humans, *C. difficile* is an important cause of enteritis in neonatal swine,[50] in horses,[51] elephants,[52] dogs,[53] ostriches,[50] and small animals, such as hampsters, mice, and rabbits are susceptible to infection and are commonly used for experimental models of CDAD. Features of the disease that are unusual (but not rare) and often mis-interpreted or overlooked by physicians are very high leucocyte counts,[54] and CDAD is one of the commonest cause of nosocomial leukemoid reaction (leukocyte count $\geq 30,000$ cells/mm$^3$) that is seen mainly in the intensive care unit (personal experience). Most of these patients have been on broad spectrum antibiotics (or recent exposure) and may or may not have diarrhea. In a previous report of an observational study of 400 in-patients with white blood cell counts (WBC) of $\geq 15,000$ cells/mm$^3$, *C. difficile* infections was present in 25% of patients with WBC counts of $>30,000$ cells mm$^3$ without hematological malignancy.[54] In recent case series of 20 patients with leukemoid reaction and CDAD (collected over 1 year), patients with leucocyte count $>35,000$ cells/mm$^3$ had a worst prognosis and higher mortality rate than controls with CDAD without a leukemoid reaction.[55]

It is not generally appreciated or recognized by clinicians that CDAD can present with obstipation (without any diarrhea), usually with distended abdomen and severe leucocytosis.[56] Even in the most recent review of CDAD in the medical literature this aspect of the disease was not mentioned.[57] This author has diagnosed about 2–4 cases per year of CDAD without diarrhea in the last several years (personal observation). Clues to the diagnosis include fever without obvious cause, unexplained leucocytosis, distended abdomen with or without generalized tenderness, recent or present antibiotics, narcotics for pain or post-operative management, and obtundation in the critical care unit. The absence of diarrhea is likely secondary to narcotics, sedatives, and paralyzing anesthetic agents. Diagnosis is usually confirmed by insertion of a rectal tube to obtain stools (with or without flushing with saline) for testing. Early recognition and treatment often result in prompt improvement but a late diagnosis is associated with toxic megacolon, colectomy, and high mortality. In a recent review of CDAD requiring colectomy, 25 of 67 patients (37%) had no history of diarrhea, and 30(45%) presented with shock.[58]

## 8.4.1 Antibiotic-Associated Diarrhea

Although, *C. difficile* is the most important cause of antibiotic-associated diarrhea (AAD), it only accounts for 20–25% of the cases. Most cases have no proven etiology but subside promptly with withdrawal of the antibiotics. Postulated causes include altered bowel flora by antibiotics, but poorly understood pathogenesis, and by the promotility effect of some agents (i.e., erythromycin). In a recent prospective study of nosocomial AAD, 4,659 in-patient fecal specimens were tested (over 11 months) for *C. difficile* cytotoxin, *Clostridium perfringens* enterotoxin, and *Staphylococus aureus*.[59] The prevalence of *C. difficile* cytotoxin was 12.7%, whereas *C. perfringens* enterotoxin was detected in 3.3% and *S. aureus* only 0.2%. The incidence of CDAD varies widely at tertiary-care centers across the United States in a study of seven centers from 2000 to 2003.[60] The mean annual case rates of CDAD were 12.1 per 10,000 patient-days (range 3.1–25.1) and 7.4 per 1,000 hospital admissions (range, 3.1–13.1). In a defined population of 274,000 (Swedish county), with one tertiary and two primary hospitals, the annual incidence of CDAD was determined over a 12-month period for the community.[61] The annual CDAD incidence in the county was 97 primary episodes per 100,000 and 78% of all episodes were classified as hospital associated with a mean incidence of 5.3 primary episodes per 1,000 admissions. The incidence among hospitalized subjects was 1,300-fold higher than that in the community, reflecting a 37-fold difference in antibiotic consumption.[61]

During a 5-year period (1995–1999) a total of 7,090 stool samples, from patients with acute diarrhea, were examined for bacterial pathogens in the Greek island of Crete.[62] *C. difficile* was isolated from 65 out of 451 diarrhea specimens (14.4%), and toxin B was detected in all cases. In a nationwide study in Sweden in 1995 the incidence of CDAD was 58 per 100,000 inhabitants per year.[63] CDAD was almost twice as prevalent as all (combined) cases of reportable bacterial and protozoal diarrhea. Age-specific incidence was increased >10-fold over the age range of 60–98 years, and 28% of all cases involved no recent hospitalization (community-acquired CDAD).[63]

CDAD is also a recognized problem in subjects with the acquired immunodeficiency syndrome (AIDS). In a previous prospective study from Peru CDAD was the most prevalent etiology of diarrhea in this group of patients, and was associated with increased mortality after adjustment for coinfection, CD4 lymphocyte count, and weight loss.[64] In a large study from CDC between 1992 and 2002, involving >100 medical facilities in nine major cities, *C. difficile* was the most common cause of bacterial diarrhea in HIV-infected subjects, 4.1 cases per 1,000 person years.[65]

A recent report from the CDC noted an increased incidence, severity, and the presence of *C. difficile* in US populations in the community, including children and persons with no history of antibiotic exposure.[66] Patients ranged in age from 6 months to 72 years, and almost 50% of patients were less than 18 years of age. Only 65% of the community-associated *C. difficile* infection had a history of antimicrobial use within 3 months before the onset of diarrhea. Three of five children with

CDAD (unrelated to antibiotics) required hospitalization, and bloody diarrhea was reported in 26%.[66] Interestingly, evidence of transmission of *C. difficile* among close contacts was noted for two children. In a prospective study at a children's hospital emergency department in St. Louis, *C. difficile* toxin was detected in 46 of 688 diarrhea specimens (6.7%) and the prevalence was greater than other bacterial pathogens individually (i.e., Shiga toxin producing *Escherichia coli*, *Salmonella* species, *Shigella* species, etc.).[67] However, causality of *C. difficile* toxin in producing diarrhea could not be proved, as children without diarrhea can have the presence of the toxins at rates equal to those with diarrhea in hospitals.[68]

Since 2000 outbreaks of severe CDAD have been reported in a number of institutions in North America and Europe.[45,47,49] These outbreaks are linked to a new strain that produces more toxin and is more resistant to fluoroquinolones. An increase in the incidence of CDAD was reported in Quebec, Canada, from 36 per 100,000 people in 1991 to 153 per 100,000 people in 2003, and a tenfold increase for persons older than 65 years age.[69] Moreover, the disease was more severe with increased rates of toxic megacolon, shock, and death. The attributable mortality to this hypervirulent strain of *C. difficile* had been estimated to be 16.7%,[70] and the disease appears more refractory to standard therapy with high rates of relapse. This is in contrast to previous studies of nosocomial CDAD from the usual strains of toxigenic *C. difficile*, where no excess mortality had been found after adjustment for age, comorbidity, and disease severity.[71] However, the data on attributable mortality is conflicting, as a previous report before 2000 noted a threefold increase in mortality in patients with CDAD, as compared to matched controls (for age, sex, and underlying disease).[72] There are also reports in the United States showing an increase in CDAD, from 82,000 cases in 1996 to 178,000 cases in 2003.[73] Furthermore, there has been an increasing trend of more severe disease with greater complications and mortality in the United States[74,75] and other areas of the world.[76]

Antibiotic-associated hemorrhagic colitis is a distinct form of AAD in which *C. difficile* is absent.[77] This form of colitis was first described in 1978, usually after a course of penicillin.[78] This condition has also been reported with quinolones and cephalosporins, and usually resolves after discontinuation of the antibiotics.[79,80] Although, *Klebsiella oxytoca* had been isolated from patients with antibiotic-associated hemorrhagic colitis, it could also be found in stools of healthy subjects[80] and the cause remained unknown until recently. In a very recent report from Austria, 22 cases of antibiotic-associated colitis (negative for *C. difficile*) and 385 healthy controls were compared for the presence of *K. oxytoca*.[81] Six patients had findings on colonoscopy consistent with antibiotic-associated hemorrhagic colitis, and five of these six cases had culture positive for *K. oxytoca* versus six (1.6%) of the healthy subjects. All the five strains of *K. oxytoca* from the patients demonstrated cytotoxic effect on monolayers of HEp-2 cells, when incubated with supernatant from the cultures.[81] Moreover, in rats given amoxicillin-clavulanate and inoculated with *K. oxytoca* produced histological changes of colitis (predominantly in the cecum) resembling those of the patients with antibiotic-associated hemorrhagic colitis.[80] Thus, *K. oxytoca* is now an established but relatively rare cause of AAD or hemorrhagic colitis.

## 8.4.2 Risk Factors for CDAD

The incidence of AAD differs with the antibiotic and varies from 5% to 25%, and CDAD occurs in 10% to 20% of all AAD.[82] The major risk factor for CDAD is the use of antibiotics, especially agents effective against anaerobes (such as clindamycin) or broad-spectrum agents including expanded-spectrum penicillins, cephalosporins, and fluoroquinolones. Epidemics of diarrhea caused by highly clindamycin-resistant strains of *C. difficile* have been reported in the United States,[83] the Netherlands,[21] and Sweden[84] related to increased clindamycin usage and controlled by hospital-wide restriction of clindamycin.[85] Similarly, hospital outbreaks of CDAD have been reported with widespread use of third-generation cephalosporins,[86–88] and newer and older fluoroquinolones.[74,89–93] The main features of these recent outbreaks are not only related to the disruption of the normal bowel flora (either as a result of broad spectrum or anaerobic activity), but also to the development of antimicrobial resistance (usually at a high level) by *C. difficile* to the offending agent.[83,84,94,95]

Nearly all cases of CDAD secondary to antibiotics are due to orally or parenterally administered agents, and there is some evidence to suggest that poorly absorbed antimicrobials have a decreased risk of AAD and CDAD.[96] Topical antimicrobials have decreased risk but a case of toxic megacolon and CDAD have been reported in a burn patient induced by silver sulfadiazine.[97] Rare cases of CDAD have also been reported with antituberculosis agents[98] and with cancer chemotherapy.[99,100] Although cancer chemotherapy commonly causes diarrhea because of toxic effect on the intestinal mucosa, CDAD may occur from poorly understood mechanism and can be fatal.[100] Some cancer chemotherapy agents have antimicrobial effects and this combined with endothelial injury may be the pathogenic mechanism.

CDAD has recently been reported by the CDC from low risk-patients without significant antibiotic exposure.[101] Eight (24%) of 33 patients reported no exposure to antimicrobial agents within 3 months before CDAD onset. Seven cases occurred in patients who had close contact with a person with diarrheal illness, two of whom had confirmed CDAD. Three (9%) of the 33 patients contracted CDAD after receiving ≤3 doses of antimicrobials and two received only one dose of clindamycin before CDAD onset.[101]

Besides exposure (ingestion) to *C. difficile* spores and recent antimicrobials other risk factors have been defined for developing CDAD. The widely varied rates of nosocomial CDAD in tertiary-care centers across the United States[60] maybe a reflection of various factors, such as presence of an antibiotic control policy, patient population demographics, and most important the assiduity and numbers of infection control staff. Nosocomial outbreak of CDAD related to a single clone of *C. difficile* is often due to lax infection control practices and this becomes evident by clustering of cases on a few units or wards. The recent outbreaks of the hypervirulent *C. difficile* strains in Quebec hospitals could be related to poor infection control practices.[102,103] Molecular characterization of *C. difficile* strains are very helpful in determining cross-infection and nosocomial spread. In a prospective study in a Swedish hospital over a year, a total of 304 cases of CDAD were diagnosed (incidence 7/1,000 admissions), but by molecular epidemiology only 32% of the nosocomial cases and 23% of all cases were of same PCR-ribotype.[104] Thus, most cases of CDAD in this hospital were caused by endogenous strains of *C. difficile* (harbored by the patients) rather than truly acquired in the hospital. Higher rates of CDAD on certain units such nephrology (37 cases/1,000 admission), hematology (30/1,000), and organ transplantation wards (21/1,000) in this report,[104] likely reflects intensive antimicrobial use and long-term hospitalization. Other studies have found prolonged hospitalization,[105] admission to the intensive care units,[106] older age,[106] total antibiotic burden,[107] decreased restriction of antibiotic use,[108] intensity of environmental contamination of rooms in hospital,[109] designated HIV units,[110] reduced mobility of patients (indication of debility and frailty),[111] nonsurgical gastrointestinal procedures, use of nasogastric tubes, and immunosuppressants[112] as risk factors for CDAD. Gastric acidity constitutes a major defence mechanism against enteric pathogens. It has been well known for decades that conditions producing hypochlorhydria predispose to gastroenteritis, and that even antacids could reduce the inoculum or the $ID_{50}$ of salmonella or shigella species. Acid-suppressive agents such as proton pumps inhibitors (PPI) and $H_2$-receptors antagonists ($H_2$ RAS) increase gastric pH, and may increase the risk of enteric infections including CDAD. Several studies of hospital and long-term care in patients[113–116] and recent community-based studies[117,118] have examined the association of PPI usage and risk of CDAD, with conflicting results.

A recent community-based study using the United Kingdom General Practice Research Database (GPRD), reported an increased of CDAD from less than 1 case per 100,000 in 1994 to 22 per 100,000 in 2004.[117] The adjusted rate ratio of CDAD was elevated with use of PPI (2.9-fold), $H_2$ RAS (2.0-fold), and nonsteroidal anti-inflammatory agents NSAIDS (1.3-fold). The 40-fold increase in incidence of CDAD from 1990–2004 could largely be artifactual from improvements in reporting.[119] Moreover, the clinical diagnosis of CDAD, by general practitioners without use of *C. difficile* toxin may be inaccurate, and a positive toxin assay alone may represent colonization. Other criticisms of this study included potential confounding of inadequately controlled variables such as antibiotic use, comorbidity, receipt of chemotherapy or immunosuppressants, and the unexpected correlation with NSAIDS may reflect detection bias.[118] The same investigators from the United Kingdom re-examined their previous data,[117] using an alternative case definition of CDAD (receipt of oral vancomycin).[120] They identified 317 cases of community-acquired CDAD treated with oral vancomycin and 3,167 matched control subjects. Exposure of PPI was associated with increased risk of CDAD (OR 3.5, 95% CI 2.5–5.2), as well as antibiotic exposure (OR 8.2, 95% CI 6.1–11.0); and 45% of the case subjects had not received antibiotics.[120] Comorbidities, associated with increased risk of CDAD included renal failure, inflammatory bowel and malignant disease, and prior infection with methicillin-resistant *Staphylococcus aureus* (MRSA). In a larger population-based study in Ontario, Canada, examining patients $\geq$66 years who were hospitalized for CDAD, 1,389 case patients and 12,303 matched control subjects were analyzed.[118] In this study case patients were no more likely than control subjects to have received a PPI in the preceding 90 days. Thus, opinions on this issue are widely polarized and it will require a large prospective, randomized, blinded, controlled trial to resolve the debate.[121]

## 8.5 Diagnosis

The diagnosis of CDAD is usually made by confirmation of *C. difficile* toxin A or B or both in the stool. Culture for the organism is not usually preformed for diagnosis as this can represent asymptomatic carriage. However, performance of toxigenic culture is useful for investigation of outbreaks and for research purposes. The "gold standard" for toxin assay is the tissue culture cytotoxicity neutralization assay for toxin B (CCNA), but this takes 24–48 h, is costly and work intensive. Most diagnostic laboratories perform a toxin enzyme immunoassay (EIA) for toxin A and B alone for investigation of CDAD, however, the sensitivity and reliability has recently been questioned. Earlier studies in the 1990s showed that rapid diagnostic tests for detection of toxin A only (immunocard, EIA, or latex agglutination) were suboptimal because of lack of sensitivity (68–72%).[122] EIAs that detect both toxins A and B are preferred by most diagnostic laboratories because of their higher diagnostic accuracy. In general, the relative sensitivity and specificity values of the various tests vary considerably. In the John Hopkins Hospitals between 2003 and 2004 the sensitivity of TOXAB-EIA (TechLab, Blacksburg, VA) and similar assays (Premier *C. difficile* Toxin A + B [Merdian Diagnostics, Cincinnatii, Ohio]) were found to be around 71%, with a specificity of 73%, unacceptably low.[123] Therefore, the John Hopkins Hospitals have evaluated and instituted a two-step algorithm. First stools were tested for *C. difficile* glutamate dehydrogenase antigen (ag-EIA-C.DIFF CHEK-60: TECHLab/Wampole), sensitivity 98%, specificity 89.3% compared to cell culture cytotoxicity neutralization assay (CCNA), with a negative predictive value of >99%[123]; and only ag-positive stools were tested for CCNA.

A new EIA for simultaneous detection of *C. difficile* common antigen and toxin A (Triage *C. difficile* panel, Biosite) is being evaluated. In a study assessing six commercial assays the Triage panel had the best sensitivity (95%), but sensitivity of the toxin detection was lower (77%) with a specificity of only 75%.[124] In a more recent study the Triage Panel and the toxigenic culture showed good agreement with 74 (92.5%) of 80 positive stool samples showing concordance.[125]

Other diagnostic tests being investigated for CDAD include a new immumochromatography assay for toxins A and B (ICTAB), and a real-time PCR on the toxin B gene. In a recent study of 367 fecal samples from 300 patients with diarrhea, 23 (6.2%) were confirmed by cell cytotoxicity assay to be CDAD, the sensitivity and specificity for the ICTAB assay was 91% and 97%, and for the PCR 87% and 96%.[126] Chromatographic assays for toxin A alone, (Clearview *C. difficile* A, Oxoid, and Color PacToxin A, Becton Dickinson) are somewhat less sensitive than the ICTAB assay, both 89% and specificity of 83–89%.[124] The real-time PCR for toxin B has been found in other recent studies to have sensitivity of 91–100%, and specificity of 94–100%.[127,128]

A toxigenic culture approach using multiplex PCR for simultaneous identification and characterization of toxin genes (tcdA and tcdB), has been developed with good diagnostic reliability.[125] A disadvantage of this technique over real-time PCR and immunoassays is a turnaround time of 36–48 h to provide a result, whereas the Triage *C. difficile* Panel provide results within 1 h. Furthermore, although PCR amplification procedures can detect the genes for toxin A and B, these methods do not directly detect either toxin in clinical specimen. Also there are no simple-to-use commercial kits and equipment for molecular applications related to *C. difficile*, making it difficult for most diagnostic laboratories.

In conclusion current EIA's for toxin A/toxin B appears to be suboptimal for maximal diagnostic accuracy of CDAD; cell culture cytotoxicity assay is cost- and labor-intensive and not available to most hospital laboratories, and this applies to most PCR methods. In centers with cell culture cytotoxicity assay available a two-step algorithm with screening with ag-EIA is more cost-effective. The two most promising rapid techniques that would be suitable for most diagnostic laboratories include the Triage *C. difficile* panel and the immunochromatographic assay (ICTAB). The disadvantage of the former is the inability to detect A–/B+ isolates. However, the prevalence and importance of these strains (A–/B+) are very diverse with various prevalence rates: 0.2% in the United States, 2.5–3% in European countries, 6.7–39% in Japan, and up to 56.5% in Israel.[125]

## 8.6 Management

In mild (≤4 stools/day) cases of CDAD simple discontinuation of the offending antibiotics maybe all that is necessary to achieve a clinical response. In hospitals and chronic care institutions contact precautions (gloves and gowns), in a single room and with unshared toilet facilities, should be instituted. Hospital personnel should wash their hands after direct contact (or with body fluids), and alcohol gel for hand sanitation is not effective in killing *C. difficile* spores. Some experts have expressed concern that increase in hospital outbreaks in recent years maybe related to the advent and popularity of alcohol gels, but there is no direct evidence to support this contention. In general anti-diarrhea agents which impede bowel motility are contraindicated in CDAD and may predispose to toxic megacolon. As previously mentioned narcotics may delay the recognition and diagnosis of CDAD due to lack or absence of diarrhea and should be avoided. Other measures in management include intravascular volume replacement with intravenous saline and correction of electrolyte imbalance.

## 8.6.1 Specific Therapy

Moderate to severe cases of CDAD should usually be treated with metronidazole or vancomycin orally. Oral metronidazole is considered the agent of first choice by most guidelines, as it is equally as effective as oral vancomycin in previous randomized studies,[129,130] much less expensive than oral vancomycin (1/200 the cost), which may predispose to development of vancomycin-resistant enterococci (VRE) colonization or infection. This latter concern has not been proven but it is reasonable to restrict the use of vancomycin. Moreover, a recent report from South Korea found a possible link between increased use of oral vancomycin and sudden increase in VRE infections.[131] *C. difficile* isolates are usually susceptible in vitro to many antimicrobial agents including vancomycin, metronidazole, bacitracin, rifampin, fusidic acid, teicoplanin, ramoplanin, tiacumarin B and C.[130] There are a few studies assessing the in vitro susceptibility of *C. difficile* to metronidazole and vancomycin in recent years from large collections of isolates. PeLáes et al.[132] in Spain collected 415 *C. difficile* isolates between 1993 and 2000, and found 6.3% was resistant to metronidazole at a breakpoint of 16 µg/ml, and 3.1% had intermediate resistance to vancomycin. In the United Kingdom a recent surveillance of isolates collected between 1995–1996 and 2000–2001 found little variation in susceptibility of either metronidazole or vancomycin to *C. difficile*, with all except one strain being susceptable.[133] Other groups have also reported very low resistance rates to metronidazole and vancomycin from France[134] and Hong Kong.[135]

Recent reports of poor clinical outcome and high recurrence rate following metronidazole therapy have raised the issue of optimal therapy for CDAD.[136,137] To date these observations are not related to development of increasing resistance to metronidazole or vancomycin. Bartlett[56] has recently suggested that oral vancomycin should be considered the agent of first choice in seriously ill patients with CDAD, because of more rapid clinical response compared to metronidazole reported in one study,[138] better pharmacologic profile with high colonic luminal concentration (100 times higher than the MIC), whereas metronidazole has low concentration in the colonic lumen. A previous study assessed metronidazole fecal concentration during 10 episodes of CDAD in 9 patients during oral ($N = 7$) or intravenous ($N = 3$) therapy.[139] Fecal metronidazole and hydroxymetabolite concentrations showed wide interpatient variation (dependent on the water content of the stools) and were similar during oral and intravenous therapy. The mean metronidazole concentration of watery stool was $9.3 \pm 7.5$ µg/g wet weight (range 6.8–24.2), semiformed samples $3.3 \pm 3.6$ µg/g wet weight, and $1.2 \pm 2.8$ µg/g for formed fecal samples.[139] A similar trend and concentrations were found for the hydroxymetabolite. This study (where all patents responded to metronidazole) demonstrate that the fecal concentration is adequate in diarrheal conditions (probably secreted directly by inflamed mucosa) and CDAD, but the concentration will decrease during recovery. The $MIC_{90}$ of *C. difficile* isolates is about 1–2 µg/ml (1–2 mg/l) to metronidazole in a recent report,[133] and thus on a average during the diarrheal phase the concentration of meronidazole should be four- to ninefold higher than the MIC. This is consistent with the observed clinical response seen in trials of CDAD with metronidazole.

In a recent Cochrane review[140] of antibiotic treatment for CDAD, nine controlled, randomized trials were reviewed, six of which compared different antibiotics. The studies differed in methods for diagnosis, exclusion/inclusion criteria and dosages of antibiotics. Metroindazole doses varied from 250 mg four times a day to 500 mg three times a day, and oral vancomycin 125 mg four times a day to 500 mg three times a day, with duration of therapy ranging from 7 to 14 days, and 10 days was most commonly used. All of the studies had relatively small sample sizes, and only two trials compared oral vancomycin to oral metronidazole with a total of 87 and 76 patients in each treatment group, respectively. There were no differences between oral vancomycin and metronidazole in terms of symptomatic cure, bacteriologic cure, or recurrences. Other antibiotics found to be as effective as vancomycin for initial symptomatic resolution of CDAD, but even smaller sample sizes, include bacitracin (only available for topical therapy), fusidic acid, rifaximin, and teichoplanin.[140] Secondary outcome measures in this review: surgery, sepsis, and death occurred infrequently in all studies. Only one placebo-controlled randomized study was performed in 1978 for post-operative pseudomembranous colitis, with vancomycin 125 mg four times for 5 days, being superior to placebo.[141] This was a study of poor quality with small number of patients (21 found to be *C. difficile* infected). No placebo-controlled study has been done for CDAD with mild diarrhea, where withdrawal of offending antibiotics usually result in resolution of symptoms (unpublished data). In a very recent randomized, controlled (single center) trial of CDAD, 66 patients received metronidazole (250 mg 4 times daily) and 69 oral vancomycin (125 mg 4 times daily) for 10 days.[142] The overall care rate was 84% for metronidazole versus 97% for vancomycin ($p = 0.06$), not significant. Relapses between the two groups were also not significantly different. However, in a subgroup analysis of severe CDAD (arbitrarily defined as endoscopic presence of pseudomembranous colitis, or treatment in the ICU, or $\geq 2$ points which included age >60 years, temperature >38.3°C, albumin level <2.5 mg/dl or white blood count >15,000 cells/mm) response appeared better with vancomycin (97% vs 76%, $p = 0.02$).[142] However, this trial involved a small number of patients and a higher dose of metronidazole 500 mg three times per day should be considered for more severe disease. Despite this some experts are now recommending oral vancomycin as first-line therapy for severe CDAD.[143,144] However, others including myself, are of the opinion that the superiority of vancomycin therapy remains to be proven,[145] and metronidazole 500 mg tid should remain the agent of choice for severe CDAD.

One of the studies excluded from the previous review was a randomized, placebo-controlled trial comparing vancomycin, or metronidazole versus placebo for treatment of asymptomatic carriers of *C. difficile*.[146] At the end of follow-up (40 to >90 days) vancomycin was significantly associated with higher *C. difficile* carriage rate (7/10) than placebo (2/10), and metronidazole only eradicated 40% (4/10). Thus, no specific therapy is required for asymptomatic carriers of *C. difficile*.

Rifampin has excellent in vitro activity against *C. difficile* and potentially could improve the response rate of CDAD when combined with oral vancomycin or metronidazole. In a prospective, randomized trial of oral metronidazole alone ($N = 20$) compared to metronidazole plus rifampin ($N = 19$) for 10 days in primary episodes of CDAD, there were no significant differences in response rate or relapse rate (both groups high, 38–42%).[147]

A novel approach to primary treatment of CDAD in progress is the use of an oral nonantibiotic polymer to bind the toxins. Tolevamer is a soluble, high-molecular weight, anionic polymer (>400 kDa) that noncovalently binds *C. difficile* toxins A and B.[148,149] In a phase II double-blind three-arm randomized study of two doses of tolevamer (3 g and 6 g/day) compared to oral vancomycin 500 mg/day for 10 days; at the higher dose tolevamer was found to be non-inferior to vancomycin (response rate 83% and 91%, respectively) for mild to moderate CDAD.[150] There was a trend for lower recurrence rate with tolevamer (6 g/day), 10% compared to 19% with vancomycin, but this polymer was associated with increased risk of hypokalemia. Cholestyramine can bind the toxins but also bind and inactivate the antibiotics used in treatment.

Nitazoxanide, an antiparasitic agent used for intestinal infections, such as giardiasis and cryptosporidiosis, by blocking anaerobic metabolism of eukaryocytes,[151,152] maybe useful for treating CDAD. Two-thirds of the drug is excreted in the feces after oral dosing,[153] and low concentration of nitazoxanide and its metabolite (tizoxanide) inhibit *C. difficile*.[154] In a recent double-blind, randomized trial nitazoxanide 500 mg twice daily for 7 days ($N = 40$) or for 10 days ($N = 36$) was compared to metronidazole (250 mg four times a day for 10 days ($N = 34$) in hospitalized patients with CDAD.[155] The response rate at 7 days of therapy were similar between metronidazole (82.4%) and nitazoxanide (89.5%), but at 31 days a sustained response was greater in the 10-day nitazoxanide group (74.3%) than in the metronidazole group (57.6%), not statistically significant.[155] Nitazoxanide is available in the United States at a wholesale price of $240 for a 10-day course (metronidazole is about $11), and is not approved by the us Food and Drug Administration (FDA) for this indication.

Severe CDAD can process to toxic megacolon, adynamic ileus, and death, and is a therapeutic challenge. A surgical consultation is essential as colectomy may be necessary but before this decision medical treatment should be instituted. Patients with toxic megacolon or ileus should be on no oral intake as a general principle, and usually require a nasogastric or nasojejunal tube drainage. Besides intravascular volume replacement, hemodynamic stabilization, and correction of electrolyte imbalance there is no consensus on the medical approach to treatment. Intravenous vancomycin does not provide any significant colonic luminal concentration. Intravenous metronidazole is secreted in the bowel lumen in the presence of colitis[138] and a case series of 10 patients with severe CDAD with vomiting, (but no toxic megacolon) showed good response in all to intravenous metronidazole monotherapy.[156] However, others have recommended vancomycin by nasogastric tube or by enema for those with severe CDAD unable to take oral medications.[156] In a case series of nine patients with CDAD and severe ileus or fulminant colitis, intravenous solution of vancomycin (0.5–1 g dissolved in 1–2 L of normal saline) by retention enema (for 60 min) with a 18-French Fohey catheter every 4–12 h (until clinical improvement), was used with good success in eight patients.[157] In another report colonoscopic decompression combined with intracolonic vancomycin in seven patients with severe pseudomembranous colitis associated with ileus and toxic colon resulted in complete resolution in four (57%) and partial resolution in one, thus avoiding colectomy in the responders.[158]

Recent surveys have indicated that fulminant life-threatening CDAD have been increasing in North America and elsewhere. In the University of Pittsburg Medical Centre life-threatening CDAD increased from 1.6% in 1989 to 3.2% in 2000.[159] Patients undergoing colectomy had an overall death rate of 57%; and predictors of death were preoperative requirements for vasopressors, older age, and immunosuppression. In Quebec, Canada, not only was there increased incidence of CDAD from 35.6 per 100,000 population in 1991 to 153.3 per 100,000 in 2003, but the proportion of complicated cases increased as well from 7.1% to 18.2%.[69] Also the 30-day mortality increased from 4.7% in 1991–1992 to 13.8% in 2003.

In conclusion for primary CDAD oral metronidazole should still be considered the agent of first choice, but oral vancomycin should be considered if there is no significant improvement after 3 days. For fulminant cases with ileus or toxic megacolon intravenous metronidazole combined with intracolonic vancomycin by retention enemas or with decompression colonoscopy seems the best choice based on limited data, before surgical intervention.

## 8.6.2 Recurrences of CDAD

The prevalence of recurrence of CDAD after primary treatment with oral vancomycin or metronidazole varies from 10% to 50%, with an average of 20–25%. Recent outbreaks with the hypervirulent strains of *C. difficile* have in general been reporting higher recurrence rates, up to 47%.[136] Among patients who experience one recurrence rates there is a higher frequency of additional recurrences (42–62%).[160–162] Factors predictive of recurrent CDAD include increasing age, general debility (decreased quality of life score),[161] prolonged hospitalization, and continued or repeated courses of antibiotics. In my experience (unpublished data) most of the recurrences are secondary to repeated or continued antibiotics after specific therapy for CDAD has been terminated. In many instances the continued or repeated courses of antibiotics were unnecessary, misguided therapy for asymptomatic bacteriuria, bacterial colonization of wounds, tracheal secretion or sputum with no evidence of clinical infection. These recurrences may occur from 1 to 12 weeks after primary therapy and varies in number of episodes, from 1 to 14 recurrences.

It is important to differentiate between relapse of the same organisms from recurrent infection with a different strain in studies and clinical trials, especially in comparative drug trials or investigation of outbreaks. A few studies have addressed this issue by molecular analysis of *C. difficile* isolates with varying results. In a report from Spain of recurrent CDAD in HIV subjects DNA analysis of isolates showed relapse accounted for 64% and reinfection was responsible for 32%, with a combination of both in 4%, in recurrent episodes.[163] Similar rates of reinfection (26–33.3%) causing recurrent CDAD have been reported as well in non-immunosuppressed patients by using molecular analysis.[164,165] In the Quebec outbreak of a hypervirulent strain of *C. difficile*, 33.3% of patients had at least a second recurrence within 60 days, most of which were considered to be reinfections rather than relapse based on clinical impressions (prolonged hospitalization being a major predictor).[166]

The mechanisms of recurrent CDAD may be a relapse from persistence of the organisms with inadequate recovery of the normal bowel flora to provide colonization resistance, or acquisition of a new strain under the same conditions. There is also evidence that the host immune response to the *C. difficile* toxins play a role in the risk for recurrent CDAD. In a previous study patients with a single episode of CDAD had higher concentration of serum IgM and IgG against toxin A than those with recurrent episodes.[167] It has also been found by the same group in a prospective study that patients with *C. difficile* intestinal colonization on antibiotic who remain asymptomatic had greater serum levels of IgG antibody against toxin A than those in whom CDAD developed.[168] Antibody responses (IgM) to surface layer proteins of *C. difficile* are also lower in patients with recurrent CDAD versus in those with a single episode, but was not different between asymptomatic carriers and those with disease.[169]

### 8.6.2.1 Management of Recurrent CDAD

The pragmatic approach to the management of recurrent CDAD should include discontinuation and avoidance of any antimicrobials, if possible, and preferably management at home if the patient is not too ill. As the two major predispositions include prolonged, recurrent antibiotics and prolonged hospitalization, if treatment with antibiotics are absolutely necessary for underlying proven infection (not colonization), then antimicrobials with reported low risk for CDAD should be chosen (i.e., nitrofurantoin, trimethoprim-sulfamethoxazole, aminoglycosides, narrow spectrum beta-lactams, doxycycline, macrolides, metronidazole, and vancomycin).[57]

The standard practice is to restart the same course of specific therapy as used for primary treatment. Although there is no data on comparison of longer duration of therapy it seems prudent to give a longer course (i.e., 3 weeks), and preferably to continue for several days beyond the offending antibiotic course, if continued. In recent outbreaks with high recurrences the values of metronidazole for re-treatment has been questioned, and some expert advocate using oral vancomycin as first choice. However, in an analysis of 154 patients with first recurrent CDAD in Quebec, metronidazole was not inferior to vancomycin for treatment.[166] Risk factors for complications (shock, megacolon, perforation, need for colectomy, or death) were older age, high leucocyte count (>20,000 WBC/mm$^3$), and renal failure.

Various attempts have been made to break the cycle of recurrent CDAD (RCDD) with no consensus as to the optimal approach. Although most patients suffering from their first episode of CDAD are cured with standard treatment, once recurrence occurs further repeated episodes are common (45–65%), and occasionally continue over a few years. It has been estimated that RCDD prevalence ranges from 1,846 to 36,620 cases/year in the United States.[162] RCDD is associated with prolongation of hospitalization, excessive health care expenditure, lost of employment days, and major inconvenience and morbidity to the patients. Treatment of these recurrent episodes required an average of 265 additional days/patient of vancomycin and almost 20 days/patients of metronidazole to treat all recurrent episodes.[161]

Most guidelines for treatment of RCDD recommended repeat courses of the standard therapy (metronidazole or oral vancomycin), which often results in further recurrences or failure. Measures used in various reports include probiotics, prolong tapering doses of vancomycin, or pulse vancomycin therapy, combination with rifampin, intravenous immunoglobulin (IVIG), and even administration of normal donor stool.

Probiotics in RCDD

Detailed discussion of probiotics will be reviewed in Chapter 9 (*Probiotics in Infectious Diseases*), and their value in CDAD will be briefly summarized in this section. The two most promising and best studied probiotics are *Saccharomyces boulardii* and *Lactobacillus rhamnosus GG*. *S. boulardii* is a nonpathogenic yeast similar to "bakers yeast" that produces an enzyme that can inactivate toxin A and B. Randomized, controlled studies on probiotics to treat or prevent RCDD have been preformed with mixed results. Recent reviews of the topic have also provided mixed interpretations. Dendukuri[170] and Johnston et al.[171] both concluded that the data is insufficient to merit routine use of probiotics for the prevention and treatment of CDAD. In contrast, McFarLand[172] and Katz[173] in recent reviews in 2006 concluded that *S. boulardii* is effective for treatment of CDAD with reduction in recurrences, when used in combination with metronidazole or vancomycin. Katz[173] also concluded that *L. rhamnosus* GG, and probiotic mixtures could prevent or reduce the development of CDAD. Another recent meta-analysis[174] also concluded that *S. boulardii* as an adjunct to antibiotics reduces the risk of AAD.

Vancomycin in RCDD

Empirical use of pulsing or tapering dose of vancomycin has been used in RCDD with reported success in uncontrolled studies. There is no satisfactory biologically plausible reason or rationale why this approach should be more effective than

## 8.6 Management

re-treatment with standard doses for the same or extended duration. Tedesco et al.[175] in 1985 treated 22 patients with multiple relapsing CDAD with 21 days of tapering dose or a pulse dose (for 21 days) of vancomycin with success, with no further relapse over 2–12 months. The regimen consisted of oral vancomycin 125 mg every 6 h for 7 days, then 125 mg every other day for 7 days, and finally, 125 mg every 3rd day for 2 weeks. The rationale for using pulse dose is that the spore forms (which are resistant to antibiotics) will germinate to the vegetative forms during the vancomycin-free period and then are killed by the pulse doses. However, this has not been proven in vitro or in vivo by any model. Vancomycin combined with rifampin has been used in seven patients with RCDD with one recurrence.[176] However, these uncontrolled experiences are difficult to assess without appropriate comparison of standard therapy. Unlike therapy with probiotics in RCDD, there are no controlled, randomized studies comparing tapering or pulse vancomycin with standard re-treatment with vancomycin or metronidazole. Also there are no controlled, randomized studies comparing longer duration of metronidazole or vancomycin versus 10–14 days for re-treatment of RCDD.

In a review of 163 cases of RCDD (defined as one or more recurrent episodes within a year after initial response) females predominated (78%), with a mean of 3.2 episodes (range 1–14), and total duration of their recurrences ranged from 20 days to 4.0 years (mean = 113 days).[162] The overall failure rate between different antibiotic treatment were not significantly different, 46.2% recurrence with vancomycin and 42.1% recurrence with metronidazole.[162] The recurrences, however, varied with vancomycin dosing regimen: 71.4% with 1 g/day for 7–14 days; 42.9% for 2 g/day (same duration); and 31% with tapering doses over 21.5 + 10 days (10 also received pulsed doses of 125–500 mg/day every 2–3 days). Seven patients receiving pulsed doses with no tapering doses had the lowest recurrences (14.3%)[162].

Passive Immunotherapy for RCDD

Intravenous immunoglobulin (IVIG) has been used for severe refractory or recurrent CDAD in isolated cases or small case series with reported success.[177,178] Population prevalence studies have detected antibodies in serum against toxins A and/or B of *C. difficile* at variable rates. In the adult hospitalized population antibodies to these toxins are present in >60%,[179] but in the general population the prevalence is much lower (24%).[180] However, pooled immunoglobulin preparations tested (9) all contained IgG against toxin A and B by ELISA, and neutralized the cytotoxic activity of *C. difficile* toxins in vitro at IgG concentration of 0.4–1.6 mg/ml.[178]

During an initial episode of CDAD the serum antibody response to toxin A is associated with protection against recurrence,[167] and an anamnestic response in asymptomatic carriers may prevent CDAD.[168] It is not clear from these reports whether or not the serum levels of IgG to toxin A or B is directly responsible for protection, or the serum concentration maybe a surrogate marker for secretory IgA in the intestines.

In recent case-series of RCDD treated with various doses of IVIG (150–500 mg/kg for one to six doses), patients had previously failed to respond to 1–4 courses of standard therapy.[181,182] In one of the reports three of five patients with recurrent (2–3 episodes) CDAD had a good response after IVIG, but one patient with intractable disease died even after six doses of IVIG.[182] The largest case series of CDAD treated with IVIG included a total of 14 patients, 6 with RCDD and 8 with severe, refractory CDAD.[182] The patients were continued on vancomycin or metronidazole until symptoms improved, and IVIG was given as a single infusion, except two patients received two doses. Of the nine (64%) patients with complete response initially to IVIG, three had recurrences of CDAD within 1 month.[182] Thus complete cure was only achieved in six (42.8%). Although these case-series suggest that IVIG can confer rapid protection from the enterotoxic and inflammatory effects of *C. difficile* toxins, controlled, randomized studies are needed to prove the efficacy. The limited availability of IVIG and expanding use of this product for unproven indications precludes its general use for severe or recurrent CDAD.

Future investigations of IVIG as adjunctive therapy for severe, refractory, and recurrent CDAD has been considered justified in prospective, randomized trial. However, enthusiasm for further large clinical trials on IVIG in severe CDAD has been dampened by a recent negative case-control study.[183] Eighteen patients with severe disease receiving IVIG were matched to 18 subjects receiving standard therapy alone. Adverse outcomes (colectomy and/or death) occurred in six IVIG recipients (33%) compared to five control subjects (28%) receiving standard therapy.[183]

Bacteriotherapy for RCDD

Suppression of the normal bowel flora by antibiotics is a key factor in the pathogenesis of CDAD. Components of the normal bowel flora such as *Lactobacillus acidophilus*, and *Bifidobacterium bifidus* have long been used empirically as therapeutic agents in gastrointestinal disorders. Fecal bacteriotherapy uses the complete normal human bowel flora as a therapeutic probiotic mixture of living organisms. This type of bactriotherapy has been used sporadically to treat severe, refractory, or recurrent CDAD as a last resort. Limited case reports in Europe and the United States have suggested that stool bacterial flora replacement maybe of value in RCDD.[184–186] However, fecal enema has been used decades before the identification of *C. difficile* for pseudomembranous colitis.[187]

Fecal flora replacement has been administered by rectal tube, colonoscopy, and via nasogastric tube. The largest case-series to date included 18 patients with RCDD treated over a 9-year period, using a standard protocol.[188] Stool donors included household members or other healthy donors, who were screened to exclude hepatitis A, B, and C viruses; HIV-1 and HIV-2; syphilis; *C. difficile* toxins; enteric bacterial pathogens and intestinal parasites. Fifteen of 18 patients had prompt and sustained response (cured), 1 patient a relapse within 90 days and 2 died of unrelated illnesses.[188]

A recent review of bacteriotherapy using fecal flora in various gastrointestinal disorders identified 17 reports involving RCDD, inflammatory bowel disease, irritable bowel syndrome, and even chronic constipation.[189] Seven of the reports were for treatment of RCDD in 57 patients using various methods of fecal implantation (retention enema, via colonoscope, via duodenal, or nasogastric tube), different dosing 10 gm to 200 ml of feces usually suspended in 200–500 ml of saline, with one single application to five daily applications. Overall 48/57 (82.4%) of the patients had prompt response with no further recurrences, and no reports of significant adverse events.[189] However, follow-up was very variable from 3 days to 1 year. Given these promising clinical results formal research into fecal bacteriotherapy is now warranted for select cases of severe, refractory, or multiple recurrent CDAD, with use of a standard protocol and appropriate controls in randomized trials. Of greater benefit and more acceptable or aesthetic would be an in vitro preparation of mixed normal bowel flora that could be marketed. Certainly more basic research is needed to determine the essential bacteria or mixture of the bowel flora that provides protection and resistance (colonization-resistant factor) against *C. difficile* and other enteric pathogens.

### 8.6.3 Prevention

An important aspect of preventative measures to reduce the prevalence and incidence of CDAD is judicious use of antibiotics. Attempts should be made by all physicians to limit the use of antibiotics both in health care institutions and the community, for likely or proven bacterial infections where clinical benefit can be expected. Several studies have shown that a restricted antibiotic policy or multidisciplinary antibiotic program can reduce the incidence of CDAD in hospitals, and also reduces resistant bacterial strains and health care costs.[85,86,108,190] In a recent study implementation of an antibiotic management program resulted in a 22% decrease of parental broad-spectrum antibiotics (despite a 15% increase in acuity patient care); and this resulted in a significant decrease in CDAD, infections by resistant *Enterobacteriaceae*, and impact on VRE and MRSA rates.[191] In another report (from Australia) changes in the antibiotic prescribing policy (restriction of third-generation cephalosporin) resulted in a >50% reduction in the incidence of CDAD.[192]

Besides restrictive antibiotic policies infection control measures have been shown to reduce the incidence of CDAD among hospitalized patients. Standard infection-control policies include contact precautions, wearing of gowns and gloves for direct and indirect contact, single room with unshared bathroom facilities, and hand washing (not alcohol gel) after direct and indirect contact. Environmental disinfectants in reducing nosocomial CDAD has been studied to a lesser extent. In areas where CDAD is highly endemic (bone marrow transplant units) the incidence rate of CDAD decreased significantly, from 8.6 to 3.3 cases per 1,000 patient-days, after environmental disinfectant was switched from quaternary ammonium to 1:10 hypochlorite solution in the rooms of patients with CDAD.[193]

As previously mentioned in section 8.6.2.1a, careful review of the literature and meta-analysis supports the efficacy of *S. boulardii*, *Lactobacillus* GG, and probiotic mixture in the prevention of CDAD.[172,173] However, routine use of these agents to prevent CDAD are generally not recommended. Further large well-designed, randomized, controlled dose-ranging, comparative trials and cost-benefit analyses are necessary before such recommendations. However, probiotics could be considered reasonable as a preventive measure in select group of high-risk patients for CDAD.

A novel approach in the prevention of CDAD in patients receiving antibiotics is dietary manipulations to increase bacterial metabolic products (volatile and nonvolatile) that may inhibit the growth of *C. difficile*. Diets supplemented with fermentable fiber (20%) were found in mice to result in elimination of *C. difficile* colonization of the bowel within 6 days.[12] High fiber diets are now recommended by nutritional guidelines as being beneficial and healthy. Thus this simple inexpensive dietary change should be explored in clinical trials to prevent CDAD. There is also evidence that non-digestible carbohydrates (oligosaccharides) enhances bacterial colonization resistance against *C. difficile*, probably both through augmentation of bifidobacteria growth and non-bifidobacteria inhibitory mechanisms.[194] These non-digestible oligosaccharides are also part of the dietary fibers which are present in whole grain (bran), legumes, vegetables, and fruits. This approach of providing the substrates (soluble fiber and non-digestible carbohydrates) for the normal bacterial flora to ferment and increase bacterial colonization resistance is now termed "prebiotic" approach.

Administration of aminoacids to the colon may be another approach to prevent CDAD. Several aminoacids, proline, and particularly cysteine, exhibit suppression of *C. difficile* toxins in vitro.[195] Cysteine derivatives such as acetyl cysteine, glutathione, and cystine effectively down-regulate toxin production (>99% suppression by cysteine in the highest toxin-producing strain).[195] An algorithm for the diagnosis, management, and prevention of CDAD is summarized in Fig. 8.1.

---

**Algorithm for CDAD**
  **Clinical Suspicion:**

1. Diarrhea after antibiotics (within 3 months)
2. Diarrhea post cancer chemotherapy
3. Leukemoid reaction on antibiotics (ICU)
4. Obstipation/fever, leucocytosis (after surgery) on narcotics and antibiotics

  **Diagnosis:** Stool/Rectal tube aspirate ± saline

  – EIA for *C. difficile* toxin A & B (75% sensitivity) (repeat if negative or sigmoidoscopy + biopsy)

---

**Fig. 8.1** An algorithm above outline an approach to the diagnosis, management and prevention of *Clostridium difficile* associated diarrhea (CDAD). *Abbreviations*: EIA – enzyme immunoassay; ag – antigen; CCNA – cell cytotoxicity neutralization assay; PCR – polymerase chain reaction; qid – every 6 h or four times per day

- EIA for Ag *C. difficile* – if negative rules out CDAD
- pos→CCNA-confirm CDAD

**Investigational:** PCR, chromatography techniques.

**Management:**

- Discontinue antibiotics if possible
- Discontinue narcotics, anti-diarrheal agents

*Mild CDAD* – observe after withdrawal of antibiotics
*Moderate* To *Severe CDAD* – Metronidazole (1–1.5 g/day) X 2 weeks orally, no improvement in 3 days – oral vancomycin (500–1,000 mg/day) X 2 weeks. Some experts recommend vancomycin as first-line therapy for severe disease.
*Patients requiring antibiotics* for proven infection:

- Switch to narrow spectrum agent, co-trimoxazole, nitrofurantoin, or macrolides if possible.
- Continue metronidazole or vancomycin for few days beyond course of antibiotics even of diarrhea resolve or >2 weeks.

**Recurrent CDAD:**

- Discontinue antibiotics
- Re-treat with metronidazole or vancomycin 2–3 weeks
- Best evidence support Saccharomyces boulardii 250–500 mg qid X 2–4 weeks.
- Biologic evidence support high fiber diet–bran, legumes, fruits, vegetables.

**Investigational:**

- Tapering or intermittent oral vancomycin for 4–6 weeks
- Bacteriotherapy (normal fecal implant)
- Intravenous Immnoglobulin (IVIG)

**Toxic Mega Colon with CDAD:**

- Naso-Gastric tube drainage (standard)
- Discontinue antibiotics and narcotics
- Decompression with rectal tube/or colonoscopy

Best evidence support: Intracolonic vancomycin solution; 0.5–1 gm in 1–2 L normal saline every 6–12 h by retention enema, or colonoscopy until clinical improvement, plus intravenous metronidazole.

**Investigational:** IVIG 0.5 gm/kg – 1–2 doses

- Last resort – colectomy.

**Fig. 8.1** (Continued)

> **Prevention of CDAD:**
> 
> - Restrict clindamycin, broad spectrum antibiotics
> - Strict contact precautions/hand washings; clean room surfaces with 1:10 bleach solution
> - Best manage at home if possible
> - High fiber diet with non-digestible oligosaccharides
> - Best evidence support *S. Boulardii*, *Lactobacilius GG*, yogurt with viable lactobacillus mixture in high-risk patients receiving antibiotics.
> 
> **Most Promising Future Treatment/Prophylaxis:**
> 
> - Severe or relapsing CDAD – immune whey – WPC-4D
> - Prevention - Active immunization with toxoid A & B
> - Purified adhesion of *B. adolescentis* 1027 for patients receiving antibiotics, bovine colostrum whey.

**Fig. 8.1** (Continued)

## 8.6.4 Future Directions

There is need for development of more effective treatment for CDAD as current therapies, in existence for nearby 30 years, are suboptimal. A new glycolipodepsipeptide, ramoplanin, shows promise in both hamster and in vitro gut model.[196] Ramoplanin was shown in these models to be as effective as vancomycin in resolving symptoms and reducing cytotoxin production but was more effective in killing *C. difficile* spores and preventing recrudescence. Thus further clinical trials were warranted with this agent.

Rifalazil, a new benzoxazinorifampin that possess activity against *Mycobacterium tuberculosis* and gram-positive bacteria, appears to be more effective than vancomycin in a CDAD hamster model, and unlike vancomycin, which is associated with relapse of *C. difficile* toxin in 10–15 days after discontinuation, there was no signs of disease or fecal toxins 30 days after cessation of rifalazil.[197] Thus this promising agent needs to be assessed in randomized, comparative trials of CDAD.

For severe refractory CDAD and presence of toxic megacolon future treatment to reduce mortality may include human monoclonal antibodies to neutralize toxins A and B. Transgenic mice carrying human immunoglobulin genes have been used to develop humanized monoclonal antibodies to *C. difficile* toxins[198]. In a stringent hamster model combination of monoclonal antibodies against toxins A and B reduced mortality from 100% to 45% ($p < 0.0001$), compared to controls.[198] Hence development of these antibodies should be tested in multicenter trials in severe CDAD, especially in the elderly and immunocompromised hosts where the mortality rate in high, and these novel therapies may obviate the need for colectomy.

## 8.6 Management

There is strong evidence that the pathogenic mechanisms of CDAD involve severe inflammation and up-regulation of pro-inflammatory cytokines and cyclo-oxygenase (Cox)-2 expression in lamina propria macrophages, with elevated prostaglandin levels. Celecoxib, a specific Cox-inhibitor, can reduce toxin A-induced prostaglandin, block histologic damage and intestinal secretion in rabbit model receiving toxin A.[199] Thus, it would be interesting and warranted to study the effect of early administration of celecoxib in human trials of CDAD.

Active immunization with inactivated toxins (toxoid) is a potential means of preventing CDAD. In the hamster model vaccination with *C. difficile* toxoid by intramuscularly (IM) immunization alone or combined with rectal immunization provided full protection from death or diarrhea after *C. difficile* infection.[200] High serum antitoxin B titers as well as toxin B-neutralizing titers were achieved with IM immunization, and passive transfer of mouse antitoxin antibodies protected hamsters from toxin-mediated mucosal disease.[200] Preliminary trial in humans have shown that a parenteral *C. difficile* vaccine containing both toxoid A and toxoid B is safe and immunogenic, and was associated with resolution of recurrent diarrhea in three patients with CDAD.[201] Larger randomized, controlled trials are needed for high-risk patients receiving antibiotics and for recurrent CDAD.

Another novel approach to prevent relapse of CDAD (or for treatment of severe cases) involve oral administration of specific secretary IgA (sIg A) antibodies to neutralize the cytotoxic effect of *C. difficile* toxins (passive immunization). Immune whey protein concentrate (40% immune WPC-40) was made from milk after immunization of Holstein-Frisian cows with *C. difficile*-inactivated toxins and killed whole-cell *C. difficile*.[202] Immune WPC-40, contain high concentration of specific sIga, with neutralizing effect of *C. difficile* cytotoxin in cell assays and protected hamsters from lethal *C. difficile* caecitas. In a preliminary study of 16 patients with CDAD (nine with relapsing RCDD), immune WPC-40 (three times daily for 2 weeks) after standard antibiotic therapy was tolerated and highly effective.[202] None of the patients suffered another episode of CDAD (follow-up median 333 days) and *C. difficile* toxins disappeared from the feces after completion of therapy in all but one case. This promising therapy should not be too expensive to produce and larger randomized, controlled studies are needed.

Attempts to prevent CDAD by blocking adhesion of *C. difficile* to intestinal epithelial cell lines in vitro have also been demonstrated, and could have therapeutic or prophylactic applications. Various concentrations of xylitol and bovine colostrum whey demonstrate dose-dependent inhibition of adhesion of *C. difficile* to Caco-2 cells.[203] In hamsters, prevention of CDAD was 100% effective by prior colonization by nontoxigenic clindamycin-resistant *C. difficile*, when challenged with a toxigenic strain after clindamycin administration.[204] This suggested that the nontoxigenic *C. difficile* colonized the intestines at a higher and faster rate than the toxigenic strains and prevented their establishment. A broader application of a probiotic derivative, purified adhesin of *Bifidobacterium adolescentis* 1,027 (*B. ado* 1,027) is possible, as this novel product can inhibit the bacterial adhesion to intestinal epithelial cell line Lovo of *C. difficile*, enterotoxigenic *Escherichia coli*, and enteropathogenic *E. coli*.[205]

Further randomized, controlled, large multicenter trials to define the most effective current therapy (metronidazole vs vancomycin) for severe CDAD is still desirable. However, an accepted standard criteria for severe disease needs to be defined by international experts. Finally, a rapid and reliable (cost-effective) diagnostic algorithm for the detection of *C. difficile* may be available for most clinical laboratories, but needs confirmation by other centers. In a most recent study from Switzerland a two-step algorithm for detection of *C. difficile* in 1,468 stool specimens using a screening antigen immunoassay (C.DIFF CHEK-60) and a rapid toxin immunoenzymatic A/B assay (TOX, A/B QUIK CHEK) allowed final results for 92% of specimens within 4 h.[206]

# References

1. Lyerly, D.M., Krivan, H.C., Wilkins, T.D., (1988), *Clostridium difficile*: its disease and toxins. Clin. Microbiol. Rev. 1:1–18.
2. Baverud, V., Gustafsson, A., Franklin, A., Aspan, A., Gunnarsson, A., (2003), *Clostridium difficile*: prevalence in horses and environment, and antimicrobial susceptibility. Equire Vet. J. 35:465–471.
3. Lyerly, D.M., Allen, S.D., (1997), The clostridia, in: Emmerson, A.M., Hawkey, P., Gillespie, S. (ed)., Principles and Practice of Clinical Bacteriology. Wiley, New York; pp. 559–623.
4. Ozaki, E., Kato, H., Kita, H., Karasawa, T., Maegawa, T., Koins, Y., Matsumoto, K., Takada, T., Nomoto, K., Tanaka, R., Nakamura, S., (2004), *Clostridium difficile* colonization in healthy adults: transient colonization and correlation with enterococcal colonization. J. Med. Microbiol. 53:167–172.
5. Kato, H., Kita, H., Karasawa, T., Maegawa, T., Koino, Y., Takakuwa, H., Saikai, T., Kobayashi, K., Yamagishi, T., Nakamura, S., (2001), Colonization and transmission of *Clostridium difficile* in healthy individuals examined by PCR ribotyping and pulsed-field gel electrophoresis. J. Med. Microbiol. 50:720–727.
6. Savariau-Lacomme, M.P., Lebarbier, C., Karjalainen, T., Collignon, A., Janoir, C., (2003), Transcription and analysis of polymorphism in a cluster of genes encoding surface-associated proteins of *Clostridium difficile*. J. Bacteriol. 185:4461–4470.
7. Lemee, L., Bourgeois, I., Ruffin, E., Collingnon, A., Lemeland, J.F., Pons, J.L., (2005) Multilocus sequence analysis and comparative evolution of virulence-associated genes and housekeeping genes of *Clostridium difficile*. Microbiology 151:3171–3180.
8. Cohen, S.H., Tang, Y.J., Silva, J.R. J., (2000), Analysis of the pathogenicity locus in *Clostridium difficile* strains. J. Infect. Dis. 181:659–663.
9. Barbut, F., Decre, D., Lalande, V., Burghoffer, B., Noussair, L., Gigandon, A., (2005), Clinical features of *Clostridium difficile*-associated diarrhea due to binary toxin (actin-specific ADP-ribosyltransferase) – producing strains. J. Med. Microbiol. 54:181–185.
10. Sehaihia, M., Wren, B.W., Mullang, P., Fairweather, N.F., Minton, N., Thomson, N.R., Roberts, A.P., Cerdeno-Tarraga, A.M., Wang, H., Holden, M.T., Wright, A., Churcher, C., Quail, M.A., Baker, S., Bason, N., Brooks, K., Chillingworth, T., Cronin, A., Davis, P., Dowd, L., Fraser, A., Feltwell, T., Hance, Z., Holroyd, S., Jagels, K., Moule, S., Mungall, K., Price, C., Rabbinowitsch, E., Sharp, S., Simmonds, M., Stevens, K., Unwin, L., Whitehead, S., Dupuy, B., Dougan, G., Barrell, B., Parkhill, J., (2006), The multidrug-resistant human

pathogen *Clostridium difficile* has highly mobile, mosaic genome. Nature Genetics; 38:779–786.
11. Clabots, C.R., Johnson, S., Bettin, K.M., Mathie, P.A., Mulligan, M.E., Schaberg, L.R., Peterson, L.R., Gerding, D.N., (1993), Development of a rapid and efficient restriction endonuclease analysis typing system for *Clostridium difficile* and correlation with other typing system. J. Clin. Microbiol. 31:1870–1875.
12. Ward, P.B., Young, G.P., (1997), Dynamics of *Clostridium difficile* infection. Control using diet. Advances Exp. Med. Biol. 412:63–75.
13. Tasteyre, A., Karjalainen, T., Avesani, V., Delmee, M., Collignon, A., Bourlioux, P., Barc, M.C., (2001), Molecular characterization of *flid* gene encoding flagellar cap and it's expression among *Clostridium difficile* isolates from different serogroups. J. Clin. Microbiol. 39:1178–1783.
14. Hennequin, C., Porcheray, F., Waligora-Dupriet, A., Collignon, A., Barc, M., Bourlioux, P., KarjaLainen, T., (2001), GroEl (Hsp60) of *Clostridium difficile* is involved in cell adherence. Microbiology 147:87–96.
15. Naaber, P., Lehto, E., Salminen, S., Mikelsaar, M., (1996), Inhibition of adhesion of *Clostridium difficile* to Caco-2cells. FEMS. Immunol. Med. Microbiol. 14:205–209.
16. Spigaglia, P., Mastrantonio, P., (2002), Molecular analysis of the pathogenicity locus and polymorphism in the putative negative regulator of toxin production (tcdc) among *Clostridium difficile* clinical isolates. J. Clin. Microbiol. 40:3470–3475.
17. Rupnik, M., Avesani, V., Janc, M., von ichel-Streiber, C., Delmée, M., (1998), A novel toxinotyping scheme and correlation of toxinotypes with serogroups of *Clostridium difficile* isolates. J. Clin. Microbiol. 36:2240–2247.
18. Sambol, S.P., Merrigan, M.M., Lyerly, D., Gerding, D.N., Johnson, S., (2000), Toxin gene analysis of a variant strain of *Clostridium difficile* that causes human clinical disease. Infect. Immun. 68:5480–5887.
19. Alfa, M.J., Kabani, A., Lyerly, D., Moncrief, S., Neville, L.M., Al-Borrak, A., Harding, G. K., Dyck, B., Olekson, K., Embil, J.M., (2000), Characterization of a toxin A-negative, toxin B-positive strain of *Clostridium difficile* responsible for a noscomial outbreak of *Clostridium difficile*-associated diarrhea. J. Clin. Microbiol. 38:2706–2714.
20. Johson, S., Kent, S.A., O'Leary, K.J., Merrigan, M.M., Sambul, S.P., Peterson, L.R., Gerding, D., (2001), Fatal pseudomembranous colitis associated with a variant *Clostridium difficile* not detected by toxin A immuno assay. Ann. Intern. Med. 135:434–438.
21. Kuijper, E.J., de Weerdt, J., Kato, H., Kato, N., van Dam, A.P., van der Vorm, E.R., Weel, J., van Rheenen, C., Dankert, J., (2001), Nosocomial outbreak of *Clostridium difficile*-associated diarrhea due to a clindamycin-resistant enterotoxin A-negative strain. Eur. J. Clin. Microbiol. Infect. Dis. 20:528–534.
22. Komatsu, M., Kato, H., Aikara, M., Aihara, M., Shimakawa, K., Iwasaki, M., Nagasaka, Y., Fukuda, S., Matsuo, S., Arakawa, Y., Watanabe, M., Iwatani, Y., (2003), High frequency of antibiotic-associated diarrhea due to toxin A negative, toxin B-positive *Clostridium difficile* in a hospital in Japan and risk factors for infection. Eur. J. Clin. Microbiol. Infect. Dis. 22:525–529.
23. Barbut, F., Lalande, V., Burghoffer, B., Thien, H.V., Grimprel, E., Petit, J.C., (2002), Prevalence and genetic characterization of toxin A variant strains of *Clostridium difficile* among adults and children with diarrhea in France. J. Clin. Microbiol. 40:2079–2083.
24. Pituch, H., van den Braak, N., Van Leeuwen, W., Van Belkum, A., Martirosian, G., Obuch-Woszczatynski, P., Luczak, M., Meisel-Mlkolajczyk, F., (2001), Clonal dissemination of a toxin-A-negative/toxin-B-positive *Clostridium difficile* strain from patients with antibiotic-associated diarrhea in Poland. Clin. Microbiol. Infect. 7:442–446.
25. Moncreif, J., Zheng, L., Neville, L.M., Lyerly, D.M., (2000), Genetic characterzarion of toxin A-negative, toxin B-positive *Clostridium difficile* isolates by PCR. J. Clin. Microbiol. 38:3072–3075.

26. Cohen, S.H., Tang, Y.J., Hansen, B., Silva, J. Jr., (1998), Isolation of a toxin B-deficient mutant strain of *Clostridium difficile* in case of recurrent *C. difficile*-associated diarrhea. Clin. Infect. Dis. 26:410–412.
27. Moncrief, J.S., Lyerly., S.D., Wilkins, T.D., (1997), Moleculer biology of the *Clostridium difficile* toxins, In: Rood, J.I., McClane, B.A., Songer, J.G., Titball, R.W. (eds), The Clostridia: Molecular Biology and Pathogenesis. Academic Press, New York, pp. 369–392.
28. Gerard, N.P., Pothoulakis, C., (1998), Neurokinin-1(NK-D) receptor is required in *Clostridium difficile*-induced enteritis. J. Clin. Invest. 101:1547–1550.
29. Na, X., Moyer, M.P., Pothoulakis, C., La-Mont, J.T., (2008), gp96 is a human colonocyte plasma membrane binding protein for *Clostridium difficile* toxin A. Infect. Immun 76: 2862–2871.
30. Rocha, M.F., Sidrim, J.J., Lima, A.A., (1999), *Clostridium difficile* as an inducer of inflammatory diarrhea. Revista SOC. Brasil. Med. Trop. 32:47–52.
31. Keel, M.K., Songer, J.G., (2006), The comparative pathology of *Clostridium difficile*-associated disease. Vet. Path. 43:225–240.
32. Alcantara, C., Stenson, W.F., Steiner, T.S., Guerrant, R.L., (2001), Role of inducible cyclooxygenase and prostaglandins in *Clostridium difficile* toxin A-induced secretion and inflammation in an animal model. J. Infect. Dis. 184:648–652.
33. Ishida, Y., Maegawa, T., Kono, T., Kimura, A., Iwakura, Y., Nakamura, S., Mukaida, N., (2004), Essential involvement of IFN-gamma in *Clostridium difficile* toxin A-induced enteritis. J. Immunol. 172:3018–3025.
34. Warny, M., Keates, A.C., Keates, S., Castagliuolo, I., Zacks, J.K., Qamor, A., Pothoulakis, C., Lamont, J.T., Kelly, C.P., (2000), p 38 MAP kinase activation by *Clostridium* toxin A mediates monocyte necrosis, 1 L-8 production, and enteritis. J. Clin. Invest. 105:1147–1156.
35. Solomon, K., Webb, J., Ali, N., Robins, R.A., Mahida, Y.R., (2005), Monocytes are highly sensitive to *Clostridium difficile* toxin A-induced apoptotic and nonapototic cell death. Infect. Immun. 73:1625–1634.
36. Stubbs, S., Rupnik, M., Gibert, M., Brazier, J., Duerden, B., Popoff, M., (2000), Production of actin-specific ADP-ribosyltransferase (binary toxin) by strains of *Clostridium difficile*. FEMS Microbiol. Lett. 186:307–312.
37. Barth, H., Aktories, K., Popoff, M.R., Stiles, B.G., (2004), Binary bacterial toxins: biochemistry, biology, and applications of common *Clostridium* and *Bacillus* proteins. Microbiol. Mol. Biol. Rev. 68:373–402.
38. Justus, P.G., Martin, J.L., Goldberg, D.A., Taylor, N.S., Bartlett, J.G., Alexander, R.W., Mathians, J.R., (1982), Myoelectric effects of *Clostridium difficile*: motility-altering factors distinct from cytotoxin and enterotoxin in rabbits. Gastro-enterology; 83:836–843.
39. Geric, B., Rupnik, M., Gerding, P.N., Grabnar, M., Johnson, S., (2004), Distribution of *Clostridium difficile* variant toxinotypes with binary toxin genes among clinical isolates in a American hospital. J. Med. Microbiol. 53:887–894.
40. Goncalves, C., Decré, D., Barbut, F., Burghoffer, B., Petit, J.C., (2004), Prevalence and characterization of a binary toxin (action-specific ADP-ribosyltransferase) from *Clostridium difficile*. J. Clin. Microbiol. 42:1933–1939.
41. Terhes, G., Urban, E., Soki, J., Hamid, K.A., Nagy, E., (2004), Community-acquired *Clostridium difficile* diarrhea caused by binary toxin, toxin A, and toxin B gene-positive isolates in Hungary. J. Clin. Microbiol. 42:4316–4318.
42. Geric, B., Johnson, S., Gerding, D.N., Grabnar, M., Rupnik, M., (2003), Frequency of binary toxin genes among *Clostridium difficile* strains that do not produce large clostridial toxins. J. Clin. Microbiol. 41:5227–5232.
43. McEllistrem, M.C., Carmen, R.J., Gerding, D.N., Genheimer, C.W., Zheng, L., (2005), A hospital outbreak of *Clostridium difficile* disease associated with isolates carrying binary toxin genes. Clin. Infect. Dis. 40:265–272.
44. Barbut, F., Decre, D., Lalonde, V., Burghoffer, B., Noussair, L., Gigandon, A., Espinasse, F., Raskine, L., Robert, J., Mangeol, A., Branger, C., Petit, J.C., (2005), Clinical features of

*Clostridium difficile*-associated diarrhea due to binary toxin (actin-specific ADP-ribosyltransferase)-producing strains. J. Med. Microbiol. 54:181–185.
45. McDonald, L.L., Gielgore, G.E., Thompson, A., Owens Jr., R.C., Kazakova, S.V., Sambol, S.P., Johson, S., Gerding, D.N., (2005), An epidemic, toxin gene-variant strain of *Clostridium difficile*. N. Engl. J. Med. 353:2433–2441.
46. Geric, B., Carmen, R.J., Rupnik, M., Genheimer, C.W., Sambol, S.P., Lyerly, D.M., Gerding, D.N., Johnson, S., (2006), Binary toxin-producing, large clostridial toxin-negative *Clostridium difficile* strains are enterotoxic but do not cause disease in hamsters. J. Infect. Dis. 193:1143–1150.
47. Loo, V.G., Poirier, L., Miller, M.A., Oughton, M., Libman, M.D., Michaud, S., Borgault, A. M., Nguyen, T., Frenette, C., Kelly, M., Vibien, A., Brassard, P., Fenn, S., Dewar, K., Hudson, T.J., Horn, R., Rene, P., Monczak, Y., Dascal, A., (2005), A predominantly clonal multi-institutional outbreak of *Clostridium difficile*–associated diarrhea with high morbidity and mortality. N. Engl. J. Med. 353:2503–2505.
48. Kuijer, E.J., van den Berg, R.J., Debast, S., Visser, C.E., Veenendaal, D., Troelstra, A., van der Kooi, T., van den Hof, S., Notermans, D.W., (2006), *Clostridium difficile* ribotype 027, toxinotype III, the Netherlands. Emerg. Infect. Dis. 12:827–830.
49. Warny, M., Pepin, J., Fang, A., Killgore, G., Thompson, A., Brazier, J., Frost, E., McDonald, L.C., (2005), Toxin production by an emerging strain of *Clostridium difficile* associated with severe disease in North America and Europe. Lancet 366:1079–1084.
50. Songer, J.G., (2004), The emergence of *Clostridium difficile* as a pathogen of food animals. Animal Health Res. Rev. 5:321–326.
51. Baverud, V., Franklin, A., Gunnarsson, A., Gustafsson. A., Hellander-Edman, A., (1998), *Clostridium difficile* associated with acute colitis in mares when their foals are treated with erythromycin and rifampicin for *Rhodococcus equi* pneumonia. Equine Vet. J. 30:482–488.
52. Bojesen, A.M., Olsen, K.E., Bertelsen, M.F., (2006), Fatal enterocolitis in Asian elephants (Elephas maximus) caused by *Clostridium difficile*. Vet. Microbiol. 116:329–335.
53. Chouicha, N., Marks, L.S., (2006), Evaluation of five enzyme immunoassays compared with the cytotoxicity assay for diagnosis of *Clostridium difficile* associated diarrhea in dogs. J. Vet. Diag. Invest. 18:182–188.
54. Wanahita, A., Goldsmith, E.A., Musher, D.M., (2002), Conditions associated with leucocytosis in a territory care hospital with particular attention to the role of infection caused by *Clostridium difficile*. Clin. Infect. Dis. 34:1585–1592.
55. Marinella, M.A., Burdette, S.A., Bedimo, R., Markert, R.J., (2004), Leukemoid reactions complicating colitis due to *Clostridium difficile* South. Med. J. 97:959–963.
56. Zachariadis, G., Connon, J.J., Fong, I.W., (2002), Fulminant *Clostridium difficile* colitis without diarrhea: Lack of emphasis in diagnostic guidelines. Am. J. Gastroent. 97:2929–2930.
57. Bartlet, J.G., (2006), Narrative review: The new epidemic of *Clostridium difficile*-associated enteric disease. Ann. Intern. Med. 145:758–764.
58. Longo, W.E., Mazuski, J.E., Virgo, K.S., Lee, P., Bahadursingh, A.N., Johnson, F.E., (2004), Outcome after colectomy for *Clostridium difficile* colitis. Dis. Colon Rectum 47:1620–1626.
59. Asha, N.J., Tompkins, D., Wilcox, M.H., (2006), Comparative analysis of prevalence, risk factors, and molecular epidemiology of antibiotic-associated diarrhea due to *Clostridium difficile*, *Clostridium perfringens*, and *Staphylococus aureus*. J. Clin. Microbiol. 44:2785–2791.
60. Sohn, S., Climo, M., Diekema, D., Fraser, V., Herwaldt, L., Marino, S., Noskin, G., Perl, T., Song, X., Tokars, J., Warren, D., Wong, E., Yokoe, D.S., Zembower, T., Sepkowitz, K.A., (2005), Varying rates of *Clostridium difficile*-associated diarrhea at prevention epicenter hospitals. Infect. Cont. Hosp. Epid. 26:676–679.
61. Noren, T., Akerlund, T., Back, E., Sjoberg, L., Persson, I., Alriksson, I., Burman, L.G., (2004), Molecular epidemiology of hospital-associated and community-acquired *Clostridium difficile* infection in a Swedish county. J. Clin. Microbiol. 42:3635–3643.

62. Maraki, S., Georgiladakis, A., Tselentis, Y., Samonis, G., (2003), A 5 year study of the bacterial pathogens associated with acute diarrhea on the island of Crete, Greece, and their resistance to antibiotics. Eur. J. Epid. 18:85--90.
63. Karlström, O., FrykLund, B., Tullus, K., Burman, L.G., and the Swedish *C. difficile* Study Group, (1998), A prospective nationwide study of *Clostridium difficile*-associated diarrhea in Sweden. Clin. Infect. Dis. 26:141–145.
64. Gottlieb, A.L., Gayles, M.K., Grahn, K.F., Chavez-Perez, V.M., Salas Apolinario, I., Gilman, R.H., (1998), Diarrhea and *Clostridium difficile* infection in Latin American patients with AIDS. Working Group on AIDS in Peru. Clin. Infect. Dis. 27:487–493.
65. Sanchez, T.H., Brooks, J.T., Sullivan, P.S., Juhasz, M., Mintz, E., Dwarkin, M.S., Jones, J.L., and the adult/adolescent spectrum of HIV Disease Study Group, (2005), Bacterial diarrhea in persons with HIV infection, United States, 1999–2002. Clin. Infect. Dis. 41:1621–1627.
66. Centers for Disease Control and Prevention, (2005), Severe *Clostridium difficile*-associated disease in populations at low risk–four states. MMWR Morb. Mortal Wkly Rep. 54:1201–1205.
67. Klein, E.J., Boster, D.R., Stapp, J.R., Wells, J.G., Qin, X., Clausen, C.R., SwerdLow, D.L., Braden, C.R., Tarr, P.I., (2006), Diarrhea etiology in children's hospital emergency department: a prospective cohort study: Clin. Infect. Dis. 43:807–813.
68. Vesikori, T., Jsolauri, E., Maki, M., Gronroos, P., (1984), *Clostridium difficile* in young children: association with antibiotic usage. Acta Paediatr. Scand. 73:86–91.
69. Pepin, J., Valiquette, L., Alary, M.E., Villemure, P., Pelletier, A., Forget, K., Pépin, K., Chouinard, D., (2001), *Clostridium difficile*-associated diarrhea in a region of Quebec from 1991 to 2003: a changing pattern of disease severity. CMAJ 171:466–472.
70. Pepin, J., Valiquette, L., Cosselte, B., (2005), Mortality attributable to nosocominal *Clostridium difficile*-associated disease during an epidemic caused by a hypervirulent strain in Quebec. CMAJ 173:1037–1042.
71. Kyne, L., Hamel, M.B., Polavaram, R., Kelly, C.P., (2002), Health care costs and mortality associated with nosocomial diarrhea due to *Clostridium difficile*. Clin. Infect. Dis. 34:346–353.
72. Erikson, S., Aronsson, B., (1989), Medical implications of nosocomial infection with *Clostridium difficile*. Scand. J. Infect. Dis. 21:733–734.
73. McDonald, L.C., (2005), *Clostridium difficile*: responding to a new threat from an old enemy. Infect. Control. Hosp. Epidemiol. 26:672–675 (editorial).
74. Dallal, R.M., Harbrecht, B.C., Boujoukas, A.J., Sirio, C.A., Farkas, L.M., Lee, K.K., Simmons, R.L., (2002), Fulminant *Clostridium difficile*: an underappreciated and increasing cause of death and complications. Ann. Surg. 235:363–372.
75. Muto, C.A., Pokrywka, M., Shutt, K., Mendelsohn, A.B., Nouri, K., Posey, K., (2005), A large outbreak of *Clostridium difficile*-associated disease with an unexpected proportion of deaths and colectomies at a teaching hospital following increased fluoroquinolone use. Infect. Control Hosp. Epidemiol. 26:273–280.
76. Owens, R.C., (2006), *Clostridium difficile*-associated disease: an emerging threat to patient safety: insights from the society of Infectious Disease Pharmacists. Pharmacotherapy 26:299–311.
77. Beaugerie, L., Metz, M., Barbut, F., Bellaiche, G., Bouhnik, Y., Raskine, L., Nicholas, J.-C., Chatelet, F.-P., Lehn, N., Petit, J.C., and the Infectious Colitis Study Group (2003), *Klebsiella oxytoca* as an agent of antibiotic-associated hemorrhagic colitis. Clin. Gastroenteriol. Hepatol. 1:370–376.
78. Toffler, R.B., Pingound, E.G., Burrell, M.I., (1978), Acute colitis related to penicillin derivatives. Lancet 2:707–709.
79. Koga, H., Aoyagi, K., Yoshimura, R., Kimura, Y., Lida, M., Fujishima, M., (1999), Can quinolones cause hemorrhagic colitis of late onset? Report of three cases. Dis. Colon Rectum 42:1502–1504.

80. Bellaiche, G., Le Pennec, M.P., Choudat, L., Ley, G., Shama, J.L., (1997), Value of rectosigmoidoscopy with bactericological culture of colonic biopsies in the diagnosis of post-antibiotic hemorrhagic colitis related to *Klebsiella oxytoca*. Gastroenterol. Clin. Biol. 21:764–767.
81. Hőgenauer, C., Langner, C., Beubler, E., Lippe, I.T., Schicho, R., Gorkiewicz, G., Krause, R., Grestgrasser, N., Krejs, G.J., Hinterleitner, T.A., (2006), *Klebsiella oxytoca* as a causative organism of antibiotic-associated hemorrhagic colitis. N. Engl. J. Med. 355:2418–2426.
82. Bergogne-Berezin, E., (2000), Treatment and prevention of antibiotic associated diarrhea. Internat. J. Antimicrob. Agents: 16:521–526.
83. Johnson, S., Samore, M.H., Farrow, K.A., Killgore, G.E., Tenover, F.C., Lyras, D., Rood, J. I., DeGirolami, P., Baltch, A.L., Rafferty, M.E., Pear, S.M., Gerding, D.N., (1999), Epidemics of diarrhea caused by clindamycin-resistant strain of *Clostridium difficile* in four hospitals. N. Engl. J. Med. 341:1645–1651.
84. Noren, T., Tang-Feldman, Y.J., Cohen, S.H., Silva, J. Jr., Olcen, P., (2002), Clindamycin resistant strains of *Clostridium difficile* isolated from cases of *C. difficile* associated diarrhea (CDAD) in hospital in Sweden. Diag. Microbiol. Infect. Dis. 42:149–151.
85. Climo, M.W., Israel, D.S., Wong, E.S., Williams, D., Coudron, P., Markowitz, S.M., (1998), Hospital-wide restriction of clindamycin: effect on the incidence of *Clostridium difficile*-associated diarrhea and cost. Ann. Interm. Med. 128:989–995.
86. Wilcox, M.H., Freeman, J., Fawley, W., Mackinlay, S., Brown, A., Donaldson, K., Corrado, O., (2004), Long-term surveillance of cefotaxime and piperacillin-tazobactam prescribing and incidence of *Clostridium difficile* diarrhea. J. Antimicrob. Chemother 54:168–172.
87. Starr, J.M., Impallomeni, M., (1997), Risk of diarrhea, *Clostridium difficile* and cefotaxime in the elderly. Biomed. Pharmacother. 51:63–67.
88. Settle, C.D., Wilcox, M.H., Fawley, W.N., Corrado, O.J., Hawkey, P.M., (1998), Prospective study of the risk of *Clostridium* diarrhea in elderly patients following treatment with cefotaxime or piperacillin-tazobactam. Aliment. Pharmacol. Ther. 12:1217–1223.
89. Yip, C., Loeb, M., Salama, S., Moss, L., Olde, J., (2001), Quinolone use as a risk factor for nosocomial *Clostridium difficile*-associated diarrhea. Infect. Control Hosp. Epidemiol. 22:572–575.
90. Ackermann, G., Tang-Feldman, Y.J., Schaumann, R., Henderson, J.P., Rodloff, A.C., Silva, J., Cohen, S.H., (2003), Antecedent use of fluoroquinolones is associated with resitance to moxifloxacin in *Clostridium difficile*. Clin. Microbiol. Infect. 9:526–530.
91. Gaynes, R., Rimland, D., Killum, E., Lowery, H.K., Johson, T.M., 2nd, Killmore, G., Tenover, F.C., (2004), Outbreak of *Clostridium difficile* infection in a long-term care facility: association with gatifoxacin use. Clin. Infect. Dis. 38:640–645.
92. Pepin, J., Saheb, N., Coulombe, M.A., Alory, M.E., Corriveau, M.P., Authier, S., Leblanc, M., Rivard, G., Bettez, M., Primeau, V., Ngugen, M., Jacob, C.E., Lanthier, L., (2005), Emergence of fluoroquinolones as the predominant risk factor for *Clostridium difficile*-associated diarrhea: A cohort study during an epidemic in Quebec. Clin. Infect. Dis. 41:1250 1260.
93. McCusker, M.E., Harris, A.D., Perencevich, E., Roghmann, M.C., (2003), Fluoroquinolone use and *Clostridium difficile*-associated diarrhea. Emerg. Infect. Dis. 9:730–733.
94. Gerding, D.N., (2005), Clindamycin, cephalosporins, fluoroquinolones, and *Clostridium difficile*-associated diarrhea: this is an antimicrobial resistance problem. Clin. Infect. Dis. 38:646–648 (editorial).
95. Pituch, H., Brazier, J.S., Obuch-Woszczatynski, P., Waltanska, D., Meissel-Mikolajczyk, F., Luczak, M., (2006), Prevalence and association of PCR ribotypes of *Clostridium difficile* isolated from symptomatic patients from Warsaw with macrolide-lincoamide-streptogramin B (MLSB) type resistance. J. Med. Microbiol. 55:207–213.
96. Surawicz, C.W., (2005), Antibiotic-associated diarrhea and pseudomembranous colitis: are they less common with poorly absorbed antimicrobials. Chemotherapy 51 (Suppl I):81–89.
97. Jennings, L.J., Hanumandass, M., (1998), Silver sulfadiazine induced *Clostridium difficile* toxic megacolon in a burn patient: case report. Burns 24:676–679.

98. Akutagawa, H., Takada, E., Egashira, Y., Adachi, G., Kurisu, Y., Edagawa, G., Hirata, I., Katsu, K., Shibayama, Y., (2004), Four cases of pseudomembranous colitis due to antituberculous agents. Jap. J. Gastroenterol. 101:890–894.
99. Kerst, J.M., Van der Lelie, J., Kuijper, E.J., (2001), Diarrhea due to *Clostridium difficile* toxin in hematooncological patients. Ned. Tijdschr. GeneesKd. 145:1137–1140.
100. Wong, A.S., Lam, C.S., Tambyah, P.A., (2001), Fatal chemotherapy associated *Clostridium difficile* infection – a case report. Singapore Med. J. 42:214–216.
101. Center for Disease Control & Prevention, (2005), Severe *Clostridium difficile*-associated disease in populations previously at low risk–four states, 2005. Morb. Montal Wkly Rep. CDC 54:1201–1205.
102. Beaulieu, M., Thirion, D.J.G., Williamson, D., Pichette, G., (2006) *Clostridium difficile*-associated outbreaks: the name of the game is isolation and cleaning. Clin. Infect. Dis. 42:725(letter).
103. Weiss, K., (2006), Poor infection control, not fluoroquinolones, likely to be primary cause of *Clostridium difficile*–associated diarrhea outbreaks in Quebec. Clin. Infect. Dis. 42:725–727 (letter).
104. Svenungsson, B.O., Burman, L.G., Jalakas-Pornull, K., Lagergren, A., Struwe, J., Akerlund, T., (2003), Epidemiology and molecular characterization of *Clostridium difficile* strains from patients with diarrhea: low disease incidence and evidence of limited cross-infection is a Swedish teaching hospital. J. Clin. Microbiol. 41:4031–4037.
105. Palmore, T.N., Sohn, S., Malak, S.F., Eagan, J., Sepkowitz, K.A., (2005), Risk factors for acquisition of *Clostridium difficile*-associated diarrhea among outpatients at a cancer hospital. Infect. Control Hosp. Epidemiol. 26:680–684.
106. Barbut, F., Corthier, G., Charpak, Y., Cerf, M., Monteil, H., Fosse, T., Trevoux, A., Barbeyrac, B., Boussougnant, Y., Tigaud, S., Tytgat, F., Sedallian, A., Duborgel, S., Collignon, A., Le Guern, M.E., Bernasconi, P., Petit, J.C., (1996), Prevalence and pathogenicity of *Clostridium difficile* in hospitalized patients. A French multicentre study. Arch. Intern. Med. 156:1449–1454.
107. Schwaber, M.J., Simhon, A., Block, C., Roval, V., Ferderber, N., Shapiro, M, (2000), Factors associated with nosocomial diarrhea and *Clostridium difficile*-associated disease on the adult wards of an urban tertiary care hospital. Eur. J. Clin. Microbiol. Infect. Dis. 19:9–15.
108. Ho, M., Yang, D., Wyle, F.A., Mulligan, M.E., (1996), Increased incidence of *Clostridium difficile*-associated diarrhea following decreased restriction of antibiotic use. Clin. Infect. Dis. 23(Suppl I): S102–S106.
109. Samore, M.H., Venkataraman, L., De Girolami, P.C., Arbeit, R.D., Karchmer, A.W., (1996), Clinical and molecular epidemiology of sporadic and clustered cases of nosocomial *Clostridium difficile* diarrhea. Am. J. Med. 100:32–40.
110. Mody, L.R., Smith, S.M., Dever, L.L., (2001), *Clostridium difficile*-associated diarrhea in a VA medical center: clustering of cases, associated with antibiotic usage, and impact on HIV-infected patients. Infect. Control Hosp. Epidemiol. 22:42–45.
111. Henoun Loukili, N., Martinot, M., Hansmann, Y., Christmann, D., (2004), Risk factors for nosocomial *Clostridium difficile* diarrhea in an infectious and tropical diseases department. Med. Malad. Infect. 34:57–61.
112. Bignardi, G.E., (1998), Risk factors for *Clostridium difficile* infection. J. Hosp. Infect. 40:1–15.
113. Cunningham, R., Dale, B., Undy, B., Gaunt, N., (2003), Proton pump inhibitors as a risk factor for *Clostridium difficile* diarrhea. J. Hosp. Infect. 54:243–245.
114. Dial, S., Alrasadi, K., Manoukian, C., Huang, A., Menzies, D., (2004), Risk of *Clostridium difficile* among hospital inpatients prescribed proton pump-inhibitors: cohort and case-control studies. CMAJ 171:33–38.
115. Shah, S., Lewis, A., Leapold, D., Dunstan, F., Woodhouse, K., (2000), Gastric acid suppression does not promote clostridial diarrhea in the elderly. Quat. J. Med. 93:175–181.

116. Al-Tureihi, F.I., Hassoun, A.,Wolf-Klein, G., Isenberg, H., (2005), Albumin, length of stay, and proton pump inhibitors: Key factors in *Clostridium difficile* associated disease in nursing home patients. J. Am. Med. Dir. Assoc. 6:105–108.
117. Dial, S., DeLaney, J.A.C., Barkun, A.N., Suissa, S., (2005), Use of gastric-acid suppressive agents and the risk of community-acquired *Clostridium difficile*-associated disease. JAMA 294:2989–2995.
118. Lowe, D.O., Mamdani, M.M., Kopp, A., Low, D.E., JuurLink, D.N., (2006), Proton pump inhibitors and hospitalization for *Clostridium difficile*-associated disease: A population based study. Clin. Infect. Dis. 43:1272–1276.
119. vanStaa, T.-P., Leufkens, H.G.M., (2006), Gastric acid-suppression agents and risk of *Clostridium difficile*-associated disease. JAMA 295:2599 (letter).
120. Dial, S., Delaney, J.A.C., Schneider, V., Suissa, S., (2006), Proton pump inhibitor use and risk of community-acquired *Clostridium difficile*-associated disease defined by prescription for oral vancomycin therapy. CMAJ 175:745–748.
121. Cunningham, R., (2006), Proton pump inhibitors and the risk of *Clostridium difficile*-associated disease: further evidence from the community. CMAJ 175:757–758.
122. Fedorker, D.P., Engler, H.D., Ó Shaughnessy, E.M., Williams, E.C., Reichelderfer, C.J., Smith, W.I. Jr., (1999), Evaluation of two rapid assays for detection of *Clostridium difficile* toxin A in stool specimens. J. Clin. Microbiol. 39:3044–3047.
123. Ticehurst, J.R., Aird, D.Z., Dam, L.M., Borek, A.P., Hargrove, J.T., Carroll, K.C., (2006), Effective detection of toxigenic *Clostridium difficile* by a two-step algorithm including tests for antigen and cytotoxin. J. Clin. Microbiol. 44:1145–1149.
124. Vanpouke, H., DeBaere, T., Claeys, G., Vaneechoutte, M., Verschraegen, G., (2001), Evaluation of six commercial assays for the rapid detection of *Clostridium difficile* toxin and/or antigen in stool specimens. Clin. Microbiol. Infect. 7:55–64.
125. Lemee, L., Dhalluin, A., Testelin, S., Mattrat, M.A., Maillard, K., Lemeland, J.F., Pons, J.-L., (2004), Multiplex PCR targeting tpi (Triose Phosphate Isomerase) tcdA (Toxin A), and tcdB (ToxinB) genes for toxigenic culture of *Clostridium difficile*. J. Clin. Microbiol. 42:5710–5714.
126. Van den Berg, R.J., Bruijnesteijn van Coppenraet, L.S., Gerritsen, H.J., Endtz, H.P., van der Vorm, E.R., Kuijper, E.J., (2005), Prospective multicenter evaluation of a new immunoassay and real-time PCR for rapid diagnosis of *Clostridium difficile*-associated diarrhea in hospitalized patients. J. Clin. Microbiol. 43:5338–5340.
127. Guilbault, C., Labbe, A.C., Poirier, L., Busque, L., Beliveau, C., Laverdiere, M., (2002), Development and evaluation of a PCR method for detection of the *Clostridium difficile* toxin B gene in stool specimens. J. Clin. Microbiol. 40:2288–2290.
128. van den Berg, R.J., Kuijper, E.J., van Coppenraet, L.E., Claas, E.C., (2006), Rapid diagnosis of toxigenic *Clostridium difficile* in faecal samples with internally controlled real-time PCR. Clin. Microbiol. Infect. 12:184–186.
129. Teasley, D.G., Gerding, D.N., Olson, M.M., Peterson, L.R., Gebhard, R.L., Schwartz, M.J., (1983), Prospective randomized trial of metronidazole versus vancomycin for *Clostridium difficile*-associated diarrhea and colitis. Lancet; 2:1043–1046.
130. Wenisch, C., Parschalk, B., Hasenhiindl, M., Hirschl, A.M., Graninger, W., (1996), Comparison of vancomycin, teichoplanin, metronidazole, and fusidic acid for the treatment of *Clostridium difficile*-associated diarrhea. Clin. Infect. Dis. 22:813–818.
131. Shin, J.W., Yong, D., Kim, M.S., Chang, K.H., Lee, K., Kim, J.M., Chong, Y., (2003), Sudden increase of vancomycin-resistant enterococcal infections in a Korean tertiary care hospital: possible consequences of increased use of oral vancomycin. J. Infect. Chemother. 9:104–105.
132. Peláez, T., Alcolá, L., Alonso, R., Rodriguez-Créixems, M., Garcia-Lechuz, Bouza, E., (2002), Reassessment of *Clostridium difficile* susceptibility to metronidazole and vancomycin, Antimicrob. Agents Chemother. 46:1647–1650.

133. Freeman, J., Stott, J., Baines, S.D., Fawley, W.N., Walcox, M.H., (2005), Surveillance for resistance to metronidazole and vancomycin in genotypically distinct and UK epidemic *Clostridium difficile* isolates in a large teaching hospital. J. Antimicrobial Chemother 156:988–989.
134. Barbut, F., Decre, D., Burghoffer, B., Lesage, D., Delisle, E., Lalande, V., Delmee, M., Avesani, V., Sano, N., Coudert, C., Petit, J.L., (1999), Antimicrobial susceptibilities and serogroups of clinical strains of *Clostridium difficile* isolated in France in 1991 and 1997. Antimicrob. Agents Chemother. 43:2607–2611.
135. Wong, S.S., Woo, P.C., Luk, W.K., Yuen, K.Y., (1999), Susceptibility testing of *Clostridium difficile* against metronidazole, and vancomycin by disc diffusion and Etest. Diag. Microbial. Infect. Dis. 34:1–6.
136. Pépin, J., Alary, M.-E., Valiguette, Raiche, E., Ruel, J., Fulop, K., Godin, D., Bourassa, C., (2005), Increasing risk of relapse after treatment of *Clostridium difficile* colitis in Quebec, Canada. Clin, Infect. Dis. 40:1591–1597.
137. Musher, D.M., Aslam, S., Logan, N., Nallacheru, S., Bhaila, I., Borchert, F., Hamill, R.J., (2005), Relatively poor outcome after treatment of *Clostridium difficile* colitis with metronidazole. Clin. Infect. Dis. 40:1586–1590.
138. Wilcox, M.H., Howe, R., (1995), Diarrhea caused by *Clostridium difficile*: response time for treatment with metronidazole and vancomycin. J. Antimicrob. Chemother. 36:673–679.
139. Bolton, R.P., Culshaw, M.A., (1986), Faecal metronidazole concentrations during oral and intravenous therapy for antibiotic associated colitis due to *Clostridium difficile*. Gut; 27:1169–1172.
140. Bricker, E., Garg, R., Nelson, R., Loza, A., Novak, T., Hansen, J., (2005), Antibiotic treatment for *Clostridium difficile*-associated diarrhea in adults. Cochrane Database Syst. Rev. CD004610.
141. Keighley, M.R., Burdon, D.W., Arabi, Y., W.Lliams, J.A., Thompson, H., Young, D., Johnson, M., Bentley, S., George, R.H., Mogg, G.A., (1998), Randomized controlled trail of vancomycin for pseudomembranous colitis and post-operative diarrhea. Brit. Med. J. 2:1667–1669.
142. Zar, F.A., Bakkanagari, S.-R., Moorthi, K.M.L.S.T., Davis, M.B., (2007), A comparison of vancomycin and metronidazole for the treatment of *Clostridium difficile*-associated diarrhea, stratified by disease severity. Clin. Infect. Dis. 45:302–307.
143. Kupers, E.J., Surawicz, C.M., (2008), *Clostriduim difficile* infection. Lancet. 371: 1486–1488.
144. Bartlett, J.G., (2008), The case for vancomycin as the preferred drug for treatment of *Clostridium difficile* infection. Clin. Infect. Dis. 46:1489–1492.
145. Pepin, J., (2008), Vancomycin for the treatment of *Clostridium difficile* infection: for whom is this expensive bullet really magic? Clin. Infect. Dis. 46:1493–1498.
146. Johnson, S., Homann, S.R., Bettin, K.M., Quick, J.N., Clabots, C.R., Peterson, L.R., Gerding, D.N., (1992), Treatment of asymptomatic *Clostridium difficile* carriers (fecal excretors) with vancomycin or metronidazole. A randomized, placebo-controlled trial. Ann. Intern Med. 117:297–302.
147. Lagrotteria, D., Holmes, S., Smieja, M., Smaill, F., Lee, C., (2006), Prospective, randomized inpatient study of oral metronidazole versus oral metronidazole and rifampin for treatment of primary episode of *Clostridium difficile*-associated diarrhea. Clin. Infect. Dis. 43:547–552.
148. Kurtz, C.B., Cannon, E.P., Brezzani, A., Pitruzzello, M., Dinardo, C., Rinard, E., Acheson, D.W., Fitzpatrick, R., Kelly, P., Shackett, K., Papoulis, A.T., Goddard, P.J., Barker, R.A. Jr., Palace, G.P., Klinger, J.D., (2001), GTIGO-246, a toxin binding polymer for treatment of *Clostridium difficile* colitis. Antimicrob. Agents Chemother. 45: 2340–2347.
149. Braunlin, W., Xu, Q, Hook, P., Fitzpatrick, R., Klinger, J.D., Burrier, R., Kurtz, C.B., (2004), Toxin binding of tolevamer, a polyanionic drug that protects against antibiotic-associated diarrhea. Biophys J. 87:534–539.
150. Louie, T.J., Peppe, J., Watt, C.K., Johnson, D., Mohammed, R., Dow, G., Weiss, K., Simon, S., John, J.F. Jr., Garber, G., Chasen-Taber, S., Davidson, D.M., for the Tolevamer Study

# References

Investigator Group, (2006), Tolevamer, a noval nonantibiotic polymer, compared with vancomycin in the treatment of mild to moderate severe *Clostridium difficile*-associated diarrhea. Clin. Infect. Dis. 43:411–420.
151. White, C.A. Jr., (2004), Nitazoxanide: a new broad spectrum antiparasitic agent. Expert. Rev. Anti; Infect. Ther. 2:43–49.
152. Fox, L.M., Saravolatz, L.D., (2005), Nitazoxanide: a new thiazolide antiparasitic agent. Clin. Infect. Dis. 40:1173–1180.
153. Broekhuysen, J., Stockis, A., Lins, R.L., De Graeve, J., Rossignol, J.F., (2000), Nitazoxanide: pharmacokinetics and metabolism in man. Int. J. Clin. Phamacol. Ther. 38:387–394.
154. Dubreuil, L., Houcke, I., Mouton, Y., Rossignol, J.F., (1996), In vitro evaluation of activities of nitazoxanide and tizoxanide against anaerobes and aerobic organisms. Antimicrob. Agents Chemother. 40:2266–2270.
155. Musher, D.M., Logan, N., Hamill, R.J., Dupont, H.L., Lentnek, A., Gupta, A., Rossignol, J.-F., (2006), Nitazoxanide for the treatment of *Clostridium difficile* colitis. Clin. Infect. Dis. 43:421–427.
156. Fiedenberg, F., Fernadez, A., Kaul, V., Niami, P., Levine G.M., (2001), Intravenous metronidazole for treatment of *Clostridium difficile* colitis. Dis. Colon Rectum; 44:1176–1180.
157. Apisarnthanarak, A., Razavi, B., Mundi, L.M., (2002), Adjunctive intracolonic vancomycin for severe *Clostridium difficile* colitis: case series and review of The Literative. Clin. Infect. Dis. 35:690–6961.
158. Shetler, K., Nieuwenhuis, R., Wren, S.M., Triadafilopoulos, G., (2001), Decompressive colonoscopy with intracolonic vancomycin administration for the treatment of severe pseudomembranous colitis. Surg. Endosc. 15:653–659.
159. Dallal, R.M., Harbrecht, B.G., Boujoukas, A.J., Sirio, C.A., Farkas, L.M., Lee, K.K., Simmons, R.L., (2003), Fulminant *Clostridium difficile*: an underappreciated and increasing cause of death and complications. Curr. Surg. 60:227–230.
160. Fekety, R., Mc Farland, L.V., Surawicz, C.M., Greenberg, R.N., Elmer, G.W., Mulligan, M. E., (1997), Recurrent *Clostridium difficile* diarrhea: characteristics of and risk factors for patients enrolled in a prospective, randomized, double-blinded clinical trial. Clin. Infect. Dis. 24:324–333.
161. McFarland, L.V., Surawicz, C.M., Rubin, M., Fekety, R., Elmer, G.W., Greenberg, R.N., (1999), Recurrent *Clostridium difficile* disease: epidemiology and clinical characteristics. Infect. Control Hosp. Epidemiol. 20:43–50.
162. McFarland, L.V., Elmer, G.W., Surawicz, C.M., (2002), Breaking the cycle: treatment strategies for 163 cases of recurrent *Clostridium difficile* disease. Am. J. Gastroenterol. 97:1769–1775.
163. Alonso, R., Gros, S., Pelaez, T., Garcia-de-Viedma, D., Rodriguez-Creixems, M., Bouza, E., (2001), Molecular analysis of relapse vs re-infection in HIV-positive patients suffering from recurrent *Clostridium difficile* associated diarrhea. J. Hosp. Infect. 48:86–92.
164. Tang-Feldman, Y., Mayo, S., Silva, J.Jr., Cohen, S.H., (2003), Molecular analysis of *Clostridium difficile* strains isolated from 18 cases of recurrent *Clostridium difficile* associated diarrhea. J. Clin. Microbiol. 41:3413–3414.
165. van den Berg, R.J., Ameen, H.A., Furusawa, T., Claas, E.C., van der Vorm, E.R., Kuijper, E. J., (2005), Coexistence of multiple PCR-ribotype strains of *Clostridium difficile* in faecal samples limits epidemiological studies. J. Med. Microbiol. 54:173–179.
166. Pepin, J., Routhier, S., Gagnon, S., Brazeau, I., (2006), Management and outcomes of a first recurrence of *Clostridium difficile* associated disease in Quebec, Canada. Clin. Infect. Dis. 42:758–764.
167. Kyne, L., Warny, M., Qamar, A., Kelly, C.P., (2001), Association between antibody response to toxin A and protection against recurrent *Clostridium difficile* diarrhea. Lancet 357:158–159.
168. Kyne, L., Warny, M., Qamar, A., Kelly, C.P., (2000), Asymptomatic carriage of *Clostridium difficile* and serum levels of IgG antibody against toxin A.N. Engl. J. Med. 342:390–397.

169. Drudy, D., Calabi, E., Kyne, L., Sougioultzis, S., Kelly, E., Fairweather, N., Kelly, C.P., (2004), Human antibody response to surface layer proteins in *Clostridium difficile* infection. FEMS Immun. Med. Microbiol. 41:237–242.
170. Dendukuri, N., Costa, V., McGregor, M., Brophy, J.M., (2005), Probiotic therapy for the prevention and treatment of *Clostridium difficile*-associated diarrhea: a systematic review. CMAJ 173:167–170.
171. Johnston, B.C., Supina, A.L., Vohra, S., (2006), Probiotics for pediatric antibiotic-associated diarrhea: a meta-analysis of randomized placebo-controlled trials. CMAJ; 175:377–383.
172. McFarland, L.V., (2006), Meta-analysis of probiotics for the prevention of antibiotic associated diarrhea and the treatment of *Clostridium difficile* disease. Am. J. Gastroenterol. 101:812–822.
173. Katz, J.A., (2006), Probiotics for the prevention of antibiotic-associated diarrhea and *Clostridium difficile* diarrhea. J. Clin. Gastroenterol. 40:249–255.
174. Mrukowicz, S.H., (2005), Meta-analysis: non-pathogenic yeast *Saccharomyces boulardii* reduces risk for antibiotic-associated diarrhea. Aliment. Pharmacol. Ther. 22:365–372.
175. Tedesco, F.J., Gordon, D., Forston, W.C., (1985), Approach to patients with multiple relapses of antibiotic-associated pseudomembranous colitis. Am. J. Gastroenterol. 80:867–868.
176. Buggy, B.P., Fekety, R., Silva, J.Jr., (1987), Therapy of relapsing *Clostridium difficile*-associated diarrhea and colitis with the combination of vancomycin and rifampin. J. Clin. Gastroenterol. 9:155–159.
177. Leung, D.Y., Kelly, C.P., Boguniewicz, M., Pothoulakis, C., Lamont, J.T., Flores, A., (1991), Treatment with intravenously administered gamma globulin of chronic relapsing colitis induced by C. *difficile* toxin. J. Pediatrics 118:633–637.
178. Salcedo, J., Keates, S., Pothoulakis, C., Warmy, M., Castagliuolo, I., Lamont, J.T., Kelly, C. P., (1997), Intravenous immunoglobulin therapy for severe *Clostridium difficile* colitis. Gut 41:366–370.
179. Viscidi, R., Laughon, B.E., Yolken, R., Bo-Linn, P., Moench, T., Ryder, R.W., Bartlett, J.G., (1983), Serum antibody response to toxins A and B of *Clostridium difficile*. J. Infect. Dis. 148:93–100.
180. Bacon, A.E., III, Fekety, R., (1994), Immunoglobulin G directed against toxin A and B of *Clostridium difficile* in the general population and patients with antibiotic-associated diarrhea. Diag. Microbiol. Infect. Dis. 18:205–209.
181. Wilcox, M.H., (2004), Descriptive study of intravenous immunoglobulin for the treatment of recurrent *Clostridium difficile* diarrhea. J. Antimicrob. Chemother. 53:882–884.
182. McPherson, S., Rees, C.J., Ellis, R., Soo, S., Panter, S.J., (2006), Intravenous immunoglobulin for the treatment of severe, refractory, and recurrent *Clostridium difficile* diarrhea. Dis. Colon Rectum 49:640–645.
183. Juang, P., Skledar, S.J., Zgheib, N.K., Paterson, D.L., Vergis, E.N., Shannon, W.D., Ansani, N.T., Branch, R.A., (2007), Clinical outcomes of intravenous immune globulin in severe *Clostridium difficile*-associated diarrhea. Am. J. Infect. Control 35:131–137.
184. Schwan, A., Sjolin, S., Trottestam, U., Aronsson, B., (1983), Relapsing *Clostridium difficile* enterocolitis cured by rectal infusion of homologous faeces. Lancet 2:845.
185. Tvede, M., Rask-Madsen, J., (1989), Bacteriotherapy for chronic relapsing *Clostridium* diarrhea in six patients. Lancet 1:1156–1160.
186. Persky, S.E., Brandt, L.J., (2000), Treatment of recurrent *Clostridium difficile*-associated diarrhea by administration of donated stool directly through a colonoscope. AM. J. Gastroenterol. 95:3283–3285.
187. Eisenman, B., Silen, W., Bascom, G.S., Kauvar, A.J., (1958), Fecal enema as an adjunct in the treatment for pseudomembranous colitis. Surgery 44:854–859.
188. Aas, J., Gessert, C.E., Bakken, J.S., (2003), Recurrent *Clostridium difficile* colitis. Case series involving 18 patients treated with donor stool administration via a nasogastric tube. Clin. Infect. Dis. 36:580–585.

189. Borody, T.J., Warren, E.F., Leis, S.M., Surace, R., Ashman, O., Siarakas, S., (2004), Bacteriotherapy using fecal flora: toying with human motions. J. Gastroenterol. 38:475–483.
190. Ludlam. H., Brown, N., Sule, O., Redpath, C., Coni, N., Owen, G., (1999), An antibiotic policy associated with reduced risk of *Clostridium difficile* associated diarrhea. Age Ageing 28:578–580.
191. Carling, P., Fung, T., Killion, A., Terrin, N., Barza, M., (2003), Favorable impact of a multidisciplinary antibiotic management program conducted during 7 years. Infect control Hosp. Epidem. 24:699–706.
192. Thomas, C., Stevenson, M., Williamson, D.J., Rily, T.V., (2002), *Clostridium difficile* associated diarrhea. Epidemiological data from Western Australia associated with a modified antibiotic policy. Clin. Infect. Dis. 35:1457–1462.
193. Mayfield, J.L., Leet, T., Miller, J., Mundy, L.M., (2000), Environmental control to reduce transmission of *Clostridium difficile*. Clin. Infect. Dis. 31:995–1000.
194. Hopkins, M.J., Macfarlane, G.T., (2003), Nondigestible oligosaccharides enhance bacterial colonization resistance against *Clostridium difficile* in vitro. Applied Environ. Microbiol, 69:1920–1927.
195. Karlsson, S., Lindberg, A., Norin, E., Burman, L.G., Akerlund, T., (2000), Toxins, butyric acid, and other shortchain fatty acids are coordinately expressed and down-regulated by cysteine in *Clostridium difficile*. Infect. Immun. 68:5881–5888.
196. Freeman, J., Baines, S.D., Jabes, D., Wilcox, M.H., (2005), Comparison of the efficacy of ramoplanin and vancomycin in both in vitro and in vivo models of clindamycin-induced *Clostriduim difficile* infection. J. Antimicrob. Chemother. 56:717–725.
197. Pothoulakis, C., (2004), Rifalazil treats and prevents relapse of *Clostridium difficile* associated diarrhea in hamsters. Antimicrob. Agents Chemother. 48:3975–3979.
198. Babcock, G.J., Broering, T.J., Hernandez, H.J., Mandell, R.B., Donahue, K., Boatright, N., Stack, A.M., Lowry, I., Graziano, R., Molrine, D., Ambrosino, D.M., Thomas, W.D., (2006), Human monoclonal antibodies directed against toxins A and B prevent *Clostridium difficile*-induced mortality in hamsters. Infect. Immun. 74:6339–6347.
199. Alcantra, C., Stenson, W.F., Steiner, T.S., Guerrant, R.L., (2001), Role of inducible cyclooxygenase and prostaglandins in *Clostridium difficile* toxin A- induced secretion and inflammation in a animal model. J. Infect. Dis. 184:648–652.
200. Giannasca, P.J., Zhang, Z.X., Lei, W.D., Boden, J.A., Giel, M.A., Monath, T.P., Thomas, W. D.Jr., (1999), Serum antitoxin antibodies mediate systemic and mucosal protection from *Clostridium difficile* disease in hamsters. Infect. Immun. 67:527–538.
201. Sougioultzis, S., Kyne, L., Drudy, D., Keates, S., Maroo, S., Pothoulakis, C., Giannasca, P.J., Lee, C.K., Warny, M., Monath, Kelly, T.P., Ciaran, P., (2003), *Clostridium difficile* toxoid vaccine in recurrent *C. difficile* associated diarrhea. Gastroenterology. 128:764–770.
202. van Dissel, J.T., de Groot, N., Hensgens, C.M., Numan, S., Kuijper, E.J., Veldkamp, P., van't Wout, J., (2005), Bovine antibody-enriched whey to aid in the prevention of a relapse of *Clostridium difficile* associated diarrhea: preclinical and preliminary clinical data. J. Med. Microbiol. 54.197–205.
203. Naaber, P., Lchto, E., Salminen, S., Mikelsaar, M., (1996), Inhibition of adhesion of *Clostridium difficile* to Ca Co-2 cells. Fems Immun. Med. Microbiol. 14:205–209.
204. Merrigan, M.M., Sambol, S.P., Johnson, S., Gerding, D.N., (2003), Prevention of fatal *Clostridium difficile* associated disease during continuous administration of clindamycin in hamsters. J. Infect. Dis. 188:1922–1927.
205. Zhong, S.S., Zhang, Z.S., Wang, J.D., Lai, Z.S., Wang, Q.Y., Ren, Y.X., (2004), Competitive inhibition of adherence of enterotoxigenic *Escherichia coli*, enteropathogenic *Escherichia coli* and *Clostridium difficile* to intestinal epithelial cell line lovo by purified adhesin of *Bifidobacterium adolescentis* 1027. World J. Gastroenterol. 10:1630–1633.
206. Fenner, L., Widmer, A.F., Goy, G., Rudin, S., Frei, R., (2008), Rapid and reliable diagnostic algorithm for detection of *Clostridium difficile*. J. Clin. Microbiol. 46:328–330.

# Chapter 9
# Probiotics in Infectious Diseases

## 9.1 Introduction

Probiotics are defined as dietary supplements of living microorganisms found in the normal flora with low or no pathogenicity, but with positive effects on the health of the host. A broader definition of probiotics proposed is "microbial cell preparations or components of microbial cells that have a beneficial effect on health, and well being of the host." The term "probiotic" is derived from the Greek meaning "for life", this strictly should be viable organisms. Commensal bacteria have coevolved with humans and the body contains tenfold as many indigenous protective microorganisms as it does eukaryotic cells. Vast numbers of microorganisms colonize the skin, mouth, gut, and all orifices without damage to the host, and some of these microorganisms protect the body from invasion by pathogens.

There is accumulating evidence that normal colonizing or resident microbial flora of the gastrointestinal tract (GI), skin, and mucosa of various orifices are necessary to maintain good health. Although these microorganisms can on occasion cause disease, mainly in the immune-compromised hosts or in the presence of indwelling foreign material, they play essential roles in maintaining the integrity of the endothelial and mucosal lining, interfere with establishment of invading pathogens, and stimulate the innate immune system. Native or resident microflora colonizes the skin, oral cavity, the GI tract, upper respiratory tract, and urogenital tract. Transient microorganisms colonize the body from the external environment and can persist if some niche is not filled with resident native flora.

The full-term infant before birth live in a "sterile" milieu, but at vaginal delivery rapidly becomes colonized by microorganisms from the birth canal of the mother and environment, including coliforms, streptococci, and gram-positive, non-spore-forming anaerobic rods. Breast-fed infants have increased number of *Bifidobacteria* but rarely have *Clostridia* colonizing the GI tract. Formula-fed infants, on the other hand, have large numbers of *Lactobaccili*, *Bacteroides*, and *Clostridia* and relatively few *Bifidobacteria* species.[1,2] When food supplements are started the microflora are similar between breast-fed and formula-fed infants with *Bacteroides* and anaerobic gram-positive cocci predominating. After 2 years of age the gut flora becomes similar to adults, with *Bacteroides* species and anaerobic gram-positive increasing to exceed *Bifidobacterium*.[2,3] The GI tract is colonized by more than 500 different bacterial species, and strict anaerobes outnumber aerobes by more than 10 to 1. The interactions between the host immune system and colonizing microflora begin in the neonate and continue throughout life.[1,2] The normal flora of the GI tract is essential for maintaining health in the host by several mechanisms, including stimulating the immune system, protecting the host from invading pathogens (bacteria, viruses, and protozoa), and aiding digestion and provision of nutrients (i.e., vitamin K).[1–3]

## 9.2 Background

The use of probiotics probably extended from ancient times when traditional medicines included fermented foods. About a century ago, Metchnikoff[4] proposed that the beneficial effect of bacteria in yogurt was responsible for the long life of Bulgarian peasants (yogurt containing *Lactobacillus* species, "produce compounds useful against premature ageing"). In the 1930s a Japanese microbiologist, Minoru Shirota, selected beneficial strains of lactic acid bacteria that could survive through the digestive system and used them to develop fermented milk products.[5] He proposed that many diseases could be prevented if an optimal gut microflora were maintained.

In the last 50 years probiotics have been proposed as beneficial for many infectious diseases and chronic conditions such as Crohn's disease. However, the literature in the past 10 years is now replete with clinical and biological studies with probiotics on various conditions. The most extensive studied conditions with probiotics include infectious diarrheas in children, antibiotic-associated diarrhea (AAD), including *Clostridium difficile* colitis (CDAD), urogenital infections in women, neonatal infections, and inflammatory bowel diseases. However, recent studies have also addressed the value of probiotics in allergy prevention, anti-tumor action in the gut and elsewhere, and effects on post-operative infectious complications, and infections associated with aging.

Interest and clinical trials have also extended (with and without probiotics) to the health benefits and prophylactic effects of dietary substances, usually nondigested carbohydrates, which stimulate the growth and metabolism of protective commensal bacteria ("prebiotics").[6,7] The combination of probiotic and prebiotic for health benefits is termed "symbiotic." Lactosucrose, fructo-oligosaccharides, inulin, bran, psyllium, and germinated barley extracts foster the growth of *Lactobacillus* and *Bifidobacterium* species and stimulate production of short-chain fatty acids, especially butyrate.[8,9] In addition, increased substrate availability and enhanced numbers of metabolically active *Lactobacilli* and *Bifidobacteria* increase bacterial fermentation, with increased butyrate production and improvement of epithelial barrier function. The net result of prebiotic administration is functionally equivalent to administering probiotic bacteria.

## 9.3 Mechanisms of Action

The intestinal mucosal barrier to microbial pathogens and their toxins is a combination of epithelial, mucosal, and immunologic luminal factors acting together to control penetration of invaders and modulate self-limited inflammation and appropriate immunologic reactions.[10] Luminal factors that control pathogenic bacterial colonization include gastric acidity to kill or decrease the inoculum of harmful microbes; mucus to trap foreign agents and toxins; digestive enzymes to hydrolyze antigens; and active peristalsis to facilitate exit and expulsion of toxins. Secretory immunoglobulins IgA and IgM released into the lumen in response to antigenic microbial stimulation agglutinate and prevent attachment and penetration of invaders across the mucosal surface. The enterocyte acts as a sensor of luminal stimuli and through signal-transduction pathways, stimulate the lymphoid tissue and immune cells to upregulate inflammatory cytokine production. The most commonly used probiotics are lactic acid producing bacteria, including species of *Lactobacilli*, *Bifidobacterium*, and *Enterococcus*; and nonpathogenic yeasts, principally *Saccharomyces boulardii*. Probiotic bacteria with desirable properties and documented beneficial effects include *L. acidophilus*, *L. casei* Shirota strain, *L. johnsonii*, LJI, *L. reuteri*, and *Bifidobacterium lactis* Bb12.[1,11] *L. rhamnosus* LGG is the most extensively studied probiotic in adults and children.[10]

Multiple mechanisms have been proposed to explain the beneficial effects of probiotics in infections and intestinal inflammation (Table 9.1).[12] These mechanisms can be broadly divided into four categories: (1) improvement of epithelial and mucosal barrier function; (2) inhibition of pathogenic microbes (colonization resistance); (3) inactivation of microbial toxins; (4) and immunomodulation. These mechanisms are inter-related and can be species-specific but the exact modes of action have not been fully elucidated for many probiotics.

### *9.3.1 Mucosal Integrity*

The means by which probiotics can improve epithelial mucosal barrier function is not well understood, but it may include production of short-chain fatty acids such as butyrate by *Lactobacillus* and *Bifidobacterium* species. Stimulation of mucins may decrease bacterial translocation, as shown in the murine model treated with *L. plantarum*[14] and in the rabbit model treated with *Lactobacillus* GG.[15] Probiotics (*L. reuteri* or VSL3) also appear to decrease mucosal permeability, thus preventing bacterial translocation and invasions in IL-10 knockout mine.[16,17] Clinical studies in critically ill patients, however, have shown no effect on intestinal permeability (measured by lactulose/rhamnose test) with administration of symbiotic containing *L. acidophilus*, *B. lactis* Bb12, *S. thermophilus*, *Lactobacillus bulgaricus*, and oligofructose.[18] It has also been postulated that probiotics may improve or maintain intestinal mucosal integrity by restoring or preventing disruption of the normal

**Table 9.1** Mechanisms of action of probiotics

- **Maintain mucosal integrity or barrier**
  - Enhance mucus production
  - Decrease mucosal permeability
  - Restoring normal microflora
  - Stimulate intestinal lactase activity
- **Colonization resistance (inhibit pathogenic bacteria)**
  - Competitive inhibition for adhesion sites
  - Decrease luminal pH
  - Secrete bacteriocins, hydrogen peroxide
  - Inhibit epithelial invasion
- **Inactivation of microbial toxins and virulence factors**
  - *S. boulardii* inactivate toxins A & B of *C. difficile*
  - Decrease toxin activity or expression
  - Down regulate virulence factors expression
- **Immunomodulation**
  - Enhance secretory immunoglobulin A production
  - Induce protective cytokines (1L-10, TGF-β)
  - Suppress proinflammatory cytokines (TNF-α)
  - Enhance expression of innate antimicrobial defense

intestinal microflora. This would be important in AAD and infectious diarrheas. The normal gut microflora provides a natural defense against invading pathogenic microorganisms and changes in the normal bacterial population can result in higher risk of infections. Human studies have demonstrated that a symbiotic (*B. bifidum*, *B. lactis*, and oligosaccharides) can increase the size and diversity of protective fecal bifidobacterial populations, which are often markedly reduced in older people.[19] It has also been shown that probiotics comprising *L. acidophilus* and *B. bifidum* can modulate the response of intestinal microflora to the effects of antibiotics.[20] In another placebo, controlled study of *L. paracasei* F19 administered twice weekly for 3 weeks in children did not after the numbers of lactobacilli (other than *Lactobacillus* F19) or bifidobacteria.[21] However, in elderly adults a fermented milk product with *Lactobacillus* F19 twice daily for 12 weeks increases the number of other lactobacilli during the adminstration.[21]

Acid-producing probiotics have been postulated to be beneficial in some types of diarrhea by partial lactose digestion and stimulation of intestinal mucosal lactase activity. Episodes of acute gastroenteritive disaccharidase activity (and temporary lactase deficiency) in the small intestine may affect the transport of monosaccharides and produce osmotic diarrhea. Lactobacilli used in fermented milk produce active β-galactosidase to decrease lactose concentration and may play a role in decreasing osmotic diarrhea with some infections such as rotavirus gastroenteritis.[22,23]

## 9.3.2 Colonization Resistance

The first step in microbial colonization or infection is adherence to microvillus glycoconjugates (terminal sugars on oligosaccharide side chain on microvillus membrane, proteins and lipids) through adhesions on the microbial surface. Different organisms have different affinity for terminal sugars; and the carbohydrate composition and glycosylation of membrane proteins and ligands may determine the type of flora that colonizes the gut. With adherence comes proliferation for the microbe to colonize the mucosal surface. The colonization bacteria through epithelial "cross-talk" uses the epithelial cell machinery to facilitate translocation.[10] For instance, *Escherichia coli* can attach to a physiologic receptor or insert its own receptor to modify the epithelial surface action composition, facilitate engulfment by enterocyte and enhance translocation by entocytosis.[24] Another example by a different mechanism is *Salmonella typhimurium*, which adheres to the epithelial growth factor receptor and by signal-transduction pathway release molecules that open tight junctions between enterocytes, and enhance paracellular translocation.[25]

There is now evidence that the normal indigenous organisms can also communicate with intestinal epithelial cells to enhance host defenses against pathogens-induced disease. The precise mechanism by which this occurs is unknown. Probiotics can protect the host from colonization by pathogenic invaders by many different means in the intestines. Competitive inhibition for microbial adhesion sites is one means by which probiotics may prevent pathogenic microorganisms from establishing a niche in the gut. For example, the probiotic may have the same preferential carbohydrates receptors as the pathogens, such as mannose for *B. profringins*, which can competitively inhibit pathogenic *E. coli*.[26] Attachment to the intestinal epithelium by probiotics can actively stimulate epithelial and lymphocyte functions,[27] enhancing the protective capacity of mucosal defences. *B. adolescentis* 1027 or its purified adhesin can inhibit the adhesion of enterotoxigenic and enteropathogenic *E. coli* and *C. difficile* to intestinal epithelial cells in vitro in a dose-dependent manner.[28] Other examples of adhesion site inhibition include *Lactobacillus* GG and *L. plantarium* blockage of enteropathogenic *E. coli* attachment to human colonic cells in vitro[29]; and the ability of *S. boulardii* to decrease attachment of *Entamoeba histolytica* trophozoites to erythrocytes.[30] In animal model *L. plantorum* 299V prevented bacterial translocation in endotoxemic rats by its capability to adhere to the intestinal mucosa.[31] *Lactobacilli*, the predominant microorganisms of the vaginal microflora, play a major role in maintenance of the healthy urogenital tract by preventing the colonization of pathogenic bacteria. This has led to the use of probiotics in the prevention of recurrent urinary tract infections (UTI) and vaginitis. In vitro adherence studies of three human urogenital pathogens (*E. coli*, *Staphylococcus aureus*, and Group B. *streptococcus*) to vaginal epithelial cells (VEC), have shown the capability of similar *Lactobacilli* species (*L. acidophilus* and *L. paracassei*) to inhibit adhesion of Group B *Streptococcus* and *S. aureus* but not *E. coli*.[32] However, *L. acidophilus* can also affect cell membrane components in *E. coli* and produces biosurfactants that inhibit their adhesion to surfaces.[33]

In addition, *Lactobacillus* RC-14 strain may protect urogenital epithelium by up-regulating mucin production which may act as a barrier to infection.[34]

The lactic acid producing bacteria of the uroepithelium and the gut can also suppress pathogens by producing antimicrobial substances, such as organic acids, free fatty acids, hydrogen peroxide, ammonia, and bacteriocins. *Lactobacillus* GG has the ability to produce a low-molecular weight antibacterial substance that inhibits both gram-positive and gram-negative enteric bacteria.[35] In vitro supernatants from *L. rhamnosus* GR-1 and *L. fementum* RC-4 also can inactivate $10^9$ particles of double-stranded DNA adenovirus and negative-stranded RNA vesicular stomatitis virus within 10 min.[36] Whether this is due to acid alone or a specific antiviral property is not clear.

## 9.3.3 Inactivation of Microbial Toxins

Several bacterial gastroenteritis are toxin-mediated such as cholera, shigellosis, travelers diarrhea from enterotoxigenic *E. coli*, and enterohemorrhagic (shiga toxin) *E. coli* colitis. However, there is no good evidence that probiotics can inactivate these toxins or are of any value in these entities. The most important cause of nosocomial diarrhea and a major problem associated with antibiotic use is *C. difficile* infection. The disease being caused by the cytotoxin and enterotoxin effects of toxin A and B.

*S. boulardii* is a nonpathogenic yeast, related to baker's yeast, that has received much attention in the treatment of severe or recurrent *C. difficile* colitis. *S. boulardii* was first shown to inhibit *C. difficile* toxin A enteritis in rats by releasing a 54-KDa serine protease which digests the toxin A molecule and its brush border receptor.[37] Subsequent investigation by the same group found that *S. boulardii* secreted protease proteolytically digests toxin A and B molecules, and reversed the toxins-induced inhibition of protein synthesis in human colonic cells.[38] Bacterial probiotics (*L. acidophilus* and *B. bifidum*) may possibly decrease *C. difficile* toxin activity or expression, as in a preliminary randomized, placebo-controlled study in the elderly ($N = 138$) they decreased the recovery of *C. difficile* toxin by about 59%.[39] Bifidobacteria colonization can also inhibit toxin production by Shiga toxin-producing *E. coli* possibly by lowering intestinal pH.[40] Some *Lactobacillus* strains can down-regulate expression of virulence factors, under control of transcriptional regulator aggR, in several enteroaggregative *E. coli* (an increasingly recognized cause of diarrhea).[41]

## 9.3.4 Immunomodulation

The development of the immune system in humans depends on the interaction with a large variety of commensal bacteria, predominantly located in the gut.[42] It was recently shown that the recognition of commensal bacteria by epithelial cells protects against intestinal injury.[43] Moreover, there is evidence that the polysaccharide of common commensal bacteria (*Bacteroides fragilis*) can mediate multiple immunomodulatory activities essential to the development of a normal immune system.[44]

It has been proposed that intestinal colonization by probiotics can strengthen the host's mucosal defenses through the enhancement of the secretory antibody response, through a tightening of the mucosal physical barrier to microorganism translocation, and by a balance in the T-helper cell response.[45–47] In support of this contention is that probiotics can enhance the immunological response to oral or systemic vaccines.[48] A number of studies showed that several probiotic agents can induce protective cytokines, including 1L-10 and transforming growth factor β, and suppress proinflammatory cytokines, such as tumor necrosis factor, in the mucosa of patients with pouchitis and Crohn's disease.[49–52] Probiotic agents can also prevent and treat colitis independently of 1L-10 induction in 1L-10-deficient mice.[53]

Viable probiotics are not essential for immunomodulation as nonviable components can mediate their effects. Both secreted proteins and DNA of *Streptococcus salivarium* species (VSL3) can block nuclear factor (NF)-KB and p38 mitogen-activated protein kinase activation and prevent apoptosis of epithelial cells.[54,55] Different effects are produced with DNA from different bacterial species within the VSL3 mixture.[54] Suppression of experimental colitis by nonmethylated DNA (CpG) from VSL3 and certain *E. coli* strain is mediated through toll-like receptor (TLR)-9, which binds CpG.[56]

In human genome microarray studies, intravaginal insertion of *L. rhamnosus* GR-I can induce over 700 gene expression changes, including innate antimicrobial defenses.[57] It appears that GR-I signaling produces factors which induce macrophage-secreted inhibitory factors suppressing *E. coli*-induced inflammatory cytokines.[57] Animal studies also showed that *L. reuteri* RC-14 can prevent *S. aureus* infection probably by blocking collagen-binding receptors, producing anti-infective signaling and modulation of immunity.[58] Different probiotics have demonstrated adjuvant-like effects on intestinal and systemic immunity with oral administration. *L. casei* GGG enhances IgM and IgA serum antibody response in acute rotavirus gastroenteritis in children,[59] and in the convalescent stage it increases the number of IgA antibody secreting cells to rotavirus.[60] Healthy adults vaccinated with oral typhoid vaccine demonstrated higher serum IgA to *S. typhi* than control when given fermented milk with *L. acidophilus* and *Bifidobacterium* species for 3 weeks.[61] A recent animal study also demonstrated that yoghurt accelerated the recovery of defense mechanisms against *S. pneumoniae* in protein-malnourished mice.[62]

Probiotics may also affect cell-mediated immunity. Oral or parenteral administration of *L. casei* can increase macrophage phagocytic activity against several intracellular bacteria in mice.[63] Lactobacilli colonizing human intestinal mucosa (especially *L. paracasei*) are strong stimulators of 1L-12 production, thereby enhancing cell-mediated immunity.[64] Increase 1L-12 may also down-regulate the Th-2 response, decreasing 1L-4 and IgE production, thus explaining the potential role of probiotics in allergy prevention.[65] Commensal lactobacilli and streptococci can also stimulate human peripheral blood mononuclear cells to produce 1L-12, 1L-18, and interferon-gamma.[66] *S. boulardii* oral ingestion can also induce complement and reticuloendothelial activation in humans.[67]

Severe sepsis is associated with dysfunction of the macrophage/monocyte, an important cellular effector of the innate immune system. A bacteria-free, lysozyme-modified probiotic component (LZMPC) of *Lactobacillus* species administered orally effectively protected rats against lethality from polymicrobial sepsis induced by cecal ligation and puncture.[68] LZMPC up-regulated the expression of cathelicidin-related antimicrobial peptide (CRAMP) in macrophages and enhanced bactericidal activity of these cells. This resulted in increased bacterial clearance in the liver.[68]

Age-related decline in lymploid cell activity (immunosenescence) is believed to account for the increased risk of infections and neoplastic diseases in the elderly. Dietary supplementation with *L. rhamnosus* HN001 or *B. lactis* HN019 for 3 weeks significantly increased natural killer (NK) cell activity in 27 healthy elderly subjects.[69] The proportion of CD56-positive lymphocytes in peripheral circulation was higher, and the ex vivo PBMC tumoricidal activity against K562 cells was increased by an average of 62% to 101%.[69] In younger adults (20–35 years of age), 8 weeks of dietary supplementation with *Bacillus polyfermenticus* (Bispan strain) had been shown, as well, to increase the percentages of $CD4^+$ helper T cells (32%), $CD8^+$ cytotoxic T cells (28%), and $CD56^+$ NK cells (35%) compared with the control group.[70] The concentration of IgG in the experimental group was also 12% higher than the placebo group.

## *9.3.5 Bacterial Translocation*

The gastrointestinal tract and the liver play major roles in the development of multiorgan failure in critically ill patients. This is an important and common complication of severe septic shock and other prolonged shock syndromes. The liver Kupffer cells and macrophages are responsible for clearance and deactivation of endotoxemia, bacteremia from the gut, cytokines, leukotrienes, and various toxins. During mesenteric hypo-perfusion the integrity of the intestinal mucosa become impaired with increased permeability to bacteria, endotoxins, and various other toxins which are transported from the lumen across the mucosa into the circulation and the lymph nodes (bacterial translocation). This results in imbalance of the cytokine cascade with greater proinflammatory activation and increased levels of TNF-alpha, 1L-1, 1L-6, and 1L-10, thus worsening the systemic inflammatory response syndrome (SIRS) and contributing to multiorgan failure. Impaired macrophage function in the liver and intestinal wall likely plays a role in bacterial translocation. Bacterial translocation is believed to be an important cause of nosocomial infection, as well, following major abdominal surgery and organ transplantation, and liver cirrhosis.

Probiotics have been tested in animal models to prevent or modify bacterial translocation. In experimental cirrhosis with ascites, rats treated with antioxidants and *Lactobacillus johnsonii* LA1 had decreased bacterial translocation and decreased endotoxemia compared to cirrhotic rats receiving water ($p < 0.05$).[71] A previous study demonstrated that the adhesive compatibility of *L. plantarum* 299V (reduced adherence of enteric bacteria) was responsible for the prevention of bacterial translocation in endotoxemic rats.[31] In rats undergoing liver resection and/or colonic anastomosis lactic acid bacteria significantly decreased bacterial translocation and bacterial concentration in the mesenteric lymph nodes,[72] In this model bacterial overgrowth in the cecum and impaired hepatic regeneration, but not histological changes or alterations of paracellular permeability, were the potential mechanisms for bacterial translocation.

## 9.4 Clinical Application of Probiotics

Probiotics have mainly been used by non-medical health care professionals such as holistic practitioners, naturopaths, chiropractors, and herbalists for many years. However, in the past several years there have been much interest in the medical and scientific community. The interest in probiotics by physicians have been generated by several factors: surging levels of multi-resistant pathogenic organisms, failures of standard therapy, consumer demand for natural substitutes for drugs, and increasing scientific and clinical evidence showing effectiveness of some probiotic strains.[73] The Food and Agriculture Organization of the United Nations (FAO) and the World Health Organization (WHO) have stated that there is adequate scientific evidence to indicate there is potential for probiotic foods to provide health benefits, and specific strains are safe for human consumption.[74]

Despite a large body of literature on probiotics and human health (over 1,000 in the past 5–8 years), a comprehensive review by the expert panel of FAO and WHO found only a small number of areas in which probiotics have proven clinical benefit.

### 9.4.1 Probiotics for Newborns and Children

#### 9.4.1.1 Necrotizing Enterocolitis

Necrotizing enterocolitis of the newborn (NEC) is a major cause of mortality and morbidity in low birth weight infants (<1,500 g) after the first week of life. The fulminant form of the disease often leads to intestinal perforation, peritonitis, bacteremia, and septic shock. The disease is characterized by presence of air in the wall of the intestines, portal venous system, or peritoneal cavity, and by necrosis of the bowel wall with mucosal sloughing.

The pathogenesis of NEC involves ischemic mucosal injury (especially to the terminal ileum) from hypoxia, hypotension, endotoxemia, and excessive epinephrine.[75] Predisposing factors include prematurity, hyaline membrane disease, exchange transfusion via the umbilical vein, and exclusive formula feeding. Bacterial colonization of the intestines by pathogens such as *Clostridium*, *Klebsiella*, certain *E. coli* strains, *Pseudomonas*, *Staphylococcus aureus*, and *Salmonella* have been implicated. NEC rarely occurs in breast-fed infants. Breast milk may play a protective role through the presence of antibodies, lysozyme, and other natural antimicrobial peptides, or cellular elements. However, breast feeding may be protective by encouraging colonization of the gut with normal commensals such as lactobacilli and bifidobacteria, which suppresses other pathogens. In a study of the enteric microflora of 25 babies with NEC compared to 23 matched controls, lactobacilli were less common in babies with NEC (12% versus 48%, $p = 0.006$).[76] These findings suggested a correlation between decreased commensal lactobacilli and bifidobacteria, and increased risk of NEC.

In a preliminary non-randomized study from Columbia newborns receiving live *Lactobacillus acidophilus* and *Bifidobacteria* ($N = 1237$) compared to historical controls ($N = 1282$), during the previous year, had a 60% reduction in NEC and overall mortality.[77] This was the initial proof of concept study. A subsequent double-blind, randomized study in Italy treated preterm infants with birthweight <1,500 g with *Lactobacillus* GG ($N = 295$) once a day until discharge (mean 47 days) or placebo ($N = 290$); however, there was no significant reduction of NEC or sepsis.[78] Two recent randomized, controlled studies of probiotic mixture in low birth weight neonates have shown beneficial effects. In a relatively small study from Israel, 72 infants received feeding supplement with *Bifidobacteria infantis*, *S. thermophilus*, and *B. bifidus* or no probiotic supplements in 73 controls.[79] The incidence of NEC was reduced in the study group (4% versus 16.4%, $p = 0.03$); NEC was also less severe in the probiotic-treated group and all NEC-related deaths occurred in control infants.[79] In a larger, single-center trial from Taiwan 180 infants received *L. acidophilus* and *B. infantis* with breast milk and 187 controls were fed breast milk alone.[80] The incidence of death or NEC was significantly lower in the probiotic-treated group. The incidence and severity of NEC were significantly reduced in the treated group.[80] Thus, these recent randomized trials indicate that probiotics mixtures with bifidobacteria are useful in decreasing the risk of NEC. However, before this can be accepted as standard therapy a larger, multi-center, randomized, preferably placebo-controlled trial should confirm these results.

### 9.4.1.2 Infectious Diarrhea in Children

Numerous trials have been conducted in infectious diarrheas in children with mixed results, but overall there have been modest benefits in mild to moderately severe diarrhea. Studies have investigated the clinical value of mostly lactobacilli and

## 9.4 Clinical Application of Probiotics

bifidobacteria, and occasionally *S. boulardii* in various settings: community acquired diarrhea, nosocomial diarrhea, viral diarrhea, and AAD.

In a recent Cochrane Database review[81] of probiotics in acute infectious diarrhea 23 studies met the inclusion criteria with a total of 1,917 participants. The trials varied with subjects studied (children and adults), probiotics tested, dosage, methodological quality, and diarrhea definitions and outcomes. Overall probiotics reduced the risk of diarrhea at 3 days (relative risk (RR) 0.66, 95% CI 0.55–0.77), and the duration of diarrhea by 30 h. Thus, probiotics appear to be useful as an adjunct to rehydration in acute infectious diarrheas in children and adults, but more research is needed to define the optimal probiotic regimens.

Similar conclusions were reached by previous meta-analysis restricted to children,[82–84] or limiting the analysis to lactobacilli.[84] Several stains of lactobacilli have been studied but the most frequently investigated is *Lactobacillus* GG, and the findings with reduced risk of infectious diarrhea are most consistent with this strain. *Lactobacillus* GG seems to be the most effective for bacterial-induced diarrhea.[85]

Based on subgroup analysis of one of the meta-analyses[84] there is a dose-dependant response to the lactobacilli in acute diarrheas, with a dose of $>10^{11}$ CFU/day during the first 48 h being the most effective. In the meta-analysis by Huang et al.,[82] *Lactobacillus* GG reduced the diarrhea of nonbacterial diarrhea by 1.2 days ($p < 0.001$), whereas other probiotics reduced diarrhea by only 0.6 days ($p < 0.001$). In a more recent single-center randomized, double-blind, placebo-controlled study to assess other lactobacilli strains, a mixture of three *L. rhamnosus* strains (Lakcid, Biomed, and Poland) was used at a dose of $1.2 \times 10^{10}$ CFU twice daily for 5 days.[86] These lactobacilli strains shorten the duration of rotaviral diarrhea by 39 h and time of intravenous rehydration, but not in other diarrheal illnesses.[86]

Two recent randomized trials in developing countries with more severe diarrhea reported no significant benefit with *Lactobacillus* GG.[87,88] The lack of efficacy in these studies may be related to several factors: (1) lower rates of rotavirus infection; (2) lower dose used $10^9$ CFU/day; (3) later administration of the probiotic after completing rehydration in one study[88] (evidence indicates early administration is more effective); and co-administration with milk formula containing lactose[88], thus possibly masking any favorable effect of the probiotic.[85]

*S. boulardii* (250 mg/day) was recently assessed in 200 children hospitalized in Turkey with acute diarrhea (41.5% due to rotavirus) versus placebo for 5 days.[89] The duration of diarrhea was significantly shorter in the treated group (4.7 versus 5.5 days, $p < 0.05$); stool frequency less after the second day of treatment ($p < 0.005$); and hospital stay significantly shorter in the *S. boulardii* group (2.9 versus 3.9 days, $p < 0.001$).

Nosocomial diarrhea in children admitted to hospital for other reasons is a significant problem with prevalence rates of 4.5–22.6 episodes per admission.[85] Rotavirus is the most common cause followed by AAD. Several randomized, controlled trials have been performed with mixed results. In one trial of 81 children *Lactobacillus* GG ($6 \times 10^9$ CFU twice a day) reduced the risk of nosocomial diarrhea compared to placebo (6.7% versus 33.3%, $p = 0.002$), as well as the risk for rotavirus illness (2.2% versus 16.7%, $p = 0.02$), the predominant etiologic agent.[90] A larger trial of 220 children failed to show a benefit of *Lactobacillus* GG $10^{10}$ CFU once per day over placebo, but breast feeding was effective.[91] The difference in the dosing (once a day versus twice a day) between the two trials could account for the conflicting results.

In another randomized, controlled trial of 55 infants admitted to a chronic-care hospital, supplementation with *B. bifidum* and *S. thermophilus* reduced the prevalence of nosocomial diarrhea compared to placebo (7% versus 31%).[92] The risk of rotavirus gastroenteritis was significantly lower in the probiotic-treated group (RR = 0.3), and there was a shorter duration of rotavirus shedding. Thus, overall the evidence for prevention of nosocomial diarrhea in children with probiotics is weak and may be dependent on dose and the combination of organisms.

Day-care setting is frequently complicated by outbreaks of infectious diseases in children and in particular respiratory and intestinal infections. Several studies over the years have investigated the benefit of probiotic milk formula as preventative measure. In a large, multicenter, placebo-controlled study over 7 months involving 571 children from 18 day-care centers in Finland, 282 received daily *Lactobacillus* GG with milk and 289 milk alone.[93] Surprisingly, the probiotic-treated group had mainly reduction in respiratory infections with complications by 17%, less antibiotic treatment for respiratory infection by 19%, and fewer absence from day care because of illness by about 1 day. In another multicenter, double-blind, randomized trial 201 children from 14 day-care centers in Israel were fed formula alone (controls, $N = 60$), or supplemented with *B. lactis* ($N = 73$), or with *L. reuteri* ($N = 68$).[94] The controls had significantly more febrile episodes and diarrhea episodes and longer duration than either probiotic. The *L. reuteri* group compared with *B. lactis* group had a significantly decrease in number of days with fever, clinic visits, child care absences, and antibiotic prescription. Unlike the Finnish study there was no effect on respiratory illness. In a somewhat different setting, residential nurseries or foster care centers, in a smaller sample size ($N = 90$ total), milk formula supplemented with *B. lactis* had no significant benefit.[95]

## 9.4.2 Antibiotic-Associated Diarrhea

Mild to severe episodes of AAD are common side effects of antibiotic therapy. The incidence of AAD differs with the antibiotic and varies from 5% to 25%.[96] *C. difficile* is the most important cause of AAD, although it accounts for only 10–25% of such episodes. *C. difficile*-associated diarrhea (CDAD), however, is responsible for the greatest proportion of mortality, morbidity, and prolonged hospital stay associated with AAD. Details of the pathogenesis, management, and prevention of CDAD and AAD were discussed in chapter 8. This section will review mainly the evidence for prevention of AAD and CDAD with probiotics.

Probiotics may offer potential preventative and therapeutic benefit for AAD by restoring the intestinal microflora. A variety of different probiotic organisms have been evaluated for primary prevention of AAD in both adults and children. However, the best-studied probiotics for prevention or treatment of AAD or CDAD are *L. rhamnosus* GG (LGG), *S. boulardii*, and probiotic mixtures.

### 9.4.2.1 Prevention of AAD with Probiotics

There are numerous trials reported on the use of probiotics to prevent AAD in both adults and children, and there are at least four meta-analyses on this topic. D'Souza et al.[98] pooled nine trials and found that probiotics significantly reduced the odds of AAD (OR = 0.37, 95% CI 0.26–0.52), but did not provide data on publication bias or heterogeneity testing. Cremonini et al.[99] analyzed seven trails and also noted that probiotics produced a pooled relative risk of 0.40 (95% CI 0.27–0.57). No significant publication bias or heterogeneity was found ($p = 0.42$). Another meta-analysis analyzed five trials restricted to use of *S. boulardii* only and found a pooled relative risk of 0.43 (95% CI 0.23–0.78).[100] No significant publication bias was found.

The most recent and comprehensive meta-analysis on this topic by McFarland[101] analyzed 25 randomized, controlled trials (RCTs) with a total of 2,810 patients. Of 16 RCTS in adults patients, 7 (44%) showed significant efficacy for probiotics. In children 6 of 9 (67%) RCTs had significant efficacy for probiotics in preventing AAD. The pooled analysis of these trials showed that probiotics significantly reduced the relative risk of AAD (RR = 0.43, 95% CI 0.31–0.58, $p < 0.001$).[101] Subgroup analysis stratified by type of probiotics (Table 9.2) showed that *S. boulardii*, LGG and probiotic mixtures were the most efficacious.[101] This meta-analysis also found a dose-response for probiotics to prevent AAD, and doses of $\geq 10^{10}$ CFU/day providing the greatest efficacy.[101] Only 9(36%) of the RCTs attempted to determine the etiologies of AAD in their trials. Four trials that stratified the *C. difficile* status reported treatment-specific efficacies, and none were significant because of inadequate sample size.

### 9.4.2.2 Probiotics and *C. difficile* Diarrhea

In McFarland's[101] review and meta-analysis six RCTs provided adequate data regarding CDAD with a total of 354 patients. All were done in adults and the three of the studies were done exclusively in patients with recurrent CDAD. Two (33%) of the six trials reported a significant reduction of recurrent CDAD with probiotics. Five of the trials were treating established CDAD and the probiotic was combined with standard therapy (metronidazole or vancomycin).

Pooled data from the six RCT's were used for the meta-analysis. There was a high degree of homogenicity between the studies and absence of publication bias.[101] The combined efficacy showed that the probiotics had a significant protective effect for CDAD, RR = 0.59, $p = 0.005$. Of the three different probiotics tested for the treatment of CDAD, only *S. boulardii* showed significant reductions on recurrences. Neither LGG, *L. plantarum* 299v nor mixture of *L. acidophilus* and

**Table 9.2**

| Clinical application of probiotics in infections | Comments |
|---|---|
| **A. Proven clinical efficacy** | |
| • *S. boulardii* in recurrent CDAD | Avoid in immunosuppression |
| • *Lactobacillus* GG in prevention of AAD in children | Safe |
| **B. Potential clinical efficacy** | Large multicenter trials needed |
| • Lactobaccili/bifidobacteria for neonatal infections (necrotising enterocolitis) | |
| • *Lactobacillus* GR-I plus L. RC-14 for recurrent cystitis in women | |
| • Lactobacilli: ($H_2O_2$ strains) for bacterial vaginosis | |
| • Surgical-related infections (post-pancreatitis, post-hepatectomy or liver transplantation) | |
| • *Helicobacter pylori* infections | |
| **B. No clinical efficacy** | |
| • Recurrent candida vaginitis | |
| • Post-antibiotic vaginal candidiasis | |
| **C. Licensed for use** | |
| • Bacteriophage for meat and poultry products to prevent listeria infections | |

*B. bifidum* showed any protective effect. In another very recent review of probiotics on AAD and CDAD a similar conclusion was reached that *S. boulardii* is effective for prevention of recurrent CDAD in adults, whereas LGG is useful in the treatment and prevention of AAD in children.[102] Not included in these reviews and meta-analysis is a recent RCT (double-blinded, single-center in Turkey) of 151 patients receiving antibiotic therapy, comparing *S. boulardii* twice daily versus placebo,[103] AAD in the control arm was greater (9%) compared to the study group (1.4%), $p < 0.05$; CDAD occurred in 2/7 patients with AAD in the placebo arm and none in the probiotic arm. Previous reviews that found insufficient evidence to support routine clinical use of probiotics to prevent CDAD, likely at the time had insufficient trials to include in their analysis.[104]

## 9.4.3 Urogenital Infections

Probiotics have been evaluated for the prevention of recurrent urogenital infections in healthy females in three main areas: (i) recurrent urinary tract infection (mainly cystitis); (ii) recurrent candida vulvovaginitis, (iii) and recurrent bacterial (nonspecific) vaginosis. For more than 30 years, urologists have recognized that urinary pathogens infect the host generally from ascension from the rectum, via the vagina (in females) to the urethra and bladder.

The microbiology of the female genital tract is very complex. In healthy women the vagina contains $10^9$ CFU/g of secretion, with a variety of aerobic and anaerobic bacteria and yeasts. The phase of the menstrual cycle, presence or absence of menstruation (menopause), sexual activity, childbirth, surgery, and antibiotics all may influence the microbial pattern of the vagina.[105] Quantitatively the most abundant isolate in vaginal cultures of healthy women is *Lactobacillus*, which plays an important role in keeping vaginal ph low (<4.5).

### 9.4.3.1 Probiotics in Urinary Tract Infection

Most females will experience one or more episodes of cystitis in their lifetime, usually when they become sexually active. The incidence of uncomplicated lower urinary tract infection (UTI) in women is estimated to be 0.5 episodes/person/year, with a recurrence rate of between 27% and 48%.[106] Although cystitis is considered a mild affliction it is responsible for significant symptomatology, morbidity, and impairment of quality of life. Moreover, it can lead to ascending infection and more serious pyelonephritis, especially in pregnancy and underlying reflux uropathy. Worldwide several hundred million women suffer from UTI annually, with an estimated cost of over $6 billion a year.[107]

The great importance of prior vaginal colonization with pathogenic coliform bacteria in women suffering from UTI, and the significance of the persistence or reappearance of these bacteria in the causation of recurrent infection have been established several decades ago by Stamey.[108] The protective effect of the normal vaginal flora, particularly lactobacilli is now well-accepted. The healthy female urogenital flora consists of many species of microorganisms, with lactobacilli being dominant in premenopausal women. *L. acidophilus* is not the main commensal but *L. crispatus, L. jejensii* and *L. iners* are the most common species.[109,110] Besides Lactobacilli other vaginal flora, such as *Atopobium* spp., *Megasphaera* spp., and *Leptotrichia* spp,[110] produce lactic acid and other substances which keep the vaginal pH low and prevent the overgrowth of pathogens. Estrogens seem to promote colonization of the vagina with lactobacilli and reduce the vaginal pH, thus controlling the establishment of coliforms and pathogens.[111] This is thought to be the main reason why postmenopausal women are more susceptible to recurrent UTI and urogenital infections than premenopausal women.

In patients with UTI the flora of the vaginal vestibule are colonized mainly by uropathogens, especially *E. coli* and other Enterobacteriaceae. The ability of these uropathogens to cause disease is associated with their adhesion to the urogenital epithelium and ability to produce other virulence factors (adhesins, hemolysin, and siderophores). Stamey and Sexton[112] noted in the early 1970s that the vaginal vestibule of women with recurrent UTI had higher incidence of colonization with Enterobacteriaceae between episodes than women without recurrent UTI.

Subsequently, the same group demonstrated that *E. coli* adheres more readily to introital epithelium in women with recurrent UTI.[113] Conversely it has been demonstrated that compared to control women without any history of UTI, lactobacilli was significantly depleted in the vagina of patients with recurrent UTI.[114] Thus it has been postulated that the lactobacilli provides a bacterial barrier to interfere with the ability of coliform pathogens to colonize the vaginal vestibule and thus reduce the risk of ascension into the bladder.[115] Recent in vitro studies have shown that specific lactobacilli strains can interfere with adherence, growth, and colonization of the human urogenital epithelium by uropathogens. *L. acidophilus* RG-14 biosurfactant "surlactin" inhibited the adhesion of the majority of bacteria from a urine suspension to silicone rubber, and was effective against *E. coli*, *Enterococcus faecalis*, and *Staphylococcus epidermidis*.[33] An anti-adhesive, surface-active protein purified from *L. fermentum* RC-14 could also prevent the adhesion of uropathogens.[116] There is considerable variation among *Lactobacillus* strains and their anti-adherence properties. Based on a combination score on adherence, exclusion, and inhibition of pathogen growth, *L casei* GR-1 had the highest score.[117]

### 9.4.3.2 Animal Studies

Chronic UTI in female rats by injecting bacteria incorporated in agar beads into the bladder have been described; and subsequent bladder inoculation with *L. casei* GR-1 can decolonize the uroepithelium within 48 h of 21 (84%) of 25 animals.[118]

Persistent vaginal colonization with a pyelonephritogenic strain of *E. coli* has been established in four adult monkeys.[119] The effect of repeated vaginal flushes of lactobacilli or vaginal fluid from healthy monkeys was tested for their ability to eradicate the *E. coli*. Lactobacilli was able to reduce vaginal *E. coli* and eliminate the uropathogen in only two of six experiments, whereas normal vaginal fluid (with mixed bacterial flora) eliminated the organism in all eight experiments.[119] Thus, the entire normal vaginal flora was much more effective in inhibiting the colonization of the vagina with *E. coli* than lactobacilli alone.

In mice it has been demonstrated that *L. casei* shirota administered intraurethrally 1 day before and daily after infection with *E. coli* could inhibit the growth of the uropathogen and the inflammatory responses in the urinary tract.[120] In another murine model of ascending infection with *Proteus mirabilis* an in indigenous *L. murimis* strain from the vaginal tract of a female mouse significantly lowered the bacterial counts in the kidney and bladder of prophylactically treated mice.[121]

*L. crispatus* CTV-05 commonly detected in the vagina of many healthy women has been assessed for safety and persistence in female primates. *Lactobacillus* intravaginal capsule was inserted into 10 female Macaca and only 3 animals had evidence of colonization with *L. crispatus* 2 days later.[122] There was no evidence of adverse effect.

### 9.4.3.3 Microbiological Studies in Healthy Women

Studies of probiotics on their ability to colonize the vaginal vestibule has been performed in women with both oral and intravaginal preparations, mainly by using lactobacilli strains. A comprehensive review of the microbiological and clinical studies was recently published.[123] Can oral probiotics result in increased colonization of lactobacilli in the vagina, or alter the vaginal flora? Reports of studies on this question have provided conflicting results.

In one study of 42 postmenopausal healthy women oral *L. rhamnosus* GG ($10^9$ CFU) in a yogurt base for one or two doses per day for 1 month resulted in the vaginal colonization of only four (9.5%) women with the same strain at a very low number of bacteria.[124] Reid et al.[125] had previously shown in asymptomatic women (with 40% having healthy vaginal flora) that oral administration of *L. rhamnosus* GR-1 and *L. fermentum* RC-14 was associated with greater restoration of normal vaginal flora than *Lactobacillus* GG (with doses of $> 8 \times 10^8$ CFU of viable bacteria). In a randomized, double-blind, placebo-controlled trial, of 64 healthy woman, half received oral capsules of *L. rhamnosus* GR-1/*L. fermentum* RC-4 ($>10^9$CFU per strain) once daily for 60 days and half received plcebo.[126] Cultures of vaginal fluid showed a significant increase in lactobacilli ($p = 0.01$), a decrease in yeast ($p = 0.01$) and a reduction of coliforms ($p = 0.01$) at day 28 in the treated group compared to placebo. Fewer coliforms remained in the lactobacilli-treated women at day 90 ($p < 0.01$) and there were no adverse effects with the probiotic. A smaller randomized study in 10 women also showed increased vaginal lactobacilli with oral administration but the increase was very small in three of eight subjects.[127]

As expected, intravaginal instillation of probiotics have resulted in more consistent and higher concentration of lactobacilli in vaginal fluid. Persistence of the lactobacilli in the vagina post-instillation has been found at 3 days (100%),[128] 7 days (80%),[129] 14 days (73% for *L. rhamnosus* GR-1/ *L. fermentum* RC-14 and 21% for *Lactobacillus GG*),[128] and at 3 weeks (20%).[129] *L. crispatus* CTV-05 has also been shown to colonize the vagina of 62% of patients versus 2% of control, 5 days ($p < 0.001$), up to 30 days after intravaginal administration.[130] The intravaginal instillation is also safe.

### 9.4.3.4 Clinical Utility in UTI

Prevention of recurrent UTIs in women has taken several different approaches with varying degrees of success. In cases where reoccurrence of UTI is correlated with sexual intercourse a single dose of antibiotic post-intercourse is usually effective. Intermittent antibiotics (three times a week) as suppressive therapy for 6–12 months also have been shown to be of value, but can result in selection of resistant bacteria and yeast superinfection. More natural ways of preventing these common reoccurrences are therefore desirable, and include consumption of cranberry juice and utilization of probiotics.

Only two double-blind, randomized, controlled trials have been reported on the impact of intravaginal lactobacilli and recurrent UTIs. In the first trial 47 women with three or more episodes of lower urinary tract symptoms in the previous year received vaginal *L. casei* var *rhamnosus* or placebo twice weekly for 6 months.[131] There was no significant difference in recurrent UTI, however, the low incidence of infection (mean 1.4 per year) was too low to show a difference with such small sample size. Moreover, the *Lactobacillus* strain used (*L. acidophilus*) was not well characterized and did not colonize the vagina.

Using different strains of lactobacilli (*L. rhamnosus* GR-1 and *L. fermentum* B-52) as vaginal suppository once weekly ($10^9$CFU), or *Lactobacillus* growth factor weekly for 1 year, Reid et al.[132] randomized 55 premenstrual women with recurrent UTIs. The UTI rate decreased from by 73% (from 6 to 1.6 episodes/year $p < 0.001$) in the first group and 79% (from 6 to 1.3 episodes/year, $p < 0.001$), in second group, using a milk-based prebiotic causing stimulation of the patients indigenous vaginal lactobacilli.[132]

Other studies with controls to assess risk of recurrence of UTI include 41 women treated for acute cystitis and those with recurrence received *L. rhamnosus* GR-1 and *L. fermentum* B 54 vaginal suppositories or skimmed milk twice weekly for 2 weeks and at the end of each of the next 2 months.[133] The recurrence of UTI over 6 months decreased to 21% in the probiotic group compared to 47% in the skimmed milk treated group.[133] In an uncontrolled pilot study of intravaginal *L. crispatus* GAI48332 nine women with frequent recurrent UTIs (3–8 episode in 1 year) were treated every 2 days for 1 year.[134] No side effects were noted and there was a significant reduction of episodes of UTI (from an average $5.0 \pm 1.6$ episodes to $1.3 \pm 1.2$, $p = 0.007$).

Various lactobacilli administered orally have also been studied to reduce recurrent UTIs. A group of 150 women treated for UTI were randomly separated into three groups: the first group received cranberry-lingoberry juice 50 ml per day for 6 months; the second group took *Lactobacillus* GG 100 ml ($4 \times 10^{10}$ CFU) 5 days per week for 1 year; and third control group received no further treatment.[135] During the 6-months period 8 (16%) in the cranberry group, 19 (39%) in the *Lactobacillus* group, and 18 (36%) in the control had at least one episode of UTI. Cranberry juice was more effective than controls ($p = 0.014$) while *Lactobacillus* GG was not.[135]

The failure of oral lactobacilli in this study may be due to the inability of *L. rhamnosus* GG to colonize the vagina,[128] thus not making it the optimal choice, as it fails to prevent uropathogens from colonizing the genital tract. A more rational choice for clinical trial would be a combination of *L. rhamnosus* GR-1 and *L. reuteri* (fermentum) RC-14, hydrogen peroxide producing strains that normalize the vaginal flora.[126]

A major complication of spinal cord injury patients is recurrent UTIs, which is related to prolonged or permanent urethral catheterization. Presently there is no effective way of adequately preventing catheter-related infections. Often recurrent or prophylactic antibiotics lead to multi-resistant bacteria or yeast colonization. A recent pilot trial in spinal cord injury patients demonstrated the ability of a non-pathogenic *E. coli* 83972 to prevent catheter-related UTI.[136] In this study 27 patients were randomized (3:1 ratio) to have their bladder inoculated with *E. coli* 83972 or sterile saline. Thirteen (62%) of 21 patients in the experimental group became colonized with *E. coli* 83972 for ≥1 month, 9 lost the inoculated organism after 3.5 months, and 4 patients remained colonized throughout the 12-month period.[136] The number of UTI episodes during the year was significantly lower in the experimental group (mean 1.6 versus 3.5 episodes, $p = 0.0.36$).

## 9.4.4 Probiotics in Vaginitis

Yeast vaginitis is extremely common in women and occasional recurrences frequently occur spontaneously, but more often after antibiotic therapy. Recurrences of candida vaginitis post-antibiotics are attributed to alteration or suppression of the normal vaginal flora. The mechanism by which normal vaginal flora suppresses yeast infection is not well understood but a number of factors could be involved. These could include competition for nutrients and mannose and hydrophobic binding to receptors,[137,138] and possibly production of a bacteriocins-like peptide that is fungistatic.[139]

Probiotics are commonly used and recommended for vulvovaginitis that develops after antibiotic treatment. In one study of 751 women with vulvovaginitis 40% has used yogurt or *Lactobacillus* orally or vaginally to prevent post-antibiotic yeast vaginitis.[140] However, no previous trials had shown the effectiveness of this treatment. In many women (60%) candida colonize the vagina and co-exist with lactobacilli, and even in the presence of yeast vaginitis lactobacilli are commonly seen on microcopy and recovered in cultures (personal experience). It has been postulated that candida may overcome normal lactobacilli flora by production of catalase which catalyzes the conversion of hydrogen peroxide (produced by lactobacilli and others) to water and oxygen.[141]

To test whether oral or vaginal lactobacilli can prevent yeast vulvovaginitis post-antibiotic therapy, a recent randomized multicenter-controlled trial was performed in Australia.[142] Lactobac (continuing *L. rhamnosus* and *B. longum*) orally or Femilac vaginal pessaries (containing *L. rhamnosus*, *L. delbrueckii*, *L. acidophilus*, and *S. thermophilus*) versus similar placebos were studied. Overall, 55/235 (23%) developed post-antibiotic yeast vulvovaginitis, and there was lack of effect with either forms of intervention.[142]

Bacterial or nonspecific vaginosis is the most common form of vaginitis that affects millions of women annually, and is associated with premature labor, pelvic inflammatory disease, and increased risk of human immunodeficiency virus acquisition. Recent studies using molecular identification techniques found that women without bacterial vaginosis (BV) had 1–6 vaginal bacterial species (mean 3.3 phylotypes) and *Lactobacillus* species were the predominant bacteria (83–100% of clones).[143] Whereas, women with BV had greater bacterial diversity, with 9–17 phylotypes (mean 12.3, $p < 0.001$), and newly recognized species were present in 32–89% of clones per sample. Women with bacterial vaginosis have complex vaginal infections with many newly recognized species, including three bacteria in the *Clostridiales* order that were highly specific for BV.[143]

There is some evidence that probiotic lactobacilli can reduce the risk of BV with either oral or vaginal administration. Hydrogen peroxide generating lactobacilli are present in the vagina of most normal women but are absent in most women with BV. Lactobacilli generation of hydrogen peroxide (particularly in the presence of peroxidase and a halide) is toxic to some of the bacteria that are prominent in BV.[144] In a pilot study of 10 women[145] and in a randomized, placebo-controlled trial of 64 women daily oral intake of *L. fermentum* RC-4, resulted in some patients with asymptomatic BV reverting to a normal lactobacilli-dominated bacterial flora (37% compared to 13% on placebo, $p = 0.02$).[146]

Two randomized, controlled trials had been conducted in the early 1990s using vaginal *Lactobacillus* to control bacterial vaginosis. In the first report 60 women with BV were randomized to receive lyophilized *L. acidophilus* as vaginal suppository or placebo.[147] Soon after completion of treatment 16/28 (57%) in the treated group had normal vaginal wet smear versus 0/29 in the control arm. However, in this short term study only three (10.7%) of the probiotic-treated women remained free of BV after subsequent menstruation.[147] In the second trial 32 nonmenopausal women with BV were randomized to receive *L. acidophilus* vaginal tablets (Gynoflor) or placebo.[148] Four weeks after the start of therapy 88% in the treated group and 22% in the placebo group were free of the BV. Thus, intravaginal administration of hydrogen peroxide generating lactobacilli appears to be more promising than oral preparation. However, larger, multicenter trials are needed in women with recurrent BV over a longer period (6–12 months) to determine the suppressive or preventative effect of one or two vaginal *Lactobacillus* suppositories to reduce recurrence.

## 9.4.5 Miscellaneous Infections

### 9.4.5.1 Candidiasis in Neonates

Preterm neonates, especially those managed in neonatal intensive care units, are susceptible to invasive candidiasis. Colonization by *Candida* species is the most important predictor of the development invasive fungal infection in preterm neonates, and the gut is the major reservoir. In a clinical trial of 80 preterm neonates with very low birth weight, during the first 3 days of life neonates were randomized to receive either oral probiotic (*L. casei* subspecies rhamnosus) added to human milk or human milk alone for 6 weeks.[149] The lactobacilli-treated group had significantly lower incidence (23.1% versus 48.8%) of enteric colonization or intensity of candida colonization than the control group, and no adverse events were reported.[149]

## 9.4.5.2 *Helicobacter pylori* Infection

*Helicobacter pylori* is the pre-eminent cause of peptic ulcer disease, and chronic infection is strongly associated with gastric carcinoma and gastric lymphomas. Evidence suggests that ingestion of lactic acid bacteria exerts a suppressive effect of *H. pylori* in animals and humans. In children with asymptomatic *H. pylori* colonization regular ingestion of viable *L. johnsonii* LAI was found to have a moderate but significant suppression effect compared to heat-killed probiotics or control vehicle in double-blind randomized, controlled study.[150] Viable *L. paracasei* STll, however, had no effect. In a more recent trial, 138 patients who failed standard triple therapy to eradicate *H. pylori* were randomized to receive 1 week of quadruple therapy with or without a 4 week pretreatment with *Lactobacillus* and *Bifidobacterium*-containing yogurt.[151] The yogurt containing regimen had a significantly higher *H. pylori* eradication rate than quadruple therapy only, 85% versus 71.1% by intention-to treat analysis, $p < 0.05$; and 90.8% versus 76.6% pre-protocol analysis, $p < 0.05$.[151]

## 9.4.5.3 Surgical-Related Infections

In recent years probiotics have been investigated on their potential benefits in prevention of surgical wound and intra-abdominal infections. Acute, severe hemorrhagic pancreatitis is one of the conditions predisposing to intra-abdominal sepsis and abscess. In a double-blind, randomized trial of 45 patients with pancreatitis 22 received viable *L. plantarum* 299 with an oat fiber substrate, and 23 controls received a similar preparation with heat-killed organisms twice daily for a week.[152] Infected necrosis and abscess occurred in 1/22 (4.5%) in the treatment group versus 7/23 (30%) in the control group, $p = 0.023$. Thus, this relatively small study needs to be confirmed by a much larger, randomized multicenter trail with use of probiotics for a longer period, at least 2 weeks. Such a trial is underway by the Dutch Acute Pancreatitis Study Group, with the aim of enrolling 200 patients with acute severe pancreatitis.[153] The result of this trial is eagerly awaited and not available at this time of writing. A rodent model of pancreatitis supports the hypotheses that modification of intestinal flora with multispecies probiotics results in reduced bacterial translocation, morbidity, and mortality.[154]

Biliary cancer surgery is associated with a high risk of post-operative infectious complications. In a recent randomized, controlled trial from Japan 101 patients were randomized before hepatectomy into a group receiving post-operative symbiotic with enteral feeding (group A), or preoperative plus post-operative symbiotic (group B).[155] The post-operative infections occurred in 12 of 40 (30%) in group A and 5 of 41 (12%) in group B, $p < 0.05$ (81 completed the trial). There was evidence of enhanced immune responses in patients treated with symbiotic pre- and post-operatively.[155]

Bacterial infections frequently occur as well early after liver transplantation. A prospective randomized, double-blind trial was undertaken in 66 liver transplant recipients in Germany.[156] Half the patients received enteral feeding immediately post-operatively with a composition of four lactic acid bacteria and four fibers, while the control group received the fibers only. The treatment started one day before surgery and continued for 14 days. The prevalence of post-operative bacterial infections was significantly reduced by the probiotics; 48% in the control arm and 3% in the treated group.[156] A previous trial by the same investigators included 172 patients undergoing major abdominal surgery including liver tranplantation.[157] The patients in that study were randomized to receive either (a) a conventional parenteral or enteral feeding, (b) enteral nutrition with fiber and *L. plantarum* 299, or (c) enteral nutrition with fiber and heat-inactivated lactobacilli (placebo). The rate of bacterial infections after liver, gastric, or pancreatic resection were 31% in the conventional group compared to 4% in the *Lactobacillus* group and 13% in the placebo group.[157] In 95 liver transplant recipients' infections developed in 34% and 48% of the placebo and conventional groups, versus only 13% of the symbiotic treated group.[157] This study demonstrated that prebiotics may have some mild benefit but greater effect was seen with the addition of the probiotic (symbiotic).

Infection is a frequent complication of severe third degree burns, and *Pseudomonas aeruginosa* is a common pathogen. Moreover, widespread use of antibiotics in burn units commonly leads to the presence of multi-resistant bacteria. Thus, a more natural way of prevention of wound infections without using topical or systemic antimicrobial would be a significant advance in the management of burn victims. A recent study demonstrated that whole cultures or culture filtrates of *L. plantarum* can inhibit the pathogenic activity of *P. aeruginosa*, both in vitro and in vivo.[158] In vitro *L. plantarum* cultures or filtrates could inhibit *P. aeruginosa* quorum-sensing signal molecules (acyl-homoserine-lactones) and two virulence factors controlled by these signals, elastase and biofilm. Using a burned-mouse model infected with *P. aeruginosa*, treatment with *L. plantarum* at 3–9 days post-infection resulted in inhibition of *P. aeruginosa* colonization, improvement in tissue repair, enhanced phagocytosis of the organism by tissue phagocytes, and a decrease in apoptosis at 10 days.[158]

### 9.4.5.4 Parasitic Infections

*Cryptosporidium parvum* is an occasional cause of self-limited diarrhea in travelers to developing countries. However, it is more important as a cause of severe protracted diarrhea in immunocompromised hosts, particularly in the acquired immunodeficiency syndrome (AIDS). In patients with AIDS there is no established effective therapy, besides immune reconstitution by treating the underlying disease. Supplementation with *L. reuteri* or *L. acidophilus* has been shown to reduce intestinal shedding of *C. parvum* oocysts in immunodeficient C57 BL/6 mice.[159] *L. acidophilus* was more efficacious than *L. reuteri* in reducing fecal shedding of the parasite. The lactobacilli supplementation reduced parasitic load by mechanisms unrelated to suppression of T-helper type 2 cytokines (1L-4, 1L-8), which are related to immunosuppression; or to restoration of T-helper type I cytokines (1L-2 and interferon γ), which are required for recovery from parasitic infections.[159] The effect of the probiotics may be mediated by factors released into the intestinal lumen by the lactobacilli and other possible host cellular mechanisms.

*Giardia lamblia* is the most common cause of parasite-related diarrhea in developed countries and a significant cause of traveler's diarrhea. Although most cases are easily treated with metronidazole, some clinical trials report therapeutic failure suggesting drug resistance. Also, in patients with AIDS recurrent or refractory giardiasis is becoming a problem (personal experience). A recent double-blinded, placebo-controlled trial with *S. boulardii* in 65 adult patients with giardiasis has been reported.[160] Thirty patients received metronidazole with *S. boulardii* (250 mg twice daily) for 10 days and 35 controls received metronidazole and placebo for the same duration. At 2 and 4 weeks post-therapy, six (17.1%) of the control group continued to excrete *G. lamblia* cysts versus none in the treated group.[160] It would be interesting to repeat this study in patients with AIDS and recurrent or refractory giardiasis. The mechanism by which *S. boulardii* enhance the clearance of *G. lamblia* is not clear from this report.

## 9.5 Probiotics as Food Additives

Probiotics which are normal human commensals may have direct clinical effects in human health, population well being by inhibiting pathogens that may contaminate our food supply. In fact the only probiotic to be licensed by the Food and Drug Administration (FDA) for human consumption is designed for this purpose. As of August 2006 a mixture of six bacteriophages as a food addictive is allowed to be sprayed on the surface of fresh meat, meat products, fresh poultry, and poultry products.[161] The rationale is for this probiotic mixture to be used as an antimicrobial agent to control *Listeria monocytogenes* (which has been related to food-borne outbreaks of illnesses, including gastroenteritis, neonatal sepsis, bacteremia in pregnancy, and meningitis) in the production of meat and poultry products.

Bacteriophages are viruses that infect only bacteria and are ubiquitous; moreover humans are routinely exposed to them at high levels through food, water, and the environment without adverse effect. Phages are also part of the normal microbial population of the human gut. The phages being used in this food addictive are lytic double-stranded DNA phages specific for *L. monocytogenes* strains known to be associated with food-borne illnesses (i.e., serotypes 1/2a, 4b, and 1/2b).[161] This may be the start of a new era to use commensal microorganisms to prevent foodborne illnesses (especially infections). Widespread use of this technology may result in marked reduction of certain diseases such as *E. coli* hemorrhagic colitis with the hemolytic uremic syndrome, which is a serious and often fatal disease in young children. Moreover, substitution of probiotics in animal feeds instead of antibiotics, to promote health and greater yield in animal farming, could theoretically lead to reduced antimicrobial resistance in the community.

## 9.6 Adverse Effects of Probiotics

In controlled prospective evaluation of probiotics in clinical trials nearly all reports found probiotics to be safe without adverse events. However, there all several case reports of fungemia associated with use of *S. boulardii* or with *S. cerevisiae* (bakers yeast). A recent review of the topic found a total of 60 cases of *S. cerevisiae* fungemia reported worldwide.[162] Overall 60% of these patients were in the ICU, and 71% were receiving enteral or parenteral nutrition. Use of probiotics was detected in 26 (43.3%) of the patients, and 17 patients (28.3%) died.[162] Thus, *S. boulardii* or *S. cerevisiae* should be carefully reassessed or used cautiously in immunosuppressed or critically ill patients.

Lactobacilli and bifidobacteria are extremely rare causes of infection in humans, as are probiotics based on these organisms. There is no evidence that ingested probiotic lactobacilli or bifidobacteria pose any risk of infection greater than that associated with commensal strains. The existing data suggest that the risk of bacteremia (most common form of infection) is <1 case per million individuals.[163] There have been a few cases of *Lactobacillus* infection where the isolate is indistinguishable from the probiotic strains recently consumed.[163] In a recent review of 89 cases of *Lactobacillus* bacteremia, in 11 patients (12.3%) the strain was identical with the probiotic *L. rhamnosus* GG.[164] In 82% of the cases, the patients had severe or fatal comorbidities. In a previous surveillance in Finland between 1995 and 2000, increased probiotic use of *L. rhamnosus* GG was not associated with increased *Lactobacillus* bacteremia.[165] Since probiotics are fermented in the colon and may have an osmotic effect in the intestines, large doses may cause bloating, abdominal discomfort, and mild diarrhea.[166]

## 9.7 Conclusion and Future Directions

Interest and clinical utilization of probiotics will likely continue to increase over the next decade. Studies have fulfilled biological plausibility and proof of concept for several different strains of probiotics in a variety of diseases. However, clinical trials have only confirmed the value of probiotics for the treatment or prevention of a few diseases. Areas where probiotics have proven clinically benefit or appears promising are summarized in Table 9.2.

Although hydrogen peroxide producing lactobacilli have been recognized in the vaginal vestibule as being essential to maintain normal homeostasis and healthy milieu for over 3 decades, there is no definite clinical proof at present that probiotics can prevent recurrent UTI or BV. These two conditions are relatively common in healthy women and large multicenter trials to establish the value of *Lactobacillus* probiotics should be feasible. A multicenter randomized, controlled trial of non-antibiotic (including probiotics) versus antibiotic prophylaxis for recurrent UTI is currently underway in the Nederlands.[167] The study consists of two interlinked randomized clinical trials. In one trial, 280 premenopausal women will receive either cranberry capsules 500 mg twice daily or trimethoprim/sulfamethoxazole once daily for 12 months. In the other trial, 280 premenopaused women will receive oral lactobacilli (*L. rhamnosus* GR-I and *L. reuteri* RC-14 > $10^9$CFU twice daily) or standard antibiotic for 12 months. Future trials in women with recurrent UTI and BV should study intravaginal preparations of probiotics once or twice weekly, which may be more convenient and likely to provide more consistent and higher concentrations of the lactobacilli in the vagina.

The benefit of *S. boulardii* in recurrent or refractory CDAD appears to be well established. Considering the biological properties of this yeast (ability to inactivate toxins A and B), further trials need to be conducted for severe, hypervirulent *C. difficile* infection to determine any clinical effect in reducing mortality or morbidity (such as need for colectomy).

## References

1. Alvarez-Olmos, M.I., Oberhelman, R.A., (2001), Probiotic agents and infectious diseases: a modern perspective on a traditional therapy. Clin. Infect. Dis. 32:1567–1576.
2. Savage, D.C., (1977), Microbiological ecology of the gastrointestinal tract. Ann. Rev. Microbiol. 31:107–133.
3. Macfarlane, G.T., Macfarlane, S., (1997), Human colonic microbiota: ecology, physiology and metabolic potential of intestinal bacteria. Scand. J. Gastroenterol. 32(Suppl 222):3–9.
4. Metchnikoff, (1907), The Prolongation of Life. London: Heinemann.
5. Cripps, A.W., Gleeson, M., (1999), Ontogeny of mucosal immunity and aging. In: Pearay, L. O. (ed), Mucosal immunology. San Diego, Academic Press, pp. 253–266.
6. Cummings, J.H., (1998), Dietary carbohydrates and the colonic microflora. Curr Opin. Clin. Nutr. Metab. Care 1:409–414.
7. Bird, A.R., Brown, IL, Topping, D.L., (2000), Starches, resistant starches, the gut microflora and human health. Curr Issues Intest. Microbiol. 1:25–37.
8. Kleessen, B., Hartmann, L., Blaut, M., (2001), Oligofructose and long-chain inulin: influence on the gut microbial ecology of rats associated with a human faecalflora. Br. J. Nutr. 86:291–3000.
9. Hopkins, M.J., Macfarlane, G.T., (2003), Nondigestible oligosaccharides enhance bacterial colonization resistance against *Clostridium difficile* in vitro. Appl. Environ. Microbiol. 69:1920–1927.
10. Walker, W.A., (2000), Role of nutrients and bacterial colonization in the development of intestinal defence. J. Pedi Gastroenterol. 30(Suppl 2): S2–S7.
11. Gorbach, S.L., (2000), Probiotics and gastrointestinal health. Am. J. Gastroenterol. 95(Suppl I):S147–S171.
12. Mack, D.R., Michail, S, Wei, S., McDougall, L, Hollingsworth, M.A., (1999), Probiotics inhibit enteropathogenic *E. coli* adherence in vitro by inducing intestinal gene expression. Am. J. Physiol. 276:G941–G950.

13. Mattar, A.F., Teitelbaum, D.H., Drongowski, R.A., Yongyi, F., Hurmon, C.M., Coran, A.G., (2002), Probiotics upregulate muc-2 mucin gene expression in a caco-2 cell culture model. Pediatr. Surg Int. 18:586–590.
14. Pavan, S., Desreumaux, P., Mercenier, A., (2003), Use of mouse models to evaluate the persistence, safety, and immune modulation capacities of lactic acid bacteria. Clin Diagn. Lab. Immun. 10:696–701.
15. Mattar, A.F., Drongowski, R.A., Coran, A.G., Harmon, C.M., (2001), Effect of probiotics on enterocyte bacterial translocation in vitro. Pediatr. Surg. Int. 17:265–268.
16. Madsen, K.L., Doyle, J.S., Jewell, L.D., Tavernini, M.M., Fedorak, R.N., (1999), *Lactobacillus* species prevents colitis in interleukin-10 gene deficient mice. Gastroenterology 116:1107–1114.
17. Madsen, K., Cornish, A., Soper, P., McKaigney, C., Jijon, H., Yachimec, C., Doyle, J., Jewell, L., De Simone, C., (2001), Probiotic bacteria enhance murine and human intestinal epithelial barrier function. Gastroenterology 121:580–591.
18. Jain, P.K., McNaught, C.E., Anderson, A.D., Macfie, J., Mitchell, C.J., (2004), Influence of symbiotic containing *Lactobacillus acidophilus* LA5, *Bifidobacterium lactis* Bb12, *Streptococcus thermophilus, Lactobacillus bulgarious* and oligofructose on gut barrier function and sepsis in critically ill patients: a randomized controlled trial. Clin. Nutr. 23:441–445.
19. Bartosch, S., Woodmansey, E.J., Paterson, J.C., McMurdo, M.E., Macfarlane, G.T., (2005), Microbiological effects of consuming a symbiotic containing *Bifidobacterium bifidum, Bifidobacterium lactis*, and oligofructose in elderly persons, determined by real-time polymerase chain reaction and counting of viable bacteria. Clin. Infect. Dis.40:28–37.
20. Madden, J.A., Plummer, S.F., Tang, J., Garaiova, I., Plummer, N.T., Herbison, M., Hunter, J. O., (2005), Effect of probiotics on preventing disruption of the intestinal microflora following antibiotic therapy: a double-blind, placebo-controlled pilot study. Internat. Immunopharmacol. 5:1091–1097.
21. Sullivan, A., Bennet, R., Viitanen, M., Palmgren, A.C., Nord, C.E., (2002), Influence of *Laclobacillus* F19 on intestinal microflora in children and elderly persons and impact on *Helicobacter pylori* infections. Microb. Ecol. Health Dis. 14(Suppl 3):17–21.
22. Mcfarlane, G., Cummings, J.H., (1999), Probiotics and prebiotics: can regulating the activities of intestinal bacteria benefit health? BMJ 318:999–1003.
23. Hozapfel, W.H., Haberer, P., Snel, J., Schillinger, U., Huis in't Veld, J.H.J., (1998), Overview of gut flora and probiotics. Int. J. Food Microbiol. 41:85–101.
24. Krogfelt, K.A., (1991), Bacterial adhesion: genetics, biogenesis and role in pathogenesis of fimbrial adhesions of *Escherichia* coli. Rev. Infect. Dis. 13:721–735.
25. Galan, J.E., Pace, J., Hayman, M.J., (1992), *Salmonella typhimurium* enter epithelial cells via the epidermal growth factor receptor. Nature 94:588–5891.
26. Insoft, R.M., Sanderson, I.R., Walker, W.A., (1996), Development of immune function in the intestine and its role in neonatal disease. Pediatr. Clin. North Am. 43:551–571.
27. Dai, D., Walker, W.A., (1999), Protective nutrients and bacterial colonization in the immature human gut. Adv. Pediatr. 46:353–382.
28. Qun-ying, Pan; L.-J., Ren, Y.-X., (2004), Competitive inhibition of adherence of enterotoxigenic *Escherichia coli*, enteropathogenic *Escherichia coli* and *Clostridium difficile* to intestinal epithelial cell line Lovo by purified adhesin of *Bifidocterium adolescentis* 1027. World J. Gastroenterol. 10:1630–1633.
29. Michail, S., Wei, S., Mack, D.R., (1997), *Escherichia coli* strain E2348169 in vitro adhesion is reduced in the presence of Lactobacillus species. Gastroenterology 112 (Suppl): A1042 (abstract).
30. Rigothier, M.C., Maccunio, J., Gayrol, P., (1994), Inhibitory activity of *Saccharomyces* yeasts on the adhesion of *Entamoeba histolytica* trophozoites to human erythrocytes in vitro. Parasit. Res. 80:10–15.

# References

31. Mangell, P., Lennernas, P., Wang, Mei, Olsson, C., Ahrne, S., Molin, G., Thorlacius, H., Jeppsson, B., (2006), Adhesive capability of *Lactobacillus plantarum* 299V is important for preventing bacterial translocation in endotoxemic rats. APMIS 114:611–618.
32. Zorate, G., Nader-Macias, M.E., (2006), Influence of probiotic vaginal lactobacilli on in vitro adhesion of urogenital pathogens to vaginal epithelial cells. Lett. Appl. Microbiol. 43:174–180.
33. Veltraeds, M.C., vander Belt, B., vander Mei, H.C., Reid, G., Buscher, H.J., (1998), Interference in initial adhesion of uropathogenic bacteria and yeasts silicone rubber by a *Lactobacillus acidophilus* biosurfactant. J. Med. Microbiol. 49:790–794.
34. Reid, G., Bruce, A.W., (2006), Probiotics to prevent urinary tract infections: the rationale and evidence. World J. Urol. 24:28–32.
35. Silva, M., Jacobus, N.V., Deneke, L., Gorbach, S.L., (1987), Antimicrobial substance from a human lactobacillus strain. Antimicrob. Agents Chemother. 31:1231–1233.
36. Cadieux, P., Burton, J., Gardiner, G., Braunstein, I., Bruce, A.W., Kang, C.Y., Reid, G., (2002), *Lactobacillus* strains and vaginal ecology. JAMA 287:1940–1941.
37. Castagliuolo, I., LaMont, J.T., Nikulasson, S.T., Pothoulakis, C., (1996), *Saccharomyces boulardii* protease inhibits *Clostridium difficile* toxin A effect in rat ileum. Infect. Immun. 6A:5225–5232.
38. Castagliuolo, I., Riegler, M.F., Valenick, L., Lamont, J.T., Pothoulakis, C., (1999), *Saccharomyces boulardii* protease inhibits the effects of *Clostridium difficile* toxins A and B in human colonic mucosa. Infect. Immun. 67:302–307.
39. Plummer, S. Weaver, M.A., Harris, J.C., Dee, P., Hunter, J., (2004), *Clostridium difficile* pilot study: effect of probiotic supplementation on the incidence of *C. difficile* diarrhea. Int. Microbiol. 7:59–62.
40. Asahara, T., Shimizu, K., Nomoto, K., Hamabata, T., Ozawa, A., Takeda, Y., (2004), Probiotic bifidobacteria protect mice from lethal infection with Shiga toxin-producing *Escherichia coli* 0157:H7. Infect. Immun. 72:2240–2247.
41. Ruiz-Perez, F., Sheikh, J., Davis, S., Boedeker, E.C., Nataro, J.P., (2004), Use of a continuous-flow anaerobic culture to characterize enteric virulence gene expression. Infect. Immun. 72:3793–3802.
42. Backhed, F., Ley, R.E., Sonnenburg, J.L., Peterson, D.A., Gordon, J.L., (2005), Host-bacterial mutualism in the human intestine. Science 307:1915–1920.
43. Rakoff-Nahoum, S., Paglino, J., Eslami-Varzaneh, E., Edberg, S., Madzhitov, R., (2004), Recognition of commensal microflora by toll-like receptors is required for intestinal homeostasis. Cell 118:229–241.
44. Mazmanian, S.K., Liu, C.-H., Tzianabos, A.O., Kasper, D.L., (2005), An immunomodulatory molecule of symbiotic bacteria directs maturation of the host immune system. Cell 122: 107–118.
45. Majamas, H., Isolauri, E., (1997), Probiotics: A novel approach in the management of food allergy. J. Allergy Clin. Immunol. 99:178–183.
46. Isolauri, E., Majamaa, H., Arvola, T., Rantala, I., Virtanen, E., Arvilommi, H., (1993), *Lactobacillus casei* strain reverses increased intestinal permeability induced by cow's milk in sucking rats. Gastroenterology 105:1643–1650.
47. Sutas, Y., Hurme, M., Isolauri, E., (1996), Down-regulation of anti-CD3 antibody-induced IL-4 production by bovine caseins hydrolyzed with Lactobacillus GG derived enzymes. Scand. J. Immunol. 43:687–689.
48. Bengmark, S., (1998), Ecological control of the gastrointestinal tract: The role of probiotic flora. Gut 42:2–7.
49. Ulisse, S., Gionchetti, P., D'Alo, S., Russo, F.P., Pesce, I., Ricci, G., Rizzello, F., Helwig, U., Cifone, M.G., Campieri, M., DeSimone, C., (2001), Expression of cytokines, inducible nitric oxide synthase, and matrix metalloproteinases in pouchitis: effects of probiotic treatment. Am. J. Gastroenterol. 96:2691–2699.

50. Pathmakanthan, S., Li, C.K., Cowie, J., Hawkey, C.J., (2004), *Lactobacillus plantarum* 299: beneficial in vitro immuno-modulation in cells extracted from inflamed human colon. J. Gastroenterol. Hepatol. 19:166–173.
51. Borruel, N., Carol, M., Casellas, F., Antolin, M., de Lara, F., Espin, E., Naval, J., Guamer, F., Malagelada, J.R., (2002), Increased mucosal tumour necrosis factor production in Crohn's disease can be downregulated ex vivo by probiotic bacteria. GU7 51–659–664.
52. Steidler, L., Hans, W., Schotte, L., Neirynck, S., Obermeier, F., Falk, W., Fiers, W., Remaut, E., (2000), Treatment of murine colitis by *Lactococcus lactis* secreting interleukin-10. Science 289:1352–1355.
53. McCarthy, J., O'Mahony, L., O'Callaghan, L., Sheil, B., Vanghan, E.E., Fitzsimons, N., Fitzgibbon, J., O'Sullivan, G.C., Kiely, B., Collins, J.R, Shanaham, F., (2003), Double blind, placebo controlled trial of two probiotic stains in interleukin-10 knockout mice and mechanistic link with cytokine balance. Gut 52:975–980.
54. Jijon, H.B., Backer, J., Diaz, H., Yeung, H., Thiel, D., McKaigney, C., De Simone, C., Madsen, K., (2004), DNA from probiotic bacteria modulates murine and human epithelial cell immune function. Gastroenterology 126:1358–1373.
55. Yan, F., Polk, D.B., (2002), Probiotic bacteria prevents cytokine-induced apoptosis in intestinal epithelial cells. J. Biol. Chem. 277:50959–50965.
56. Rachmilenitz, D., Katakara, K., Karmeli, F., Hayashi, T., Reinus, L., Akira, S., Lee, J., Takabayshi, K., Takeda, K., Raz, E., (2004), Toll-like receptor 9 signaling mediates the anti-inflammatory effects of probiotics in murine experimental colitis. Gastroenterology 126:520–528.
57. Reid, G., Kim, S.O., Kőhler, G.A., (2006), Selecting, testing and understanding probiotic microorganisms. FEMS Immunol. Med. Microbiol. 46:149–157.
58. Gan, B.S., Kim, J., Reid, G., Cadieux, P., Howard, J.C., (2002), *Lactobacillus fermentum* RC-14 inhibits *Staphylococcus aureus* infection of surgical implants in rats. J. Infect. DIS. 185:1369–1372.
59. Kaila, M., Isolauri, E., Soppi, E., Virtanen, E., Laine, S., Arvilommi, H., (1992), Enhancement of the circulating antibody secreting cell response in human diarrhea by a human lactobacillus strain. Pediatri Res. 32:141–144.
60. Kaila, M., Isolauri, E., Maija, S., Arvilommi, H., Vesikari, T., (1995), Viable versus inactivated lactobacillus strain GG in acute rotavirus diarrhea. Arch. Dis. Child. 72:51–53.
61. Link-Amster, H., Rochat, F., Saudan, K.Y., Mignot, O., Aeschlimann, J.M., (1994), Modulation of a specific humoral immune response and changes in intestinal flora mediated through fermented milk intake. FEMS Immunol. Med Microbiol. 10:55–64.
62. Villena, J., Racedo, S., Aguero, G., Alvarez, S., (2006), Yoghurt accelerates the recovery of defence mechanisms against *Streptococcus pneumoniae* in protein-malnourished mice. Brit. J. Nutr. 95:591–602.
63. Perdigon, G., de Macias, M.E., Alvarez, S., Oliver, G., de Ruiz Holgado, A.A., (1986), Effect of periorally administered lactobacilli on macrophage activation in mice. Infect. Immun. 53:404–410.
64. Hessle, C., Hanson, L.A., Wold, A.E., (1999), Lactobacilli from human gastrointestinal mucosa are strong stimulators of IL-I2 production. Clin. Exp. Immunol. 116:276–282.
65. Murosaki, S., Yamamoto, Y., Ito, K., Inokuchi, T., Kusaka, H., Ikeda, H., Yoshikai, Y., (1998), *Lactobacillus planatarum* L-137 suppress naturally fed antigen-specific IgE production by stimulation of 1L-12 production in mice. J. Allergy Clin. Immunol. 102–57–64.
66. Miettinen, M., Matikainen, S., Vuopio-Varkila, J., Pirhonen, J., Varkila, K., Kurimoto, M., Julkunen, I., (1998), Lactobacilli and streptococci induce interleukin-12 (IL-12), IL-18, and gamma interferon production in human peripheral blood mononuclear cells. Infect. Immun. 66:6058–6062.
67. Caetano, J.A., Parames, M.T., Babo, M.Y., Santos, A., Ferreira, A.B., Freitas, A.A., Coelho, M.R., Mateus, A.M., (1986), Immunopharmacological effects of *Saccharomyces boulardii* in healthy volunteers. Int. J. Immunopharmacol. 8:245–259.

68. Bu, H.F., Wang, X., Zhu, Y.Q., Williams, R.Y., Hsueth, W., Zheng, X., Rozenfeld, R.A., Zuo, X.L., Tan, X.D., (2006), Lysozyme-modified probiotic components protects rats against polymicrobial sepsis: role of macrophages and cathelicidin-related innate immunity. J. Immun. 177:8767–8776.
69. Gill, H.S., Rutherfurd, K.J., Cross, M.C., (2001), Dietary probiotic supplementation enhances natural killer cell activity in the elderly: an investigation of age-related immunological changes. J. Clin. Immunol. 21:264–271.
70. Kim, H.S., Park, H., Cho, I.Y., Paik, H.D., Park, E., (2006), Dietary supplementation of probiotic *Bacillus polyfermentus*, Bispain strain, modutales natural killer cell and T cell subject population and immunoglobulin G levels in human subjects. J. Medicinal Food 9:321–327.
71. Chiva, M., Soriano, G., Rochat, I., Peralta, L., Rochat, F., Llovet, T., Mirelis, B., (2002), Effect of *Lactobacillus johnsonii* and antioxidants on intestinal flora and bacterial translocation in rats with experimental cirrhosis. J. Hepatol. 37:456–462.
72. Seehofer, D., Rayes, N., Schiller, R., Stockmann, M., Muller, A.R., Schirmeir, A., (2004), Probiotic partly reverse increased bacterial translocation after simultaneous liver resection and colonic anastomosis in rats. J. Surg. Res. 117:262–271.
73. Reid, G., Jass, J., Sebulsky, M.T., McCormick, J.K., (2003), Potential uses of probiotics in clinical practice. Clin. Microbiol. Rev. 16:658–672.
74. Food and Agriculture Organization of the United Nations and World Health Organization, (2001), Regulatory and clinical aspects of dairy probiotics. Food and Agriculture Organization of the United Nations and World Health Organization of the United Nations and World Health Organization Working Group Report (Online).
75. Guerrant, R.L., Lima, A.A.M., (2000), Inflammatory enteritides, in: Principles and Practice of Infectious Diseases, 5th edition, Mandell, G.L., Bennett, J.E., Dolin, R., (eds.), Churchhill Livingstone, Philadelphia, pp. 1126–1136.
76. Blakey, J.L., Lubitz, L., Campbell, N.T., Gillan, G.L., Bishop, R.F., Barnes, G.L., (1985), Enteric colonization in sporadic neonatal necrotizing enterocolitis. J. Pediatr. Gastroenterol. Nutr. 4:591–595.
77. Hoyos, A.B., (1999), Reduced incidence of necrotizing enterocolitis associated with enteral administration of *Lactobacillus acidophilus* and *Bifidobacterium infantis* to neonates in an intensive care unit. Int. J. Infect. Dis. 3:197–202.
78. Dani, C., Biadaioli, R., Bertini, G., Martelli, E., Rubaltelli, F.F., (2002), Probiotic feeding in prevention of urinary tract infection, bacterial sepsis and necrotizing enterocolitis in preterm infants. A prospective double-blind study. Biol. Neonate; 82:103–108.
79. Bin-Nun, A., Bromiker, R., Wilschanski, M., Kaplan, M., Rudensky, B., Caplan, M., Hammerman, C., (2005), Oral probiotics prevent necrotizing entercolitis in very low birth weight neonates. J. Pediatr. 147:143–146.
80. Lin, H.C., Su, B.H., Chen, A.C., Lin, T.W., Tsai, C.H., Yeh, T.F., Oh, W., (2005), Oral probiotics reduce the incidence and severity of necrotizing enterocolitis in very low birth weight infants. Pediatrics 115:1–5.
81. Allen, S.J., Okoko, B., Martinez, E., Gregorio, G., Dans, L.F., (2007), Probiotics for treating infectious diarrhea. Cochrane Systematic Rev. Access. No. 00075320–100,000,000–02019.
82. Huang, J.S., Bousvaros, A., Lee, J.W., Diaz, A., Davidson, E.J., (2002), Efficacy of probiotic use in acute diarrhea in children: a meta-analysis. Dig. Dis. Sci. 47:2625–2634.
83. Szawska, H., Mrukowicz, J.Z., (2001), Probiotics in the treatment and prevention of acute infectious diarrhea in infants and children: a systematic review of published randomized double-blind, placebo-controlled trials. J. Pediatr. Gastroenterol. Nutr. 33(Suppl):s17–s25.
84. Van Niel, C.W., Feudtner, C., Garrison, M.M., Christakis, D.A., (2002), Lactobacillus therapy for acute infectious diarrhea in children: a meta-analysis. Pediatrics. 109:678–684.
85. Guandalini, S., (2006), Probiotics for children: use in diarrhea. J. Clin. Gastroenterol. 40:244–248.

86. Szymanski, H., Pejcs, J., Jarvien, M., Chmierlarczyk, A., Strus, M., Heczko, P.B., (2006), Treatment of acute infectious diarrhea in infants and children with a mixture of three *Lactobacillus rhamnosus* strains – a randomized double-blind, placebo-controlled trial. Alimentary Pharmacol. Ther. 23:247–253.
87. Costa-Ribeiro, H., Ribeiro, T.C., Maltos, A.P., Valois, S.S., Neri, D.A., Almeida, P., Cerqueira, C.M., Ramos, E., Young, R.J., Vanderhoof, J.A., (2003), Limitations of probiotic therapy in acute, severe dehydrating diarrhea. J. Pediatr. Gastroenterol. Nutr. 36:112–115.
88. Salazar-Lindo, E., Miranda-Langschwager, P., Campos-Sanchez, M., Chea-Woo, E., Sack, R.B., (2004), *Lactobacillus casei* strain GG in the treatment of infants with acute watery diarrhea: a randomized, double-blind, placebo controlled clinical trial. BMC Pediatr. 4:18.
89. Kurugol, Z., Koturoglu, G., (2005), Effects of *Saccharomyces boulardii* in children with acute diarrhea. Acta Paediatr. 94:44–47.
90. Szajewska, H., Kotowska, M., Mrukowicz, J.Z., Armaska, Mikolajczyk, W., (2001), Efficacy of *Lactobacillus* GG in prevention of nosocomial diarrhea in infants. J. Pediatr. 138:361–365.
91. Mastretta, E., Longo, P., Laccisaglia, A., Balbo, L., Russe, R., Mazzaaccara, A., Gianino, P., (2002), Effect of *Lactobacillus* GG and breast-feeding in the prevention of rotavirus nosocomial infection. J. Pediatr. Gastroenterol. Nutr. 35:527–531.
92. Saavedra, J., Bauman, N.A., Oung, I., (1994), Feeding of *Bifidobacterium bifidum* and *Streptococcus thermophilus* in hospital for prevention of diarrhea and shedding of rotavirus. Lancet 344:1046–1049.
93. Hatakka, K., Savilahti, E., Ponka, A., Meurman, J.H., Poussa, T., Nase, L., Soxelin, M., Korpela, R., (2001), Effect of long term consumption of probiotic milk on infections in children attending day care centres: double blind, randomized trial. BMJ (Clin. Res. ed) 322:1327.
94. Weizman, Z., Asli, G., Alsheikh, A., (2005), Effect of a probiotic infant formula on infections in child care centers: comparison of two probiotic agents. Pediatrics 115:5–9.
95. Chouraqui, J.P., Van Egroo, L.D., Fichot, M.C., (2004), Acidified milk formula supplemented with *Bifidobacterium lactis*: impact on infant diarrhea in residential care settings. J. Pediatr. Gastroenterol. Nutr. 38:288–292.
96. Bergogne-Berezin, E., (2000), Treatment and prevention of antibiotic associated diarrhea. Int. J. Antimicrob. Agents 16:521–526.
97. Elmer, G.W., McFarland, L.V., (2001), Biotherapeutic agents in the treatment of infectious diarrhea. Gastroenterol Clin. North Am. 30:837–853.
98. D' Souza, A., Chakravarthi, R., Cooke, J., Bulpitt, C.J., (2002), Probiotics in prevention of antibiotic associated diarrhea: meta-analysis. BMJ 321:1–6.
99. Cremonini, F., DiCarso S., Nista, E.C., Bartolozzi, F., Capello, G., Gasbarrini, G., Gasbarrini, A., (2002), The effect of probiotic administration on antibiotic-associated diarrhea. Aliment. Pharmacol. Ther. 16:1461–1467.
100. Szajewska, H., Mrukowicz, J., (2005), Meta-analysis: non-pathogenic yeast *Saccharomyces boulardii* in the prevention of antibiotic-associated diarrhea. Aliment. Pharmacol. Ther. 22:365–372.
101. McFarland, L.V., (2006), Meta-analysis of probiotics for the prevention of antibiotic-associated diarrhea and the treatment of *Clostridium difficile* disease. Am. J. Gastroenterol. 101:812–822.
102. Katz, J.A., (2006), Probiotics for the prevention of antibiotic-associated diarrhea and *Clostridium difficile* diarrhea. J. Clin. Gastroenterol. 40:249–255.
103. Can, M., Besirbellioglu, B.A., Avci, I.Y., Beker, C.M., Pahsa, A., (2006), Prophylactic *Saccharomyces boulardii* in the prevention of antibiotic-associated diarrhea: a prospective study. Med. Sci Monitor. 12: pI 19–22.
104. Dendukuri, N., Costa, V., Mc Gregor, M., Brophy, JM., (2005), Probiotic therapy for the prevention and treatment of *Clostridium difficile*-associated diarrhea: a systematic review. CMAJ 173:167–170.

105. Sweet, R.L., Gibbs, R.S., (eds), (1990), Clinical microbiology of the female genital tract. 2nd edition, Williams & Wilkins, , Baltimore, MD, pp. 2–10.
106. Hooton, T.M., Scholes, D., Hughes, J.P., Winter, C., Roberts, P.L., Stapleton, A.E., Stergachis, A., Stamm, W.E., (1996). A prospective study of risk factors for symptomatic urinary tract infection in young women. N. Engl. J. Med. 335:468–474.
107. Foxman, B., Barlow, R., D'Arcy, H., Gillespice, B., Sobel, J.D., (2000), Urinary tract infection: self-reported incidence and associated costs. Ann. Epidemiol. 10:509–515.
108. Stamey, T.A., (1973), The role of Enterobacteriaceae in recurrent urinary infections. J.Urol. 109:467.
109. Antonio, M., Hawes, S., Hillier, S., (1999), The identification of vaginal Lactobacillus species and the demographic and microbiologic characteristics of women colonized by these species. J. Infect. Dis. 180:1950–1956.
110. Zhou, X., Bent, S.J., (2004), Characterization of vaginal microbial communities in adult healthy women using cultivation-independent methods. Microbiology 150:2565–2573.
111. Stamm, W., Raz, R., (1999), Factors contributing to susceptibility of postmenopausal women to recurrent urinary tract infections. Clin. Infect. Dis. 28:723–725.
112. Stamey, T.A., Sexton, C.C., (1975), The role of vaginal colonization with Enterobacteriaceae in recurrent urinary infections. J. Urol. 113:214–217.
113. Fowler, J.E., Stamey, T.A., (1997), Studies of introital colonization in women with recurrent urinary-infection. VII. The role of bacterial adherence. J. Urol. 117: 472–473.
114. Bruce, A.W., Chadwick, P., Hassan, A., VanCott, G.F., (1973), Recurrent urethritis in women. CMAJ 108:973–976.
115. Bruce, A.W., Reid, G., (2003), Probiotics and the urologists. Can. J. Urol. 10:1785–1789.
116. Heineman, C., van HylckamaVlieg, J.E., (2000), Purification and characterization of a surface-binding protein from *Lactobacillus fermentum* RC-14 that inhibit adhesion of *Enterococcus faecalis* 1131. FEMS Microbiol Lett. 190:177–180.
117. Reid, G., Cook, R.L., A.W., (1987), Examination of strains of lactobacilli for properties that may influence bacterial interference in the urinary tract. J. Urol. 138:330–335.
118. Reid, G., Chan, R.C., Bruce, A.W., Costerton, J.W., (1985), Prevention of urinary tract infection in rats with indigenous *Lactobacillus casei* strain. Infect. Immun. 49:320–324.
119. Herthelius, M., Gorbach, S.L., (1989), Elimination of vaginal colonization with *Escherichia coli* by administration of indigenous flora. Infect. Immun. 49:320–324.
120. Asahara, T., Nomoto, K., Watanuki, M., Yokokura, T., (2001), Antimicrobial activity of intraurethrally administered probiotic *Lactobacillus casei* in marine model of *Escherichia coli* urinary tract infection. Antimicrob. Agents. Chemother. 45:1751–1760.
121. Fraga, M., Scavore, P., Zunino, P., (2005), Preventative and therapeutic administration of an indigenous *Lactobacillus* sp: strain against *Proteus mirabilis* ascending urinary tract infection in a mouse model. Antonie van Leeuwenhoek 88:25–34.
122. Patton, D.L., Cosgrove Sweeney, Y.T., Antonio, M.A., Rabe, L.K., Hillier, S.L., (2003), *Lactobacillus crispatus* capsules: single-use safety study in the Macaca nemestrina model. Sex Transm. Dis. 30:568–570.
123. Falagas, M.E., Betsi, G.I., Tokas, T., Athanasiou, S., (2006), Probiotics for prevention of recurrent urinary tract infections in women.A review of the evidence from microbiological and clinical studies. Drugs 66:1253–1261.
124. Colodner, R., Edelstein, H., Chazan, B., Raz, B., (2003), Vaginal colonization by orally administered *Lactobacillus rhamnosus* GG. Israel Med. Assoc. J. 5:767–769.
125. Reid, G., Beuerman, D., Heinemann, C., Bruce, A.W., (2001), Probiotic lactobacillus dose required to restore and maintain a normal vaginal flora. FEMS. Immunol. Med. Microbiol. 32:37–41.
126. Reid, G., Charbonneau, D., Erb, J., Kochanowski, B., Beuerman, D., Poehner, R., Bruce, A. W., (2003), Oral use of *Lactobacillus rhamnosus* GR-1 and *L. fermentum* RC-14 significantly alters vaginal flora: randomized, placebo-controlled trial in 64 health women. FEMS Immunol. Med. Microbiol. 35:131–134.

127. Morelli, L., Zonenenschain, D., DelPiano, M., Cognein, P., (2004), Ulitization of the intestinal tract as a delivery system for urogenital probiotics. J. Clin. Gastroenterol. 38 (Suppl):S107–S110.
128. Cardieux, P., Burton, J., Gardiner, G., Braunstein, I., Bruce, A.W., Kang, C.Y., Reid, G., (2002), *Lactobacillus* strains and vaginal ecology. JAMA 287:1940–1941.
129. Burton, J., Cardieux, P., Reid, G., (2003), Improved understanding of the bacterial vaginal microbiota of women before and after probiotic instillation. Appl. Environ. Microbiol. 69:97–101.
130. Hoesl, C.E., Altwein, J.E., (2005), The probiotic approach: an alternative treatment option in urology. Eur. Urol. 47:288–296.
131. Baerheum, A., Larsen, E., Digranes, A., (1994), Vaginal application of lactobacilli in the prophylaxis of recurrent urinary tract infection in women. Scand. J. Prim Health Care 12:239–243.
132. Reid, G., Bruce, A.W., Taylor, M., (1995), Instillation of lactobacilli and stimulation of indigenous organisms to prevent recurrence of urinary tract infections. Microecol. Ther. 23:32–45.
133. Reid, G., Bruce, A.W., Taylor, M., (1992), Influence of 3-day antimicrobial therapy and lactobacillus suppositories on recurrence of urinary tract infection. Clin. Ther. 14:11–16.
134. Wehara, S., Mondon, K., Nomoto, K., Seno, Y., Kariyama, R., Kumon, H., (2006), A pilot study evaluating the safety and of *Lactobacillus* vaginal suppositories in patients with recurrent urinary tract infection. Int. J. Antimicrob. Agents 28(Suppl):S30–S34.
135. Kontiokari, T., Sundqvist, K., Nuutinen, M., Pokka, T., Koskela, M., Uhari, M., (2001), Randomized trial of cranberry-lingoberry juice and *Lactobacillus* GG drink for the prevention of urinary tract infections in women. BMJ 322:1–5.
136. Darouiche, R.O., Thornby, J.I., Cerra-Stewart, C., Donovan, W.H., Hull, R.A., (2005), Bacterial interference for prevention of urinary tract infection: a prospective, randomized, placebo-controlled, double-blind pilot trial. Clin. Infect. Dis. 41:1531–1534.
137. Braun, P.C., (1999), Nutrient uptake by *Candida albicans*: the influence of cell surface mannoproteins. Can. J. Microbiol. 45:353–359.
138. Masuoka, J.C., Hazen, K., (1999), Differences in the acid-labile component of *Candida albicans* mannan from hydrophobic and hydrophilic yeast. Glycobiology 9:1281–1286.
139. Okkers, D.J., Dicks, L.M., Silvester, M., Joubert, J.J., Odendall, H.J., (1999), Characterization of pentocin TV35b, a bacteriocin-like peptide from *Lactobacillus pentosus* with a fungistatic effect on *Candida albicans*. J. Appl. Microbiol. 87:726–734.
140. Pirotta, M., Gunn, J., Chondros, P., (2003), "Not thrush again". Women's experience of post-antibiotic vulvovagintis. Med. J. Aust. 179:43–46.
141. Nakagawa, Y., Koide, K., Watanabe, K., Morita, Y., Mizuguchi, I., Akashi, T., (1999), The expression of the pathogenic yeast *Candida albicans* catalase gene in response to hydrogen peroxide. Microbiol. Immunol. 43:645–651.
142. Pirotta, M., Gunn, J., Chondros, P., Grover, S., O'Malley, P., Hurley, S., Garland, S., (2004), Effect of lactobacillus in preventing post-antibiotic vulvovaginal candidiasis: a randomized controlled trial. BMJ, doi:10.1136/bmj.38210.494977.DE.
143. Fredricks, D.N., Fiedler, B.S., Marrazzo, J.M., (2005), Molecular identification of bacteria associated with bacterial vaginosis. N. Engl. J. Med. 353:1899–1911.
144. Klebanoff, S.J., Hillier, S.L., Escheinbach, D.A., Waltersdorph, A.M., (1991), Control of the microbial flora of the vagina by $H_2O_2$-generation lactobacilli. J. Infect. Dis. 164:94–100.
145. Reid, G., Bruce, A.W., Fraser, N., Heinemann, C., Owen, J., Henning, B., (2001), Oral probiotics can resolve urogenital infections. FEMS Microbiol. Immunol. 30:49–52.
146. Reid, G., Charbonneau, D., Erb, J., Kochanowski, B., Beuerman, D., Poehner, R., Bruce, A. W., (2003), Oral use of *Lactobacillus rhamnosus* GR-1 and *L. fermentum* RC-14 significantly alters vaginal flora: randomized, placebo-controlled trial in 64 healthy women. Fems Immunol. Med. Microbiol. 35:131–134.

147. Hallen, A., Jarstrand, C., Pahlson, C., (1992), Treatment of bacterial vaginosis with lactobacilli. Sex. Transm. Dis.19:146–148.
148. Parent, D., Bossens, M., Bayot, D., Kirkpatrick, C., Graf, F., Wilkinson, F.E., Kaiser, R.R., (1996), Therapy of bacterial vaginosis using exogenously-applied *Lactobacilli acidophili* and low dose of estriol: placebo-controlled multicentric clinical trial. Arzneimittelforschung 46:68–73.
149. Manzoni, P., Mostert, M., Leonessa, M.L., Priolo, C., Farina, D., Monetti, C., Latino, M.A., Gomirato, G., (2006), Oral supplementation with *Lactobacillus casei* subspecies *rhamnosus* prevents enteric colonization by *Candida* species in preterm neonates: a randomized study. Clin. Infect. Dis. 42:1735–1742.
150. Cruchet, S., Obregon, M.C., Salazar, G., Diaz, E., Gotteland, M., (2003), The effect of the ingestion of a dietary product containing *Lactobacillus johnsonii* LA1 on *Helicobacter pylori* colonization in children. Nutrition 19:716–721.
151. Sheu, B.S., Cheng, H.C., Kao, A.W., Wang, S.T., Yang, Y.J., Yang, H.B., Wu, J.J., (2006), Pretreatment with lactobacillus-and bifidobactrerium containing yogurt can improve the efficacy of quadruple therapy in eradicating residual *Helicobacter pylori* infection after failed triple therapy. Am. J. Clin. Nutr. 83:864–869.
152. Kecskes, G., Belagyi, T., Olah, A., (2003), Early jejunal nutrition with combined pre-and probiotics in acute pancreatitis – prospective, randomized, double-blind investigations. Magyar Sebeszet 56:3–8.
153. Besselink, M.G.H., Timmerman, H.M., Buskens, E., Nieuwenhuijs, V.B., Akkermans, L.M. A., Gooszen, H.C., and members of the Dutch Acute Pancreatitis Study Group, (2004), Probiotic prophylaxis in patients with predicted severe acute pancreatitis (PROPATRIA): design and rationale of a double-blind, placebo-controlled randomized multicenter trial. BMC Surg. 4:12 (http://www.biomedcentral.com./1471–2482/4/12).
154. van Minnen, L.P., Timmerman, H.M., Lutgendorff, F., Verheem, A., Harmsen, W., Konstantinov, S.R., Smidt, H., Visser, M.R., Rijkers, G.T., Gooszen, H.G., Akkermans, L.M.A., (2007), Modification of intestinal flora with multispecies probiotics reduces bacterial translocation and improves clinical course in a rat model of acute pancreatitis. Surgery 141:470–480.
155. Sugawara, G., Nagino, M., Nishio, H., Ebata, T., Takagi, K., Asahara, T., Nomoto, K., Nimura, Y., (2006), Perioperative symbiotic treatment to prevent postoperative infectious complications in biliary cancer surgery: a randomized controlled trial. Ann. Surg. 244:706–714.
156. Rayes, N., Seehofer, D., Theruvath, T., Schiller, R.A., Langrehr, J.M., Jonas, S., Bengmark, S., Neuhaus, P., (2005), Supply of pre-and probiotics reduces bacterial infection rates after liver transplantation – a randomized, double-blind trial. Am. J. Transplant. 5:125–130.
157. Rayes, N., Seehofer, D., Muller, A.R., Hansen, S., Bengmark, S., Neuhaus, P., (2002), Influence of probiotics and fibre on the incidence of bacterial infections following mayor abdominal surgery – results of a prospective trial. Zeitschrift Gastroenterol. 40:869–876.
158. Valdez, J.C., Peral, M.C., Rachid, M., Santana, M., Perdigon, G., (2005), Interference of *Lactobacillus plantorum* with *Pseudomonas aeruginosa* in vitro and in infected burns: the potential use of probiotics in wound treatment. Clin. Microbiol. Infect. 11:472–479.
159. Alak, J.I., Wolf, B.W., Mdurvwa, E.G., Pimentel-Smith, G.E., Kolavala, S., Abdelrahman, H., Suppiramanian, V., (1999), Supplementation with *Lactobacillus reuteri* or *L. acidophilus* reduced intestinal shedding of *Cryptosporidium parvum* oocysts in immunodeficient C57BL/6mice.Cell. Mole. Biol. 45:855–863.
160. Besirbellioglu, B.A., Ulcay, A., Can, M., Erdem, H., Tanyuksel, M,. Avci, I.Y., Araz, E., Pahsa, A., (2006), *Saccharomyces boulardii* and infection due to *Giardia lamblia*. Scand. J., Infect. Dis. 38:479–481.

161. Department of Health and Human Services, Food and Drug Administration, (2006), Food additives permitted for direct addition to food for human consumption: bacteriophage preparation 21 CFR Part 172 (docket no.2002F-0316).http://www.fda.gov./docket/98Fr/cfo559.pdf.
162. Munoz, P., Bouza, E., Cuenca-Estrella, M., Eiros, J.M., Perez, M.J., Sanchez-Somolinos, M., Rincon, C., Hortal, J., Pelaez, T., (2005), *Saccharymes cerevisciae* fungemia: an emerging infectious disease. Clin. Infect. Dis. 40:1635–1637.
163. Borriello, S.P., Hammes, W.P., Holzapfel, W., Marteau, P., Schrezenmeir, J., Vaara, M., Valtonen, V., (2003), Safety of probiotics that contain lactobacilli or bifidobacteria. Clin. Infect. Dis. 36:775–780.
164. Salminen, M.K., Rautelin, H., Tynkkynen, S., Poussa, T., Saxelin, M., Valtonen, V., Jarvinen, A., (2004), *Lactobacillus* bacteremia, clinical significance, and patient outcome, with special focus on probiotic *L. rhamnosus* GG. Clin. Infect. Dis. 38:62–69.
165. Salminen, M.K., Tynkkynen, S., Rautelin, H., Saxelin, M., Vaara, M., Ruutu, P., Sarna, S., Valtonen, V., Jarvinen, A., (2002), Lactobacillus bacteremia during a rapid increase in probiotic use of *Lactobacillus rhamnosus* GG in Finland. Clin. Infect. Dis. 35:1155–1160.
166. Marteau, P., Seksik, P., (2004), Tolerance of probiotics and prebiotics. J. Clin. Gastroenterol. 38(Suppl 6):s67–s69.
167. Beerepoot, M.A.J., Stobberingh, E.E., Geerling, S.E., (2006), A study of non-antibiotic VERSUS antibiotic prophylaxis for recurrent urinary tract infections in women. Nederlands Tijdschrift voor GeneesKunde 150:574–575.

# Chapter 10
# Device-Related Infections

## 10.1 Introduction

Device-related or foreign-body-related infection is a complication of medical progress, which has progressively increased over the past three decades and will continue to rise for the foreseeable future. We can only hope to limit the rates of infection per device and reduce the consequences from prompt and appropriate management, but absolute prevention will be unattainable. As technological advances in medicine continue to progress, there will be new and innovative devices implanted in patients to prolong and improve the quality of life, and with these new techniques it is predictable that there will be novel infections associated with their implantation.

There are numerous devices inserted in the human body for various conditions, and the scope of this chapter is not to review all foreign-body-related infections, but the most frequent and troublesome conditions. Devices that are most prone to infections are usually meant for temporary use but have become long term or permanent due to special needs. These usually involve catheters communicating with a normally sterile site with the surface of the body, i.e., urethral catheters and intravascular catheters. Table 10.1 lists devices and risk of infection.

Exposure to invasive medical devices is one of most important risk factor for nosocomial infections and occurs in more than two million patients annually with an annual cost of about US$11 billion.[1] It is estimated that 45–50% of all nosocomial infections are related to devices. Devices predispose to infections by breaking or invading the cutaneous or mucosal barriers and by supporting growth of microorganisms. Presence of foreign material impairs the host defense mechanisms locally, and infection or colonization result in chronic infection or tissue necrosis. The extent of the problem can be appreciated with the knowledge that more than 30% of hospitalized patients have one or more vascular catheters inserted; more than 10% of hospitalized patients have indwelling urinary catheters; total hip replacement worldwide exceeds one million a year, and knee replacement more than 250,000.[1]

**Table 10.1** Devices and risk of infection

| A Devices with external communication | Infection |
|---|---|
| 1) Urogential Devices | High risk >7 days |
|    i) urethral catheter | UTI |
|    ii) suprapubic bladder catheter | UTI |
|    iii) nephrostomy catheter | pyelonephritis |
|    iv) ureteric stents | pyelonephritis |
| 2) Intravascular catheters | Moderate risk >10 days |
|    i) central venous catheters | Bacteremia |
|    ii) tunneled venous catheters | Bacteremia |
|    iii) arterial catheters | Bacteremia |
|    iv) peripheral venous catheters | Septic phlebitis/cellulitis |
| 3) Temporary draining catheters | Low risk within 10 days |
|    i) Intrapleural catheter | Empyemia |
|    ii) Intraperitoneal catheter | peritonitis |
|    iii) ventricular drain | meningitis |
| 4) Permanent indwelling catheters | Low risk <1 month |
|    i) peritoneal dialysis catheter | peritonitis |
|    ii) peraitaneous bite dust catheter | cholangitis |
| **B Implanted devices** | |
| 1) Ventricular shunts (peritoneal, atrial, pleural) | meningitis (10%) |
| 2) Intracardiac | – |
|    i) prosthetic valves | endocarditis 11 |
|    ii) pacemaker and implantable cardioverter - defibrillator | bacteremia, endocarditis (1–3% at 60 months) |
|    iii) ventricular assist device | insertion site infection -common/duration dependent |
|    iv) Coronary artery stents | rare |
| 3) Intraocular lens | endopththalmitis (<1%) |
| 4) Vascular grafts | Risk 1–6% |
|    i) aortic graft | – bacteria, mycotic aneurysm; enteric fistula |
|    ii) periyphreal vascular graft | – wound drainage, pseudoaneurysm, hemorrhage, occlusion |
|    iii) arterio-venous graft | – bacteremia, local abscess |
| 5) Orthopedic prosthesis | Risk 0.5–2% |
|    i) hip prosthesis | – local joint and bone (<3%) |
|    ii) knee prosthesis | 0.39–1.0% |
|    iii) spinal prosthesis | 0.39–1.0% |
|    iv) arterial fixation of fractures (screws/plates) | Chronic osteomyelitis |
|    v) other prosthetic joints | |
| 6) Miscellaneous Devices | |
|    i) Inferior vena cava filter | persistent bacteremia (rare) |
|    ii) intrabiliary stents | cholangitis (common with obstruction) |
|    iii) breast implants | mastitis (2–2.5%) |
|    iv) penile implants | 2–8% risk |
|    v) transjugular intrahepatic portosystemic shunt (TIPS) | endotipsitis (1.3–1.7%) Bacteremia |
|    vi) Cochlear implants | meningitis (rare) |
|    vii) ventral hernia mesh | wound infection |
|    viii) oral implants | perimplantitis/osteomyelitis |
|    ix) maxillo-facial prosthesis | low rates |
|    x) voice-prosthesis | |

## 10.2 Pathogenesis of Device-Related Infections

Acute epidemic bacterial infectious diseases are caused by free-floating (planktonic) microorganisms, which cause diseases in healthy individuals and usually run their courses until the hosts become immune. However, in device-related and certain chronic infections (as in the cystic fibrosis, chronic otitis media with cholesteatoma, etc.) the organisms grow in biofilms.[2] More than 99.9% of bacteria grow in biofilms on a wide variety of surfaces in industrial and environmental ecosystems. A biofilm is a "microbiologically derived sessile community characterized by cells that are irreversibly attached to a substratum or interface or to each other, are embedded in a matrix of extracellular polymeric substances that they have produced, and exhibit a altered phenotype with respect to growth rate and gene transcription."[3] Examination of natural biofilms show that the sessile populations consists of mushroom-like microcolonies, which are much more active metabolically than their planktonic counter parts.[4] The biofilm microcolonies are composed of cells ($\simeq$15% by volume) embedded in matrix material ($\simeq$85% by volume), with ramifying channels to conduct water and nutrients to the community.[4] The microcolonies are viscoelastic and deformable in high-shear stress, and can creep across surfaces. The biofilms constitute the most defensive life strategy adopted by prokaryotic cells, and represent an evolutionary adaptation to hostile environments in nature. Fragments of the biofilms can break off or detach when the shear forces exceed their tensile strength, as an example the detachment of vegetations that form on native heart valves in a high-shear environment.

Planktonic bacteria adhere to surfaces and initiate biofilm formation preferentially in very high-shear environment, and smooth surfaces are colonized as easily as rough surfaces. When planktonic bacteria transform to biofilm communities, depending on nutrient and other advantages and if condition favors permanent settlement, the adherent cells upregulate the genes involved in matrix production and the process of biofilm formation begins.[5] Both biofilm formation and detachment are under the regulatory control of molecules (same chemical signals that regulates quorum sensing) that guide formation of slime-enclosed microcolonies and water channels.[2] Thus, quorum-sensing molecules discovered in planktonic bacteria may have evolved to control biofilms and many other bacterial functions and behavior. Unlike planktonic bacteria, biofilm microorganisms are inherently resistant to antibiotics and to virtually all antibacterial agents.[5] Resistance to antibacterial agents is not just due to diffusion limiation[6] but based on change in cellular characteristics.[7] Bacteria adopt a much different phenotype when they adhere to foreign surfaces to form biofilms, and the resistance to antibiotics is related to different set of genes expressed in biofilm from those expressed in the corresponding planktonic cells.[8]

Implant infections are extremely resistant to antibiotics and host defences and frequently persist until the device is removed, which is the standard therapy. Tissue damage caused by surgery and foreign body implantation further increased the susceptibility to infection, activation of host defences, and stimulation or up-regulation of proinflammatory cytokines by bacterial products and toxins. The molecular mechanisms of antibacterial resistance by biofilm colonies may include repressed growth within the biofilm, physiochemical interaction of "slime" (glycocalyx and exopolysaccharides) with some antibiotics (via dipole, H, ionic bonds, complexes) and changes in the cell envelope following adhesion to foreign bodies.[1] "Slime" which consists of thick, hydrated, polyanionic-gelled polysaccharides and glycoproteins act like exchange resins, thus absorb and adhere to certain cationic antibiotics (i.e., aminoglycosides) and saturating the binding sites.[9] Thus, the combination of dormancy, cell wall alterations and binding of antibiotics to "slime" all may explain resistance of implant infection to antimicrobial therapy until the foreign body is removed.[10]

## 10.2.1  Impairment of Local Defence

A notable feature of implant-related infections is the high frequency of low-virulent, non-pathogenic microorganisms which are usually normal skin commensals. The mere presence of a foreign body in the human host lowers the threshold of bacterial infection and induces local immunosuppression. The mechanism of device-related infections involves defects in both host's humoral and cellular defences.[11]

Foreign body surfaces reduce the killing capacity of phagocytes by triggering slow burst of superoxide and weaken a secondary burst of phagocytes.[12] Neutrophils surrounding teflon material for instance, exhibited decreased bactericidal activity and reduced superoxide production.[13,14] The production of extracellular slime and the relatively poor immunogenicity of the cell wall proteins of the biofilm bacteria may increase these defects.[15,16] Decreased opsonic antibody response to biofilm cell envelope proteins[17] and generation of bacterial neutrophil inhibitor[18] can further impair phagocytosis and microbial killing. Both crude preparations of bacterial slime and S*taphylococcus epidermidis* isolates from implant-related infections have been shown to produce a neutrophil inhibitory factor.[16,18]

The extracellular slime substance from *S. epidermidis* can also inhibit lymphocyte activity and impair cell-mediated function.[19] Repeated macrophage stimulation by biomaterial particles can also cause macrophage exhaustion, production of reactive oxygen intermediates and result in adjacent tissue damage.

Thus, the implant material is effectively surrounded by a fibro-inflammatory zone with impaired defences, which does not become incorporated as part of the normal host tissue.[1] The perpetuating stimulation of cellular immune responses results in superoxide radical and cytokine-mediated damage, further increases susceptibility to infection and eventually results in fibrosis around the implant (i.e., breast implant), osteolysis and loosening around orthopedic endo-prosthesis, and failure of the implant. The inflammatory responses around the foreign body may cause degradation of the biomaterial itself (via oxidative products) and enhance the susceptibility to infection.[20]

In a murine model of graft infection the expression of major histocompatibility complex (MHC) class II by neutrophils, monocytes, and lymphocytes was suppressed compared to sterile controls.[21] There is also some evidence that prostaglandin $E_2$ modulates the monocyte MHC-II suppression in biomaterial infection.[22] Defects in opsonic activity and macrophage bacterial clearing capability, related to decreased production of interferon (IF) – γ and interleukin (IL) – 1 by peritoneal mononuclear immune cells have been detected in patients with dialysis catheter-related peritonitis.[1] There is also evidence that cardiac circulatory devices can induce aberrant T-cell activation with higher surface expression of CD4's marker that leads to programmed cell death of CD4+ − T cells.[23] This defect in cellular immunity may predispose to fungal infections, which has been noted with these devices. Cellular immune defect in recipient of these cardiac devices has also been demonstrated by cutaneous anergy to recall antigens and lower than normal T-cell proliferative responses after activation via the T-cell receptor complex.[24] Stimulation of T-cell activation and decrease of Th1-cytokine producing CD4 T cells can result in B-cell hyperactivity and dysregulation of immunoglobulin synthesis by Th2 cytokines.[25] Hence, resulting in excessive production of autoimmune antibodies, including those directed at human leucocyte antigen (HLA) and phospholipids antigens. These antibodies may increase organ allograft rejection after subsequent cardiac transplantation.

Physical factors such as high physiologic shear stress on surfaces of arterial grafts and cardiac valves may also impair local immune defences, by preventing circulating leucocytes to adhere to biomaterial and interact with adherent bacteria.[26] Furthermore, host proteins such as fibrinogen and fibronectin that absorb to implant surfaces can influence the acute inflammatory response because of proinflammatory properties.

## 10.2.2 Resistance to Antimicrobial Agents

As previously mentioned it is well-documented that biofilm organisms are inherently resistant to antibiotics, disinfectants or germicides compared to planktonic bacteria. The susceptibility of the same organisms in the planktonic phenotype compared to the biofilm phenotype varies from 20- to 1,000-fold.[27] Table 10.2 summarizes data on selected antibiotics susceptibility against some planktonic and biofilm bacteria.[28–31]

Antibiotic resistance mechanisms of biofilm organisms are different from planktonic bacteria, and do not involve modifying enzymes, target mutations, or efflux pumps. The resistance in biofilm bacteria seems to depend on multicellular strategies.[32] Biofilm bacteria on dispersal to the planktonic form rapidly revert to the more antibiotic susceptible phenotype, which is against acquired resistance from mutation, plasmic, or translocation of genetic elements.

There are three main proposal mechanisms for biofilm antibiotic resistance: (1) slow penetration and failure of antibiotic to penetrate beyond the surface layers, (2) resistant, phenotype, and (3) altered microenvironment.[32] There is no generic barrier to the diffusion of antibiotic solutes through the biofilm matrix, and some antibiotics permeate the bacterial biofilm readily.[7] Some antibiotics (aminoglyco-

**Table 10.2** Differences in susceptibility of planktonic vs Biofilm bacteria

| Organisms | Antibiotic | MIC or MBC (g/ml) Planktonic | Biofilm | Reference |
|---|---|---|---|---|
| S. aureus | vancomycin | 2 (MBC) | $20^a$ | 24 |
| P. aeruginosa | imipenem | 1 (MIC) | $>1024^b$ | 25 |
| E. coli | ampicillin | 2 (MIC) | $512^b$ | 25 |
| S. sanguis | doxycycline | 0.063 (MIC) | $3.15^c$ | 26 |
| P. pseudomallei | ceftazidime | 8 (MBC) | $800^d$ | 27 |
| K. pneumoniae | ciprofloaxacin | 0.18 (MIC) | $1.8^e$ | 28 |

a = concentration required for 99% reduction
b = minimal biofilm eradication concentration
c = concentration required for >99.9% reduction
d = concentration required for ~99% reduction
e = log reduction after 4 and 24 h only 1.02 CFU for biofilm vs 4.4 CFU for planktonic bacteria

sides) with positive charge bind to negative charged polymers in the biofilm[33] and retard or slow the penetration.[34] The role of diffusion in antibiotic resistance of biofilms is controversial and may not be sigificant.[4]

The second postulate that the biofilm forms represent a unique and highly protected phenotypic state, a cell differentiation similar to spore formation, with expression of different sets of genes has become the current in vogue hypothesis.[4] The current antibiotics were selected on their ability to kill or inhibit planktonic bacteria, and are inactive on the multicellular microcolonies of the biofilm communities. There is some evidence from a dose-response study of antibiotic resistance in *P. aeruginosa* biofilm that most bacteria in the biofilm are rapidly killed with antibiotics but survivors represent a small population of superresistant cell fraction.[35] In normal circumstances the host immune system would eliminate the small remaining population of planktonic cells, but in biofilm the cells are protected by the matrix and allow regrowth of the superresistant cells after antibiotic treatment.

Another possible mechanism for biofilm resistance depends on an altered chemical microenvironment. Concentration gradients of nutrients and metabolic products exist across the layers or zones of biofilms. Oxygen maybe completely consumed in the surface layer resulting in an anaerobic environment in the deeper layers of the biofilm.[36] Marked pH difference between the surface fluid and the interior may result from accumulation of acid waste products, causing antagonism of some antibiotic action.[37] Aminoglycoside for example are 8- to 60-fold less active in an acidic or anaerobic medium than in an alkaline medium. Experimental evidence reveal zones of metabolic inactivity within biofilms, which reflect dormant bacteria (in non-growing state) resulting from a combination of nutrient depletion or inhibition by toxic wastes.[38] Generally dormant bacteria are more resistant to antibiotics than actively growing organisms. Increased osmotic concentration within the interior of the biofilm can also influence antimicrobial activity, by changes in relative proportions of porins that affect cell wall permeability to antibiotics.[32]

Biofilm-associated cells grow significantly slower than planktonic cells and as a result take up antibiotics more slowly. Cell culture techniques designed to assess rate of growth on resistance have found that the slow-growing *Escherichia coli* cells within a biofilm were the most resistant to cetrimide.[38] Similar results have been found for *S. epidermidis* biofilm, where growth rates strongly influenced susceptibility.[39] It has also been shown that younger *P. aeruginosa* biofilms (2 days old) are much more susceptible to antibiotic inactivation than older (10 days old) chemostat-grown *P. aeruginosa* biofilms.[40]

There appears to be a relationship between physiological microenvironmental conditions biofilm formation and rate of growth. Nutrient limitation, build up of toxic metabolites and environmental stresses, by synthesizing sigma factors that under control of the RPOs regulon regulate the transcription genes, favor formation of biofilms and slowing of bacterial growth rate.[3] It has been shown that bacterial adherence to surfaces result in the repression or induction of genes that results in a number of physiological responses.[41]

## 10.3 Specific Device-Related Infections

### 10.3.1 Intravascular Devices

The numbers and diversity of intravascular devices (IVDs) used for vascular access have dramatically increased over the past 30 years in modern health care centers across the world. The utilization of short-term central venous catheters (CVCs) of different types (uncuffed, nontunnel triple lumen catheter, pulmonary artery catheter, short-term uncuffed hemodynamic monitoring) are now standard in most modern intensive care units (ICUs).

Moreover, there has been a great increase as well in the use of long-term or indefinite IVDS in hospitals and out-patient settings. These include devices for home antibiotic therapy, such as peripherally inserted central venous catheters (PICCs), surgically implanted cuffed and tunneled CVCs for long-term or permanent total parenteral nutrition (as in short gut syndrome), chemotherapy for cancers, and chronic out-patient hemodialysis.

The tremendous increase of utilization of these various IVDs have been accompanied over the years with substantial rise in infectious complications, particularly bloodstream infections. Intravascular devices are now the single most important cause of health care associated bacteremia or bloodstream infections (BSI).[42,43] It has been estimated that 250,000 to 500,000 IVD-related BSIs occur each year in the United States.[13] There is general agreement that IVD-related BSIs are associated with longer hospital stay (from 10 to 20 days), and excess health are costs (from US $4,000 to US$56,000 per episode).[43–47] However, the impact of IVD-related BSIs on attributable mortality is controversial,[44–47] and this may largely be due to the dilutional effect of low-virulent organisms (coagulase negative staphylococci), accounting for the majority of BSIs.

**Table 10.3** Rates of IVD-related blood stream infections

| Catheter | Incidence rate (Per 100 IVDs, %) | No. 1000 IVD Days |
|---|---|---|
| Peripheral IV | 0.1% | 0.5 |
| Midline IV | 0.4% | 0.2 |
| Noncuffed CVC | 4.4% | 2.7 |
| Arterial | 0.8% | 1.7 |
| PICC | 2.4% | 2.1 |
| Cuffed/tunneled CVC* | 22.5% | 1.6 |
| Central venous ports* | 3.6% | 0.1 |

IV = intravenous
CVC = central venous catheter
PICC = peripherally inserted central catheter
* = Surgically implanted long-term devices

The rates of BSIs vary with the type and reason for the IVD, among other factors to be discussed later, but also with the method of calculating rates of infection. Previous analysis of the risk of BSIs per 100 devices would clearly show greater risk of infection for longer-term catheters, with very low risk for peripheral intravenous catheters which would normally last for 3–5 days. In more recent years it has been widely recommended for calculating and reporting infectious rates as BSIs per 1000 catheter days.[48] A recent systematic review of 200 published prospective studies evaluating risk of bloodstream infection in adults with different intravascular devices have been reported.[49] In general the use of cuffed and tunneled dual lumen CVCs, compared to noncuffed, nontunneled catheters for temporary use and CVCs with anti-infective surfaces, was associated with significantly lower rates of catheter-related BSI.[49] Table 10.3 summarizes the incidence of blood stream infection for different types of intravascular catheters.

### 10.3.1.1 Mechanism of IVD-Related BSI

Microorganisms may infect or colonize intravascular catheters by a few routes: (1) at the interface between the catheter and the patient's skin (believed to be the most frequent site of access); (2) intraluminally through the connecting ports of the catheter; (3) and through contamination of the infusate (the least common route). For the first two mechanisms the source of the microorganisms are predominantly resident flora or colonization organisms on the patients skin, and less frequently organisms residing on the hands of health care workers. The leading pathogens of intravascular catheter-related infections are coagulase-negative staphylococci, *S. aureus*, enterococcus, gram-negative bacilli (predominantly from ICUs), candida species and diphtheroids. Experiments of catheter infection using coagulase-negative staphylococci demonstrate by scanning electron microscopy show the following sequence: adherence to the catheter surface followed by cell proliferation (even in the absence of enteral nutrient source), possibly breakdown of catheter components, and production of a slime (biofilm) covering the bacterial colonies.[50]

Different bacterial species may utilize separate mechanisms for adherence and colonization of catheters or devices in general. *S. epidermidis* achieve attachment to surface of devices that is mediated either by nonspecific factors (such as surface tension, hydrophobicity, and electrostatic forces) or by specific adhesins (proteinaceous autolysin encoded by the altE gene and the capsular polysaccharide adhesin, likely encoded by the ica operon).[51,52] The accumulative phase during which the bacteria adhere to each other and form a biofilm, is mediated by the polysaccharide intercellular adhesin encoded by the ica operon.[53] However, the ica genes are associated with initial colonization and not persistence.[54] Most recently, Sar Z (a transcriptional regulator) was found to be a key regulator of *S. epidermidis* biofilm formation and virulence.[55] Sar Z gene influence the transcription of the biosynthetic operon for biofilm exopolysaccharide, and the expression of virulence genes controlling regulations of lipases, proteases, resistance to antimicrobial peptides, and hemolysis.[55] Adherence of *S. aureus*, on the other hand, is more dependent on the presence of host-tissue ligands, such as fibronectin, fibrinogen, and collagen. *S. aureus* adheres to the host-tissue ligands by microbial surface proteins, such as FnbpA and FnbpB which bind to fibronectin; clumping factor which binds to fibrinogen; and collagen adhesin which binds to collagen.[56,57] However, strains of *S. aureus* lacking these surface proteins likely can cause device infections with a heavy inoculum.[57]

Infusion of contaminated fluid is an occasional source of catheter-related BSIs. These episodes often are recognized after local outbreaks of bacteremias with the same strain of organism in clusters (point-source out breaks). The implicated microorganisms usually can survive and multiply in nutritionally poor fluids (i.e., saline) or at refrigerated temperatures used to store blood products. Noscomial outbreaks of *Enterobacter* species bacteremia have been reported with contaminated intravenous saline and 5% dextrose,[58–60] and human albumin.[61] Bacteremias secondary to contaminated blood products maybe under-recognized and under-reported, and could be misdiagnosed as a blood, or blood-product reaction. Whole blood components or red blood cells are stored at 1–6°C and common blood contaminants (*Staphylococcus* or *Propionibacterium* spp) generally proliferate poorly at these temperatures. Clinical infection or sepsis from contaminated blood transfusion are rare events, and involve a variety of gram-negative bacilli which are capable of growth at 1–6°C, such as *Yersinia enterocolitica* and *Serratia liquefaciens*.[62] Transfusion of platelet concentrates poses a greater risk for BSIs as platelets are stored at 20–24°C to preserve function. Thus such storage allows excellent growth medium for a broad spectrum of bacteria. Surveillance studies have demonstrated that 1 in 1,000 to 2,000 platelet units are bacterially contaminated, and clinical sepsis would be expected in at least 1 in 10 to 2 in 5 contaminated transfusion (200–1,600 cases annually).[62] Surveillance studies from the United States, the United Kingdom, and France shows that gram-positive organisms were implicated in 71% of platelet transfusion related sepsis, but gram-negative *Enterobacteriae* account for the majority of fatalities.[62]

In recent years needle-less access systems have been widely introduced throughout the health care system to improve health care worker safety from blood-borne pathogen exposure. However, the use of intravascular needle-less catheter valves has been associated with 2.7-fold increased bloodstream infections, with subsequent decrease following removal of the device.[63] Contamination of these valves were found in 24.3%, predominantly coagulase negative staphylococci, resulting in colonization of the port of central venous catheters.[63]

### 10.3.1.2 Diagnosis of IVD-Related Bloodstream Infection

Central venous catheters of all types are the most frequent cause of nosocomial bloodstream infection, and about 250,000 to 500,000 episodes occur in the United States annually.[64] Early and accurate diagnosis is important for appropriate management and timely removal (or avoidance of unnecessary removal) of these central venous or arterial catheters. Several techniques have been developed to confirm the diagnosis of IVD-related bacteremia. Methods that require removal of the catheters (qualitative, semiqualitative, or quantitative catheter segment cultures) are not commonly used anymore as this results in unnecessary removal of non-infected catheters.

Methods that require retention of the catheter until the diagnosis is confirmed are more popular and cost-effective, unless there is obvious clinical evidence of IVD-related infection (which is uncommon). Growth of microorganisms from blood cultures obtained via the central catheters is sensitive but not specific, as bacteremias from other sources will often be positive as well. Paired quantitative blood cultures drawn through the catheter-port and percutaneously, once considered the gold standard, is considered diagnostic of IVD-related BSIs when the concentration of organisms is three- to fivefold greater from the device than in the peripherally drawn blood. However, this technique is time-consuming and expensive, thus not suitable for routine use in most hospitals.

Direct visualization of any microorganisms from blood aspirated from the catheter, by staining lysed and centrifuged blood cells with acridine orange (acridine orange leucocyte cytospin technique[65]), is a rapid but insensitive method. Paired conventional blood cultures drawn from the catheter and percutaneously can be assessed semiquantitatively by determination of differential time to become positive (time of incubation to show positive growth by a automated continuous monitoring culture system, which is now popular in most modern urban hospitals). Catheter-drawn blood culture which turns positive $\geq 2$ h earlier than peripherally drawn culture is indicative of IVD-related BSI.[66] In a recent meta-analysis of 51 studies, assessing eight diagnostic methods, paired quantitative blood culture was the most accurate diagnostic test of IVD-related BSI,[67] but the least practical and most expensive method. Paired blood cultures with differential time to positivity is an acceptable, less expensive, and more practical alternative, with pooled sensitivity of 89% (short term) and 90% (long term) and pooled specificity of 87% (short term) and 72% (long term). The overall sensitivity and specificity of the acridine orange leucocytospin test were 72% and 91%, respectively.[66]

In a more recent prospective, randomized study of three procedures (semiquantitative superficial swab culture from hub and insertion site, differential quantitative blood cultures, and differential time to positivity) were compared.[67] The sensitivity, specificity, and accuracy of superficial cultures were 78.6%, 92.0%, and 90.2%, respectively; differential quantitative blood cultures, 71.4%, 97.7%, and 94.1%, respectively, and differential time to positivity, 96.4%, 90.3%, and 91.2%, respectively. Although the investigators recommend superficial semiquantitatives and peripheral blood culture to screen for catheter-related BSI, because of low cost, ease of performance and wide-availability, this study is of limited size, 204 episodes of suspected IVD-related BSI but only 28 confirmed,[68] and further larger studies are needed. If anything, this study confirms the acceptable accuracy of differential time to positivity of paired diagnostic test in centers with automated continuous monitoring culture system. A recent review of this diagnostic method has also confirmed the usefulness, high sensitivity, and specificity of this technique.[69]

### 10.3.1.3 Management of Intravascular-Catheter-Related BSI

The majority of BSIs secondary to intravascular catheters have mainly fever with no focal inflammatory signs at the catheter site. On occasion there is evidence of inflammation and pus oozing from the insertion site (exit-site infection), with or without surrounding cellulitis. In surgically implanted long-term catheters there may be signs of inflammation, induration, and tenderness along the tunnel (tunnel infection). Presence of these signs is an indication for immediate removal of these catheters.

The principles of management of intravascular-catheter-related infections involve removal of the device and specific antimicrobial therapy. Dispute exists for both forms of therapy but guidelines have been published based on expert opinions,[70] rather than results of clinical controlled, randomized trials, or even large case-control studies. A major issue with these guidelines (not based on solid evidence) is that they become standard of care, which can lead to medico-legal litigations when not being followed.

The approach to management of intravascular-catheter-related suspected infections should depend on the severity of illness and risk for such complications, as well as investigations to exclude other sources of infection such as pneumonia, urinary tract, and intra-abdominal site. Current (but imperfect) evidence and most expert opinions recommend removal of intravascular non-tunneled catheters (peripheral or central venous or arterial) when there is proven evidence of microbial infection, or clinical signs of exit site, tunnel infection, or surrounding cellulitis of insertion site. With permanent surgically implanted catheters (tunneled-devices) there is some evidence that they can be salvaged in certain circumstances.

In critically ill patients with severe sepsis or all patients with septic shock syndrome it is reasonable to remove possible infected catheters immediately before confirmation of IVD-related BSI, regardless of absence of clinical signs and especially when the catheter had been in place for more than 3 days. In these circumstances the catheter tip should be cultured besides obtaining paired blood cultures. Empirical broad-spectrum antibiotics are recommended in these circumstances after obtaining cultures, the choice should be dependent on the local resistance patterns in the institution. Further adjustment in therapy should be made based on the microorganism and susceptibility.

### 10.3.1.4 Contentious Issues in Management of IVD Infections

Certainly when there is evidence of metastatic infection such as osteomyelitis, septic arthritis, or endocarditis, treatment and duration should follow the usual standards for these conditions (3–6 weeks duration). Collaborative guidelines by the Infectious Disease Society of America, Society of Critical care medicine, and the Society for Healthcare Epidemiology of America recommends removal of non-tunneled catheters; antibiotics for 10–14 days for gram-negative bacilli; 14 days for *S. aureus* (perform a transesophageal echocardiogram [TEE]); 14 days of antifungal therapy for *Candida* spp; after last positive blood culture (provided no evidence of visceral involvement, i.e., *Candida retinitis*); and 5–7 days of vancomycin for coagulase-negative staphylococci.[69]

There are reasonably good evidence to support the recommendations for *S. aureus* and *Candida* spp catheter-related BSIs. However, there is no evidence to support any antimicrobial therapy for coagulase-negative staphylococci uncomplicated catheter-related infection; and poor evidence for the prolonged therapy for gram-negative bacilli bacteremia once the source (catheter) have been removed. These guidelines may be contributing to the overuse of antimicrobials and for unnecessary duration, which often can lead to multiresistant gram-negative bacilli, and vancomycin-resistant enterococci (VRE), vancomycin intermediate-resistant staphylococci (VIRS). Moreover, unnecessary or prolonged used of these antibiotics often predispose to *Clostridium difficile* colitis, adverse reactions and increased health are costs.

Coagulase-negative *Staphylococcus* (CoNS) bacteremia are often skin contaminants and were previously ignored and considered benign. However, these low-virulent organisms can be associated with prosthetic value endocarditis, vascular-graft infections, and rarely native valve endocarditis in patients with significant cardiac valvular disease. Other prosthetic devices such as orthopedic prosthesis or intracranial ventricular shunts are usually infected by these skin commensals by direct inoculation at the time of surgical implantation. CoNS rarely causes septic syndrome in patients with bacteremia, and the mortality associated with this catheter-related bacteremia is quite low (~0.7%).[70] Vancomycin or any antibiotics have not been established as being necessary to treat catheter-related BSIs with CoNS as an evidence-based therapy, and removal of the catheter alone is usually adequate therapy (personal experience).

There is also no evidence that gram-negative bacteria from intravascular catheters, once removed and the patient is afebrile, requires more than 5–7 days of antibiotic therapy. Recent evidence shows that even in patients with ventilation-associated pneumonia, with or without gram-negative bacteremia, no more than 8 days therapy is needed (with the exception of *Pseudomonas aeruginosa*).[71] Also in patients with intra-abdominal sepsis (with or without gram-negative bacteremia), 5–7 days of antibiotic is considered adequate once the source have been removed and adequately drained, the peripheral white blood cell count returns to normal, and the subject remains afebrile for at least 1–2 days.[72] Thus, the current guidelines by these societies should be revisited and revised.

### 10.3.1.5 Antibiotic Lock Therapy

These is some evidence that tunneled long-term intravascular catheters can be salvaged even when infected or associated with BSIs. A previous review in 2001[69] noted that 66.5% of infected tunneled catheters could be salvaged by antibiotic therapy, especially with the antibiotic lock or dwell technique. There was evidence that response to conservative management was better with exit-site infection or bacteremia without any clinical signs, but tunnel infection or pocket infection would require removal of the device. In addition the response to antibiotic lock therapy (ALT) was dependent on the micro-organism, good response with CoNS but poor response with *S. aureus* and *P. aeuroginosa*.[70] The previous review in 2001 of seven open studies with ALT (with or without systemic antibiotics) found response and catheter salvage in 138 (82.6%) of 167 episodes.[70] Compared to parenteral therapy alone treatment with ALT was significantly more likely to result in catheter salvage (RR 1.24, $p = 0.001$).[70]

The antibiotic lock or dwell technique involves injection of pharmacologic concentrations of antibiotics (most commonly vancomycin or aminoglycoside) in the hub and lumen of the catheter (without infusion or flushing) to dwell locally for 8–24 h, for several days; plus additional systemic therapy via a different route. The concept is to achieve local concentration of the antibiotic in the catheter lumen 100–1,000 times the usual MIC to kill biofilm sessile bacteria. This therapy is based on the assumption that most tunneled-catheter infection are initiated by contamination of the hub, and not from the skin-catheter interface.

The use of tunneled Broviac-Hickman type catheters and totally implantable venous access devices (ports) have greatly increased in the past decade. Attempts to salvage infected catheters are appealing to reduce the morbidity and costs of replacement, and moreover there may be limited venous access sites available. The majority of reports on efficacy of antibiotic lock therapy have been on open observational case series in patients receiving long-term parenteral nutrition,[74–78] and some studies on hemodialysis[79–81] and onco-hematological patients.[82,83] In a recent review of four studies in the hemodialysis population, ALT with systemic antibiotics resulted in successful catheter salvage in about 69% of the cases, with the remainder removed after lack of improvement in 48 h.[84] In recent prospective evaluation of ALT in the management of catheter-related bacteremias, associated with cancer chemotherapy or parenteral nutrition in a Spanish hospital over 44 months, 801 long-term intravascular devices were placed in 105 patients.[85] Of the 127 episodes of bacteremia documented 92 (72.4%) were catheter-related. However, only 48 episodes met the criteria for analysis, with 19 treated with ALT plus systemic antibiotics and 29 episodes treated only with systemic antibiotics. Isolated microorganisms were similar in the two groups. The catheter had to be removed in one episode in the ALT group and seven episodes in the controls. Overall successful treatment was achieved in 84% and 65% of the ALT group and control group, respectively ($p = 0.27$).[85] Failure to demonstrate a statistical significant difference likely was due to insufficient sample size.

An area of uncertainty and under-investigated is the need for treatment of an IVC colonized with *S. aureus* but with negative blood cultures. This is often recognized when the removed catheter tip reveals significant growth ($\geq 15$ CFU). It is believed that catheter colonization with bacteria will eventually lead to bacteremia if not removed, and is strongly associated with concomitant bacteremia. However, it is not clear whether antibiotic treatment is necessary or not once the catheter is removed. There have been two recent studies addressing this issue. In the first report of a retrospective cohort of 77 patients with CVC- tip positive for *S. aureus* (without concomitant bacteremia), 9 (12%) subsequently developed *S. aureus* bacteremia at a median time of 4 days after removal.[86] No antibiotic therapy was an independent risk factor for the subsequent bacteremia. In a more recent retrospective study of 184 patients with *S. aureus* catheter tip colonization (CVCs and arterial catheters), 14 (7.6%) subsequently developed bacteremia (median time 3 days after removal, range 2–25 days).[87] Twelve (24%) of 49 patients who did not receive antibiotic therapy developed subsequent *S. aureus* bacteremia, versus 2 (4%) of the 50 treated patients (intravenous or oral antistaphylococcal agent for a minimum of 3 days).[86] Antibiotic therapy within 1–2 days after removal of the CVC was associated with an 83% lower risk of subsequent bacteremia in this latter study,[87] and a 91% reduction in the first study.[86] Thus, current evidence (albeit weak) supports a course of short-term therapy for *S. aureus* colonization of CVCs or arterial catheters until further prospective randomized trials are conducted.

### *10.3.2 Prevention of Central versus Catheter Infections*

It is estimated that more than 15% of patients who receive central vascular catheters have complications.[88] Infectious complications occur in 5–26%, mechanical complications in 5–19% and thrombotic complications in 2–26%.[88] Factors that influence the risks of infectious complications include site of insertion, insertion technique (including skin preparation), level of experience by the physician, duration of catheterization, method of maintenance of the insertion site and catheter, frequency of manipulation (multipurpose or single-purpose), level of urgency of insertion (likely related to insertion technique), and sites of infection elsewhere that may cause hematogenous seeding to the catheter.

Selection of the subclavian site appears to be the preferred site for central venous catheter insertion to minimize the risk of infectious complications. In a randomized study subclavian versus femoral venous catheterization was associated with significantly less infectious complications, and a trend to decreased catheter-related bacteremias (1.2 infection versus 4.5 infections per 1,000 catheter days, $p = 0.07$).[89] Accumulated experience (non-randomized) suggests that subclavian catheterization is less likely to result in catheter-related infection than internal jugular vein catheterization.[88,90]

Preparation of the site with maximal aseptic technique (including mask, sterile gowns, and a large sterile drape) has been shown to reduce the risk of catheter-related infection and to be cost saving (about US$167) per catheter inserted.[91] Chlorhexidine for skin preparation is more effective than povidone-iodine in reducing catheter colonization and is the preferred antiseptic of choice.[92]

In a recent large multicenter cohort study involving 103 ICUs in 67 hospitals with more than 375,000 catheter-days observation, a combination of evidence-based intervention resulted in a large and sustained (up to 66%) reduction in rates of catheter-related bloodstream infection throughout the 18-month study period.[93] Five evidence-based procedures recommended by the CDC were the target interventions. The recommended procedures include: (1) hand washing, (2) using full-barrier precautions, (3) cleaning the skin with chlorhexidine, (4) avoiding the femoral site if possible, and (5) removing unnecessary catheters. Despite lack of randomization the result of this large well-conducted study is compelling, and the costs and efforts minor to implement that these five simple procedures should be universally adopted.[94]

Several studies have demonstrated that prophylactic antibiotics, especially by antibiotic lock, are effective in reducing catheter-related infections. Six studies in the hemodialysis population have shown that prophylactic ALT prevented catheter-related bacteremias by an overall 64–100% reduction in the frequency.[72] Other studies in the oncology population have shown similar protective efficacy.[95–97] However, the use of prophylactic antibiotics is discouraged because of the concern of encouraging antibiotic-resistant bacteria.[89]

It has been estimated that about 50% of the catheter-related infections result from microbes gaining access via the cutaneous surface, whereas the remainder arise from contamination of the hub and infusate. To reduce cutaneous mode of infection attempts have been made to apply topical antibiotics or antiseptic ointments to the catheter exit-site. Antibiotic ointments (bacitracin, neomycin, and polymyxin) to catheter-insertion site increases the rate of catheter colonization by fungi, promotes the emergence of antibiotic-resistant bacteria, does not lower catheter-related bloodstream infections, and are thus not recommended.[88] Mupirocin is a topical antibacterial ointment with demonstrated efficacy in eradicating *S. aureus* colonization (including MRSA). Several trials have been performed in the hemodialysis population with catheter-exit-site application or intranasally in patients with *S. aureus* colonization or in all subject, single-application regimens, or maintenance continuously or intermittently. In a recent meta-analysis of pooled trials with mupirocin in hemodialysis subjects, rate of *S. aureus* infections was reduced by 80% and *S. aureus* bacteremia by 78%.[98] Although both weekly mupirocin therapy for all patients undergoing dialysis and 3 monthly therapy targeting only patients with *S. aureus* nasal colonization can be cost saving (US$748,000–$1,000,000 per 1,000 patients on hemodialysis annually),[99] widespread use is not an accepted practice because of the risk of mupirocin resistance. Long-term continuous use of mupirocin should be discouraged as resistance emergence is a problem[100]; but targeted 3 monthly therapy with patients recurrently colonized should be more acceptable and needs further study. Povidone-iodine ointment topical application at the catheter-insertion site in hemodialysis have also been shown in a randomized trial to decrease catheter-related *S. aureus* infection and bacteremia,[101] and resistance development may not be a problem, but there is limited studies on this application. Use of silver-impregnated subcutaneous cuffs has been shown not to reduce catheter-related bloodstream infection and is not recommended.[88] Optimal dressing changes and most desirable dressing (gauze vs transparent material) are controversial with no set guidelines.[88] It has been my personal experience that the transparent dressings are associated with local blood collection at the insertion site (lack of pressure effect), and therefore more potentially at risk for exit-site infections.

There is much debate and controversy on the value of antimicrobial impregnated CVC in the prevention of catheter-related bloodstream infections. There are two commercially available antimicrobial impregnated CVCs; one uses a combination of minocycline and rifampin, and the other a combination of chlorhexidine and silver sulfadiazine. A previous meta-analysis[102] concluded that CVCs impregnated with chlorhexidine and silver sulfadiazine was efficacious in preventing bloodstream infection, and a further analysis demonstrated that their use was cost-effective.[103] Although use of antimicrobial impregnated CVCs have been recommended by the Hospital Infection Control Advisory Committee[104] for high-risk, prolonged use, concerns and debate continues over cost, emergence of antimicrobial resistance and questionable efficacy rates.

In a recent review of the benefit of antimicrobial impregnated CVCs McConnell et al.[105] found several methodological flaws of 11 trials and concluded that their clinical benefits are unproven, and that more rigorous studies were needed. Crinch and Makii[106] on the other hand, argued that there is sufficient scientific evidence from 19 randomized, controlled trials, 3 meta-analysis, and 2 cost-benefit analysis to support the clinical benefit of antimicrobial impregnated CVCs. Thus, they would recommend selective use of these specialized CVCs in situations or areas where catheter-related bloodstream infection remains high despite adherence to strict infection control practices.

There is some but limited data that antiseptic containing hubs can decrease the risk of CVC-related bacteria.[107,108] It is important that all catheters be removed as soon as it is no longer needed (not remain for convenience), as infection increases over time especially after 5–7 days. Routine changing of CVCs at fixed schedules (either over a guide wire or at a different site) is not recommended, as it has not been shown to reduce the infectious complications.[88]

## 10.4 Cardiovascular Device Infectious

### 10.4.1 Cardiac Devices and Infections

Implantation of various cardiac devices have increased dramatically in the past decade, as the mean age of the population increases and people live longer and are prone to increased cardiac diseases. These cardiac devices have been found to reduce symptoms and mortality rates in appropriate populations, and infectious complications are being recognized more frequently which are challenging and often difficult to treat. In a recent study from a large population-based database cardiac device implantation rates increased from 3.26 per 1,000 Medicare beneficiaries in 1990 to 4.64 implantation per 1,000 beneficiaries, an increase of 42% in 10 years ($p < 0.001$).[109] Cardiac device infections showed a larger increase, from 0.94 device infections per 1,000 beneficiaries in 1990 to 2.11 device infections per 1,000 beneficiaries in 1999, an increase of 124%.[109]

The variety of cardiac devices are also increasing over the years with advances in biotechnology, and infections of the following devices will be reviewed in this chapter; prosthetic heart values, pacemakers, implantable cardioverter defibrillator (ICD), and implantable left ventricular assist device (LVAD).

### 10.4.2 Trends in Prosthetic Valve Endocarditis

The incidence of prosthetic valve endocarditis (PVE) is increasing and represents 20–30% of all cases of infective endocarditis in large series.[110] The risk of PVE is estimated at 12 months to be 1%, and 2–3% at 60 months.[111] Bioprosthetic and mechanical valves are at similar risk of infection after 5 years, but mechanical valves maybe at a greater risk in the first 3 months after surgery.[112]

The largest database on PVE has recently been reported from an international prospective observational study conducted at 61 medical centers in 28 countries over 5 years.[113] Definite PVE (using Duke University diagnostic criteria) was present in 556 (20.1%) of 2,670 patients with infective endocarditis. *S. aureus* was the most common organism (23.0%), followed by CoNS (16.9%); which is in contrast to previous estimates that found CoNS as the most common cause of PVE.[114] Early cases of PVE (within 2 months of surgery) are usually hospital acquired and result from inoculation at surgery, or following catheter-related infections in the ICU. Microorganisms causing early PVE were (in earlier studies) most frequently CoNS, followed by *S. aureus*, *Enterococcus* spp, and gram-negative bacteria.[110] In the recent prospective cohort study, however, *S. aureus* was the commonest organism (35.9%) in early PVE, followed by CoNS (17.0%), culture negative (17.0%), *Enterococcus* spp. (7.5%), fungi (9.4%), gram-negative bacteria (5.6%), and streptococci (3.7%).[113]

Late PVE occurs at least 12 months after surgery, although some studies classify late PVE as occurring >2 months after surgery, are largely community acquired and similar in causation as native valve endocarditis. Intermediate occurring PVE between 2–12 months after surgery are a mixture of hospital and community-acquired episodes. In the large prospective cohort study[113] streptococci as a group caused (21.1%) of late PVE (predominantly *Viridans streptococci* and *Streptococcus bovis*), followed by CoNS (19.9%), *S. aureus* (18.4%), enterococcus spp. (12.7%), culture negative (12.4%), fungi (3.3%), and gram-negative bacilli were rare (1.2%).

Health care-associated infections have recently been found to significantly influence the clinical characteristics, microbial etiology, and outcome of PVE.[113] Health care-associated PVE was found in 36.5% of the overall cohort, and 71% of these cases occurred within the first year of valve implantation (the majority within 60 days).[113] Most cases of health care-associated PVE are nosocomial in origin (69.5%), and intravascular device infection probably accounted for just under half (42.9%). The etiology of health care-associated PVE shows a predominance of *S. aureus* (34%) and CoNS (25.6%), with low rates of enterococcal (9.4%) and viridans streptococcal (4.9%) infections,[113] as expected.

In PVE most series find that the aortic valve is involved most frequently, with both aortic valve and mitral valves affected in about 15% of cases.[110] Peri-annular extension and abscess formation are very common in PVE (50–100%), and are predictive of higher mortality, congestive heart failure, and the need for cardiac surgery. In the large international cohort study prosthetic aortic valve was infected in 69.1% and prosthetic mitral valve or ring in 50.4% of patients.[113]

Management of PVE can be difficult and often require a combination of medical and surgical therapy, especially in cases occurring <12 months after surgical implantation. No comparative studies exist to determine the most effective antimicrobial therapy for even the commonest causes of PVE. Guidelines have been published by the American Heart Association[115] and European Society of Cardiology[116] for treatment of PVE, for specific microorganisms based on in vitro susceptibility and limited animal models. It should be noted that the animal models on foreign-body-related infection are really soft tissue implantations, and no adequate or valid PVE animal model exits. In cases of strongly suspected or proven (by Duke's criteria) of PVE empiric therapy is often started with a combination of vancomycin, gentamicin, and oral rifampin until identification and susceptibility are available (especially in cases occurring <12 months after surgery).

Surgical management of PVE is a contentious issue in certain areas, but should be considered and discussed with the cardiovascular surgeon soon after the diagnosis. In the recent international cohort study of PVE[113] surgery was performed in 48.9% of patients during the index hospitalization, and the in-hospital mortality was 22.8%. The strongest predictors of mortality were persistent bacteremia (>7 days), heart failure, intracardiac abscess, stroke, and older age. Mortality was also greater in cases with *S. aureus* infection (adjusted O R, 1.73) and highest in the early PVE

(<2 months) and similar thereafter (personal communication with Andrew Wang). The guidelines for surgical therapy by the American Heart Association[114] did not differentiate between native valve and PVE, whereas the guidelines by the European Society of Cardiology[115] provided separate guidelines for PVE, which are somewhat different. The guidelines for surgical therapy for bacterial infective endocarditis in general are summarized in Table 10.4. The European guidelines[116] for surgical intervention in the management of PVE also include early PVE (<12 months after surgery), which is a contentious issue and not included as a primary indication in the American Heart Association guidelines.

Early PVE, especially caused by *S. aureus*, are commonly complicated by annular abscesses, severe vascular dysfunction or dehiscence, stroke, and congestive heart failure. Delaying surgery for the usual indications may result in poor operative risk and higher mortality, thus earlier surgical therapy has been proposed for *S. aureus* PVE. A previous retrospective study of 33 *S. aureus* PVE reported a survival benefit of early surgery regardless of the presence of cardiac complications.[117] However, in a recent analysis of 61 *S. aureus* PVE from merged database of an international collaboration, the overall mortality was 47.5%, early valve replacement was not

**Table 10.4** Indications for surgery in infective endocarditis (IE)

**Definite Indications**
- Severe refractory CHF; aortic or mitral insufficiency with ventricular failure
  (class I, level B evidence)
- Persistent bacteremia after 1 week of adequate therapy
  (class I, level B)
- 1 embolic events during the first 2 wks of therapy
  (class I, level B)
- Echo evidence of valve dehiscence, perforation, fistula or abscess ($\geq$ 1 cm), and periannular extension with conduction abnormalities
  (class I, level B)
- Fungal endocarditis (especially on left side) (class I, level C)
- Obstructive vegetations (class I, level C)

**Relative Indications**
- Left-sided IE with aggressive bacteria that respond poorly to antibiotics
  (*ie Serratia marcecens, Pseudomonas* spp., Q-fever etc)
- Large vegetations (>1 cm) on anterior mitral leaflet during the first 2 wks of therapy; or an increase in vegetation size with appropriate antibiotics (class II$_{a/b}$, level B/C)
- Severe acute aortic insufficiency without CHF, surgery within 6 months
- Persistent vegetations after systemic embolisation
- Tricuspid vegetations >2 cm after recurrent pulmonary emboli
- Early PVE (<12 months) with *S. aureus*
  Class II b, level controversial

The above guidelines are based on combination of the American Heart Association and European Society of Cardiology guidelines.[109,110] CHF = congestive heart failure; class I: conditions for which there is evidence and or general agreement; class II: conflicting evidence, and or divergence of opinion; class II a: weight of evidence/opinion in favor; class II b: usefulness less established by evidence/opinion. Level of evidence: level B – data derived from nonrandomized studies; level C = consensus opinion of experts associated with a significant survival benefit in the whole population.[118] But patients who developed cardiac complications and underwent early valve replacement had the lowest mortality rate (28.6%).

Since there has been no randomized, controlled study to assess the benefit of surgical therapy in infective endocarditis in general, recently propensity analyses have been used to control for bias in treatment assignment and prognostic imbalances to evaluate the value of surgical intervention. This type of analysis was recently applied to assess the impact of valve surgery in adults with complicated left-sided native valve endocarditis.[119] In this study surgical therapy was significantly associated with lower mortality and patients with moderate to severe congestive heart failure showed the greatest reduction in mortality (14% vs 51%, $p = 0.001$).[119] A similar propensity analysis has now been preformed on an international cohort of 367 patients with PVE.[120] Surgical therapy was preformed in 148 (42%) of patients, and in hospital mortality was similar for patients treated with surgery compared to medical therapy above (25% and 23.4%, respectively). After adjustment for factors related to surgical intervention, brain embolism and *S. aureus* were independently associated with mortality, with a trend toward benefit for surgery (OR 0.56, 95% CI 0.23–1.36).[120] Timing of the survival end-points (in hospital vs 90 days, respectively) may have affected the outcome, as in another single center study of 66 patients a survival benefit of surgery for PVE was apparent only in long-term follow-up (survival at 10 years was 28% in the medically treated group versus 58% in the surgically treated groups ($p = 0.04$).[121] Progressive prosthesis dysfunction and valve failure at a later date appears to account for a major proportion of the later high mortality in the medically treated group.

There has been no significant progress for prevention of PVE in the past several decades. Although antibiotic prophylaxis is still recommended for dental procedure to prevent PVE,[122] there is no proof of benefit and it would not likely decrease the rates of PVE. It has been recommended that before prosthetic valve implantation to optimize dental hygiene and health. Since perioperative wound infection is a significant risk factor for PVE,[123] and likely catheter-related infections – methods to reduce these complications should be maximized. Recently, the artificial valve Endocarditis Reduction trial (AVERT) was designed to compare a new silzone sewing ring, designed to reduce infection, with the standard sewing ring on a ST – Jude mechanical heart valve.[124] This was the largest heart valve randomized, controlled trial ever planned (4,400 valve patients followed for 4 years), but it was stopped prematurely because of increased para-valvular leak associated with the silzone-coated mechanical valves.[124] The medical management of PVE with combination of antibiotics is discussed in Chapter 12.

### 10.4.3 Infections of ICD, LVAD and Pacemakers

The incidence of non-valvular cardiac device-related infections varies widely according to the device. Even for pacemaker-related infections the incidence varies from 0.13% to 19.9%, yet ICD (which is similar in many respects to pacemaker) rates of infections is only 0.0–3.2%.[125] Several factors that may account for wide-variation in the incidence of these infections include technical expertise and experience of the surgeons, selection of patients and age-related comorbidities, and site of implantation.

Worldwide there are estimated to be over 3.25 million patients with permanent pacemakers, with infections of up to 19.9% with abdominal implantation and only 0.13% with prepectoral implantation.[126] Pacemaker-infective endocarditis is rare and in a population-based study in France is estimated to be 550 cases/million recipients per year.[127] Rates of ICD infection (0.7–1.2%) are also lower with prepectoral as compared to abdominal generator placement.[125] The rate of ICD infection appears to be increasing higher than the number of ICD implantations,[126] but this may be secondary to increased recognition and improved survival of recipients resulting in more days at risk for infection.

In the pediatric population, for instance, in a study of 385 pacemakers (224 epicardial and 181 endocardial) there were 30 (7.8%) pacemaker infections and 2 (0.5%) bacteremias.[128] The large majority of cardiac device infections are likely due to pocket site contamination with skin colonizing bacteria at the time of surgical placement. Hematogenous seeding from a distant focus, particularly *S. aureus*, can account for late onset infection. Pacemaker and ICD infections can present with local manifestation (signs and symptoms of inflammation at the site of device placement) with or without systemic symptoms of fever. Systemic manifestation of fever alone is the usual hallmark of pacemaker or ICD lead-electrode infection, associated with continuous bacteremia and related to endocarditis and/or septic phlebitis.

The majority of patients with pacemaker or ICD infection present with local findings (erythema, tenderness, and/or drainage) confined to the generator pocket (69%), 20% with local and systemic symptoms, and 11% with systemic symptoms alone.[126] Pacemaker or electrode endocarditis has been reported in approximately 10% of the cases of pacemaker/ICD-related infections.[125] However, electrode-lead endocarditis occurs in less than 1% of pacemaker or ICD implants (0.58% and 0.65%, respectively in a recent study).[129]

Superficial cellulitis of the wound (implantation site) usually occur within the first two weeks after surgery, usually no drainage is present and blood cultures are negative, and the infection generally resolve with intravenous antibiotics (narrow spectrum cephalosporin or beta-lactamase-resistant penicillin).[126] Pocket infection of the pulse generator or battery-pack typically develops within the first 6 months of implantation, or after device manipulation. Even though the infection may manifest itself several months after implantation, there is evidence the organism (usually CoNS or diphtheroids) was inoculated at the time of surgery.[130] Infection with more-virulent pathogen such as *S. aureus* usually present much earlier after surgery. Pocket infection occurring after 1 year of implantation is often associated with recent surgical revision (i.e., battery change), erosion through the skin from inadequate fixation, and occasionally bacteremia from another source. Pocket infection, unlike superficial cellulitis, requires removal of the lead-generator plus antibiotics, and a new pacemaker/ICD in a remote location (opposite chest wall) after resolution of the local wound infection.

Microorganism from the pacemaker/ICD pocket can spread along the electrode tip and adjacent endocardium. Thus, pocket infection is the most common factor leading to pacemaker/ICD endocarditis, with similar organisms (staphylococci and corynebacteria). Late onset electrode endocarditis can also result from hematogenous seeding of *S. aureus*, streptococci (including viridans group), enterococci, and rarely gram-negative coliforms.[122] Clinical manifestations are mainly fever with or without pulmonary infiltrates (as seen with usual right-sided endocarditis), with persistent bacteremia and 60% of patient have no focal signs of pocket infection.[131] In a recent prospective study of 224 patients suspected with pacing system-related infections S. *epidermidis* and other CoNS caused 66.9% and 29.5% of the infections, respectively.[132] Thirty-three patients had positive blood cultures (Duke Criteria for endocarditis) and 30 had the same organisms on the lead culture. Twenty-five percent had >1 microorganisms from the lead cultures.[132] The diagnosis can be confirmed by positive blood cultures (three or more separated by hours), and echocardiogram often demonstrates a vegetation on the tip of the electrode and sometimes on the adjacent endocardium and valves.[125] TEE is much more sensitive (>95%) than transthoracic echocardiography (TTE) (<30%) in detecting vegetations.[125]

Management of pacemaker/ICD endocarditis is with appropriate bactericidal intravenous antibiotics (according to susceptibility results) for 4–6 weeks, and removal of the entire device. Although there are no comparative prospective trials on medical versus medical/surgical therapy, the overall data from retrospective and prospective observational studies shows high failure or relapse rate without complete removal of the hardware. Furthermore, patients receiving medical therapy alone compared to those treated medically and surgically have a higher mortality rate.

In a previous retrospective case series of 123 patients with pacemaker/ICD infection (97% intravenously implanted leads), only (0.86%) of 117 patients who underwent removal of the entire system had infection relapse versus 3 of 6 (50%) without complete hardware removal had relapse ($p = 0.03$).[133] In a smaller prospective study of 31 patients with pacemaker/ICD endocarditis the only prognostic factor for failure of treatment or mortality was the absence of surgical treatment ($p = <0.0001$).[129] Failure to remove infected pacemaker/ICD has been associated with almost threefold (47.6% vs 16.7%) increased risk of dying.[131] In an earlier review it was found that the mortality rate in patients with pacemaker/ICD endocarditis treated with antibiotics alone range from 31% to 66% versus 13–33% (mean 18%) in those treated with combined antibiotics and electrode removal.[134]

In patients with pacemaker/ICD for decades the electrode can become embedded and fixated by fibrocollagenous tissue. Several different techniques for electrode extraction are now available, rather than cardiotomy which carries a higher surgical risk. The options now include "locking stylet" affixed close to the distal end of the electrode, telescoping sheath to disrupt fibrous attachment mechanically and laser sheath to photo-ablate the fibrous attachment. These techniques result in lead extraction of 81–93%, and major complications (such as tamponade) can occur in up to 3.3%.[135] In a randomized trial comparing laser sheath to non-laser telescoping sheath for lead extraction in 301 patients, complete lead removal was achieved in 94% in the laser group, and only 64% in the non-laser group ($p = 0.001$).[136] However, potentially life-threatening complications occurred in three patients in the laser group and none in the non-laser group (not statistically significant). The present data indicate that transvenous pacemaker-lead removal is safe even in large vegatations.[137]

Patients with removal of pacemaker/ICD should have re-evaluation to determine need for re-implantation, as a significant proportion (13–52%) may no longer require pacing support.[125] Those requiring re-implantation of the device should be done at a separate site when the patient is afebrile and no longer bacteremic.

Although antibiotic prophylaxis is commonly used for pacemaker/ICD implantation there are no large multicenter randomized, controlled trials to prove the efficacy. In a meta-analysis of 7 randomized trials with 2,023 patients (new implants or replacements) systemic antibiotic prophylaxis (semi-synthetic penicillin or cefazolin), appeared to have a consistent protective effect ($p = 0.0046$) in preventing short-term pocket infection, skin erosion, or septicemia.[138]

As more patients require heart transplantation and with the limited availability of organs, a growing number of patients require the implantation of mechanical assist device. Left ventricular assist device (LVAD) is now used routinely in several centers, pending organ transplantation. High rates of infection (25–70%) and recurrent infections have limited the long-term use of these devices. The risk of infection of LVAD increased with the duration of use and in one review of 46 cases it was 85% after >2 weeks.[139] In a relatively large study of 88 LVAD implanted in 82 patients over a 6.5 year period, duration ranged from 0 to 434 days, 66% had infectious complication but only 38% were device-related (pocket of the device, device itself, or from the driveline).[140]

Another series of 36 LVADs implanted in 35 patients, with a mean duration of 73 ± 60 days, reported surgical site infections in 16 (45.7%) with a rate of 6.2 infections per 1,000 LVAD days; and 9 (56.2%) were deep tissue or organ space infections; and 2 bloodstream infections (0.8 cases per 1,000 LVAD days).[141] In a retrospective series of 39 patients with LVAD implantation 31 (79.5%) developed 99 nosocomial infections (4.9 per 100 support days).[142] The lungs were the most frequently involved site (31.3%), septic shock occurred in 8 (25.8%) of 31 infected patients with 26.2% episodes of bacteremia (14 primary bloodstream infections), and 20.3% developed canula infections.[142] In a randomized prospective study of long-term LVAD (68 patients) versus optimal medical therapy (61 patients) in subjects with end-stage heart failure, within 3 months after transplantation infection of the pulsatile assist device occurred in 28%.[143] Although most of the infections were in the driveline and pocket and were treated with local measures and antibiotics, fatal sepsis was common. Sepsis caused 41% of the 41 deaths in the LVAD group, but only one (2%) of 54 deaths among the controls. Drive-line or pocket infection occurred at a rate of 0.41 per patient year and pump/internal lining at a rate of 0.23

per patient year.[143] However, the current pulsatile volume-displacement devices have limitations (including large pump size, which may increase the potential for infections, and limited long-term mechanical durability). Development of a smaller continuous-flow pumps are a new type of LVAD that can provide effective hemodynamic support for at least 6 months. In a recent prospective (uncontrolled) study of 133 patients implanted with these new LVADs, localized infections not related to device implantation occurred in 28% of patients, whereas device-related infection was observed in 14% of patients, with all infections involving the percutaneous lead and none involving the pump pocket.[144] Five (20%) of the 25 patients that died in the first 180 days after device implantation was secondary to sepsis.

Infections of LVADs can manifest in three different ways[125]: (1) driveline infection, the most common type present with local inflammation and drainage at the exit site; (2) pocket site infection which causes local inflammation; (3) LVAD endocarditis (least frequent) is infection of the valves and/or the internal lining of the device, associated with continuous bacteremia. Patients may present with mixed infections involving more than one part of the device. The most common microorganisms causing infections of LVAD are *Staphylococcus* species, *Enterococcus* spp., gram-negative bacilli, and *Candida* spp.

Drive-line infection may or may not be associated with systemic signs of inflammation, but usually there are local inflammation and drainage at the exit site. Usually management consists of local therapy (with antiseptics) and systemic antibiotics.[145] Refractory exit-site infection can be managed by replacing the distal portion of the driveline in a new tunnel, and aggressive surgical excision of the neoepithelialized drainage tract has been proposed.[146]

Pump pocket infection can be indolent with CoNS infection with local fluid collection, slight tenderness with or without much erythema, and low-grade fever. However, persistent drainage from the drive-line exit site can be a sign of deeper pocket infection. More acute symptoms with florid signs of inflammation over the pocket with fever are more common with virulent organisms such as *S. aureus* or gram-negative bacilli infection. Ultrasound of the pocket and aspiration or drainage of any infected fluid should be performed. Optimal management should consist of systemic antibiotics, deplanting the device, and relocation of a new pump at a different site. Attempts to salvage the device with conservative management including drainage and irrigation of the pocket with implantation of antibiotic impregnated beads in the pocket,[143] chronic suppressive systemic antibiotic therapy, muscle flap, and omental and pectoralis transposition flaps have been used with variable temporary success until cardiac transplantaioin.[140,147]

Infection of the blood contacting surfaces or LVAD endocarditis is the least common but most life-threatening complication of LVAD. The major clues to the diagnosis of LVAD endocarditis include persistent or continuous bacteremia or fungemia, septic embolization often without evidence of vegetations on the native heart valves, new incompetence of the pump inflow or outflow valves, and absence of other sources for bacteremia or fungemia. Management includes specific systemic antimicrobial therapy and removal/replacement of the entire mechanical circulatory device if feasible (often not an option) or urgent cardiac transplantation, if a suitable donor is available. Available evidence indicate that persistent bacteremia or fungemia is not a contradiction to cardiac transplantation.[125,145]

## 10.5 Vascular Grafts

It is estimated that about 450,000 vascular grafts are inserted annually in the United States, with a projected 16,000 infected implants annually.[148] The estimated average cost for each infected implant is around $40,000 (US) or US$640,000,000 per year combined. The rates of infection and complications differ according to the three main types of prosthetic vascular grafts (arteriovenous, femoropopliteal, and aortic). More than 5% of arteriovenous grafts for hemodialysis become infected, and in some series up to 35% of hemodialysis with polytetrafluoroethylene grafts lose their access secondary to infection.[149] *S. aureus* is the most common causative agent and the risk increases in patients with chronic nasal colonization. Typically treatment consists of systemic antibiotics and removal of the AV graft, temporary venous access for dialysis and placement of another graft elsewhere. Since many hemodialysis dependent patients have limited venous access, in situ cryopreserved human vein allograft in one operative procedure has been used with low incidence of reinfection.[149] Partial graft excision of infected grafts is associated with much higher recurrent infection than total graft excision (19.8% vs 0%, $p = 0.03$).[150]

Infection of femoropopliteal graft occurs in about 4% of patients[148] and can result in loss of limb and life. Most patients do not have fever or bacteremia but they commonly present with local wound drainage, inflammation or abscess, local hematoma, or pseudoaneurysm and thrombosis. Usual implicated organisms include *Staphylococcus* species, *Enterococcus* spp, gram-negative bacilli, and sometimes mixed coliforms with anaerobes. Traditionally, femoropopliteal graft infection was treated with intravenous antibiotics for 4–6 weeks and a two-stage surgical procedure. This consisted of removal of the entire graft, with an axillary-femoral venous graft as temporary measure until a permanent new graft could be inserted after resolution of the infection. More recently a one-stage procedure for graft excision and revascularization with autologous venous conduits, prosthetic grafts, or cryopreserved homograft has been performed.[148,151] Femoral graft infection limited at a unilateral groin can also be managed by excision of the infected graft material at the groin and using a femoro-femoral bypass with an infrascrotal perineal approach.[152] Unfortunately no prospective comparative trials have compared the various surgical treatments of the different types of vascular-graft infection.

The mortality rates associated with infected aorto iliac or aortofemoral bypass grafts ranged from 25% to 75% and is higher than femoropopliteal graft infection.[153] Overall the incidence of infection of these more proximal grafts is 1–6%. Similar principles of medical and surgical therapy apply to these grafts as in femoropopliteal infected grafts. In selected cases of infected aorto-iliac or aortofemoral grafts (especially with low-virulent organisms such as CoNS and diphtheroids) graft salvage have been accomplished with muscle flap surgery and systemic intravenous antibiotics.[153,154]

Infection of aortic grafts occur in 1–2% of patients and can result from implantation of bacteria at the time of surgery, subsequently from hematogenous seeding of bacteria from another source, and occasionally from communication with the small or large bowel. These infections are associated with high mortality and morbidity, and are a challenge to diagnose and manage. Most patients with infected aortic grafts will have constitutional symptoms of fever, malaise, poor appetite, abdominal discomfort and weight loss. However, confirmation of diagnosis is often difficult and bacteremia may or may not be present (no more than 50% of patients). Patients with abdominal aortic graft presenting with upper or lower gastrointestinal hemorrhage should be suspected to have graft infection and enteric fistula. Investigations to confirm aortic graft infection (besides multiple blood cultures), include computerized tomography (CT), magnetic resonance (MR), and upper or lower intestinal endoscopy for those presenting with gastrointestinal bleeding; duplex ultrasonic scanning and arteriography. CT and MR have high sensitivity and specificity in advanced graft infections but are considerably lower in early and low-grade infections.[155] Findings on imaging indicative of graft infection include ectopic gas collection around the graft, perigraft fluid collection (especially if increasing), and pseudoaneurysm. Perigraft fluid persistence beyond 3 months after surgery is suspicious of infection. In cases of graft-enteric fistula, the prosthetic material or fistulous tract can sometimes by visualized at gastroduodenoscopy. Nuclear imaging has also been used to diagnose infected abdominal vascular graft. In the last 10 years most studies have used technician ($^{99m}$Tc) labeled leucocyte scan with the best results (sensitivity 53–100%, and specificity 85–100%), as compared to CT imaging with sensitivity of 75% and specificity of 56.6%.[156] Removal of the infected aortic graft and performing extra-anatomic bypass, with prolonged systemic antibiotics for 6–12 weeks or longer, results in acceptable outcomes, but mortality rates are high because of persistent infection or aortic stump rupture. In-situ prosthetic graft replacement or omental transposition has been used but control of the infection has occasionally been achieved. In-situ replacement with a cryopreserved aortic allograft considered to be resistant against infection has recently been performed.

In a case series of 68 patients with abdominal infected aortic graft the early postoperative (within 30 days) mortality was 16%, and later mortality (after 30 days) of 25%.[157] The presence of aortoenteric fistula was a predictor of early perioperative mortality. Eleven patients were treated with fresh and 57 with cryopreserved homograft. At 36 months after surgery the actuarial survival was 57% and the actuarial patency of the allograft was 41%.[157] There was no difference in outcome between fresh versus cryopreserved homograft, but the sample size was too small. A systematic review and meta-analysis of treatments for aortic graft infection recently analyzed pooled results of 37 clinical studies.[158] After adjustment for tests of heterogeneity the following outcomes were reported for different modalities of surgical intervention: (1) extra-anatomic bypass ($N = 459$) resulted in 8% amputation, 25% conduit failure, 6% reinfection, 18% early mortality, and 24%

late mortality; (2) rifampin-bonded prosthesis ($N = 96$) resulted in 0% amputation, 2% conduit failure, 7% reinfection, 7% early mortality, and 16% late mortality; (3) cryopreserved allograft ($N = 616$) resulted in 3% amputation, 9% conduit failure, 3% reinfection, 14% early mortality, and 14% late mortality; autogenous vein resulted in 8% amputation, 17% conduit failure; 1% reinfection, 10% early mortality, and 14% late mortality.[158] The results of this review suggest that extra-anatomic bypass should not remain as the standard surgical treatment. Although there are not much differences between the other procedures the greater experience with cryopreserved allograft would lend support for using this as the preferred choice. More data and experience is needed for the rifampin-bonded prosthesis as the results to date looks very promising.

Other conservative surgical management for infected aortic graft has been reported in small numbers of selected patients. This include complete or partial graft preservation with infrarenal aorto-iliac grafts with use of surgical drainage and irrigation with or without subtotal graft excision, and 6 weeks intravenous antibiotics with good results in 7 of 9 patients after a mean follow-up of 7.6 years.[159] Another report of salvage surgery in 9 patients with ascending aortic graft infection utilized muscle flap to wrap around the infected grafts and fill the dead space, and were able to clear the infection in all patients but with two later deaths.[160]

Endovascular grafts are becoming more popular especially for high surgical risk patients with abdominal aortic aneurysm. A recent review and survey of 40 international centers of vascular and endovascular surgery identified 62 cases of aorto-iliac infected endovascular grafts (0.4% frequency of endograft infection).[161] In 35% of patients the presenting symptoms were vague and nonspecific, and 63% eventfully presented with abdominal abscess, groin fistula, and septic embolization. The majority (49.79%) of patents were treated with surgical excision and antibiotics with an operative mortality of 16.3%. Conservative management (without surgical excision) was performed on 11 patients with mortality of 36.4%.[161] *S. aureus* was the most common infecting organism (54.5%) and the mean follow-up was ≤48 weeks.

## 10.6 Future Directions

The ideal vascular-graft material that would mimic native blood vessels, thus have low risk of infection with greater chance of cure with conservative management, has been widely sought. Autologous tissue-engineered blood vessels with physiologic mechanical properties have been developed using a technique termed sheet-based tissue engineering.[162] The vessels are created with the use of autologous fibroblasts and endothelial cells harvested from a small biopsy specimen of skin and superficial vein, with no synthetic or foreign materials.

Preliminary report on the use of these tissue-engineered blood vessels in ten patients on hemodialysis for arteriovenous sheets appears to be promising.[163] This pilot study demonstrated that tissue-engineered blood vessels could withstand the stress of arterial produced by arteriovenous fistula for at least 3 months and up to 13 months. This is an important milestone for cardiovascular engineering and larger, longer-term studies are eagerly awaited.

Traditional treatment of infections based on compounds that kill or inhibit bacterial growth are often ineffective in chronic and foreign-body-related infections. The discovery of bacterial communication system (quorum-sensing systems), which orchestrate important temporal events during the infection process, offers future means of therapy for biofilm infection other than microbial growth inhibition.[164] Natural compounds are available to over-ride bacterial signaling that are unlikely to pose selective pressure for development of resistant mutants. Recent animal experiments (mouse pulmonary model of chronic *P. aeruginosa* infection) have shown promising results of interruption of quorum signaling by a furanone compound (reduced bacterial load and improved clearing).[164] A synthetic antimicrobial peptide, bactericidal peptide 2, is also a promising novel agent for future studies as it showed potent in vivo activity in a murine model of *S. epidermidis* biomaterial-associated infection.[165]

# References

1. Schierholz, J.M., Beuth, J., (2001), Implant infections: A haven for opportunistic bacteria. J. Hosp. Infect. 49: 87–93.
2. Costerton, J.W., Stewart, P.S., Greenberg, E.P., (1999), Bacterial biofilms: A common cause of persistent infections. Science 284: 1318–1322.
3. Donlan, R.M., Costerton, J.W. (2002), Biofilms: Survival mechanisms of clinically relevant microorganisms. Clin. Microbiol. Rev. 15: 167–193.
4. Costerton, W., Veeh, R., Shirtliff, M., Passmore, M., Post, C., Ehreich, G., (2003), The application of biofilm science to the study and control of chronic bacterial infections. J. Clin. Invest. 112: 1466–1477.
5. Davies, D.G., Geesey, G.G., (1995), Regulation of alginate biosynthesis gene algc in *Pseudomonas aeruginosa* during biofilm development in continuing culture. Appl. Environ. Microbiol. 61: 866–867.
6. Suci, P.A., Mittelman, M.W., Yu, F.P., Geesey, G.G., (1994), Investigation of ciprofloxacin penetration into *Pseudomonas aeruginosa* biofilms. Antimicrob. Agents Chemother. 38: 2125–2133.
7. Stewart, P.S., (1996), Theoretical aspects of antibiotic diffusion into microbial biofilms. Antimicrob. Agents Chemother. 40: 2517–2522.
8. Sauer, K., Camper, A.K., Ehrlich, G.D., Costerton, J.W., Davies, D.G., (2002), *Pseudomonas aeruginosa* displays multiple phenotypes during development as a biofilm. J. Bacteriol. 184: 1140–1154.
9. Wagman, G.H., Bailey, J.V., Weinstein, M.J., (1975), Binding of aminoglycoside antibiotics to filtration materials. J. Antimicrob. Agents Chemother. 7: 316–319.
10. Schierholz, J.M., Beuth, J., Pulveren, G., (1999), Adherent bacteria and activity of antibiotics. J. Antimicrob. Chemother. 43: 158–160.
11. Kaplan, S.S., Basfort, R.E., Kormos, R.L., (1990), Biomaterial-associated impairment of local neutrophil function. Am. Soc. Artificial Int. Organ Transplant. J. 36: M 172–175.
12. Zimmerli, W., Lew, P.D., Waldvogel, F.A., (1984), Pathogenesis of foreign body infections: evidence of a local granulocyte defect. J. Clin. Invest. 73: 1191–1200.

13. Shanbhag, A., Yang, J., Lilien, J., Black, J., (1992), Decreased neutrophils respiratory burst on exposure to cobaltchrome alloy and polysterene in vitro. J. Biomed. Mat. Res. 26: 185–195.
14. Zimmerli, W., Waldvogel, F.A., Vaudaux, P., Nydegger, U.F., (1982), Pathogenesis of foreign bosy infection: description and characteristics of an animal model. J. Infect. Dis. 146: 187–197.
15. Myrvik, Q.N., Wagner, W., Barth, E., Wood, P., Gristina A.G., (1989), Effects of extracellular slime produced by *Staphylococcus epidermidis* on oxidative responses of rabbit alveolar macrophages. J. Invest. Surg. 2: 381–389.
16. Johnson, G.M., Lee, D.A., Regelmann, W.E., Gray, E.D., Peters, G., Quie, P.G., (1986), Interference with granulocyte function by *Staphylococcus epidermidis* slime. Infect. Immun. 54: 13–20.
17. Modun, B., Williams, P., Pike, N.J., (1992), Cell envelope proteins of *S.epidermidis* grown in vivo in a peritoneal chamber implant. Infect. Immune. 60: 2551–2553.
18. Noble, M.A., Grant, S.K., Hajen, E., (1990), Characterization of a neutrophils inhibitor factor from clinically significant *S epidermidis* infection.. J. Infect. Dis. 162: 909–913.
19. Gray, E.D., Verstegen, M., Peters, G., Regelman, W.E., (1984), Effect of extracellular slime substance from *Staphylococcus epidermidis* on the human cellular response. Lancet 1: 365–367.
20. Tang, L., Eaton, J.W., (1995), Inflammatory responses to biomaterials. Am. J. Clin. Pathol. 103: 466–471.
21. Henke, P.K., Bergamini, T.M., Garrison, J.R., Brittian, K.R., Peytom, J.C., Lam, T.M., (1997), *Staphylococcus epidermidis* graft infection is associated with locally suppressed major histocompatibility complex class II and elevated MAC-1 expression. Arch. Surg. 132: 894–902.
22. Henke, P.K., Bergamini, T.M., Brittian, K.R., Polk, H.C.Jr., (1997), Prostaglandin $E_2$ modulates monocyte MH-II(Ia) suppression in biomaterial infection. J. Surg. Res. 69: 372–378.
23. Ankersmit, H.J., Edwards, N.M., Schuster, M., John, R., Kocher, A., Rose, E.A., Oz, M., Itescu, S., (1999), Quantitative changes in T-cell population after left ventricular assist device implantation: Relationship to T-cell apoptosis and soluble CD95. Circulation 100 (Suppl 19): II211–II215.
24. Rothenburger, M., Wilhelm, M., Hammel, D., Schmid, C., Plenz, G., Tjan, T.D.T, Baba, H., Schlter, B., Scheld, H.H., Deng, M.C., Erren. M., (2001), Immune response in the early postoperative period after implantation of a left-ventricular assist device system. Transplant. Proc. 33: 1955–1957.
25. Itescu, S., Ankersmit, H.J., Kocher, A.A., Schuster, M.D., (2000), Immunobiology of left ventricular assist devices. Prog. Cardiovasc. Dis. 43: 67–80.
26. Sapatnekar, S., Kao, W.J., Anderson, J.M., (1997), Leucocyte-biomaterial interactions in the presence of *Staphylococcus epidermidis*: Flow cytometric evaluation of leukocyte activation. J. Biomed. Mater. Res. 1535: 409–420.
27. Ceri, H., Olson, M.E., Strenich, C., Read, R.R., Morck, D, Buret, A., (1999), The Calgary Biofilm Device: new technology for rapid determination of antibiotic susceptibies of bacterial biofilms. J. Clin. Microbiol. 37: 1771–1776.
28. Williams, I., Venables, W.A., Lloyd, D., Paul, F., Critchley, I., (1997), The effects of adherence to silicone surfaces on antibiotic susceptibility in *Staphylococcus aureus*. Microbiology 143: 2407–2413.
29. Larsen, T., Fiehn, N.E., (1996), Resistance of *Streptococcus sanguis* biofilms to antimicrobial agents. APMIS 104: 280–284.
30. Vorachit, M., Lam, K, Jayanetra, P., Costerton, J.W., (1993), Resistance of *Pseudomonas pseudomallei* growing as a biofilm on silastic disks to ceftazidime and cotrimoxazole. Antimicrob. Agents Chemother. 37: 2000–2002.

31. Anderl, J.N., Franklin, M.J., Stewart, P.S., (2000), Role of antibiotic penetration limitation in *Klebsiella pneumoniae* biofilm resistance to ampicillin and ciprofloxacin. Antimicrob. Agents Chemother. 44: 1818–1824.
32. Stewart, P.S., Costerton, J.W., (2001), Antibiotic resistance of bacteria in biofilms. Lancet; 358: 135–138.
33. Nichols, W.W., Dorrington, S.M., Slack, M.P.E. Walmsley, H.L., (1988), Inhibition of tobramycin diffusion by binding to alginate. Antimicrob. Agents Chemother. 32: 518–523.
34. Shigeta, M., Tanaka, G., Komatsuzawa, H., Sugai, M., Suginaka, H., Hsui, T., (1997), Permeation of antimicrobial agents through *Pseudomonas aeruginosa* biofilms: A simple method. Chemotherapy; 43: 340–345.
35. Brooun, A., Liu, S., Lewis, K., (2000), A dose-response study of antibiotic resistance in *Pseudomonas aeruginosa* biofilms. Antimicrob. Agents Chemother. 44: 640–646.
36. de Beer, D., Stoodley, P., Roe, F., Lewandowski, Z., (1994), Effects of biofilm structure on oxygen distribution and mass transport. Biotechnol. Bioeng. 43: 1131–1138.
37. Zhang, T.C., Bishop, P.L., (1996), Evaluation of substrate and pH effects in a nitrifying biofilm. Wat. Environ. Res. 68: 1107–1115.
38. Evans, D.J., Allison, D.G., Brown, M.R.W., Gilbert, P., (1990) Effect of growth-rate on resistance of gram-negative biofilms to cetrimide. J. Antimicrob. Chemother. 26: 473–478.
39. DuGuid. I.G., Evans, E., Brown, M.R.W., Gilbert, P., (1990), Growth-rate-dependent killing by ciprofloxacin of biofilm-derived *Staphylococcus epidermidis*: Evidence for cell-cycle dependency. J. Antimicrob. Chemother. 30: 791–802.
40. Anwar, H., Strap, J.L., Chen, K., Costerton, J.W., (1992), Dynamic interactions of biofilms of mucoid *Pseudomonas aeruginosa* with tobramycin and piperacillin. Antimicrob. Agents Chemother. 36: 1208–1214.
41. Dagostino, L., Goodman, A.E., Marshall, K.C., (1991), Physiological responses induced in bacteria adhering to surfaces. Biofouling 4: 113–119.
42. Crnich, C.J., Maki, D.G., (2001), The role of intravascular devices in sepsis. Curr. Infect. Dis. Rep. 3: 496–506.
43. Crnich, C.J., Maki, D.G., (2005), Infections caused by intravascular devices: epidemiology, pathogenesis, diagnosis, prevention, and treatment. In: APIC text of Infection Control and Epidermiology. Vol. I, 2nd ed. Washington, DC: Association for Professionals in Infection Control and Epidemiology, pp. 2421–2426.
44. Pittet, D., Tarara, D., Wenzel, R.P., (1994), Nosocomial bloodstream infection in critically ill patients: Excess length of stay, extra costs, and attributable mortality. JAMA 271: 1598–1601.
45. Renaud, B., Brun-Bruisson, C., ICU-Bacteremia Study Group, (2001), Outcomes of primary and catheter-related bacteremia: a cohort and case control study in critically ill patients. Am. J. Respire. Crit. Care Med. 163: 1584–1590.
46. Orsi, G.B., Di Stefano, C., Noah, N., (2002), Hospital acquired, laboratory confirmed bloodstream infections: increased length of stay and direct costs. Infect. Control Hosp. Epidemiol. 23: 190–197.
47. Blot, S.I., Depuydt, P., Annemans, L., Benoit, D., Hoste, E., De Waele, J.J., Decruyenaere, J., Vogelaers, D., Colardyn, F., Vanderwoude, K.H., (2005), Clinical and economic outcomes in critically ill patients with nosocomial catheter-related bloodstream infections. Clin. Infect. Dis. 41: 1591–1598.
48. National Nosocomial Infection Surveillance, (2002), National nosocomial infection surveillance (NNIS) system report, data summary from January 1992 to June 2002, issued August 2002. Am. J. Infect. Control. 30: 458–475.
49. Maki, d.G., Kluger, D.M., Crnich, C.J., (2006), The risk of bloodstream infection in adults with different intravascular devices: a systematic review of 200 published prospective studies. Mayo Clin. Proc. 81: 1159–1171.
50. Peters, G., Locci, R., Pulverer, G., (1982), Adherence and growth of coagulase-negative staphylococci on surfaces of intravenous catheters. J. Infect. Dis. 146: 479–482.

51. Rupp, M.E., Ulphani, J.S., Fey, P.D., Bartscht, K., Mack, D., (1999), Characterization of the importance of polysaccharide intercellular, hemagglutinin of *Staphylococcus epidermidis* in the pathogenesis of biomaterial-based infection in a mouse foreign body infection model. Infect. Immun. 67: 2627–2632.
52. Darouiche, R.O., (2001), Device-associated infections: A macroproblem that starts with microadherence. Clin. Infect Dis. 33: 1567–1572.
53. Galdbart, J.-O., Allignet, J., Tung, H.-S., Ryden, C. E.L., Solh, N., (2000), Screening for *Staphylococcus epidermidis* markers discriminating between skin-flora strains and those responsible for infections of joint prosthesis. J. Infect. Dis. 182: 351–355.
54. Vandescastede, S.J., Peetemans, W.E., Merckx, R., Van Eldere, J., (2003), Expression of biofilm-associated genes in *Staphylococcus epidermidis* during in vitro and in vivo foreign body infections. J. Infect. Dis. 188: 730–737.
55. Wang, L., Li, M., Dong, D., Bach, T.-H.L., Sturdevant, D.E., Vuong, C., Otto, M., Gao, Q., (2008), SarZ is a key regulator of biofilm formation and virulence in *Staphylococcus epidermidis* J. Infect. Dis. 1971: 1254–1262.
56. Darouiche, R.O., Landon, G.C., Patti, J.M., Nguyen, L.L., Fernau, R.C., Mc Devitt, D., Greene, C., Foster, T., Klima, M., (1997), Role of *Staphylococcus aureus* surface adhesions in orthopedic device infection. J. Med. Microbiol. 46: 75–79.
57. Green, C., Mc Devitt, D., Francois, P., Vaudaux, P.E., Lew, D.P., Foster, T.J., (1995), Adhesion properties of mutants of *Staphylococcus aureus* defective in the fibronecting-binding proteins and studies on the expression of fnb genes. Mol. Microbiol. 17: 1143–1145.
58. Matsaniotis, N.S., Syriopoulou, V.P., Theodoridou, M.C., Tzanetou, K.G., Mostrou, G.I., (1984), Enterobacter sepsis in infants and children due to contaminated intravenous fluid. Infect. Control 5: 471–477.
59. Centers for Disease Control and Prevention, (1998), *Enterobacter cloucae* blood stream infections associated with contaminated prefilled saline syringes—California, November 1998. MMWR. Morb. Mortal. Wkly Rep. 47: 959–960.
60. Maki, D.G., Rhame, F.S., Mackel, D.C., Bennett, J.V., (1976), Nationwide epidemic of septicemia caused by contaminated intravenous fluid. 1. Epidemiological and clinical features. Am. J. Med. 60: 471–485.
61. Wang, S.A., Tokars, J.L., Bianchine, P.J., Carson, L.A., Arduino, M.J., Smith, A.L., Hansen, N.C., Fitzgerald, E.A., Epstein, J.S., Jarvis, W.R., (2000), *Enterobacter cloacue* bloodstream infections traced to contaminated human albumin. Clin. Infect. Dis. 30: 35–40.
62. Brecher, M.E., Hay, S.N., (2005), Bacterial contamination of blood components. Clin. Microbiol. Rev. 18: 195–204.
63. Rupp, M.E., Sholtz, L.A., Jourdan, D.R., Marion, N.D., Tyner, L.K., Fey, P.D., Iwen, P.C., Anderson, J.R., (2007), Outbreak of bloodstream infection temporally associated with the use of an intravascular needle-less valves. Clin. Infect. Dis. 44: 1408–1414.
64. Raad, I., (1998), Intravascular-catheter-related infections. Lancet 351: 893–898.
65. Kite, P., Dobbins, B.M., Wilcox, M.H., McMahon, M.J., (1999), Rapid diagnosis of central-venous catheter-related bloodstream infection without catheter removal. Lancet 354: 1504–1507.
66. Blot, F., Nitenberg, G., Chachaty, E., Raynard, B., Germann, N., Antoun, S., Laplanche, A., Brun-Buisson, C., Tancrède, C., (1999), Diagnosis of catheter-related bacteremia: a prospective comparison of the time to positively of hub-blood versus peripheral blood culture. Lancet 354: 1071–1077.
67. Safdar, N., Fine, J.P., Maki, D.G., (2005), Meta-analysis: methods for diagnosing intravascular device-related blood stream infection. Ann. Intern. Med. 142: 451–466.
68. Bouza, E., Alvarado, N., Alcala, L., Pérez, M.J., Ricon, C., Muñoz, P., (2007), A randomized and prospective study of 3 procedures for the diagnosis of catheter-related bloodstream infection without catheter withdrawal. Clin. Infect. Dis. 44: 820–826.

69. Raad, T., Hanna, H.A., Alakech, B., Chatzinikolaou, I., Johnson, M.M., Tarrand, J., (2004), Differential time to positivity: a useful method for diagnosing catheter-related bloodstream infections. Ann. Intern. Med. 140: 18–25.
70. Mermel, L.A., Farr, B.A., Sherertz, R.J., Raad, I.I., O'Grady, N., Harris, J.S., Craven, D.E., (2001), Guidelines for the management of intravascular catheter-related infections. Clin. Infect. Dis. 32: 1249–1272.
71. Chastre, J., Wolff, M., Fagon, J.Y., Chevret, S., Thomas, F., Wermert, D., Clenenti, E., Gonzalez, J., Jusserand, D., Asfar, P., Perrin, D., Fieux, F., Aubas, S., Pneuma Trial Group, (2003), Comparison of 8 vs 15 days of antibiotic therapy for ventilator-associated pneumonia in adults. JAMA 290: 2588–2598.
72. Bohnen, J.M., Solomkin, J.S., Dellinger, E.P., Bjornson, H.S., Page, C.P., (1992), Guidelines for clinical care: anti-infective agents for intra-abdominal infection. A surgical Infection Society Policy Statement. Arch. Surg. 127: 83–89.
73. Manierski, C., Besarab, A., (2006), Antimicrobial locks: putting the lock on catheter infection. Adv. Chronic Kid. Dis. 13: 245–258.
74. Messing, B., Peitra-Cohen, S., Debure, A., Beliah, M., Bernier, J.J., (1998), Antibiotic-lock technique: a new approach to optimal therapy for catheter-related sepsis in home-parenteral nutrition patients. J PEW J. Parenter. Enteral Nutr. 12: 185–189.
75. Benoit, J.L., Carandang, G., Sitrin, M., Arnow, P., (1997), Intraluminal antibiotic treatment of central venous catheter infection in patients receiving parenteal nutrition at home. Clin. Infect. Dis. 24: 743–744.
76. Krzywda, E.A., Andris, D.A., Edmiston, C.E. Jr, Quebbeman, E.J., (1995), Treatment of Hickman catheter sepsis using antibiotic-lock therapy. Infect. Control Hosp. Epidemiol. 16: 596–598.
77. Cuntz, D., Michaud, L., Guimber, D., Husson, M.O., Gottrand, F., Turck, D., (2002), Local antibiotic-lock for the treatment of infection related to central catheters in parenteral nutrition in children. J PEN J. Parenter. Enteral. Nutr. 28: 104–108.
78. Reimund, J.M., Arondel, Y., Finck, G., Zimmermann, F., Duclos, B., Baumann, R., (2002), Catheter-related infection in patients on home parenteral nutrition: Results of a prospective survey. Clin. Nutr. 21: 33–38.
79. Capdevila, J.A., Segarra, A., Planes, A.M., Ramirez-Arellano, M., Pahissa, A., Piera, L., Martinez-Valzquez, J.M., (1993), Successful treatment of hemodialysis catheter-related sepsis without catheter removal. Nephrol. Dial. Transplant. 8: 231–234.
80. Krishnasami, Z., Carlton, D., Bimbo, L., Taylor, M.E., Balkovetz, D.F., Barker, Allon, M., (2002), Management of hemodialysis catheter-related bacteremia with an adjunctive antibiotic-lock solution. Kidney Int. 61: 1136–1142.
81. Poule, C.V., Carlton, D., Bimbo, L., Allon, M., (2004), Treatment of catheter-related bacteremia with an antibiotic-lock protocol: effect of bacterial pathogen. Nephrol. Dial. Transplant. 19: 1237–1244.
82. Bernardi, M., Cavaliere, M., Cesaro, S., (2005), The antibiotic-lock therapy in oncohematology pediatric unit. Assist. Inferm. Ric. 24: 127–131.
83. Sanchez-Muñoz, A., Aguado, J.M., Lopez-Martin, A, López-Medrano, F., Lumbreras, C., Rodriquez, F.J., Colomer, R, Lortes-Funes, F.J. (2005), Usefulness of antibiotic-lock technique in management of oncology patients with uncomplicated bacteremia related to tunnel catheters. Eur. J. Clin. Microbiol Infect. Dis. 24: 291–293.
84. Manierski, C., Besarab, A., (2006), Antibiotic-locks: putting the lock on catheter infections. Adv. Chronic Kid. Dis. 13: 245–258.
85. Fortún, F., Grill, F., Martin-Dávila, P., Blázquez, J., Tato, M., Sánchez-Corral, J., Garcia-San. Miguel, L., Moreno, S., (2006), Treatment of long-term intravascular catheter-related bacteremia with antibiotic-lock therapy. J. Antimicrob. Chemother. 58: 816–821.
86. Ruhe, J.J., Menon, A., (2006), Clinical significance of isolated *Staphylococcus aureus* central venous catheter tip cultures. Clin. Microbiol. Infect. 12: 933–936.

87. Ekkelonkamp, M.B., van der Bruggen, T., van der Vijven, D.A.M.C., Wolfs, T.F.W., Bonten, M.J.M., (2008), Bacteremic complications of intravascular catheters colonized with *Staphylococcus aureus*. Clin. Infect. Dis. 46: 114–118.
88. McGee, D.C., Gould, M.K., (2003), Preventing complications of central venous catheterization. N. Engl. J. Med..348: 1123–1133.
89. Merrer, J., DeJonghe, B., Golliot. F., Lefrant, J.Y., Raffy, B., Barre, E., Rigaud, J.P., Casciani, D; Misset, B., Bosquet, C, Outin, H., Brun-Buisson, C, Nitenberg, G; French Catheter Study Group in Intensive Care (2001), Complications of femoral and subclavian venous catheterization in critically ill patients: A randomized controlled trial. JAMA 286: 700–707.
90. McKinley, S., Mackenzie, A., Finfer, S., Ward, R., Penfold, J., (1999), Incidence and predictors of central venous catheter-related infection in intensive care patients. Anaesth. Intensive Care 27: 164–169.
91. Raad, I, I., Hohn, D.C., Gilbreath, B.J., Suleiman, N., Hill, L.A., Bruso, P.A., Marts, K., Mansfield, P.F., Bodey, G.P., (1994), Prevention of central venous catheter-related infections by using maximal sterile barrier precautions during insertion. Infect. Control Hosp. Epidemiol. 15: 231–238.
92. Maki, D.G., Ringer, M., Alvarado, C.J., (1991), Prospective randomized trial of povidone-iodine, alcohol, and chlorhexidine for prevention of infection associated with central venous and arterial catheter. Lancet 338: 339–343.
93. Pronovost, P., Needham, D., Berenholtz, S., Sinopoli, D., Chu, H., Cosgrove, S., Sexton, B., Hyzy, R., Welsh, R., Roth, G., Bander, J., Kepros, J., Goeschel, C., (2006), An intervention to decrease catheter-related bloodstream infections in the ICU. N. Engl. J. Med. 355: 2725–2732.
94. Wenzel, R.P., Edmond, M.B., (2006), Team-based prevention of catheter-related infections (editorial). N. Engl. J. Med. 355: 2781–2783.
95. Raad, I.I., Hachem, R.Y., Abi-Said, D., Rolston, K.V., Whimbey E., Buzaid, A.C., Legha, S., (1998), A prospective cross-over randomized trial of novobiocin and rifampin prophylaxis for the prevention of intravascular catheter infections in cancer patients treated with interleukin -2. Cancer 82: 403–411.
96. Henrickson, K.J., Astell, R.A., Hoover, S.M., Kuhn, S.M., Pritchett, J., Kehl, S.C., Klein, J.P., (2000), Prevention of central venous catheter-related infections and thrombotic events in immunocompromised children by the use of vancomycin/ciprofloxacin/heparin flush solution: a randomized, multicenter, double-blind trial. J. Clin. Oncol. 18: 1269–1278.
97. Bock, S.N., Lee, R.E., Fisher, B., Rubin, J.T., Schwartzentruber, D.J., Wei, J.P., Callender, D.P., Yang, J.C., Lotze, M.T., Pizzo, P.A., (1990), A prospective randomized trial evaluating prophylactic antibiotics to prevent triple-lumen catheter-related sepsis in patients treated with immunotherapy. J. Clin. Oncol. 8: 161–169.
98. Tacconelli, E., Carmeli, Y., Aizer, A., Ferreira, G., Foreman, M.G., D'Agata, E.M.C, (2003), Mupirocin prophylaxis to prevent *Staphylococcus aureus* infection in patients undergoing dialysis: a meta-analysis. Clin. Infect. Dis. 37: 1629–1638.
99. Bloom, B.S., Fendrick, A.M., Chernew, M.E., Patel, P., (1996), Clinical and economic effects of mupirocin calcium on preventing *Stayphylococcus aureus* infection in hemodialysis patients: a decision analysis. Am. J. Kidney Dis. 27: 687–698.
100. Perez-Fontan, M., Rosales, M., Rodriguez-Carmona, A., Falcon, T.G., Valdes, F; (2002), Mupirocin resistance after long-term use for *Staphylococcus aureus* colonization in patients undergoing chronic peritoneal dialysis. Am. J. Kidney Dis. 39: 337–341.
101. Levin, A., Mason, A.J., Jindal, K.K., Fong, I.W. Goldstein, M.B., (1991), Prevention of hemodialysis subclavian vein catheter infections by topical povidine-iodine. Kidney Internat. 40: 834–938.
102. Veenstra, D.L., Saint, S., Saha, S., Lumley, T., Sulivan, S.D., (1999), Efficacy of antiseptic impregnated central venous catheters in preventing catheter-related bloodstream infection: A meta-analysis. JAMA 281: 261–267.

103. Veenstra, D.L., Saint, S., Sullivan, S.D., (1999), Cost-effectiveness of antiseptic-impregnated central venous catheters for the prevention of catheter-related bloodstream infection. JAMA 282: 554–560.
104. Pearson, M.C., (1996), Guidelines for prevention of intravascular device-related infections. Hospital Infection Control Practices Advisory Committee. Infect. Control. Hosp. Epidemiol. 17: 391–402.
105. McConnell, S.A., Gubbins, P.O., Anaissie, E.J., (2003), Do antimicrobial-impregnated central venous catheters prevent catheter-related bloodstream infection? Clin. Infect. Dis. 37: 65–72.
106. Crnich, C.J., Maki, d.G., (2005), Are antimicrobial-impregnated catheters effective? When does repetition reach the point of exhaustion? Clin. Infect. Dis. 41: 681–685.
107. Halpin, D.P., O'Byrne, P., McEntee, G., Hennessy, T.P., Stephens, R.B., (1991), Effect of a betadine connection shield on central venous catheter sepsis. Nutrition; 7: 33–34.
108. Segura, M., Alvarez-Lerma, F., Tellado, J.M. Jiménez-Oms, L., Rello, J., Baró, T., Sanchez, R., Morera, A., Mariscal, D., Marrugat, J., Sitges-Serra, A., (1996), A clinical trial on the prevention of catheter-related sepsis using a new hub model. Ann Surg. 223: 363–369.
109. Cabell, C.H., Heidenreich, P.A., Chu, V.H., Moore, C.M., Stryjewski, M.E., Corey., G.R., Fowler, V.G.Jr., (2004), Increasing rates of cardiac device infections among Medicare beneficiaries: 1990–1999. Am. Heart J. 147: 582–586.
110. Hill, E.E., Herijgers, P., Herregods, M.-C., Peetermans, W.E., (2006), Evolving trends in infective endocarditis. Clin. Microbiol. Infect. 12: 5–12.
111. Devlin, R.K., Andrews, M.M., von Reyn, C.F., (2004), Recent trends in infective endocarditis: influence of case definitions. Curr. Opin. Cardiol. 19: 134–139.
112. Moreillion, P., Que, Y.A., (2004), Infective endocarditis. Lancet; 363: 139–149.
113. Wang, A., Athan, E., Pappas, P.A., Fowler, V.G., Olaison, L., Paré, C., Almirante, B., Muñoz, P., Logar, M., Tattevin, P., Iarussi, D.L., Selton-Suty, C., Jones, S.B., Casabé, J., Morris, A., Corey, G.R., Cabell, C.H., for the International Collaboration on Endocarditis-Prospective Cohort Study Investigators, (2007), Comtemporary clinical profile and outcome of prosthetic valve endocarditis. JAMA 297: 1354–1361.
114. Mylonakis, E., Calderwood, S.B., (2001), Infective endocarditis in adults. N. Engl. J. Med. 345: 1318–1330.
115. Baddour, L.M., Wilson, W.R., Bayer, A.S., Fowler, V.G. Jr., Bolger, A.F., Levison, M.E., Ferrieri, P., Gerber, M.A., Tani, L.Y., Gewitz, M.H., Tong, D.C., Steckelberg, J.M., Baltimore, R.S., Shulman, S.T., Burns, J.C., Falace, D.A., Newburger, J.W., Pallasch, T.J., Takashashi, M., Taubert, K.A., (2005), Infective endocarditis: diagnosis, antimicrobial therapy, and management of complications: a statement for healthcare professionals from the Committee on Rheumatic fever, Endocarditis, and Kawasaki Disease, Council on Cardiovascular Disease in the young, and the Councils on Clinical Cardiology, Stroke, and Cardiovascular Surgery and Anesthesia, American Heart Association; endorsed by the Infectious Diseases Society of America. Circulation; 111: e394–e434.
116. Horstkotte, D., Follath, F., Gutschik, E., Lengyet, M., Oto, A., Pavie, A., Soler-soler, J., Thienne, G., von Graeventitz: The Task Force on Infective Endocarditis of the European Society of Cardiology, (2004), Guidelines on prevention, diagnosis and treatment of infective endocarditis – executive summary. Eur. Heart. J. 25: 267–276.
117. Malcolm, D.V.J., Hibberd, P.L., Karchmer, A.W., Sleeper, L.A., Calderwood, S.B., (1998), *Staphylococcus aureus* prosthetic valve endocarditis: Optimal management and risk factors for death. Clin. Infect. Dis. 26: 1302–1309.
118. Chirouze, C., Cabell, C.H., Fowler, V.G. Jr., Khayat, N., Olaison, L., Miro, J.M., Habib, G, Abrutyn, E., Eykyn, S., Corey, G.R., Selton-Suty, C., Hoen, B, and the International Collaboration on Endocarditis Study Group, (2004), Prognostic factors in 61 cases of *Staphylococcus aureus* prosthetic valve infective endocarditis from the International Collaboration on endocarditis merged database. Clin. Infect. Dis. 38: 1323–1327.

119. Vikram, H.R., Buenconsejo, J., Hasbun, R., Quagliarello, V.J., (2003), Impact of valve surgery on 6-month mortality in adults with complicated, left-sided native valve endocarditis. JAMA 290: 3207–3214.
120. Wang, A., Pappas, P., Anstrom, K.J., Abrutyn, E., Fowler, V.G. Jr., Hoen, BN., Miro, J.M., Corey, G.R., Olaison, L., Stafford, J.A., Mestres, C.A., Cabell, C.H., and the International Collaboration on Endocarditis Investigators, (2005), The use and effect of surgical therapy for prosthetic valve endocarditis: A propensity analysis of a multicenter, international cohort. Am. Heart J. 150: 1086–1091.
121. Akowuah, E.F., Davies, W., Oliver, S., Stephens, J., Riaz, I., Zadik, P., Cooper, G., (2003), Prosthetic valve endocarditis: early and late outcome following medical or surgical treatment. Heart 89: 269–272.
122. Wilson, W., Taubert, K.A., Gewitz, M., Lockhart, P.B., Baddour, L.M., Levison, M., Bolger, A., Cabell, C.H., Takahashi, M., Baltimore, R.S., Newburger, J.W., Strom, B.L., Tani, L.Y., Gerber, M., Bonow, R.O., Pallasch, T., Shulman, S.T., Rowley, A.H., Burns, J.C., Ferrieri, P., Gardner, T., Goff, D., Durack, D.T., (2007), Prevention of infective endocarditis. Guidelines from the American Heart Association. A guideline from the American Heart Association Rheumatic Fever, Endocarditis, and Kawasaki Disease Committee, Council on Cardiovascular Disease in the Young, and the Council on Clinical Cardiology, Council on Cardiovascular Surgery and Anesthesia, and the Quality of Care and Outcomes Research Interdisciplinary Working Group. Circulation; 115: http://circahajournals.org.
123. Grover, F.L., Cohen, D.J., Oprian, C., Henderson, W.G., Sethi, G, Hammermeister, K.E., Participants in the Department of Veterans Affair Cooperative Study in Valvular Heart Disease, (1994), Determinants of the occurrence of and survival from prosthetic valve endocarditis. Experience of the Veterans Affairs Cooperative Study on Valvular Heart Disease. Cardiovasc. Surg. 108: 207–214.
124. Schaff, H.V., Carrel, T.P., Jamieson, W.R., Jones, K.W., Rufilanchas, J.J., Cooley, D.A., Hetzer, R., Stumpe, F., Duveau, D., Moseley, P., van Boven, W.J., Grunkemeir, G.L., Kennard, E.D., Holubkov, R., Artificial Valve Endocarditis Reduction Trial, (2002), Paravalvular leak and other events in silzone-coated mechanical heart valves: a report from AVERT. Ann. Thorac. Surg. 73: 785–792.
125. Baddour, L.M., Bettman, M.A., Bolger, A.F., Epstein, A.E., Ferrieri, P., Gerber, M.A., Gewitz, M. H. Jacobs, A.K., Levison, ME., Newburger, J.W., Pallasch, T.J., Wilson, W.R., Baltimore, R.S., Falace, D.A., Shulman, S.T., Tani, L.Y., Taubert, K.A., (2003), Nonvalvular cardiovascular device-related infections. Circulation 108: 2015–2031.
126. Uslan, D.Z, Baddour, L.M., (2006), Cardiac device infection: Getting to the heart of the matter. Curr. Opin. Infect. Dis. 19: 345–348.
127. Duval, X., Selton-Suty C., Alla, F., Salvador-Mazeng, M., Bernard, Y., Weber, M., Lacassin, F., Nazeyrolas, P., Chidac, C., Hoen, B, Leport, C., for the Association pour L'Etude et la prevention de L'Endocarditis Infectieuse, (2004), Endocarditis in patients with a permanent pacemaker: a 1 – year epidemiological survey on infective endocarditis due to valvular and for pacemaker infection. Clin. Infect. Dis. 39: 68 74.
128. Cohen, M.I., Bush, D.M., Gaynor, J.W., Vetter, V.L., Tanel, R.E., Rhodes, L.A., (2002), Pediatric pacemaker infection: Twenty years experience. J. Thorac. Cardiovasc. Surg. 124: 821–827.
129. del Rio, A., Anguera, I., Miro, J.M., Mont, L., Fowler, V.G. Jr., Azqueta, M., Mestres, C.A., Hospital Clinic Endocarditis Group, (2003), Surgical treatment of pacemaker and defibrillator lead endocarditis: The impact of electrode lead extraction on outcome. Chest 124: 1451–1459.
130. Da Costa, A., Lelievre, H., Kirkorian, G., Celard, M., Chevalier, P., Vandenesch, F., Etienne, J., Touboul, P., (1998), Role of the preaxillary flora in pacemaker infections: A prospective study. Circulation 97: 1791–1795.
131. Chamis, A.L., Peterson, G.E., Cabell, C.H., Corey, G.R., Sorrentino, R.A., Greenfield, R.A., Ryan, T, Rellar, L.B., Fowler, V.G.Jr., (2001), *Staphylococcus aureus* bacteremia in patients

with permanent pacemakers or implantable cardioverter-defibrillators. Circulation 104: 1029–1033.
132. Klug, D., Wallet, F., Kacet, S., Courcol, R.J., (2005), Detailed bacteriologic tests to identify the origin of transvenous pacing system infections indicate a high prevalence of multiple organisms. Am. Heart J. 149: 322–328.
133. Chau, J.D., Wilkoff, B.L. Lee, I., Juratli, N., Longworth, P.L., Gordon, S.M., (2000), Diagnosis and management of infections involving implantable electrophysiologic cardiac devices. Ann. Intern. Med. 133: 604–608.
134. Cacoub, P., Leprince, P., Nataf, P., Hausfater, P., Dorent, R., Wechsler, B., Bors V., Pavie, A., Piette, J.C., Gandjbakhch, I., (1998), Pacemaker infective endocarditis. Am. J. Cardiol. 82: 480–484.
135. Bracke. F.A., Meijer, A., van Gelder, L.M., (2001), Pacemaker lead complications: when is extraction appropriate and what can we learn from published data? Heart; 85: 254–259.
136. Wilkoff, B.L., Byrd, C.L., Love, C.J., Hayes, D.L., Sellers, T.D., Schaerf, R., Parsonnet, V., Epstein, L.M., Sorrentino, R.A., Reiser, C., (1999), Pacemaker lead extraction with the laser sheath: results of the pacing lead extractions with the excimer sheath (PLEXES) trial J. Am. Coll. Cardiol. 33: 1671–1676.
137. Ruttmann, E., Hangler, H.B., Kilo, J., Hofer, D., Muller, L.C., Hintringer, F., Muller, S., Laufer, G., Antretter, H., (2006), Transvenous pacemaker lead removal is safe and effective even in large vegetations: An analysis of 53 cases of pacemaker lead endocarditis. Pacing Clin. Electrophysiol. (PACE) 29: 231–236.
138. Da Costa, A., Kirkorian, G., Cucherat, M., Delahaye, F., Chevalier, P., Cerisier, A., Isaaz, K., Touboul, P., (1998), Antibiotic prophylaxis for permanent pacemaker implantation. A meta-analysis. Circulation 97: 1796–1801.
139. Sirvaratnam, K., Duggan, J.M., (2002), Left ventricular assist device infections: three cases and a review of the literature. ASAI OJ; 48: 2--7.
140. Hutchinson, O.Z., Oz, M.C., Ascherman, J.A., (2001), The use of muscle flaps to treat left ventricular assist device infections. Plastic Reconstrut. Surg. 107: 364–373.
141. Malani, P.N., Dyke, D.B., Pagani, F.D., Chenoweth, C,E., (2002), Noscomial infections in left ventricular assist deivce recipients. Clin. Infect. Dis. 34: 1295–1300.
142. Mekontso-Dessap, A., Kirsch, M., Vermes, E., Brun-Buisson, C., Loisance, D., Houël, R., (2002), Nosocomial infections occurring during receipt of circulatory support with para-corporal ventricular assist system. Clin. Infect. Dis. 35: 1308–1315.
143. Rose, E.A., Gelijns, A.C., Moskowitz, A.J., Heitjan, D.F., Stevenson, L.W., Dembitsky, W., Long, J.W., Ascheim, D.D., Tierney, A.R., Levitan, R.G., Watson, J.T., Meier, P., for the Randomized Evaluation of Mechanical Assistance for the treatment of Congestive Heart Failure (Rematch) Study Group, (2001), Long-term use of a left ventricular assist device for end-stage heart failure. N. Engl. J. Med. 345: 1435–1443.
144. Miller, L.W., Pagani, F.D., Russell, S.D., John, R., Boyle, A.J., Aaronson, K.D., Conte, J.V., Naka, Y., Mancini, D., Delgado, R.M., MacGillivray, Farrar, D.J., Frazier, O.H., for the Heart Mate II Clinical Investigators, (2007), Use of a continuous-flow device in patients awaiting heart transplantation. N. Eng. J. Med. 357: 885–896.
145. Holman, W.L., Rayburn, B.K., McGiffin, D.C., Foley, B.A., Benza, R.L., Bourge, R.C., Pinderski, L.J., Kirklin, J.K., (2003), Infection in ventricular assist devices: prevention and treatment. Ann. Thorac. Surg. 75 (Suppl): s48–s57.
146. Pasque, M.K., Hanselman, T., Shelton, K., Kehoe-Huck, B.A., Hedges, R., Cussivi, S.D., Ewald, G.A., Rogers, J.G., (2002), Surgical management of Novacor drive-line exit site infections. Ann. Thorac. Surg. 74: 1267–1268.
147. Saijjadian, A., Valero, I.L., Acurturk, O., Askari, M.A., Sacks, J., Kormos, R.L., Manders, E. K., (2006), Omental transposition flap for salvage of ventricular assist devices. Plast. Reconstr. Surg. 118: 919–926.
148. Darouiche, R.O., (2004), Treatment of infections associated with surgical implants. N. Engl. J. Med. 340: 1422–1429.

149. P.H., Brinkman, W.T., Terramani, T.T., Lumsden, A.B., (2002), Management of Infected hemodialysis access grafts using cryopreserved human vein allografts. Am. J. Surg. 184: 31–36.
150. Schutte, W.P., Helmer, S.D., Salazar, L., Smith, J.L., (2007), Surgical treatment of infected prosthetic dialysis arteiovenous grafts: Total versus partial graft excision. Am. J. Surg. 193: 385–388.
151. Chiesa, R., Astore, D., Piccolo, G., Melissano, G., Jannello, A., Frigerio, D., Agrifoglio, G., Bonalumi, F., Corsi, G., Costantini Brancadoro, S., Novali, C., Locati, P., Odero, A., Pirrelli, S., Cugnasca, M., Biglioli, P., Sala, A., Polvani, G., Guarino, A., Biasi, GM., Mingazzini, P., Scalamogna, M., Mantero, S., Spina, G., Prestipino, F., et al., (1998), Fresh and cryopreserved arterial homografts in the treatment of prosthetic graft infections: experience of the Italian Collaboration Vascular Homograft Group. Ann. Vasc. Surg. 121: 457–462.
152. Illuminati, G., Calio, F.G., D'Urso, A., Giacobbi, D., Papaspyropoulos, V., Ceccanei, G., (2004), Infrascrotal, perineal, femorofemoral bypass for arterial graft infection at the groin. Arch. Surg. 139: 1314–1319.
153. Seify, H., Moyer, H.R., Jones, G.E., Busquets, A., Brown, K., Salam, A., Losken, A., Culbertson, J., Hester, T.R., (2006), The role of muscle flaps in wound salvage after vascular graft infections: The Emory experience. Plast. Reconstr. Surg. 117: 1325–1333.
154. Graham, R.G., Omotoso, P.O., Hudson, D.A., (2002), The effectiveness of muscle flaps for the treatment of prosthetic graft sepsis. Plast. Reconstr. Surg. 109: 108–113.
155. Chambers, S.T., (2005), Diagnosis and management of staphylococcal infections of vascular grafts and stents. Intern. Med. J. 35 (Suppl 2): s72–s78.
156. Annovazzi, A., Bagni, B., Burroni, L., D'Alessandrla, C. Signore, A., (2005), Nuclear Medicine imaging of inflammatory infective disorders of the abdomen. Nucl. Med. Commun. 26: 657–664.
157. Chiesa, R., Astore, D., Frigerio, S., Garriboli. L., Piccolo, G., Castellano, R., Scalamogna, M., Odero, A., Pirrelli, S., Biasi, G., Mingazzini, P., Biglioli, P., Poloani, g., Guarino, A., Agrifoglio, G., Tori, A., Spina, G., (2002), Vascular prosthetic graft infection: Epidermiology, bacteriology, pathogenesis and treatment. Actu Chirugica Belgica 102: 238–247.
158. O'Connor, S., Andrew, P., Batt, M., Becquemin, J.P., (2006), A systematic review and meta-analysis of treatments for aortic graft infection. J. Vasc. Surg. 44: 38–45.
159. Calligaro, K.D., Veith, F.J., Yuan, J.G., Gargiulo, N.J., Dougherty, M.J., (2003), Intra-abdominal aortic graft infection: complete or partial graft preservation in patients at very high risk. J. Vasc. Surg. 38: 1199–1205.
160. Mitra, A., Spears, J., Perrotta, V., McClurkin, J., Mitra, A., (2005), Salvage of infected prosthetic grafts of the great vessels via muscle flaps reconstruction. Chest 128: 1040–1043.
161. Fiorani, P., Speziale, F., Calisti, A., Misuraca, M., Zaccagnini, D., Rizzo, L., Giannoni, M.F., (2003), Endovascular graft infection: preliminary results of an international enquiry. J. Endovasc. Therapy 10: 919–927.
162. L'Heureux, N., Dusserre, N., Konig, G., Victor, B., Keire, P., Wight, T.N., Chronos, N.A., Kyles, A.E., Gregory, C.R., Hoyt, G., Robbins, R.C., McAllister, T.N., (2006), Human tissue-engineered blood vessels for adult revascularization. Nat. Med. 12: 361–365.
163. L'Heureux, N., McAllister, T.N., de La Fuente, L.M., (2007), Tissue-engineered blood vessel for adult arterial revascularization. N. Engl. J. Med. 357: 1451–1453.
164. Hentzer, M., Givskor, M., (2003), Pharmacological inhibition of quorum sensing for the treatment of chronic bacterial infections. J. Clin. Invest. 112: 1300–1307.
164. Kwakman, P.H., te Velde, A.A., Vandenbroucke-Grauls, C.M., van Deventer, S.J., Zaat, S. A., (2006), Treatment and prevention of *Staphylococcus epidermidis* experimental biomaterial-associated infection by bactericidal peptide 2. Antimicrob. Agents Chemother. 50: 3977–3983.

# Chapter 11
# Current Concepts of Orthopedic Implants and Prosthetic Joint Infections

## 11.1 Introduction

It is estimated that approximately two million fracture-fixation devices (intramedultory nails, external-fixation pins, plates, and screws) and about 600,000 joint prosthesis are inserted annually in the United States.[1] Projected infections of joint prosthesis (average rate of 2%) is 12,000 and fracture-fixation devices (average 5%) is 1,000,000 annually. Infections of these orthopedic devices causes substantial morbidity and health care expenditure, with an estimated average cost for combined medical and surgical treatment of US$30,000 for an infected prosthesis, and US $15,000 for an infected fracture-fixation device.[1] Hence a conservative estimate of US$1.8 billion is spent annually for the management of infected orthopedic implants in the United States.

Although progress has been made in the last decade on the pathogenesis of this biofilm infection, there is still considerable debate and lack of standardization on the diagnosis, methods to establish the bacteriology and management. Despite the enormity of the problems posed by these orthopedic implant infections in developed countries, there is a lack of proper controlled, randomized trials on medical and surgical therapy.

The pathogenesis of biofilm infections as outlined in Chapter 10 also applies to orthopedic device infections and will not be reiterated in this chapter.

## 11.2 Microbiological Aspects

The use of perioperative antimicrobial prophylaxis and laminar air-flow surgical environment has reduced the risk of post-operative infection to less than 1% for hip and shoulder replacement and to less than 2% for knee replacement.[2–4] It is generally acknowledged that bacteria-causing infection are usually colonizing skin flora introduced at the time of surgery. However, late infections can occur from bacteremia originating elsewhere and can occur any time during the entire lifetime of the implant. In one study 15 of 44 (34%) patients with prosthetic joints developed implant-associated infection following *Staphylococcus aureus* bacteremia, but only 1 of 15 (7%) patients with other (nonarticular) orthopedic devices became infected.[5] In a prospective study the overall risk of hematogenous seeding to prosthetic joints from all pathogens was very small (0.3% for an average period of 6 years).[6] Although diagnosis of prosthetic joint infection within 1 year of placement has been widely used to arbitrarily differentiate between primary or hematogenous origin, occasionally primary infections are diagnosed more than 1 year after implantation[7].

The most commonly cultured microorganisms associated with prosthetic joint infections are coagulase negative staphylococci (CoNS) in 30–43% of cases, *S. aureus* (12–23%), mixed flora (10–11%), *Streptococci* (9–10%), gram-negative bacilli (3–6%), enterococci (3–7%), and anaerobes (2–4%).[8] However, up to 11% or more of clinically infected prosthetic joints fail to grow any microorganisms. This raises the issue of the sensitivity of routine microbiological methods in biofilm-related infections. Specificity of periprosthetic-tissue cultures can also be a problem, especially with normal skin flora such as CoNS and diphtheroids (i.e., *Propionibacterium acnes*), which may be either contaminants or pathogens. Lack of a standardized criteria for diagnosing orthopedic device infection has limited the microbiological diagnosis.

Ideally the device itself should be cultured for various microorganisms, including fastidious bacteria. However, most joint prostheses when removed for suspected infection or assumed aseptic loosening are not cultured directly, presumably because of the size of the prosthesis and risk of contamination. Fixation devices such as screws and small plates are more amenable to direct culture in a broth medium. Visualization of bacteria on gram stain from synovial fluid or periprosthetic tissue have high specificity ($\geq 97\%$) but low sensitivity ($<26\%$).[9] In aspirated synovial fluid of infected joint prosthesis the pathogen can be detected in 45–100% of cases.[9] Wound or sinus cultures are difficult to interpret because of colonizing skin flora and are best avoided. Swab cultures even intraoperatively have low sensitivity and should not be used alone. Most guidelines recommend culture of at least three (up to six) periprosthetic-tissue samples for culture.[81,110] Normally if only one of the specimens are positive for a normal skin bacteria this would likely represent contamination, and two or more specimens with the same organism represent a true pathogen. The sensitivity of these cultures ranges from 64% to 94%, depending on the definition of infection.[9]

Concerns about the sensitivity and specificity of periprosthetic-tissue cultures in biofilm infection has led some investigators to assess the role of sonicate-fluid of removed prostheses for routine microbiological culture, or molecular techniques using polymerase chain reaction (PCR) on either the sonicate-fluid or scrapings from the prosthesis. In a recent prospective evaluation of 91 consecutive patients undergoing revision total hip or knee arthroplasty synovial fluid was collected intraoperatively and analyzed by broad-range PCR assay for detection of bacterial

DNA.[12] Using a combination of clinical assessment, laboratory results, and multiple tissue cultures and histology, infection was diagnosed in 12 (13%) patients but the PCR was positive in 32 cases. Thus, PCR led to a large number of false positive results with a low positive predictive value of 34%.[12] A previous smaller study of 22 patients undergoing joint replacement for suspected infection compared routine prolonged culturing of tissue samples versus culturing scrapings from the biomaterial surface.[13] Bacterial growth was observed in 14 (64%) of cases from periprosthetic tissues, whereas scrapings showed bacterial growth in 19 (86%) of patients. In addition, confocal laser scanning microscopy detected biofilm bacteria on the surfaces of these explanted prostheses.[13]

Previous studies using bath sonication of prosthetic joints to dislodge biofilm bacteria found improved bacterial recovery[14] but increased contamination because the prosthetic components were placed in bags that leaked.[15] To overcome this problem processing of removed implants in solid containers and vortexing the contents has been used. In a recent prospective study of 331 patients undergoing knee or hip revision arthroplasty, the modified sonication method with routine culture was compared to conventional culture of synovial fluid and multiple periprosthetic tissues.[16] A standardized non-microbiologic criterion was used for diagnosis of prosthetic joint infection if one or more of the following was present: visible pus in the synovial fluid or surrounding the prosthesis, acute inflammation on histopathology, or a sinus tract communicating with the prosthesis. A total of 252 patients had aseptic failure and 79 (23.8%) had prosthetic joint infection. The sensitivities of periprosthetic-tissue and sonicate-fluid cultures were 60.8% and 78.5% ($p < 0.001$), respectively, and the specificities were 99.2% and 98.8%.[16] In patients receiving antimicrobial therapy within 14 days of surgery the difference in sensitivity was even greater, 45% (periprosthetic tissues) and 75% (sonicate) $p < 0.001$. A notable finding of this study is the striking effect of prior preoperative antibiotics on the sensitivity of tissue and sonicate-fluid culture. For tissue culture the sensitivity decreased from 76.9–47.8% to 41.2% as the antimicrobial-free interval before surgery decreased from greater than 14 days, to 4–14 days, to 0–3 days, respectively.[16] For sonicate-fluid culture, the sensitivity was 82.1–87.0% and 58.8% for the same intervals, respectively. This result indicates that the usual practice of stopping antibiotics 2 weeks before surgery may still result in false-negative cultures.

There are some limitations of the above study, which also applies to other previous studies, the main one being the absence of a "gold standard" and accepted criteria for diagnosis of prosthetic joint infection or aseptic loosening. Since the diagnosis of aseptic loosening was based on conventional clinical criteria these prostheses may not be really sterile, as other methods such as molecular techniques or examination of the surfaces with confocal laser microscopy were not examined.[17] Other limitations include failure to use newer microbiological techniques, including special cultures for fungi and mycobacteria, and this method can only be used when the prosthesis is being removed, and does not aid in the microbiologic diagnosis when explantation of the prosthesis is not an option. Although the clinical diagnosis of aseptic prosthetic joint failure may be over-diagnosed, as prospective studies showed positive bacterial culture in up to 76%,[18] it is uncertain what proportions is due to contamination versus represent true pathogen. There are also practical restrictions that would limit the general applicability of sonicate-fluid culture in the routine microbiology laboratory, including need for ultrasound equipment, some of the prostheses were too large to fit in the containers, and risk of contamination would be greater with this procedure.

## 11.3 Diagnosis

The diagnosis of infected orthopedic devices is often challenging as there is no uniform accepted criteria, and diagnostic tests are inaccurate.[16] Blood tests such as blood leukocyte count, erythrocyte sedimentation rate (ESR), and C-reactive protein (CRP) are insensitive or nonspecific for diagnostic purposes, but serial values may be helpful in assuming response to therapy. A combination of normal ESR and CRP, however, is reliable for predicting the absence of infection. Imaging studies can be helpful and plain radiographs should be used initially (least expensive), although not highly sensitive serial studies over time after implantation are useful.[19]

Loosening or displacement of the implant and periprosthetic osteolysis can occur with or without infection, but new subperiosteal bone growth and transcortical sinus tracts are more specific for infection. Sinogram and arthrogram are used occasionally and can be useful for detecting implant loosening, pseudo-bursae, and abscesses.[8] Technicium bone scan has very high sensitivity but low specificity, as the scan can remain positive more than a year after implantation due to periprosthetic bone remodeling.[20] The addition of gallium-67 improves the accuracy of bone scintigraphy to only 70–80%. Techicium – 99 m – antigranulyte monoclonal antibody fragment Fab[1] 2 scan has improved specificity and diagnostic accuracy (89% and 87%, respectively but decreased sensitivity (80%), [21] and has replaced indium – 111 – labeled leucocyte scan (labor-intensive and expensive) in Europe. A recent meta-analysis of the diagnostic accuracy of antigranulocyte scintigraphy (AGS) with monoclonal antibodies in identification of prosthetic joint infection assessed 13 studies with 522 implants.[22] The sensitivity was 83–90% and specifity 80% depending on the type of analysis. In one study of 59 infected joint prostheses (hip and knee) a combined 111-labelled leucocyte/ 99 m Tc – sulfur colloid marrow imaging was found to be 100% sensitive and 91% specific,[23] but larger studies need to confirm these results. Positron-emission tomography (PET) with 18F-fluoro-deoxyglucose (FDG) has produced mixed results in investigations of suspected prosthetic joint infection. An earlier study reported specificity of only 55% in detecting implant infection,[24] but a more recent study of 63 patients with 92 prostheses found the PET imaging to have sensitivity of 94% and specificity of 95% (using qualitative and not quantitative criteria), and triple phase bone scanning (TPBS) was only 68% sensitive and 76% specific.[25] Similar results with the FDG

PET in a smaller study on 22 patients with 29 implants in trauma patients were found: sensitivity of 100%, specifity of 87.5–93.3% and accuracy of 95–97%, with infection definition based on microbiological evaluation of surgical specimens and intraoperative findings.[26]

The majority of medical centers performing orthopedic implants do not have the availability of these newer imaging techniques. Computed tomography is often used to provide greater anatomical details and provides better contrast between normal and abnormal tissue compared to plain radiographs, however, imaging artifacts caused by metals limit its value. Magnetic resonance imaging (MRI) is arguably the "gold standard" for diagnosis of osteomyelitis without prosthesis, but only newer prosthesis composed of titanium or tantalum is safe with MRI. Future studies need to assess the diagnostic accuracy of MRI in prosthetic joint and orthopedic fixation device infections.

A simple blood test with high sensitivity to assess for possible implant infection would be useful but none of the laboratory tests are consistently reliable, or can accurately indicate infection before revision arthroplasty. Interleukin - 6 (IL-6), a proinflammatory cytokine produced by monocytes and macrophages, maybe a valuable maker in implant infection. Recently, it was found that serum IL-6 levels quickly return to normal after total joint surgery and are not elevated in patients with aseptic loosening.[27] In a recent study to assess the value of IL-6 serum levels 58 patients undergoing revision arthroplasty (17 infected by histopathological criteria and bacterial culture from periprosthetic tissues) were analyzed.[28] Although the ESR, CRP and IL-6 were significantly associated with infected prosthesis, an elevated IL-6 ($>10$ pg/ml) had the best diagnostic accuracy with sensitivity of 100%, specificity 95%, and accuracy 97%. A limitation of this assay is that IL-6 is commonly elevated in chronic inflammatory or infectious conditions (rheumatoid arthritis, multiple sclerosis, Paget disease of bone, acquired immunodeficiency syndrome, etc.) and these conditions were excluded.[28] Thus this test would be useful mainly for patients with underlying degenerative disease (the vast majority of patients with prosthetic joints) without infection or inflammation elsewhere. A large multicenter study is needed to confirm the diagnostic value of serum IL-6.

Histopathological examination of periprosthetic tissues is often used to confirm prosthetic joint infections in conjunction with cultures. In a study of 523 cases of aseptic loosening and 79 confirmed infection the presence of 2 + or more (mean of $\geq 1$ neutrophil polymorph per high power field (x 400) of at least 10 high-power fields) had a diagnostic sensitivity of 100%, specificity 97%, and accuracy of 99%.[29] However, others have found histopathology to have a sensitivity of no more than 80% and a specificity of no more than 90%.[9] Although earlier investigations found frozen sections useful at the time of revision arthroplasty to predict infection, more recent studies found limitations. A positive frozen section defined as $>10$ neutrophils per high-power field was found to have a sensitivity of 67% and specificity of 93% for all joint arthroplasties with infection, but sensitivity was higher for knee and lower for hip prosthesis.[30]

## 11.4 Clinical Presentation

Infections associated with prosthetic joints are usually classified as early (occurring within 3 months of surgery), delayed (3 to 24 months after surgery), or late (more than 24 months after surgery).[8] Early and delayed infections are usually acquired during surgery and late infections are acquired mainly from hematogenous seeding (from skin, respiratory tract, dental, and urinary tract). In a case series of 63 consecutive episodes of prosthetic hip infection observed over a 16-year period, 29% were early, 41% delayed, and 30% late infections; 57% of the infections were exogenously and 43% hematogenously acquired.[31] Early infections usually manifest as a wound infection or with acute onset of joint pain, with erythema, increased warmth, evidence of effusion and fever, and are more commonly caused by virulent organisms such as *S. aureus* and coliforms. Delayed infections are caused mainly by low virulent organisms such as CoNS and *P. acnes*.[32]

Spinal fusion implants have dramatically increased over the past decade (rose by 77% between 1996 and 2001), with annual growth rate of 18–20%, and annual budget of $2 billion in the United States for spinal devices.[33] It is estimated that infections occur in about 3% of spinal fusion.[33] Investigators have classified spinal implant infection as early onset (within 30 days of surgery) or late onset (after 30 days). In a case series of 81 patients with spinal implant infection over 8 years 37% were early onset and 63% late onset.[34] The microbiological etiology was similar to prosthetic joint infection, except *S. aureus* was the most common agent, both for early-onset (33%) or late-onset infections (22%), and polymicrobial infection was common (23% and 24%).[34] Most early infections present with increasing pain, wound drainage and erythema, with or without fever; but late infections may present with increasing pain, with or without fever and evidence of epidural or psoas muscle abscess.

Risk factors for prosthetic joint infection have been studied by several investigators using retrospective data, case-controls, observational cohort, and prospective cohort. Postoperative surgical site (wound) infection not involving the prosthesis and superficial carries a high risk of deep implant infection in prospective and matched control studies, with odds ratio (OR) of >35.[35,36] The National Nosocomial Infection Surveillance (NNIS) system surgical risk index score has been shown to be a better predictor of surgical site infection than individual components of the score. This risk index consists of scoring each operation by adding the number of risk factors among three measurements: intrinsic host risk (diabetes, rheumatoid arthritis, renal insufficiency, malnutrition, immunosuppression, etc.), surgical wound classification, and duration of the operative procedure. For 5,696 patients undergoing hip or knee total arthroplasties the NNIS system surgical patient risk index could identify patients at high risk for surgical site and prosthetic joint infection.[37] Similarly in a large case control study the NNIS system risk index score of >1 was a significant risk factor for prosthetic joint infection (even after adjustment for superficial wound infection), and a score of ≥2 had an OR 3.9.[36] Prosthetic replacement following excision of bone cancer is associated with a high risk of prosthetic implant infection (11%).[38] Systemic malignancy not involving the joint is also associated with increased risk of prosthetic joint infection (OR = 3.1).[36] History of prior joint arthroplasty on the index joint has been consistently recognized as a risk factor for prosthetic joint infection, up to eightfold greater than those with primary arthroplasty.[36,39] Nasal carriage of *S. aureus* is also a major risk factor for surgical site infections in orthopedic surgery,[40] and is likely to be important for orthopedic implant infections. The mortality and complication rates of many surgical procedures are inversely related to hospital procedure volume. In an analysis of 58,521 hip replacement, patients at hospitals and by surgeons with lower annual caseloads of primary and revision total hip replacement had higher mortality rates and selected complications, but infection of prosthetic joint was not significantly increased.[41] Risk factors for postoperative spinal infections (not limited to spinal implants) have been reported to include age, posterior instrumented fusion, high allogenic blood transfusion rates, and suboptimal sheet and dressing changing conditions.[42]

## 11.5 Management

The main objectives of treatment are to eradicate infection, restore function to the joint or bone, and to eliminate symptoms and improve quality of life. Management should be a team effort with co-ordination by the orthopedic surgeon with consultation to an Infectious Disease specialist, physiotherapist, and rehabilitation team. Approach to management may differ between practice in North America and Europe, as there are no large randomized control trials with either medical or surgical treatment to provide standardized guidelines. Most of the available data on management consists of retrospective case series from a single center usually with no controls for comparison. These observational case series mainly involve therapy of infected prosthetic hip and knee arthroplasties, with much less data on spinal implants or fracture-fixation devices.

As discussed in Chapter 9 foreign body or implant infections are extremely resistant to antibiotics and host defenses and frequently persist until the implant is removed, which is the standard therapy. However, this approach is not always possible, and it is time-consuming and the functional result may be suboptimal due to delayed reimplantation of the prosthesis (usually after $\geq 6$ weeks antibiotic therapy).

### *11.5.1 Basis of Medical Therapy*

Traditionally treatment of bacterial infections are based on in vitro susceptibility, animal models, then clinical trials, or clinical case series, observational or case control cohort studies for uncommon conditions where multi-center comparative studies are not feasible or difficult to perform. In general there has been lack of controlled randomized studies for therapy of osteomyelitis, orthopedic-related or implant infections.

In vitro susceptibility results by standard technique of planktonic bacteria do not correlate with susceptibility of the organism grown in a biofilm environment, which are usually 10- to 1,000-fold more resistant.[43,44] Furthermore, standard susceptibility tests do not correlate with treatment success of device-related infection,[45] unless the foreign body is removed. Whereas, drug efficacy on stationary and adherent microorganisms (to mimic biofilm) using only bactericidal effect (not minimal inhibitory concentration [MIC]) predicted the outcome of device-related infections.[45] In this animal model using a teflon tissue cage, rifampin was the most efficacious drug in any experimental test to cure the infection with *Staphylococcus epidermidis*.[45] However, rifampin, although the most potent anti-staphylococcal agent available should not be used alone, as a one-step mutation with rapid development of resistance will occur.

Combination antimicrobial therapy with rifampin is commonly used to treat chronic *S. aureus* osteomyelitis or staphylococcal prosthetic device infections, despite lack of proof of efficacy by controlled randomized studies (tier I standards). Earlier animal models of *S. aureus* chronic osteomyelitis in rabbits demonstrated that single-drug regimens used for 28 days were relatively ineffective (bone sterilization rate, 5–55%).[46] Combination of rifampin with other agents (aminoglycoside, cephalosporin, or trimethoprim) were more effective (bone sterilization rate 75–100%).[46] However, this model did not assess the effect of an implant or foreign body. Although animal models of osteomyelitis with internal fixation devices were developed in rabbits and guinea pigs over 2 decades ago, these models were used mainly to investigate the pathogenesis and not therapeutics.[47–49] Similarly, experimental hip and knee arthroplasty infection model in the rabbit had been developed[50,51]; but only with limited therapeutic application with short-term single agents (quinolones and glycopeptides) effect on decreasing the density of bacteria recovered from bone.[52,53] Thus previous animal model studies of orthopedic device or prosthetic infection were not adequately designed to provide guidelines for management of human infection.

An in vitro model of antibiotic efficacy or bactericidal effect on adherent bacteria as biofilm on sinter glass beads, incubated for 48 h, has been found to correlate with animal tissue cage model results.[54] In this system rifampin combinations with either vancomycin, teicoplanin, fleroxacin, or ciprofloxacin were significantly more bactericidal against adherent *S. aureus* or *S. epidermidis* than netilmicin combinations with vancomycin or daptomycin. However, although rifampin in combination with other antibiotics has been used successfully in the treatment of serious staphylococcal infections the mechanism of efficacy has been unclear.

Most nosocomial strains and a significant proportion of community *S. epidermidis* or CoNS are methicillin-resistant. In a previous study assessing the combination of rifampin with cephalothin, nafcillin, gentamicin, or vancomycin against ten strains of methicillin-resistant *S. epidermidis* (MRSE), both in vitro

## 11.5 Management

synergy (time kill and checkerboard studies on planktonic bacteria) and in vivo (rabbit endocarditis model) studies were performed.[55] The results of the checkerboard and time-kill studies did not support a role for true synergic in antibiotic combinations containing rifampin. Rather, the antibacterial activity of rifampin was enhanced by the prevention of the emergence of rifampin-resistant mutants.[55] Another study on MRSE experimental endocarditis also found that rifampin-resistant mutants could be prevented with vancomycin or gentamicin, allowing bactericidal killing by rifampin (as no synergy was found with time-kill studies).[56]

Although quinolones in combination with rifampin have bactericidal effect against adherent staphylococcal species,[54] and earlier clinical studies showed promising results in orthopedic implant infections their efficacy and reliability is now in doubt, because of increasing resistance of staphylococcal species to fluoroquinolones. Most strains of MRSA and MRSE and significant proportion of methicillin sensitive staphylococci are resistant to quinolones. In our hospital clinical microbiology laboratory over 1,300 CoNS were tested in vitro for susceptibility (presumed invasive isolates) in 2006, of these strains 65% were resistant to levofloxacin or ciprofloxacin. The most consistently active agents (standard in vitro susceptibility) were vancomycin (99%), rifampin (94%), doxycycline or tetracycline (92%), and cotrimoxazole (56%) (unpublished data, St. Michaels' Hospital Microbiology Laboratory report 2007). Thus combination of rifampin with quinolones would likely lead to failure and development of rifampin resistance in most cases of staphylococcal orthopedic implant infection. Since most clinical microbiology laboratories are unable to do in vitro susceptibility on adherent (biofilm) bacteria (also no standardized, approved method is available), standard in vitro methods are still considered the "gold standard" for guiding antimicrobial therapy. Based on current knowledge, when rifampin is used for device-related infection it should be combined with another antimicrobial to which the organism is sensitive.

Are antibiotics necessary once the prosthesis or foreign body is removed? Clinical experience and experimental studies strongly indicate that even after removal of foreign devices infection will persist in the surrounding bone, and antibiotics for weeks or months are necessary to eradicate the infection. In a rabbit model of chronic osteomyelitis following insertion of a intramedullary steel rod, removal of the foreign body and debridement of the marrow cavity did not cure the established infection.[57]

Can antibiotics alone (without surgical intervention) cure orthopedic implant infections? The paradigm for effective management includes a combination of surgical and antibiotic therapy. There are occasional reports of "cure" with antibiotics alone, or use of chronic suppressive antimicrobial therapy in elderly debilitated patients with poor surgical risk. However, these practices should be discouraged for routine management and represent exceptional circumstances, and can predispose to development of resistant strains with increased risk of adverse effects from prolonged antibiotic exposure, including *Clostridium difficile* colitis which is associated with considerable morbidity and mortality in the elderly.

## 11.5.2 Principles of Surgical Management

Traditionally removal of all infected foreign body with subsequent replacement, if necessary, once the infection is eradicated was considered the mainstay of surgical treatment. However, over the years more conservative approach has been developed to salvage prosthetic arthroplasties with some success. Four possible surgical approaches for the treatment of infected joint prosthesis include: debridement with retention of the prosthesis, removal of the infected implant without replacement or joint arthrodesis, one-stage replacement, and two-stage replacement.[1,8] Debridement involves excision of devitalized bone and soft tissue, drainage or irrigation of pus, removal of hematoma, fibrous membranes and sinus tracts. This approach with retention of the prosthesis has been recommended for select patients with early post-operative (<3 months) or acute hematogenous late (>2 years) infection, if the duration of clinical symptoms and signs is less than 3 weeks, the implant is stable, the soft tissue is in good condition, and an agent with activity against biofilm organisms is available.[8] Success rate of 80% or above has been reported in a few centers,[31,58,59] but lower success rates below 35–50% have been reported by others with less standardized selection criteria for this conservative approach.[60–66] Although Zimmeli et al,[8] guidelines for debridement with retention surgical approach include symptoms or signs less than 3 weeks, this is an area of contention. In a case series of 33 prosthetic joint infections with *S. aureus*, debridement after 2 days onset of symptoms were associated with a higher probability of treatment failure than those débrided within 2 days of onset (RR = 4.2).[61] Others have also found that this therapeutic approach was primarily effective when the duration of symptoms was <5 days.[60] Two recent reports from the Mayo Clinic have dampened the optimistic outlook or enthusiasm for debridement and retention of infected arthroplasties. Berbari et al.[67] analyzed outcome of prosthetic joint infections in 200 episodes of 160 patients with rheumatoid arthritis (37% due to *S. aureus*). The type of surgical procedure was the only clinical variable that was associated with treatment failure ($p < 0.001$). Rates of 5-year survival free of treatment failure for patients treated with debridement and retention of components were 32%, two-stage exchange 79%, and resection arthroplasty without delayed reimplantation (one-stage exchange) 61%.[67] In the second study reported by Marculeescu et al.[68] 99 episodes of prosthetic joint infection in 91 patients were treated with debridement and retention of components. *S. aureus* and CoNS were the predominant pathogens, 32% and 23%, respectively. Intravenous antibiotic therapy was given for a median of 28 days, and oral antimicrobial suppression was used in 89% for a median of 541 days. The 2-year survival rate free of treatment failure was 60%, but treatment failure occurred in 53 episodes (53.5%) of the entire cohort. Risk factors independently associated with treatment failure include presence of a sinus tract and duration of symptoms prior to surgery of ≥8 days. Moreover, whereas the proportion of episodes treated successfully was high for CoNS (61%) and *Streptococci* (78.5%), it was poor for *S. aureus* (12.5%) with a 2-year survival rate free of infection of only 22%.[68] This is similar to another report which showed that *S. aureus* was less likely cured (8%) than CoNS or *Streptococci* (56%), $p = 0.007$, with this limited surgical therapy.[65] In contrast a recent study from Spain of 60 patients with staphylococcal prosthetic joint infections (35% *S. aureus* and 65% CoNS) treated with levofloxacin – rifampin (minimum 3 months) and debridement – retention of prosthesis showed failure rates were similar between the different species of *Staphylococci*.[69] However, higher failure rates were found with MRSA, knee versus hip infections (42.8% vs 28.1%) and symptoms greater than 1 month.[69] The main limitation is that the follow-up period of 1 year in this study is certainly too short to define cure, as relapse can occur after 12 months. Penicillin-susceptible streptococcal prosthetic joint infection, with short duration of symptoms (mean 4 days), however, have a good prognosis with debridement and retention of hardware, with only 2 failures (10.5%) of 19 cases followed for a median of 3.9 years.[70]

The main limitation of these reports which could account for differences in results reported from different centers (partially or entirely) was the lack of standardization of medical and surgical therapy, without a strict selection criteria for debridement and retention surgical approach.[71] The only randomized controlled study reported to date used revision-debridement in all 33 patients with staphylococcal implant infection with 2 weeks intravenous antibiotics (flucloxacillin or vancomycin), then oral ciprofloxacin ($N = 15$) or ciprofloxacin – rifampin ($N = 18$) for 3 months with hip prosthesis and fixation devices and 6 months for knee prosthesis.[58] Only 24 patients completed the study (24 months follow up) with cure rate in all 12 patients (100%) receiving rifampin combination, compared to 7 (57%) of 12 in the ciprofloxacin placebo group ($p = 0.02$).[58] There are several limitations of this study including very small sample size and high drop-out rate (almost 30%); and the results only reveal that ciprofloxacin (a weak anti-staphylococcal agent) is ineffective for maintenance therapy, and rifampin (a potent anti-staphylococcal agent) is necessary to augment the effectiveness when a quinolone is used. Furthermore, this pilot study should not be used by itself to endorse neither the surgical nor medical therapeutics, but should be considered an initial proof of concept study.

Immediate one-stage exchange arthroplasty, the infected prosthesis is exchanged for a new one in a single surgery, is becoming popular as a surgical management. This procedure is more convenient than a two-stage exchange arthroplasty, as it involves only one major surgery and avoids a long immobilization period and hospital stay. If the organism in known pre-operatively from a joint aspirate parenteral antibiotics could be given for 2–3 weeks before the prosthesis exchange procedure. Antibiotic-impregnated cement or beads is commonly used by surgeons but the value has not been established for infected prosthesis. Two-stage procedure involves initial surgery to remove the infected implant and all necrotic dead tissue, sinus tract and pus, along with placement of a antibiotic coated spacer. The spacer avoids limb shortening and allows some mobility but is prone to dislocation and can be painful. Antibiotic coating may possibly prevent re-infection and new biofilm on this foreign body. Usually parenteral and oral antibiotics are given for 6–8 weeks, and re-implantation of a new prosthesis when there is evidence of clinical eradication of the infection. This may be assessed by following the ESR and CRP, and obtaining an aseptic aspirate for culture at least 2 weeks after completion of the antibiotics and before re-implantation. This is the procedure of choice when there are sinus tracts or deep abscesses and in the presence of multi-resistant organism (MRSA, gram-negative bacilli) or very virulent organisms. Long-term follow-up has shown a cure rate above 80%,[72] and this approach is more suitable for patients with relatively long life expectancy.

There is no randomized study to compare results of one-stage versus two-stage arthroplasties. A French multicenter study involving 127 one-stage prosthesis exchanges and 222 two-stage exchanges (82% followed for at least 2 years) found similar rates of infection control, 88% and 85%, respectively.[73] However, cases treated by one-stage exchange were more low grade or moderate infections (24% MRSA, 14% draining sinus). Thus, one-stage exchanges in moderate infections achieved the same control as two-stage exchanges in severe prosthetic joint infection.

In a recent review of 29 publications reporting on 1,757 infected total hip arthroplasties, four types of surgical treatments were assessed.[74] Hips treated with one-stage exchange without local antibiotics achieved infection control rates of 59%, and 86% with antibiotic cement (AC). Using two-stage exchanges achieved 86% without AC and 93% infection control rate with AC.[74] These results suggest that AC may have an adjuvant effect by achieving high local antibiotic levels, and improves the outcome in moderate infection treated with a one-stage procedure. Also a previous review on one-stage arthroplasty for infected hip prosthesis analyzed 12 reports involving 1,299 cases followed for an average of 4.8 years (range 0.1–17.1 years).[75] There was a wide variation in duration of parenteral antibiotics (24 h to 8 weeks) and chronic oral antimicrobials (none to 8 months after parenteral). Although success (free of infection at last follow-up) was reported in 1,077 (83%) patients, this is likely an over-estimation as the analysis should have been restricted to those cases followed for at least 2 years. Since AC was used in 99% of the cases this adjuvant modality of therapy could not be properly assessed. Factors associated with success of a direct (one-stage) exchange included: (1) no polymicrobial infection; (2) general good health of the patient; (3) methicillin sensitive CoNS, *S. aureus*, and streptococcus species; and (4) an organism that was sensitive to the antibiotic mixed into the bone cement.[75] If cases are selected for one-stage direct exchange based on these favorable factors this would limit the role of direct exchange arthroplasty in the treatment of infected hip prosthesis or other orthopedic implants. Most CoNS and increasing number of *S. aureus* are methicillin-resistant, more-over high rates of aminoglycoside resistance are present among staphylococci causing prosthetic joint infections,[76] and this class of antibiotic is most commonly used for impregnation of the cement. Furthermore, patients with comorbidities and lower life expectancy who would benefit more from one-stage versus two-stage procedures fall into the unfavorable prognostic category.

A similar review was reported for direct exchange or debridement with retention of components for infected total knee arthroplasty.[77] Infection was controlled in 33 of 37 infected total knee arthroplasties (89.2%) treated by exchange arthroplasty, in only 173 of 530 infected prosthetic knees (32.6%) treated by open debridement and retention of components, and 12 of 23 infected total knee arthroplasties (52.6%) treated by arthroscopic debridement.[77] Factors associated with successful direct exchange included infections by gram-positive organisms, absence of sinus formation, use of antibiotic-impregnated bone cement for the new prosthesis, and 12 weeks of antibiotic therapy. Factors associated with successful debridement and retention of prosthesis included symptoms less than 4 weeks, less than 4 months after the index procedure, antibiotic sensitive gram-positive organisms, no radiological evidence of loosening or osteitis, and young healthy patients.

Permanent resection arthroplasty without replacement (i.e., Girdlestone procedure) is a last resort that will result eradication of the infection but poor limb function. This option is usually undertaken when there is severe loss of bone stock with high risk of recurrent infection or poor general health that precludes implantation of a new prosthesis.

Fracture-fixation devices with bone infection usually cannot be cured without removal of the foreign body, and predispose to non-union of the fracture site which itself leads to persistent infection. The approach to surgical intervention in patients with infected fracture-fixation devices depends on the presence or absence of bone union, the comorbidities and general health of the patients, and type of device. Removal of infected hardware (plates, screws and pins) is the best solution when bone union has occurred, but in the presence of non-union the options involve removal of the device(s) with external-fixation, or insert new pins at a distant site or fuse the bone. Prolonged course of systemic antibiotics with retention of devices can sometimes be tried in patients with poor surgical risk, or until bone union occurs.

Spinal implant infection is one of the most significant complication of spinal fusion and is challenging to diagnose and manage. Again there is no consensus on preferred medical or surgical therapy. Early onset infections within 30 days implant have largely been treated with debridement, implant retention systemic antibiotic therapy for weeks or months with variable success, from $<50\%$[78] to $100\%$.[79] Previous reports of high success rate with conservative surgical therapy probably over-estimate eradication of infection, because of short-term follow-up. Relapse can be seen even up to 2 years after therapy. In a recent retrospective study of 81 spinal implant infections from the Mayo Clinic 30 patients had early-onset infection and 51 patients had late-onset ($>30$ days after implant) infection.[34] The estimated 2-year probability survival free of treatment failure with early-onset infection was 71% (28 of 30 [93%] treated with debridement, implant retention, and antibiotics). Receiving prolonged oral antibiotics ($\geq 6$ months) was associated with increased probability of survival free of infection at 2 years. Thirty-two of 51 patients with late-onset infection were treated with implant removal, with a 2-year success of 84%; but for those without implant removal the success rate was only 36%.[34] Thus, for spinal implant infection debridement with prolonged antimicrobial suppression until spinal fusion occurs is the preferred approach in early infections, but late-onset infection is best managed by removal of the implant.

## 11.5.3 Treatment Algorithm

A proposed algorithm has been developed in Switzerland for the rational surgical and medical treatment strategy for infected total hip arthroplasty.[80] The criteria for the decision of surgical approach are based on postoperative lag time, the type of infection, the condition of the implant and the soft tissue, as well as the comorbidity. The treatment options proposed were debridement with retention, one-stage and two-stage replacement. In a cohort study of 63 consecutive episodes of infected total prosthetic hips prospectively followed for 28 months, the investigators of the center validated their algorithm.[31] Patients treated according to the algorithm had a better outcome with an overall success rate of 88% (44/50) than the others 63%(8/13), $p < 0.03$. In another report by the same group outcome of 40 consecutive episodes of prosthetic knee infection was managed successfully in >80% with the same strategy.[81]

A previous study using the Markov model to simulate patient's projected lifetime clinical course in hypothetical cohorts of 65-year-old and frail 80-year-old patients, assessed the clinical and cost-effectiveness of two management strategies for infected prosthetic hip.[82] The conclusion by this analysis was that prompt debridement and retention is a reasonable strategy for older, frail patients with staphylococcal, or streptococcal infection and a non-loosened prosthesis. For younger healthier adults or *S. aureus* infection with delayed treatment two-stage exchange would be more clinical and cost-effective.[82]

Based on our current knowledge and in the absence of any randomized study a proposed algorithm for management of infected prosthetic joints is outlined in Fig. 11.1. Table 11.1 summarizes criteria that should be used for selecting patients for debridement and retention of components, and Table 11.2 criteria for those best suited for one-stage direct exchange arthroplasty. Table 11.3 outline preferred choices of antimicrobial therapy but this should be based on antimicrobial susceptibility of the organisms isolated, and the local pattern of resistance for empiric therapy should be taken into consideration.

For patient undergoing two-stage exchange it is commonly recommended to aspirate the affected joint for culture 2–4 weeks after systemic antibiotics (commonly 6 weeks) before re-implantation of a new prosthesis. The second-stage implantation should only be done in those with negative cultures, and for patients with persistent infection repeat debridement and course of systemic antibiotics should be reinstituted. In a prospective study of two-stage re-implantation for infected knee arthroplasty, 35 patients (group 1) had reimplantation without repeat aspirate, and 34 patients (group II) had joint aspirates for culture 4 weeks post-antibiotic therapy.[83] Pre-revision aspiration and culture before reimplantation was found to be useful in identifying patients with persistent infections and altered the therapeutic management and outcome. Routine aspiration of the hip joint before revision total hip arthroplasty (not two-stage re-implantation) has also been advocated but remains controversial. In a retrospective review of 142 consecutive total hip arthroplasty routine preoperative aspiration for culture was performed on 128

## 11.5 Management

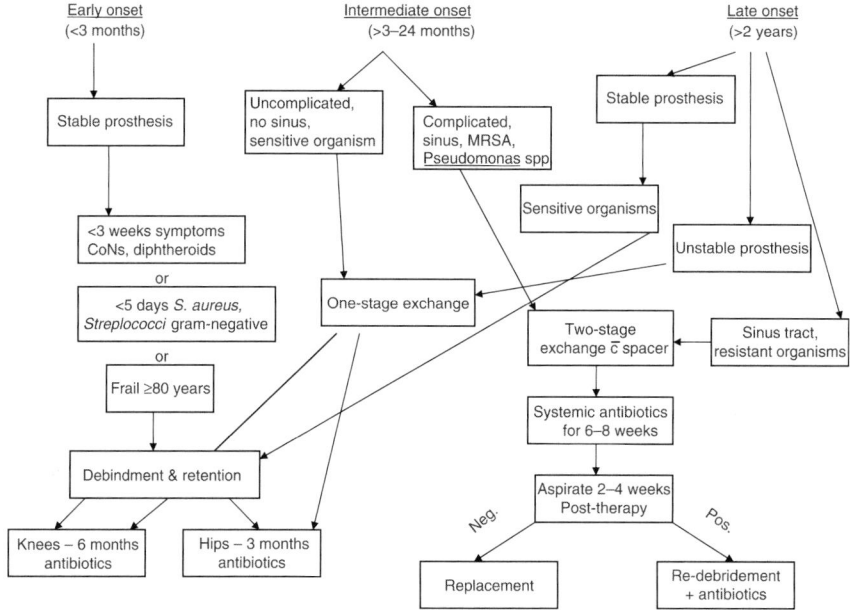

**Fig. 11.1** Algorithm for management of infected prosthetic joint

**Table 11.1** Criteria for debridement and retention of prosthesis

- Stable implant
- Absence of sinus or abscess
- Duration of symptoms less than 3 weeks for low virulent organisms (CoNS, *P. acnes*)
- Duration of symptoms less than 5 days (preferably ≤2 days) for *S. aureus*, gram-negative bacilli
- Penicillin susceptible *Streptococcus* sp. with short duration of symptoms (≤5 days)
- Early-onset infection (<3 months after surgery) or late-onset infection (>2 years)
- Pathogen susceptible to available antimicrobials.

cases.[84] Twenty-one (15%) of the 142 hips were infected, as demonstrated by intraoperative cultures. The hip aspiration-cultures preoperative were found to have high sensitivity (92%) and specificity (97%) with an accuracy of 96%.[84]

### 11.5.4 Issues with Antimicrobial Therapy

There is no consensus as regards specific antibiotics for specific organisms, bactericidal versus bacteristatic agents; intravenous versus oral agents, and duration of

**Table 11.2** Criteria for one-stage direct exchange

- Absence of wound complication after initial arthroplasty
- Methicillin sensitive *S. aureus* (absence of MRSA)
- Organism sensitive to antibiotic mixed in bone cement
- No polymicrobial infection
- No resistant gram-negative bacilli, i.e., *Pseudomonas* sp.
- Good general Health
- Absence of sinus

therapy for orthopedic implant infections. Most guidelines are based on investigators experience, in vitro activity and limited partly relevant animal models, and mostly empiricism.

Agents with excellent oral bioavailability where the blood and tissue levels are similar between parenteral and oral administration (such as the fluoroquinolones, trimethoprim-sulfamethoxazole (cotrimoxazole), rifampin, and metronidazole) can all be used orally for the entire course of treatment. Although some investigators recommend bactericidal agents there is no evidence to support this recommendation in any orthopedic infections. Moreover, most antibiotics are not bactericidal at achievable concentrations against biofilm bacteria, except for rifampin against staphylococci. Once the foreign body is removed, then any antibiotic effective against the planktonic bacteria should be effective. Rifampin is now commonly used in combination therapy for implant infections with staphylococci. However, in vitro susceptibility against the organisms should be confirmed before it is used. Since many staphylococci are now resistant to the fluoroquinolones, combination with rifampin for these infections will lead to rapid resistance as expected with rifampin monotherapy. Other potential disadvantages of quinolones for long-term therapy include selection of coliform resistance in the bowel flora, predisposition to hypervirulent *Clostridium difficle* colitis (see Chapter 8), and increased risk of Archilles tendonitis and rupture. The fluoroquinolones cause changes in extracellular matrix, signaling proteins, with concentration dependent increases of matrix metalloproteinase (especially MMP-3) as well as the apoptosis marker caspase - 3, which causes decrease type I collagen and are the likely mechanisms for the tendinopathy.[85,86] It should be noted that these signaling proteins and the metalloproteinases are involved in the pathophysiology of osteogenesis and bone remodeling after fractures.[87] Thus, the fluoroquinolones may potentially affect these processes adversely. However no clinical studies or animal models have addressed these issues, to determine whether prolonged use of the quinolones could be associated with increased periprosthetic loosening or non-union of fractures with fixation devices.

The long-acting tetracyclines (minocycline and doxycycline) have more favorable features suited for long-term oral therapy (preferably in combination with rifampin) for chronic maintenance oral therapy for staphylococcal orthopedic

## 11.5 Management

**Table 11.3** Antimicrobial choices

- *Methicullin-susceptible Staphylococci* (MSSA, MSSE)
    (i) I.V. semisynthetic Penicillins (nafcillin, cloxacillin, etc.) −6–8 gm/day; or cefazolin 3–6y/day 2–4 weeks; plus oral rifampin 300–450 mg twice daily
    (ii) Then oral cloxacillin or cephalexin 1 g 4X a day; with rifampin (for retained devices) for 1–6 months. Depending on retention of prosthesis, hip or knee arthroplasty
- *Methicullin-resistant Staphylococci* (MRSA, MRSE)
    (i) I.V. Vancomycin 1–1.5 g every 12 h plus oral rifampin 300–450 mg twice daily 2–4 weeks. (For rare contraindications to vancomycin or vancomycin intermediate resistance can use linezolid, tigecycline, or daptomycin)
    (ii) Then oral doxycycline plus rifampin 1–6 months (if resistant or intolerant to doxycycline can substitute with cotrimoxazole, levofloxacin, fusidic acid [if susceptible in vitro])
- *Streptococci and Propionibacterium acnes*
    (i) I.V. Penicillin 3–4 million units every 4 h or cefazolin (mild allergy); or clindamycin or vancomycin (for severe allergy) 2–4 weeks.
    (ii) Then oral amoxicillin 1–2 gm every 8 h or cephalexin 1 g 4Xper day; or clindamycin or marcobide (severe penicillin allergy) 1–6 months
- Enterococcal species

    A. *E. faecalis*
    (i) I.V. Ampicillin 2–3 g every 6 h 2–4 weeks; some guidelines add gentamicin 3 mg/kg/day −7–14[†] days (provided no renal, auditory-vestibular, disturbance)
    (ii) (For penicillin allergy: Vancomycin 1–1.5 g every 12 h)
    (iii) Then oral amoxicillin 1–2 g every 6 h 1–6 months (for penicillin allergy linezolid orally 600 mg every 12 h X 1 month, monitor complete blood count)

    B. *E. faecuim*
    (i) I.V. vancomycin 1.0–1.5 g every 12 h 2–4 weeks ± gentamicin 3 mg/kg/day 7–14[†] days
    (ii) Then oral linezolid 600 mg every 12 h x 1 month, for VRE can be used from the onset; other alternatives include tigecycline, dalfopristin-quinupristin (I.V. only).

    *Gram-negative bacilli*
    (i) *Aerobic coliforms* – antibiotic should depend on susceptibility. Initial intravenous therapy for 2–4 weeks when a cephalosporin, or broad spectrum penicillin is used; subsequent oral therapy for 1–6 months, could use an oral agent in the same class or a quinolone.
    (ii) If the organism is susceptible to cotrimoxazole (trimelhoprim/sulfamethazole) or a quinolone (ciprofloxacin, levofloxacin, etc.) these agents can be used orally from the onset for the entire course as the bioavailability are excellent.

    *Aerobic Diphtheroids (Corynebacterium spp.)*
    Test for susceptibility (tube dilation or E. test), automated methods not approved.
    If susceptible to penicillin use same regimen as for *P. acnes*
    Penicillin resistant strains usually susceptible to vancomycin may also be susceptible to doxycycline. Doxycycline + rifampin a suitable oral combination if susceptible.

[†] = A recent retrospective cohort study of enterococcal prosthetic joint infection found no evidence of superiority of combination with aminoglycoside versus monotherapy and greater risk of ototoxicity.[118]

device infections (especially for CoNS including MRSE, and as well for MRSA). In our hospital clinical microbiology laboratory cumulative susceptibility data for 2006, 92% of 1,384 strains of CoNS and 95% of 2,013 strains of *S. aureus* (including MRSE and MRSA) were susceptible to tetracycline or doxycycline (unpublished data). Tetracyclines belong to the class of "bone seeking agents" that are characterized by high affinity for bone, and are deposited in bone for prolong periods of time despite low serum concentrations.[88] Radiolabeled tetracycline has long been used as an excellent marker in preclinical studies of bone resorption. Tetracycline is deposited in metabolically reactive bone by chelating to calcium during bone formation process, and 3–6% is retained in the skeleton after a single dose.[88] The irreversible removal of tetracycline from bone occurring primarily through bone resorption.

Sub-antimicrobial concentration of doxycycline and non-antimicrobial tetracycline deactivates have anti-inflammatory effects by inhibiting matrix metalloproteinases (MMP), and can reduce periodontal breakdown (gingival inflammation and alveolar bone resorption) and extra-oral bone loss.[89,90] Of the tetracycline analog used in studies to ameliorate the effect of osteopenia associated with inflammatory arthritis, the most effective MMP inhibitors have been minocycline and doxycycline and a non-antibiotic derivative (4-de-demethylaminotetracline[91,92]). Although the main positive effect of tetracyclines on bone and cartilage is secondary to the anti-MMP activity, other complementary effects may include activation of osteoblasts[93] and inhibition of osteoclastic activity.[94] In an arthritis rat model tetracycline derivative positively influence bone mechanical integrity compared to untreated controls, and this was associated with inhibition of collagen breakdown.[95]

It is surprising that despite the favorable characteristics of the long-acting tetracyclines for treatment of bone infection (with or without implants), there is no formal study to assess their clinical efficacy in orthopedic infections. A review of the use of doxycycline or minocycline (with or without rifampin) for MRSA or MSSA for various infection (predominantly skin and skin-structure infections and a few osteomyelitis), reported clinical cure rate of 83%.[96] Thus, this is an area where clinical trials are warranted.

## 11.6 Prevention of Orthopedic Device Infections

Small numbers of bacteria can cause orthopedic implant infections and the source can arise from the air, the patient's skin and the surgical team. Periprosthetic infection rates have shown correlation with the number of airborne bacteria within 30 cm of the wound.[97] Impressions of the gloved hands of surgical team performing total hip arthroplasties have found contamination in 9%, predominantly CoNS, diphtheroids, micrococcus, and *S. aureus* (skin colonizing flora that commonly cause device-related infections).[98] To minimize postoperative implant infections strategies include use of ultraclean air, ultraviolet radiation, different types of surgical clothing, prophylactic systemic antibiotic, and local antibiotic-impregnated cement.

In a systemic review of 25 randomized, controlled trials (RCTs) of antimicrobial prophylaxis for total hip replacement, the surgical wound infection rates were statistically significantly reduced by systemic antibiotics compared with placebo.[99] However, there was inconclusive evidence on the optimal antimicrobial prophylaxis regimen. A first or second generation cephalosporin was most commonly used.

Prophylaxis for ≤24 h is just as effective as for several days, thus prophylaxis should not exceed 1 day. For patients severely allergic to penicillin or with cephalosporin allergy alternative prophylactic agents include one or two doses of clindamycin or vancomycin or teicoplanin. Even in countries with relatively high MRSA colonization/infection rates glycopeptide prophylaxis have not been shown to be superior to a cephalosporin. For patients colonized with MRSA decolonization with mupirocin nasal ointment with antiseptic liquid soap (1% triclosan or chlorhexidine) should be attempted >7–10 days before surgery, preferably with repeat cultures showing clearance prior to the operation. Routine use of topical mupirocin to all patients before orthopedic surgery has not been shown to reduce surgical site infection.[101] In case of emergency surgery patients colonized with MRSA vancomycin prophylaxis should be considered. For all types of surgical antibiotic prophylaxis the antimicrobial should best be given 30–60 min before incision, a second dose may be given intraoperatively for prolonged surgery (≥3 h), but post-operative doses are not recommended.

Antibacterial prophylaxis has also been shown to be of value in closed fractures of long bones with internal fixation devices. In a meta-analysis of 22 RCTs with 8,307 patients there was a significant decrease in deep wound and other infections in the antibiotic prophylactic treated patients (RR = 0.40).[102]

There is evidence as well that antibiotic-loaded bone cement can prevent deep surgical, perioperative, site infection in randomized, controlled trials,[103,104] but not late hematogenous-seeded prosthetic joint infections.[105] Large observational data from the Swedish registry with 215,000 total hip replacement found that antibiotic-impregnated cement reduced the incidence of surgical site infection by twofold lower than systemic antibiotic prophylaxis.[106] Similarly, Norwegian data with 22,150 hip arthroplasties found that antibiotic-cement reduced infection rate from 0.7% (systemic prophylaxis only) to 0.4% (combined local and systemic prophylaxis, $p = 0.001$[107])

Prophylactic antibiotics to prevent late hematogenous seeding to prosthetic joints following dental or urologic procedures have not been proven. Although, hematogenous seeding can occur at any time after the procedure the risk appears to be highest within the first two years. The American Dental Association/Academy of Orthopedic Surgeons do not recommend antibacterial prophylaxis routinely for these procedures, but suggest consideration of prophylaxis for high risks groups (within a year of implantation and in immunocompromised patients[109,110]). Recent review of the need for antibiotic prophylaxis for dental procedures has concluded that the risk, of an artificial joint becoming infected from a bacteremia of oral origin is exceeding low whereas the risk of an adverse reaction to the antibiotic prophylaxis is higher than the risk of infection.[111] It was estimated that if all patients with prosthetic joints were to receive dental antibiotic prophylaxis more subjects would die from anaphylaxis than develop infections.

As previously mentioned the greatest risk of hematogenous seeding to a prosthetic joint is from documented *S. aureus* bacteremia (34%). Although no studies have addressed the issue of duration of therapy for *S. aureus* bacteremia (from other sources) in patients with joint prosthesis it may be prudent to use prolonged therapy (4–6 weeks) even if investigation fails to reveal an infected device.

## 11.7 Future Directions

Ideally prospective, multicenter, randomized trials should be performed at different stages (early, delayed, and late) of prosthetic joint infections to determine the best surgical approach (debridement with retention, one-stage or two-stage procedures). The probability of this occurring, however, seems remote. A prospective, multicenter trial with standardized criteria for diagnosis, surgical and medical therapy according to stage of infection, using an algorithm and with long-term follow-up (at least 2–3 years, and preferably 5 years) would also be desirable and may have a greater chance of being completed than a randomized, multicenter trial.

Methods to prevent orthopedic device infection to even lower limits are still being explored, and they may have greater application in high risk patients – i.e., those with previous arthroplastics (especially infected), obese subjects, diabetics and debilitated patients or immunocompromised hosts. Laboratory studies and clinical trials have suggested that hydroxyapatite coating improves the osteointegration of various orthopedic implants. This could result in reduced loosening of fixation pins and pin-track infection. In a preliminary randomized trial of 46 patients undergoing segmental transplant or lengthening of the tibia half received standard titanium pins and half received hydroxyapatite-coated stainless-steel pins.[112] In the control group 13% developed loosening and infection at the site, compared to no loosening or infection in the hydroxyapatite group. Thus, further large multicenter, randomized trials are needed to confirm this result.

Another approach is to coat the titanium surface of prosthesis and fixation devices with antimicrobials effective against the commonest organisms that can be implanted at surgery (staphylococci, diphtheroids, etc.). A novel approach is to tether covalently vancomycin to metal (titanium) surface, with retained bactericidal activity.[113] This approach needs to be tested in large randomized trials, but the risk of encouraging vancomycin resistant staphylococci and enterococci would be a primary concern.

Incorporation of local antibiotics into bone cement or the prosthetic material (titanium) itself can lead to resistance; as shown by a report where 19 of 28 bacterial strains cultured directly from clinically retrieved gentamicin-loaded cement were gentamicin-resistant.[114] Pharmacokinetic studies have also found that gentamicin-impregnated cement or beads release less than 50% of the antibiotics into the surrounding tissues within 4 weeks, and no continuous release thereafter.[115] Simple chemical modification of surface treated titanium with an external layer of anatase titanium dioxide ($TiO_2$), which can decrease bacterial adhesion and produce photocatalytic bactericidal effects is more appealing.[116] Another innovative generation of coatings utilizes a staphylolytic endopeptidase (lysostaphin) active on staphylococci even if antibiotic resistant.[117]

Comparative trials of antimicrobial agents (combined with rifampin) for prolong oral therapy 1–6 months, after initial induction with vancomycin/rifampin for 2 weeks, for staphylococcal implant infections would be interesting and desirable. Especially to compare doxycycline plus rifampin versus levofloxacin plus rifampin (or cotrimoxazole for quinolone resistant strains) with 3 years follow-up to assess relapse of infection, periprosthetic loosening and non-union of fractures with internal fixation devices.

Although new anti-staphylococcal agents with MRSA and VRE activity are now available, such as linezolid, quinupristin/dalfopristin, tigecycline, and daptomycin, they will have limited role to play in treatment because of their expense, side-effect profile and poor oral bioavailability (except for linezolid).

## 11.8 Conclusion

Treatment and prophylaxis for orthopedic device infections have improved over the past decade. However, there is still controversy and lack of standardization with regards to diagnosis, surgical and medical therapy. Although the general principles of a foreign device-related infection mandate removal of the device to achieve optimum cure, there is some evidence that early debridement with device retention and prolonged antibiotics in selected patients can achieve acceptable cure rates. However, selection criteria, choice of antimicrobials and duration of therapy need to be better defined. Although rifampin seems to have an important therapeutic role to play for staphylococcal infections (once the organism is susceptible) the ideal partner to use in combination is undefined. Quinolones does not appear to be the best partner agent, theoretically long-acting tetracyclines (doxycycline or minocycline) are more suitable choices but more clinical trials are needed.

## References

1. Darouiche, R.O. (2004). Treatment of infections associated with surgical implants. *N Engl J Med* 350:1422–1429.
2. NIH Consensus Development Panel on Total Hip Replacement (1995), NIH consensus conference: total hip replacement. *JAMA* 273:1950–1956.
3. Harris, W.H., Sledge, C.B. (1990). Total hip and total knee replacement. *N Engl J Med* 323:801–807.
4. Sperling, J.W., Kozak, T.K., Hanssen, A.D., Cofield, R.H. (2001). Infection after shoulder arthroplasty. *Clin Ortho* 382:206–216.
5. Murdoch, D.R., Roberts, S.A., Fowler, V.G. Jr., Shah, M.A., Taylor, S.C., Morris, A.J., Corey, G.R. (2001). Infection of orthropedic prostheses after *Staphylococcus aureus* bacteremia. *Clin Infect Dis* 32:647–649.
6. Ainscow, D.A., Denham, R.A., (1984). The risk of hematogenous infection in total joint replacements. *J Bone Joint Surg Br* 66:580–582.

7. Schmalzried, T.P., Amstutz, H.C., Au, M.K., Dorey, F.J. (1992). Etiology of deep sepsis in total hip arthroplasty: the significance of hematogenous and recurrent infections. *Clin Orthop* 280:200–207.
8. Zimmerli, W., Trompuz, A., Ochsner, P.E. (2004), Prosthetic joint infections. *N Engl J Med* 351:1645–1654.
9. Trampuz, A., Steckelberg, J.M., Osmon, D.R., Cockervill, F.R., Hanssen, A.D., Patel, R. (2003). Advances in the laboratory diagnosis of prosthetic joint infection. *Rev Med Microbiol* 14:1–14.
10. Pandey, R., Berandt, A.R., Athanason, N.A. (2000). Histological and microbiological findings in non-infected and infected revision arthroplasty tissues. *Arch Orthop Trauma Surg* 120:570–574.
11. Spangehl, M.J., Masri, B.A., O'Connell, J.X., Duncan, C.P. (1999). Prospective analysis of preoperative and intraoperative investigations for the diagnosis of infection at the sites of two hundred and two revision total hip arthroplasties. *J Bone Joint Surg Am* 81:672–683.
12. Panousis, K., Grigoris, P., Butcher, I., Rana, B., Reilly, J.H., Hamblen, D.L. (2005). Poor predictive value of broad-range PCR for the detection of arthroplasty infection in 92 cases. *Acta Orthop* 76:341–346.
13. Neut, D., van Horn, J.R., van Kooten, T.G., van der Mei, H.C., Busschet, H.J. (2003). Detection of biomaterial-associated infections in orthopaedic joint implants. *Clin Orthop Related Res* 413:261–268.
14. Tunney, M.M., Patrick, S., Gorman, S.P., Sean, P., Nixon, J.R., Anderson, N., Davis, R.J., Hanna, D., Ramage, G. (1998). Improved detection of infection in hip replacements: a currently underestimated problem. *J Bone Joint Surg Br* 80:568–572.
15. Trampuz, A., Piper, K.E., Hanssen, A.D., Osmon, D.R., Cockerill, F.R., Steckelberg, J.M., Patel, R. (2006). Sonication of explanted prosthetic components in bags for diagnosis of prosthetic joint infection is associated with risk of contamination. *J Clin Microbiol* 44:628–631.
16. Trampuz, A., Piper, K.E., Jacobson, M.J., Hanssen, A.D., Unni, K.K., Osman, D.R., Mandrekar, J.W., Cockerill, F.R., Steckelberg, J.M., Greenleaf, J.F., Patel, R. (2007). Sonication of removed hip and knee prosthesis for diagnosis of infection. *N Engl J Med* 357:654–663.
17. Walvogel, F.A. (2007). Ultrasound – now also for microbiologists? (Editorial). *N Engl J Med* 357:705–706.
18. Perdreau-Remington, F., Stefanik. D., Peters, G., Ludwig, C., Rutt, J., Wenzel, R., Pulverer, G. (1996). A four-year prospective study on microbial ecology of explanted prosthetic hips in 52 patients with "aseptic" prosthetic joint loosening. *Eur J Clin Microbiol Infect Dis* 15:160–165.
19. Tiggers, S. Stiles, R.G., Roberson, J.R. (1994). Appearance of septic hip prosthesis on plain radiographs. *AJR Am J Roentgenol* 163:377–380.
20. Smith, S.L., Wastie, M.L., Forster, I. (2001). Radionuclide bone scintigraphy in the detection of significant complications after total knee joint replacement. *Clin. Radiol.* 56:221–224.
21. Vicente, A.G., Almoguerra, M., Alonso, J.C., Hefferman, A.J., Gomez, A., Contreras, P.I., Martin-Comin, J. (2004). Diagnosis of orthopedic infection in clinical practice using Tc-99 sulesomab (antigranulocyte monoclonal antibody fragment Fab'2). *Clin Nuclear Med* 29:781–785.
22. Pakos, E.E., Trikalinos, T.A., Fotopoulos, A.D., Ioannidis, J.P. (2007). Prosthesis infection: diagnosis after total joint arthroplasty with antigranulocyte scintigraphy with 99mTc-labelled monoclonal antibodies – a meta-analysis. *Radiology* 242:101–108.
23. Lowe, C., Marwin, S.E., Tomas, M.B., Krauss, E.S., Tronco, G.G., Bhargava, K.K., Nichols, K.J., Palestro, C.J. (2004). Diagnosing infection in the failed joint replacement: a comparison of coincidence detection 18F-FDG and 111In-labelled leukocyte/99mTc-sulfur colloid marrow imaging. *J Nuclear Med* 45:1864–1871.

24. Lowe, C., Pugliese, P.V., Agriyie, M.O., Tomas, M.B., Marwin, S.E., Palestro, C.J. (2000). Utility of F-18 FDG imaging for diagnosing the infected joint replacement. *Clin Positron Imaging* 3:159.
25. Reinartz, P., Mumme T., Hermanns, B., Cremerius, U., Wirtz, D.C., Schaefer, W.M., Niethard, F.U., Buell, U. (2005). Radionuclide imaging of the painful hip arthroplasty: positron-emission tomography versus triple-phase bone scanning. *J Bone Joint Surg Brit* 87:465–470.
26. Schiesser, M. Stumpe, K.D.M., Trentz, O., Kossmunn, T., Von Schulthess, G.K. (2003). Detection of metallic implant-associated infections with FDG PET in patients with trauma: correlation with microbiologic results. *Radiology* 226:391–398.
27. Wirtz, D.C., Heller, K.D., Miltner, O., Zilkens, K.W., Wolff, J.M. (2000). Interleukin-6: a potential inflammatory marker after total joint replacement. *Int Orthop* 24:194–196.
28. Dicesare, P.E., Chang, E., Preston, C.F., Liu, C.J. (2005). Serum interleukin-6 as a marker of periprosthetic infection following total hip and knee arthroplasty. *J Bone Joint Surg Am* 87:1921–1927.
29. Panday, R., Drakoulakis, E., Athanasou, N.A. (1999). An assessment of the histological criteria used to diagnose infection in hip revision arthroplasty tissues. *J Clin Path* 52:118–123.
30. Banit, D.M., Kaufer, H., Hartford, J.M. (2002). Intraoperative frozen section analysis in revision total joint arthroplasty. *Clin Orthop Related Res* 401:230–238.
31. Giulieri, S.G., Graber, P., Ochsner, P.E., Zimmerli, W. (2004). Management of infection associated with total hip arthroplasty according to a treatment algorithm. *Infection* 32:222–228.
32. Trampuz, A., Widmer, A.F. (2006). Infections associated with orthopedic implants. *Curr Opin Infect Dis* 19:349–356.
33. Deyo, R.A., Nachermson, A., Mirza, S.K. (2004). Spinal fusion surgery – the case for restraint. *N Engl J Med* 350:722–726.
34. Kowalski, T.J., Berbari, E.F., Huddleston, P.M., Steckelberg, J.M., Mandrekar, J.N., Osmon, D.R. (2007). The management and outcome of spinal implant infections: contemporary retrospective cohort study. *Clin Infect Dis* 44:913–920.
35. Wymenga, A.B., van Horn, J.R., Theeuswes, A., Muytjens, H.L., Slaoff, T.J. (1992). Perioperative factors associated with septic arthritis after arthroplasty. Prospective multi-center study of 362 knee and 2651 hip operations. *Acta Orthop Scand* 63:665–671.
36. Berbari, E.F., Hanssen, A.D., Duffy, M.C., Steckelberg, J.M., Ilstrup, D.M., Harmsen, W.S., Osmon, D.R. (1998). Risk factors for prosthetic joint infection: case control study. *Clin Infect Dis* 27:1247–1254.
37. Culver, D.H., Horan, T.C., Gaynes, R.P., Martone, W.J., Jarvis, W.R., Emori, T.G., Banerjee, S.N., Edwards, J.R., Henderson, T.S. (1991). Surgical wound infection rates by wound class, operative procedure, and patient risk index. National Nosocomial Infections Surveillance System. *Am J Med* 91 (Suppl 3B):152S–157S.
38. Jeys, L.M., Grimer, R.J., Carter, S.R., Tillman, R.M. (2005). Periprosthetic infection in patients treated for an orthopedic oncological condition. *J Bone Joint Surg (Am)* 87A:842–849.
39. Ahnfelt, L., Herberts, P. Malchau, H., Anderson, G.B. (1990). Prognosis of total hip replacement. A Swedish multicenter study of 4664 revisions. *Acta Orthop Scand* 238 (Suppl):1–26.
40. Kalmeijer, M.D., van Nieuwland-Bollen E., Bogaers-Hofman, D., de Baere, G.A.J., Kluytmans, J.A.J (2000). Nasal carriage of *Staphylococcus aureus* is a major risk factor for surgical site infections in orthopedic surgery. *Infect Control Hosp Epidemiol* 21:319–323.
41. Katz, J.N., Losina, E., Barrett, J., Phillips, C.B., Mahomed, N.N., Lew, R.A., Guadagoni, E., Harris, W.H., Poss, R., Baron, J.A. (2001). Association between hospital and surgeon procedure volume and outcomes of total hip replacement in the United States Medicare population. *J Bone Joint Surg (AM)* 83A:1622–1629.

42. Christodoulou, A.G., Givissis, P., Symeonidis, P.D., Korataglis, D., Pournaras, J. (2006). Reduction of post-operative spinal infections based on etiological protocol. *Clin Orthop Related Res* 444:107–113.
43. Stewart, P.S., Costerton, J.W. (2001). Antibiotic resistance of bacteria in biofilms. *Lancet* 358:135–138.
44. Donlan, R.M., Costerton, J.W. (2002).Biofilms: survival mechanisms of clinically relevant microorganisms. *Clin Microbiol Rev* 15:167–193.
45. Widmer, A.F., Frei, R., Rajacic, Z., Zimmerli, W. (1990). Correlation between in vivo and in vitro efficacy of antimicrobial agents against foreign body infections. *J Infect Dis* 162:96–102.
46. Norden, C.W. (1983). Experimental chronic staphylococcal osteomyelitis in rabbits: treatment with rifampin alone and in combination with other antimicrobial agents. *Rev Infect Dis* 5 (Suppl 3):s491–s494.
47. Andriole, V.T., Nagel, D.A., Southwick, W.O. (1973). A paradigm for human chronic osteomyelitis. *J Bone Joint Surg Am* 55:1511–1515.
48. Passl, R., Mÿller, C., Zienlinski, C., Eibl, M.M. (1984). A model of experimental post-traumatic osteomyelitis in guinea pigs. *J Trauma* 24:323–326.
49. Worlock, P., Slack, R., Harvey, L., Mawhinney, R. (1988). An experimental model of post-traumatic osteomyelitis in rabbits. *Br J Exp Pathol* 69:235–244.
50. Southwood, R.T., Rice, J.L., McDonald, P.J., Hakendorf, P.H., Rozenbilds, M.A. (1985). Infection in experimental hip arthroplasties. *J Bone Joint Surg Br* 37:229–231.
51. Belmatoug, N., Crèmieux, A.C., Bleton, R., Volk, A., Saleh-Mghir, A., Grossin, M., Garry, L., Carbon, C. (1996). A new model of experimental prosthetic joint infection due to methicillin-resistant *Staphyloccus aureus*: a microbiologic, histopathologic and magnetic resonance imaging characterization. *J Infect Dis* 174:414–417.
52. Crimieux, A.C., Saleh-Mghir, A., Bleton, R., Manteau, M., Belmatoug, N., Massias, L., Garry, L., Sales, N., Maziere, B., Carbon, C. (1996). Efficacy of sparfloxacin and autoradiography diffusion pattern of [$^{14}$C] sparfloxacin in experimental *Staphylococcus aureus* joint prosthesis infection. *Antimicrobial Agents Chemother* 40:2111–2116.
53. Saleg-Mghir, A., Cremieux, A.C., Bleton, R., Manteau, M., Massias, L, Garry, L., Sales, N., Maziere, B., Carbon, C. (1996). Autoradiographic of $^{14}$C-teicoplanin and efficacy of teichoplanin in an experimental staphylococcal infection. In Program and abstracts of the 36th ICAAC (New Orleans) [abst. A38]: Am Society Microbiol, Washington, DC.
54. Blaser, J., Vergeres, P., Widmer, A.F., Zimmerli, W. (1995). In vivo verification of in vitro model of antibiotic treatment of device-related infection. *Antimicrob Agents Chemother* 39:1134–1139.
55. Archer, G.L., Johnston, J.L., Vasquez, G.I., Haywood III, H.B. (1983). Efficacy of antibiotic combinations including rifampicin against methicillin-resistant *Staphylococcus epidermidis* in vitro and in vivo studies. *Rev Infect Dis* 5(Suppl 3):s538–s547.
56. Lowry, F.D., Wexler, M.A., Steigbigel, N.H. (1982). Therapy of methicillin-resistant *Staphylococcus epidermidis* experimental endocarditis. *J Lab Clin Med* 100:94–104.
57. Eerenberg, J.P., Patka, P., Haarman, H.J., Dwars, B.J. (1994). A new model for post-traumatic osteomyelitis in rabbits. *J Invest Surg* 7:453–465.
58. Zimmerli, W., Widmer, A.F., Blatter, M., Frei, R., Ochsner, P.E. for the Foreign-Body Infection (FBI) Study Group (1998). Role of rifampin for treatment of orthopedic implant-related staphylococcal infections: a randomized controlled trial. Foreign Body Infection (FBI) Study Group. *JAMA* 279:1537–1541.
59. Trebse, R., Pisot, V., Trampuz, A. (2005). Treatment of retained implants. *J Bone Joint Surg Br* 87:249–256.
60. Tattevin, P., Cremieux, A.C., Pottier, P., Huten, D., Carbon, C. (1999). Prosthetic joint infection: when can prosthesis salvage be considered? *Clin Infect Dis* 29:292–295.
61. Brandt, C.M., Sistrunk, W.W., Duffy, M.C., Hanssen, A.D., Stecklberg, J.M., Ilstrup, D.M., Osmon, D.R. (1997). *Staphylococcus aureus* prosthetic joint infection treated with debridement and prosthesis retention. *Clin Infect Dis* 24:914–919.

62. Tsukayama, D.T., Wicklund, B., Gustilo, R.B. (1991). Suppressive antibiotic therapy in chronic prosthetic joint infections. *Orthopedics* 14:841–844.
63. Tsukuyama, D.T., Estrada, R., Gustilo, R.B. (1996). A study of the treatment of one hundred and six infections. *J Bone Joint Surg Am* 78:512–523.
64. Schoifet, S.D., Morrey, B.F. (1990). Treatment of infection after total knee arthroplasty by debridement with retention of the components. *J Bone Joint Surg Am* 72:1383–1390.
65. Deirmengian, C., Greenbaum, J., Locke, P.A., Booth, R.E. Jr., Lonner, J.H. (2003). Limited success with open debridement and retention of components of acute *Staphylococcus aureus* infection after total knee arthroplasty. *J Arthroplasty* 18(7 Suppl I):22–26.
66. Crockarell, J.R., Hanssen, A.D., Osmon, D.R., Morrey, B.F. (1998). Treatment of infection with debridement and retention of the components following hip arthroplasty. *J Bone Joint Surg Am* 80:1306–1313.
67. Berbari, E.F., Osmon, D.R., Duffy, M.C.T., Harmssen, W., Mandrekar, J.N., Hanssen, A.D., Steckelberg, J.M. (2006). Outcome of prosthetic joint infection in patients with rheumatoid arthritis: the impact of medical and surgical therapy in 200 episodes. *Clin Infect Dis* 42: 216–223.
68. Marculescu, C.E., Berbari, E.F., Hanssen, A.D., Steckelberg, J.M., Harmsen, S.W., Mandrekar, J.N., Osmon, D.R. (2006). Outcome of prosthetic joint infections treated with debridement and retention of components. *Clin Infect Dis* 42:471–478.
69. Barberàn, J., Aguilar, L., Carroquino, G., Gimenez, M.J., Sanchez, B., Martinez, D., Prieto, J. (2006). Conservative treatment of staphylococcal prosthetic joint infections in elderly patients. *Am J Med* 119:993e7–993e10.
70. Meehan, A.M., Osmon, D.R., Duffy, M.C.T., Keating, M.R. (2003). Outcome of penicillin-susceptible streptococcal prosthetic joint infection treated with debridement and retention of the prosthesis. *Clin Infect Dis* 36:845–849.
71. Zimmerli, W. (2006). Prosthetic joint infections. *Best Prac Res Clin Rheum* 20:1045–1063.
72. Windsor, R.E., Insall, J.N., Urs, W.K., Miller, D.V., Brause, R.D. (1990). Two-stage reimplantation for the salvage of total knee athroplasty complicated by infection. Further follow-up refinement of indications. *J Bone Joint Surg Am* 72:272–278.
73. Vielpeau, C. (2002). The management of infected hip prosthesis – a multicenter study of 563 cases: conclusions about surgical treatment. *Rev Chir Orthop* 88: (Suppl 5):214–216.
74. Langlais, F., Belot, N., Ropars, Thomazeau, H., Lambote, J.C., Cathelineau, G. (2006). Antibiotic cements in articular prosthesis: current orthopedic concepts. *Internal J Antimicrob Agents* 28:84–89.
75. Jackson, W.O., Schmalzried, T.P. (2000). Limited role of direct exchange arthroplasty in the treatment of infected total hip replacements. *Clin Orthop Relat Res* 381:101–105.
76. Anguita-Alonso, P., Hanssen, A.D., Osmon, D.R., Trampuz, A., Steckelberg, J.M., Patel, R. (2005). High rate of aminoglycoside resistance among staphylococcus causing prosthetic joint inflammation. *Clin Orthop Relat Res* 439:43–47.
77. Silva, M., Tharani, R., Schmalzried, T.P. (2002). Results of direct exchange or debridement of the infected total knee arthroplasty. *Clin Orthop Relat Res* 404:125–131.
78. Sponsellar, P.D., La Port, D.M., Hungerford, M.W., Eck, K., Bridewell, K.H., Lenke, L.G. (2000). Deep wound infections after neuromuscular scoliosis surgery: a multicenter study of risk factors and treatment outcomes. *Spine* 25:2461–246.
79. Glassman, S.D., Dimar, J.R., Puno, R.M., Johnson, J.R. (1996). Salvage of instrumental lumbar fusions complicated by surgical wound infection. *Spine* 21:2163–2169.
80. Zimmerli, W., Ochsner, P.E. (2003). Management of infection associated with prosthetic joints. *Infection* 31:99–105.
81. Laffer, R.R., Graber, P., Ochsner, P.E., Zimmerli, W. (2006). Outcome of prosthetic knee-associated infection: evaluation of 40 consecutive episodes at a single center. *Clin Microbiol Infect* 12:433–439.

82. Fisman, D.N., Reilly, D.T., Karchmer, A.W., Goldie, S.J. (2001). Clinical effectiveness and cost-effectiveness of 2 management strategies for infected total hip arthroplasty. *Clin Infect Dis* 32:419–430.
83. Mont, M.A., Waldman, B.J., Hungerford, D.S. (2000). Evaluation of preoperative cultures before second-stage reimplantation of a total knee prosthesis complicated by infection. A comparison-group study. *J Bone Joint Surg Am* 82-A:1552–1557.
84. Lachiewicz, P.F., Rogers, G.D., Thomason, H.C. (1996). Aspiration of the hip joint before revision arthroplasty. Clinical and laboratory factors influencing attainment of a positive culture. *J Bone Joint Surg Am* 78:749–751.
85. Sendzik, J., Shakibaei, M., Schäfer-Korting, M., Stahlmann, R. (2005), Fluoroquinolones cause changes in extracellular matrix, signaling proteins, metalloproteinases and caspase-3 in cultured human tendon cells. *Toxicology* 212:24–36.
86. Corps, AN, Harrall, R.L., Curry, V.A., Fenwick, SA., Hazleman, B.L., Riley, G., (2002), Ciprofloxacin enhances stimulation of matrix metalloproteinase 3 expression by interleukin-1β in human tendon-derived cells. A potential mechanism of fluoroquinolone-induced tendinopathy. *Arth Rheumatol* 46:3034–3040.
87. Lehmann, W., Edgar, C.M., Wang, K., Cho., F.J., Barnes, G.L., Kakar, S., Graves, D.T., Rueger, J.M., Gerstenfeld, L.C., Einhorn, T.A. (2005), Tumor necrosis factor alpha (TNF-α) coordinately regulates the expression of specific matrix metalloproteinases (MMPS) and angiogenic factors during fracture healing. *Bone* 36:300–310.
88. Stepensky, D., Kleinberg, L., Hoffman, A. (2003), Bone as an effect compartment. Models for uptake and release of drugs. *Clin Pharmacokinet* 42:863–881.
89. Lee, H.M., Ciancio, S.G., Tiiter, G., Ryan, M.E., Komaroff, E., Golub, L.M., (2004), Subantimicrobial dose doxycycline efficacy as a matrix metalloproteinase inhibitor in chronic periodontitis patients is enhanced when combined with a non-steroidal anti-inflammatory drugs. *J Periodontal* 75:453–463.
90. Golub, L.M., Ramamuthy, N.S., Llavaneras, A., Ryan, M.E., Lee, H.M., Liu, Y., Bain, S., Sorsa, T. (1999), A chemically modified nonantimicrobial tetracycline (CMT-8) inhibits gingival matrix metalloproteinases, periodontal breakdown, and extra-oral bone loss in ovariectomized rats. Ann. N.Y. *Acad. Sci* 878:290–310.
91. Greenwald, R.A., Moak, S.A., Ramamurthy, N.S., Golub, L.M. (1992), Tetracyclines suppress matrix metalloproteinases activity in adjuvant arthritis and in combination with flurbiprofen, ameliorate bone damage, *J Rheumatol* 19:927–938.
92. Golub, L.M., Greenwald, R.A., Ramanurthy, N.S., McNamara, T.F., Rifkin, B.R. (1991), Tetracyclines inhibit connective tissue breakdown: new therapeutic implications for an old family of drugs. *Crit Rev Oral Biol Med* 2:297–321.
93. Sasaki, t., Kaneko, H., Ramamurthy, N.S., Golub, L.M. (1991), Tetracycline administration restores osteoblast structure and function during experimental diabetes. *Anat Rec* 231:25–34.
94. Rifkin, B.R., Vernillo, A.T., Golub, L.M., Ramamurthy, N.S. (1994), Modulation of bone resorption by tetracyclines. Ann. N.Y. Acad. Sci. 732:165–180.
95. Zernicke, R.F., Wohl, G.R., Greenwald, R.A., Moak, S.A., Leng, W., Golub, L.M. (1997), Administration of systemic matrix metalloproteinase inhibitors maintains bone mechanical integrity in adjuvant arthritis. *J Rheumatol* 24:1324–1231.
96. Ruhe, J.J., Monson, T., Bradsher, R.W., Menon, A. (2005), Use of long-acting tetracyclines for methicillin-resistant. *Staphylococcus aureus* infection: case series and review of the literature. *Clin Infect Dis* 40:1429–1434.
97. Gosden, R.E., MacGowan, A.P., Bannister, G.C. (1998), Importance of air quality and related factors in the prevention of infection in orthopedic implant surgery. *J Hosp Infect* 39:173–180.
98. Al-Maiyah, M., Hill, D., Bajwa, A., Slater, S., Patil, P., Port, A., Gregg, P.J. (2005), Bacterial contaminants and antibiotic prophylaxis in total hip arthroplasty. *J Bone Joint Surg Br* 87: 1256–1258.

99. Glenny. A.M., Song, F. (1999), Antimicrobial prophylaxis in total hip replacement: a systemic review. *Health Technol Assess* 3(21).
100. Suter, F., Avai, A., Fusco, U, Gerundini, M., Caprioli, S., Maggiolo, F. (1994), Teichoplanin versus cefamandole in the prevention of infection in total hip replacement. *Eur J Clin Microbial Infect Dis* 13:793–796.
101. Kalmeijer, M.D., Coertjens, H., van Nieuwland-Bollen, P.M., Bogaers-Hofman, D., deBaere, G.A.J., Stuur-man, A., van Belkum, A., Kluytmans, J.A.J.W. (2002), Surgical site infections in orthopedic surgery: the effect of mupirocin nasal ointment in a double-blind, randomized, placebo-controlled study. *Clin Infect Dis* 35:353–358.
102. Gillespie, W.J., WalenKamp, G. (2001), Antibiotic prophylaxis for surgery for proximal femoral and other closed long bone fractures. *Cochrane Database Syst Rev* (1):CD00–0244.
103. Josefsson, G., Gudmundsson, G., Kolmert, L., Wijkstrom, S. (1990), Prophylaxis with systemic antibiotics versus gentamicin bone cement in total hip arthroplasty. A five-year survey of 1688 hips. *Clin Orthop* 253:173–178.
104. Chiu, F.Y., Chen, E.M., Lin, C.F., Lo, W.H. (2002), Cefuroxime-impregnated cement in primary total knee orthoplasty: a prospective, randomized study of three hundred and forty knees. *J Bone Jt Surg Am* 84:759–762.
105. Josefsson, G., Kolmert, L. (1993), Prophylaxis with systemic antibiotics versus gentamicin bone cement in total hip arthroplasty. A ten-year survey of 1688 hips. *Clin Orthop* 292: 210–214.
106. Herberts, P., Malchau, H., Garrelick, G., Swedish National Hip Arthroplasty Register. (2004), Annual Report 2004 (242,393 primary THR). Swed. Nat. Hip. Register. http://www.jru.orthop.gu.se.
107. Engesaeter, L.B., Lie, S.A., Espehaug, B., Furnes, O., Vollset, S.E., Havelin, L.I. (2003), Antibiotic prophylaxis in total hip arthroplasty: effects of antibiotic prophylaxis systemically and in bone cement on the revision rate of 22,170 primary hip replacements followed 0–14 years in the Norwegian Arthroplasty Register. *Acta Orthop Scand* 74:644–651.
108. Tramprz, A., Zimmerli, W. (2006), Antimicrobial agents in orthopedic surgery: Prophylaxis and treatment. *Drugs* 66:1089–1105.
109. American Academy of Orthopedic Surgeons. (2006), Antibiotic prophylaxis for dental patients with total joint replacements (Doc.no.-1014). Available from URL:http//www.aaos.org/wordht-ml/papers/advistmt./1014.htm.
110. American Academy of Orthopedic Surgeons. (2006), Antibiotic prophylaxis for urological patients with total joint replacements. (Doc. No. 1023). Available from URL: http://www.aa-os.org//wordhtml/papers/advistmt/1023.htm.
111. Scott. J.F., Morgan, D., Avent, M., Graves, S., Goss, A.N. (2005), Patients with artificial joints: do they need antibiotic cover for dental treatment? *Austral Dent J* 50 (4 Suppl 2): s45–s53.
112. Pommer, A., Muhr, G., David, A. (2002), Hydroxyapatate-coated Schanz pins in external fixations used for distraction osteogenesis: a randomized, controlled trial. *J. Bone Jt Surg Am* 84-A:1162–1166.
113. Parvizi, J., Wickstrom, E., Zeiger, A.R., Adams, C.S., Shapiro, I.M., Purtill, J.J., Sharkey, P. F., Hozak, W.J., Rothman, R.H., Hickok, N.J. (2004), Frank Stinchfield Award. Titanium surface with biologic activity against infection. *Clin Orthop Relat Res* 429:33–38.
114. Neut, D., Van de Belt, H., Stokroos, I., Van Horn, J.R., Van der Mei, H.C., Busscher, H.J. (2001), Biomaterial-associated infection of gentamicin-loaded PMMA beads in orthopedic revision surgery. *J Antimicrob Chemther* 47:885–891.
115. Wu, P., Grainger. D.W. (2006), Drug/device combination for local drug therapies and infection prophylaxis. *Biomaterials* 27:2450–2467.
116. Campoccia, D., Montanaro, L., Arciola, C.R. (2006), The significance of infection related to orthopedic devices and issues of antibiotic resistance. *Biomaterials* 27:2331–2339.

117. Shah, A., Mond, J., Walsh, S. (2004), Lysostaphin-coated catheters eradicate *Staphylococcus aureus* challenge and block surface colonization. *Antimicrob Agents Chemother* 48: 2704–2707.
118. El Helou, O.C., Berbari, E.F., Marculescu, C.E., El Atrouni, W.I., Razonable, R.R., Steckelberg, J.M., Hanssen, A.D., Osmon, D.R, (2008), Outcome of enterococcal prosthetic joint infection: is combination systemic therapy superior to monotherapy. *Clin Infect Dis* 47:903–909.

# Chapter 12
# Combination Antimicrobial Therapies

## 12.1 Introduction

Combination of antimicrobial agents for various infectious diseases including bacterial, viral, parasitic, and fungal infections have proliferated in the past 50 years. For several conditions, combination of antimicrobial agents is established as first line of defense (such as *Mycobacterium tuberculosis*, human immunodeficiency virus [HIV], and malaria, etc.). However, much controversy exists for combination therapy for several bacterial infections and new emerging data on invasive fungal infections. This chapter will not delve into the well-established proven combinations above, but will discuss combinations, which are more controversial and are emerging issues.

The rationale for using combination over single chemotherapeutic agent varies with the infection being treated, but include: (i) delaying or prevention of resistant mutants; (ii) broaden spectrum of activity especially for infection with mixed microorganisms; (iii) enhance activity to achieve additive or synergistic effect; (iv) sequential activity on different stages of the organism; (v) utilizing different mechanism of action (lysis versus protein synthesis inhibition) to impair toxin release by the microorganism. The combination of three or four drugs for *M. tuberculosis* and HIV infection are paradigms for the first instance. With *M. tuberculosis*, mutation occurs at a low but constant rate so that treatment with a single drug, however powerful, will eventually lead to selection of resistant mutants.[1] The problem of treatment failure due to emergence of drug resistance became evident soon after the introduction of anti-tuberculosis therapy and led to the development of multiple drug regimens. Similarly, single and dual antiretroviral agents (ARVs) resulted in failure to control HIV infection with development of resistant mutants from incomplete viral suppression. Resistance mutations to ARVs may arise spontaneously as a result of error-prone replication of HIV-1 and, in addition, are selected in vitro and in vivo by pharmacological pressure.[2] The high rate of spontaneous mutation in HIV-1 has been attributed to the absence of a $3'$–$5'$ exonuclease proof-reading mechanism; and can be as high as $800 \times 10^{-4}$ per nucleotide.

Combination of antibiotics can be used to broaden the spectrum of coverage as typically found with intraabdominal sepsis, or empiric therapy of severe sepsis in the critical care unit. However, there is no evidence that the combinations are superior to single agents with a similar spectrum of antibacterial activity. In cases of empiric therapy for sepsis, single antimicrobials can be substituted once the organism has been identified with the susceptibility profile.

Using two classes of antibiotics with different mechanisms of action to obtain additive or synergistic effect was the argument commonly used for the popular use of combinations in many instances of bacterial infection. However, there was little evidence to support this contention except for enterococcal bacterial endocarditis. This issue will be further discussed with specific diseases.

The classic example of sequential therapy for different stages of the life cycle of microorganisms is *Plasmodium vivax* or *P. ovale* malaria. Initially, chloroquine is used to clear the trophozoites in red blood cells then followed soon after by primaquine to eradicate the chronic hepatic stage. However, combination therapy has become the new standard for chloroquine-resistant *P. falciparum*, with artemisinin-based combination therapies (despite absence of a chronic hepatic stage) because of emerging resistance to several antimalarial drugs.[3]

This chapter will not discuss fixed combinations such as trimethoprim-sulfamethoxazole or quinupristin-dalfopristin, where each individual component has bacteriostatic activity but together the combination exhibits synergy, leading to bactericidal activity.

## 12.2 Bacterial Infections

### 12.2.1 Bacterial Infective Endocarditis

Combination of antibiotics, mainly a beta-lactam agent with an aminoglycoside has been used to treat bacterial endocarditis for several decades but with little solid evidence (from controlled randomized trials) to establish their superiority over monotherapy. Utilization of these combinations is predominantly based on in vitro testing showing synergistic killing of the usual etiologic bacteria. The clinical merit of combination over monotherapy varies with the type of infection.

In *Streptococcus viridans*, and right-sided *Staphylococcus aureus* infections, where the cure rates are high and mortality rates low (<5%) with 4 weeks monotherapy, the value of combination therapy is mainly to shorten the duration of parenteral therapy to 2 weeks. Whereas in *S. aureus* left-sided endocarditis and enterococcal infection, the mortality rates vary from 25% to 47% and 15% to 25%, respectively.[4] Thus, the use of rapidly bactericidal synergistic combination is appealing to optimize therapy with the aim of potentially reducing the mortality and complications.

## 12.2.2 In Vitro Testing of Synergy

By definition, synergy is the working together of two or more drugs to produce an effect greater than the sum of their individual effects. However, to define synergy by laboratory methods has been contentious and to prove this effect clinically is even more difficult. The broth microdilution checkerboard technique is a popular method used for in vitro testing, which defines synergy in two-dimensional, serial twofold dilutions of drug combinations over wide antibiotic ranges. Synergistic interaction is calculated by the fractional inhibitory concentration (FIC) or fractional bactericidal concentration (FBC) indices are $\leq 0.5$, determined usually at 24 h of incubation. Disadvantages include labor intensiveness, indistinct visual endpoints (FIC), and inability to assess rapidity of bactericidal effect of the antibiotic combinations.[5]

The time-kill curve method can assess rapidity of bactericidal effect of antibiotics alone or in combination by subcultures of broth tubes containing organisms usually over a 24 h incubation period. Quantitative counts of control growth tubes are compared to the antibiotic-containing tubes. A differential decrease in counts of $\geq$to 2 $\log_{10}$/cfu caused by the drug combination compared to the most active single agent after 24 h is considered a synergistic combination. For clinical interpretation, the drug concentration used in these assays should be readily achieved in serum and sub-MIC concentrations may best be tested to optimally define synergy. In experimental models of infective endocarditis (IE), the time-kill assay provides better prediction of bacteriologic outcome than the checkerboard technique.[6]

The mechanism for bactericidal synergy has been delineated for enterococci but probably is similar for *viridans* streptococci and *S. aureus*, with combination of beta-lactam agents and aminoglycosides. Enterococci are relatively resistant to penicillin G and ampicillin (MIC $\wedge$ 2 µg/ml) and vancomycin (MIC 2–5 µg/ml) with each agent exhibiting bacteriostatic activity. In general, the aminoglycosides penetrate poorly intracellularly into enterococci or streptococci, and the cell wall active agents (penicillins, vancomycin) facilitate enhanced intracellular uptake of the aminoglycosides to produce bactericidal effect. Enterococci and streptococci are resistant to aminoglycosides at usual serum concentrations (as single agent), but synergy is still present with penicillin or vancomycin unless there is high-level of resistance with an MIC $\geq$500 µg/ml to gentamicin or >1,000 µg/ml to streptomycin. High-level aminoglycoside resistance among enterococci is increasing (~40% to gentamicin) and is associated with aminoglycoside-modifying enzymes.[7] Strains of enterococci with high-level resistance fail to show synergistic killing with combinations of aminoglycoside and penicillin or with a combination of aminoglycoside or vancomycin. In vitro susceptibility or resistance to gentamicin can predict bacteriologic outcome in experimental enterococcal endocarditis.[8] There is also clinical data (case series) that correlate aminoglycoside susceptibility and outcome in enterococcal endocarditis.[9,10]

Numerous in vitro studies have confirmed the synergy of penicillin G, ampicillin, or vancomycin with aminoglycosides against enterococci. To attain synergistic killing requires sustained levels of penicillin G $\geq$5 µg/ml[9] plus a gentamicin level of 3 µg/ml (which is as effective as 5 µg/ml) or a streptomycin peak level of 20 µg/ml.[10]

Strains of enterococci that have high-level gentamicin resistance may be susceptible to high levels of streptomycin and should be tested as synergy would occur with this agent. However, in vitro susceptibility to amikacin is not predictable of synergistic killing.[5]

In vitro synergistic effect of two β-lactams can also be demonstrated against enterococci. For 48 of 50 strains of *E. faecalis*, the MIC of amoxicillin decreased from 0.5 to 0.06 μg/ml in the presence of 4 μg/ml of cefotaxime.[11] This phenomenon may be explained by partial saturation of penicillin-binding proteins (PBPs) 4 and 5 by amoxicillin combined with the total saturation of PBPs 2 and 3 by cefotaxime, despite the intrinsic resistance of enterococci to all cephalosporins. Using a multidrug-resistant *Enterococcus faecium* (MIC 16 μg/ml of ampicillin and 512 μg/ml of vancomycin), time-kill curves demonstrated that the combination of ampicillin (8 μg/ml) with either imipenem (4 μg/ml) or vancomycin (4 μg/ml) was synergistically inhibitory.[12] However, only the triple combination of the three agents was bactericidal in vitro. In another study of 10 strains of *E. faecalis* with high aminoglycoside resistance time-kill studies with ampicillin and ceftriaxone compared to ampicillin demonstrated $\geq 2 \log_{10}$ decrease in CFU/ml at 24 h with the combination over monotherapy.[13] Although 70% of the strains showed this effect, only in 36% of the *E. faecalis* had adequate killing with this combination ($\geq 3 \log_{10}$ killing with respect to initial inoculum).[13]

Unlike enterococci, sensitive strains of streptococci and *S. aureus* are rapidly killed by the penicillins and cephalosporins. However, several in vitro studies have demonstrated enhanced killing with the combination of an aminoglycoside. Coagulase-negative staphylococci (CoNS), especially *S. epidermidis*, is a major cause of prosthetic valve endocarditis. Many of these strains, up to 80% of hospital-acquired strains, are resistant to β-lactam agents and sensitive mainly to vancomycin or other glycopeptides. However, for all strains, even when susceptible, there is poor bactericidal effect of any single agent (mainly bacteriostatic effect), similar to enterococci. *S. epidermidis* recovered from patients with prosthetic valve IE have reported resistance to semisynthetic penicillins of 63–80% and combination with vancomycin have been recommended.[14] Several in vitro studies have demonstrated some synergistic effect of combinations with vancomycin, gentamicin, and rifampicin against CoNS. Studies using microtiter checkerboard method and liberal definition of synergism (FIC <1.0 instead of 0.5) found synergistic activity with this triple antibiotic combination in 7 of 10 *S. epidermidis* recovered from patients with documented prosthetic valve IE.[15] As mentioned in Chapter 10, time-kill studies with CoNS from biofilms found no true synergism with combinations with rifampin, but rather rifampin (a potent anti-staphylococcal agent) produced most of the rapid killing effect and the other agents help prevent rifampin-resistant mutants from developing.[16]

## 12.2.3 *Animal Models of Infective Endocarditis*

Experimental models of IE using rats or rabbits have been established by insertion of a polyethylene catheter across the aortic or tricuspid valve, then intravenous injection of bacteria results in valvular vegetations. Combination of agents has been used to measure the rapidity and degree of bactericidal effect by quantitative cultures of the vegetations at sacrifice. In vivo synergism (or enhanced killing) occurs when there is a greater reduction of CFU/g of tissue with the combination than the most active single agent.

Many studies have demonstrated superior in vivo efficacy of combinations of cell wall active agents (β-lactams, vancomycin) with aminoglycoside against enterococci, *S. viridans*, *S. aureus*, and CoNS.[17] For enterococcal IE, both penicillin-streptomycin or penicillin-gentamicin exhibit enhanced killing over penicillin alone with sensitive strains, but not against penicillin-resistant or highly aminoglycoside-resistant strains.[17] Against a strain of *E. faecium* with low-level vancomycin resistance, there was increased killing in the endocarditis model with vancomycin or teicoplanin combined with gentamicin over monotherapy.[18] With a high-level vancomycin-resistant *E. faecium* (high-level gentamicin-susceptible), the triple combination of penicillin, vancomycin, and gentamicin produced a synergistic effect in the same model.[19] However, high-dose penicillin with gentamicin produced the same effect despite moderate penicillin resistance (MIC 32 µg/ml). In another report of *E. faecium* with high-level resistance to vancomycin and moderate resistance to ampicillin, the combination of ampicillin with imipenem was highly active (an additional 5 $\log_{10}$ reduction in CFU/g of vegetation compared with the most active single agent), but addition of vancomycin was not any more effective.[12] The combination of ampicillin plus ceftriaxone has also been tested in the rabbit model with high-resistant aminioglycoside *E. faecalis* infection.[13] Using doses to simulate human-like pharmacokinetics, the animals were treated for 3 days then sacrificed. The combination of ampicillin with ceftriaxone was significantly more effective than ampicillin in reducing the number of bacteria in the vegetations (5.3 +/− 0.6 $\log_{10}$ CFU vs 7.9 +/− 1.7 $\log_{10}$ CFU/g, $p = 0.0001$).[13] Unfortunately, there is no longer-term study to determine whether this is a transient effect, and whether sterilization is possible with the 2-β-lactam combination. In another study of ampicillin-cefotaxime combination for *E. faecalis* experimental endocarditis, no synergy was observed in vivo.[20]

Current guidelines for treatment of CoNS (methicillin-resistant) prosthetic valve endocarditis (PVE) advocate triple combination of vancomycin, rifampin, and gentamicin.[21] However, there is a lack of experimental or robust clinical data to support this recommendation. There is no prosthetic valve experimental endocarditis model that mimics or represents clinical PVE. Experimental models of CoNS endocarditis utilize the same rabbit model previously mentioned for native value IE (NVE). This model, however, is more representative of PVE than soft tissue cage models often referred to by guidelines. In PVE and NVE, the vegetations represent biofilm growth of sessile bacterial colonies,[22,23] and unlike chronic catheters and soft tissue prosthesis, the valves are not covered in part or whole by slime (exopolysaccharide) except for the vegetations. The superiority of three-drug combination over two-drug combination is debatable, and models of MRSE and MRSA experimental IE have produced conflicting results. Vancomycin was evaluated with and without gentamicin and/or rifampin in therapy for MRSE IE in a rabbit model by Kobasa et al.[24] Vancomycin plus rifampin or vancomycin plus gentamicin were significantly more effective than vancomycin alone. However, the three-drug combination vancomycin-gentamicin-rifampin was more effective than any two-drug combination. A subsequent study from the same center compared vancomycin to teicoplanin with and without gentamicin and/or rifampin for experimental MRSE IE.[25] Teicoplanin was just as effective as vancomycin when used in combinations. Addition of rifampin alone or gentamicin plus rifampin was significantly more effective than addition of gentamicin alone. However, addition of rifampin compared with addition of gentamicin plus rifampin did not differ significantly.[25] Lowry et al.[26] reported similar findings in therapy of MRSE endocarditis rabbit model. Three-drug combination of vancomycin-rifampin-gentamicin was not significantly different from vancomycin plus rifampin in reducing the bacterial counts of vegetation with a very brief course of therapy. In vitro killing studies also demonstrated that the combination of antibiotics with rifampin or gentamicin did not alter the killing rate significantly but prevented emergence of resistant subpopulations,[26] similar to the report by Archer et al.[16]

Studies of in vitro and in vivo bactericidal interactions of vancomycin plus rifampin against *S. aureus* have yielded conflicting results. Whereas vancomycin plus rifampin in vitro when tested by the timed-kill curve technique showed synergistic killing, the checkerboard technique indicated the two drugs were antagonistic.[27] However, in an experimental aortic valve IE due to MRSA, the combination of vancomycin plus rifampin was significantly more effective than the single-drug regimen in reduction of mean vegetation CFU/g and rate of sterilization of the valves.[27] The use of vancomycin prevented the in vivo development of resistance to rifampin. Surprisingly, in animals not sacrificed at predetermined times, vancomycin alone was as effective as the combination in reducing mortality and sterilizing renal abcesses.[27] In a similar study of MRSA experimental IE with a gentamicin-resistant strain, vancomycin as monotherapy was as efficacious as the triple combination (vancomycin-netilmicin-rifampin); and no resistance to rifampin or netilmicin developed.[28]

Earlier studies had demonstrated that nafcillin-gentamicin enhanced in vivo bactericidal activity compared to nafcillin alone in methicillin-sensitive *S. aureus* (MSSA) IE.[29] Rifampin plus cloxacillin was also more effective than cloxacillin in experimental MSSA endocarditis despite antagonism in bactericidal serum titers.[30]

## *12.2.4 Clinical Trials in Bacterial Endocarditis*

### 12.2.4.1 Streptococcal Endocarditis

In cases of penicillin susceptible streptococcal IE penicillin G intravenously for 4 weeks is the therapy of choice with cure rates above 90%.[31] However, these is good evidence (non-randomized observational studies) that shows similar response (>90% cure) with two weeks combination of intravenous penicillin with intramuscular streptomycin[32] or gentamicin/netilmicin intravenously with ceftiaxone or penicillin.[32–35] The combination allows shortening of the parenteral therapy due to more rapid killing of the organisms in the vegetations and thus quicker sterilization of the valves. The obvious advantages of short-term combination therapy in decades were shortened hospitalization course, with only abbreviated attachment to an intravenous catheter and shorter exposure to antibiotics. However, in recent years, home parenteral therapy has allowed abridged hospital course for uncomplicated cases of IE. Thus, the main advantages presently are primarily for convenience. The disadvantages include the potential toxicity of the 2-week course of aminoglycosides, which include 5–10% risk of renal impairment, auditory, and vestibular disturbances. Therefore, this combination should be used only cautiously in the elderly and preferably not at all in patients with underlying renal and auditory impairment or dizziness. In this author's experience over the past 20 years, when the potential benefits and risks of combination therapy were explained to patients with penicillin-susceptible streptococcal IE, over 90% opt for the longer course of monotherapy. Although there is no comparative clinical study, it has been recommended that IE due to relative penicillin-resistant streptococci (MIC > 0.1–0.5 µg/ml) be treated with 2 weeks of gentamicin and 4 weeks of penicillin G.[21] An alternative based on in vitro susceptibility could be 4 weeks of ceftriaxone for patients with increased risk of aminoglycoside toxicity.

### 12.2.4.2 Enterococcal Endocarditis

Traditionally, enterococcal IE has been treated with combination of intravenous penicillin G or ampicillin with streptomycin or gentamicin for 4–6 weeks, with an aminoglycoside for at least 4 weeks. This was based on clinical experience with high failure rates to monotherapy and retrospective case series showing good response with combination therapy.[36–38] Six-week course therapy is preferable for patients with symptoms of infection ≥3 months (especially mitral valve involvement),[38] or patients with PVE. Since enterococcal IE is higher in the older subjects, they are at particular risk for aminoglycoside toxicity, which can be permanent, gentamicin (most common aminoglycoside used in combination) toxicity ranges from 20% to 100% after a month's therapy. The lower rate is seen with 3 mg/kg/day and higher rate with higher doses,[38] and the response to therapy is similar in enterococcal IE. Recent prospective observational study on the largest reported series of enterococcal IE have challenged the need for ≥4 weeks aminoglycoside.[39] A nationwide prospective study in Sweden from 1995 to 1999 identified 93 cases of enterococcal IE, representing 11% of 881 definite episodes of IE.[39] Study patients had a median duration of aminoglycoside for 15 days and total antibiotic duration of 42 days. The overall cure rate was 81%, with 16% mortality and 3% relapse, similar to results from previous studies with combination of 4–6 weeks.[36–38] The cure rate in patients with mitral valve IE (54 [82%] of 66) and PVE (21 [78%] of 27) was similar. Thus, based on our current knowledge without a randomized, prospective trial 2 weeks of gentamicin with 4–6 weeks high-dose penicillin or ampicillin should be considered preferred therapy for enterococcal IE.

Experimental endocarditis of *E. faecalis* due to high-level resistance to aminoglycoside have been treated with two β-lactams with enhanced bactericidal activity in one study,[13] moreover, ampicillin-ceftriaxone was just as effective as ampicillin-gentamicin for 3 days in reducing bacterial concentration in a model of aminoglycoside-susceptible enterococcal IE.[40] In a small observational multicenter trial from Spain, 21 patients with high-level aminoglycoside-resistant (HLAR) *E. faecalis* IE and 22 patients with non-HLAR *E. faecalis* endocarditis were treated with 6 weeks course of intravenous ampicillin (2 g every 4 h) plus ceftriaxone, 2 g every 12 h.[41] The clinical cure rate at 3 months was 67.4% (29 of 43 patients) with 28.6% mortality of patients HLAR *E. faecalis* and 18.2% of patients with non-HLAR *E. faecalis* IE (infection-related causes). Among the 21 patients with HLAR *E. faecalis* IE, 11 (52%) were cured with the antibiotic combination alone.[41] Unfortunately, there was no concurrent or historical controls receiving a similar dose and course of ampicillin monotherapy for comparison. There have been a few case reports of HLAR *E. faecalis* IE treated with ampicillin monotherapy and surgery with success. By default or lack of sufficient data, the combination of ampicillin-ceftriaxone may become preferred therapy for HLAR enterococcal IE.

### 12.2.4.3 Staphylococcal Endocarditis

*S. aureus* IE can be present primarily on the right side of the heart (mainly with intravenous drug abuse [IVDA]) with a very good prognosis and response to therapy, and on the left side with a worse prognosis and greater risk for severe heart failure and systemic emboli. Prolonged intravenous therapy with single agents has been difficult to accomplish in IVDA because of poor compliance and poor venous access. Previously, a small randomized study of 25 IVDA with *S. aureus* IE (5 with left-sided involvement) found no benefit of adding gentamicin to 4 weeks of a β-lactam antibiotic.[42] In a subsequent study from San Francisco, 53 IVDA with right-sided *S. aureus* IE were enrolled in a prospective open study to receive nafcillin and tobramycin for 2 weeks, and vancomycin for penicillin-allergic patients.[43] Forty-seven of 50 patients (94%) treated with nafcillin and tobramycin were cured, whereas only 1 of 3 (33%) receiving vancomycin-tobramycin was cured.[43] As a result of this study, it became standard practice to use combined β-lactam-aminoglycoside for 2 weeks for right-sided *S. aureus* IE.

However, in an open-randomized study from Spain, 34 of 38 patients (89%) with *S. aureus* right-sided endocarditis receiving cloxacillin alone for 2 weeks were cured versus 31 of 36 (86%) patients who received cloxacillin plus gentamicin for the same period.[44] Another report from Spain in a small study randomized 31 IVDA with *S. aureus* right-sided IE to cloxacillin-gentamicin ($N = 11$), vancomycin-gentamicin ($N = 10$) and teicoplanin-gentamicin ($N = 10$) for 14 days.[45] Cure was achieved in all patients treated with cloxacillin-gentamicin but in only 60% of the vancomycin and 70% of the teicoplanin groups. Thus, it would appear that short-term (14 days) therapy with a semisynthetic penicillin with or without gentamicin is highly effective for *S. aureus* right-sided endocarditis, but short-term glycopeptide even with gentamicin is very ineffective.

Right-sided *S. aureus* endocarditis is not only less aggressive but easier to cure than left-sided staphylococcal endocarditis. There is some data that combined oral quinolone with rifampin is also effective for right-sided *S. aureus* IE. In a randomized study of 85 IVDA with right-sided *S. aureus* IE, there was no significant difference in response in patients receiving ciprofloxacin-rifampin orally (18 of 19) or intravenous oxacillin or vancomycin with gentamicin for 5 days (22 of 25) – all treated for 28 days.[46] Besides the small sample size, only 44 of 85 subjects completed the evaluation, thus casting doubt on the reliability of the results. An earlier pilot study on this oral combination reported successful outcome on 14 IVDA with right-sided staphylococcal endocarditis.[47] However, only 10 of 14 (71.4%) patients completed the full course of therapy and in actuality, the cure rate by intention to treat analysis would be 71%. There are several concerns with the oral regimen used for IE including small numbers of patients treated and poor compliance of this group of subjects to adhere to therapy for 28 days as outpatient. The data on short-term intravenous β-lactam agent alone or with gentamicin is more robust, and should remain preferred treatment for right-sided staphylococcal endocarditis.

The benefit of combination therapy with an aminoglycoside for left-sided staphylococcal IE is even less certain and has not been well-established despite the guidelines and recommendations by various medical societies. Two separate multicenter prospective trials were reported as a single communication, comparing 6 weeks of nafcillin (9–12 g/day) alone versus nafcillin for 6 weeks plus gentamicin (3 mg/kg/day) for 2 weeks, in 48 IVDA (30 with only right-sided IE) and 30 non-addicts (3 with only right-sided IE).[48] The cure rate and complications of the IE or need for surgery were similar for drug addicts and non-addicts for monotherapy or combination-therapy. In addicts, patients receiving combination therapy became afebrile more rapidly than those on monotherapy (by 1 day, mean 4.8 vs 5.8 days) and in those with only right-sided endocarditis, the duration of bacteremia on treatment was also shortened only by 1 day with the combination therapy (mean 2.6 vs 3.6 days). In non-addicts, the eradication of bacteremia was significantly faster with combination therapy (but only by 1.3 days, mean 2.8 vs 4.1 days), but duration of fever was similar between the treatment groups (mean 7.6 vs 7.7 days).[48] Significantly, greater renal dysfunction occurred in non-addicts receiving 2 weeks of gentamicin in combination. Hence, guidelines have recommended administering gentamicin for only 3–5 days to reduce the potential for nephrotoxicity.

A recent meta-analysis of comparative trials to assess the role of aminoglycoside in combination with β-lactam for treatment of bacterial endocarditis has been reported.[49] Five comparative trials (four randomized) were analyzed, with four studies on *S. aureus* native-value IE ($N = 261$ patients) and one study with *S. viridans* IE. There was no significant difference between monotherapy and combination with aminoglycoside regarding mortality, treatment success, or relapse of endocarditis.[49] Nephrotoxicity was more common with the combination of aminoglycoside than monotherapy (OR 1.72, $p = 0.020$).

### 12.2.4.4 Prosthetic Valve Endocarditis

Recent international prospective observational database from 61 medical centers in 28 countries has identified *S. aureus* (23.0%) as the most common cause of prosthetic valve endocarditis (PVE), followed by CoNS (16.9%) from a cohort of 556 cases.[50] Seventy-one percent occurred within the first year of valve implantation, and the majority of cases occurred after the early (60-day) period. Complications of PVE are common including: heart failure (32.8%), stroke (18.2%), intracardiac abscess (29.7%), and persistent bacteremia (8.8%). Surgery was required in 272 (48.9%) during the index hospitalization and in-hospital death occurred in (22.8%),[50] despite usual standard combination therapy. Unfortunately, details of medical therapy was not provided in this report but most centers have been using combination of β-lactam agent (for methicillin-sensitive strains) or vancomycin combined with rifampin and gentamicin for staphylococcal PVE-based on current guidelines.[21] Previous reports have also found that mortality rates of *S. aureus* (47%) and CoNS (36%) are significantly higher than viridans streptococcal PVE.[51] However, current guidelines for therapy of staphylococcal PVE are based on small, retrospective data predominantly from a study in the early 1980s.[52]

Karchmer et al.[52] reported their experience on 75 episodes of CoNS PVE, 80% of which were methicillin-resistant. Cure was achieved in 21 of 26 (80.7%) cases treated with vancomycin and only 10 of 20 (50%) treated with a β-lactam antibiotic. Failure of the β-lactam therapy was largely due to heterogenous methicillin-resistant strains. Further analysis of monotherapy (vancomycin) versus combination therapy in the MRSE PVE cases showed cure with vancomycin alone in three of six cases (50%), vancomycin plus rifampin in seven of eight (87.5%), vancomycin plus gentamicin in five of five (100%), and vancomycin, rifampin plus gentamicin in six of seven (85.7%) of cases.[52] Thus, this data would suggest that vancomycin alone is inadequate for MRSE PVE but the combination with rifampin or gentamicin would be preferable. This small retrospectively collected data does not support or suggest superiority of triple therapy (vancomycin-gentamicin-rifampin) over double therapy (vancomycin-rifampin), and 2 weeks of gentamicin (as recommended) would increase the risk for nephrotoxicity and ototoxicity. Although it may be argued that gentamicin may decrease the risk of development of rifampin-resistant mutants (as shown in a small study published in abstract form[53]), there is no clinical evidence of this being significant. In a prospective, randomized treatment trial of MRSE PVE comparing vancomycin-rifampin to triple therapy with gentamicin, no difference in cure rates (78%) were noted although rifampin resistance developed in 37% of the dual therapy and none in the triple therapy group.[53]

There is no data to support triple combination in *S. aureus* PVE in clinical trials, and the recommendations are based on strategy for CoNS PVE and experimental soft tissue foreign body related infections. However, this model is not directly applicable to PVE. In a rat model of implanted subcutaneous teflon tissue-cage infection with MRSA, treatment with vancomycin and rifampin for 6 days resulted in rifampin resistance in four of 25% (16%) of animals.[54] In a subsequent study by the same group using a similar model of experimental MRSA foreign body infection, triple therapy (vancomycin-rifampin-fleroxacin) decreased bacterial counts more rapidly than two-drug therapy.[55] However, unlike their previous study, no rifampin-resistant mutants developed with dual therapy (vancomycin-rifampin).

## 12.2.5 Gram-Negative Bacilli Infections

A significant number of gram-negative bacterial infections are difficult to treat and combination therapy (usually aminoglycosides plus a β-lactam agent) are often used. Combination therapy was initially recommended for severe pseudomonas sepsis because of poor outcome to aminoglycoside monotherapy (often because of inadequate dosing as a result of narrow therapeutic/toxic ratio) and modest activity of earlier anti-pseudomonal β-lactams (carbenicillin, ticarcillin). However, with the advent of more potent drugs (ceftazidime, piperacillin-tazobactam), there is no good evidence of the superiority of combination over monotherapy (see Chapters 6 and 7).

Besides, pseudomonas species, other difficult-to-treat microorganisms include *Enterobacter*, *Serratia*, *Klebsiella*, and *Acinobacter* species, which are associated with nosocomial outbreaks and high-level resistance to most antimicrobials. Whether combination antimicrobial therapy is more efficacious than monotherapy, or can prevent emergence of resistance still remain unproven and controversial. In a recent meta-analysis of eight RCTs comparing aminoglycoside and β-lactam combination therapy versus β-lactam monotherapy, there was no associated beneficial effect on the development of antimicrobial resistance.[56] In effect, β-lactam monotherapy was associated with fewer superinfections and surprisingly fewer treatment failures (OR, 0.62). A similar recent meta-analysis of 64 trials, randomizing 7,586 patients, compared β-lactam-aminoglycoside combination versus β-lactam monotherapy for severe sepsis.[57] There was no difference in all cause fatality and clinical failure, nor differences in rate of resistance development, but combination therapy resulted in greater nephrotoxicity. In yet another meta-analysis of 17 studies (10 retrospective cohort studies included) assessing effect of combination versus monotherapy on mortality in gram-negative bacteremia, no mortality benefit was found with combined therapy.[58] Sub-group analysis of *Pseudomonas aeroginosa* bacteremias showed a significant mortality benefit (OR 0.50, 95% CI 0.30–0.79), but this was likely due to inclusion of earlier retrospective studies which may introduce bias.

Pseudomonas pneumonia, especially in critical care units on ventilated patients, has been associated with high mortality and combination therapy had been considered optimal or preferred management. In a recent retrospective multicenter, observational study in Spain of 183 episodes of pseudomonas ventilator-associated pneumonia, initial use of combination reduces the likelihood of inappropriate therapy (which is associated with higher mortality).[59] However, administration of one effective antimicrobial or combination therapy provided similar outcomes.

## 12.2.6 Community-Acquired Pneumonia

In the past 7 years, a number of studies have suggested that combination antimicrobial (β-lactam plus macrolide) therapy may be superior to β-lactam monotherapy for severe pneumococcal pneumonia.[60,61] These studies were retrospective or uncontrolled in design and suffered from major limitations. In a prospective, multicenter, international study of 592 adults with severe illness due to *Streptococcal pneumoniae* bacteremia, the 14-day mortality was not significantly different between combination and monotherapy.[62] In a subgroup of 94 patients critically ill (defined by the Pitt bacteremic score), combination therapy was superior to monotherapy (14-day mortality 23.4% vs 55.3%, $p < 0.008$). The difference in mortality was independent of in vitro activity, class of antibiotics, ICU support or country.[62]

These results should be interpreted with caution and larger, randomized controlled, multicenter prospective trials in critically ill patients with pneumococcal sepsis are warranted. There are several possible explanations for the findings including: (i) epiphenomenon, which can be a problem with small sample size especially with subgroup analysis; (ii) bias because of unblinded, non-randomized nature of the study; (iii) a true effect because of obscure, unrecognized biological effect of the combination. It is possible that macrolides used in combination may have microbial effect on unrecognized atypical pathogens (as in mixed infections), or exert a nonspecific anti-inflammatory effect, which modulated excessive cytokine response in sepsis. At present, severe pneumococcal pneumonia or sepsis still should be treated with penicillin G (if MIC $< 4.0$ μg/ml) or ceftriaxone or newer quinolone or vancomycin for highly resistant strains (MIC $\geq 4.0$ μg/ml)

## 12.3 Fungal Infections and Combination Therapy

Invasive fungal infections are associated with high morbidity and mortality in certain high-risk patients despite standard antifungal therapy. With the proliferation of new antifungals that have become available in recent years, there has been interest and research in the use of combination of agents with different target sites (Fig. 12.1) to maximize antifungal effect. To date and for the past 3 decades, the only established antifungal combination has been amphotericin B combined with flucytosine for cryptococcal meningitis. Despite improvement in our present antifungal armamentarium, optimal therapy for invasive aspergillosis, disseminated mucormycosis, disseminated fusariosis, and other filamentous fungal infections are unknown and standard therapy often results in unsatisfactory outcome. This chapter will review evidence for combination antifungals by in vitro methods, animal models, and clinical experience.

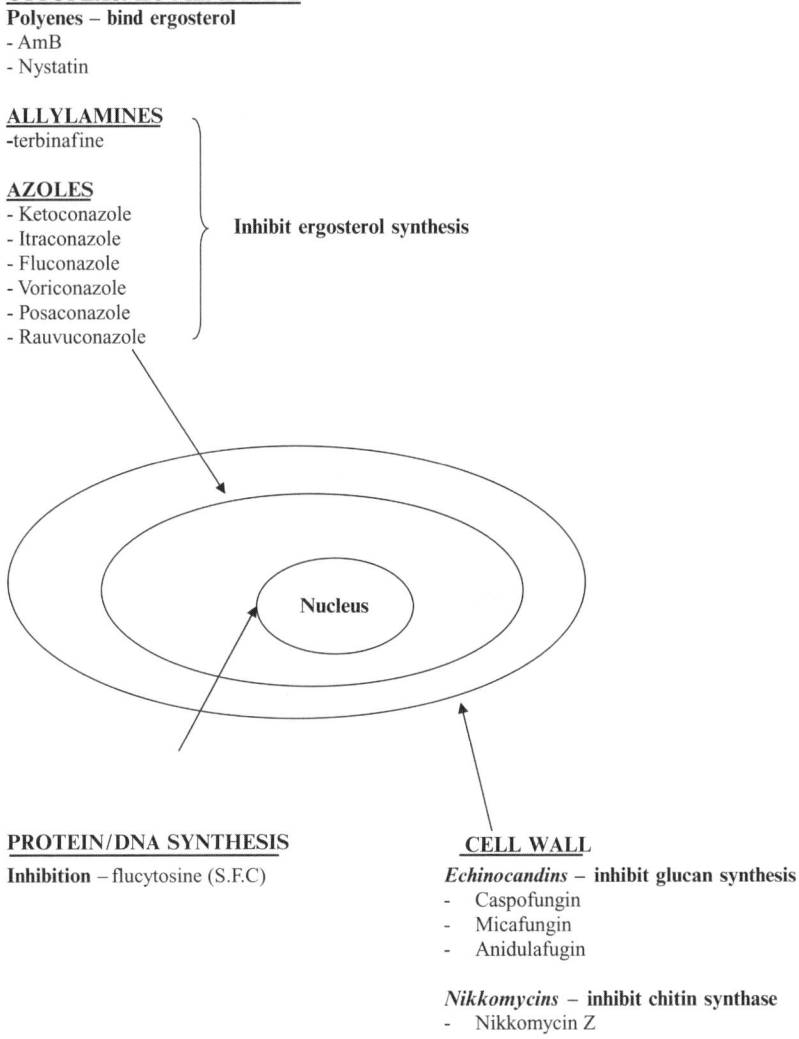

**Fig. 12.1** *Azoles and polyenes can inhibit or bind to ergosterol, leading to cell lysis and allowing 5-FC to enter the cell and inhibit nucleic acid synthesis.
*Candins and Nikkomycins cause disruption of cell wall allowing the antifungals (polyenes, azoles, 5-FC) to enter

## 12.3.1 In Vitro Antifungal Combination Assays

In vitro susceptibility assays have been standardized for fungi over the past decade or more but these tests are highly dependent on fungal species, incubation temperature and duration, media and other method-dependent factors. Standardization and reproducibility have best been defined for yeast forms (Candida species), especially for single antifungal agents.[63] Recommendations for determination of minimal inhibitory concentration (MIC) of single antifungals for yeasts and mold are currently available.[63–65] The MIC is the minimum concentration of the drug inhibiting 80% (or 50% in some cases) of fungal growth relative to the control (with no drug exposure). Although antifungal susceptibility can be used to guide therapy (often in retrospect), susceptibility of an organism does not predict successful outcome, and resistance in vitro should often predict therapeutic failure, but host factors are often more important than susceptibility results in predicting outcome.

Combination of antifungal agents (mainly two drugs) to assess enhanced or synergistic fungistatic or fungicidal activity can be determined in vitro by the checkerboard method, time kill method or Epsilometer test (E-test).[66] These methods are based on static drug concentrations and interaction at a single time point and direct correlation between in vitro and in vivo interactions is not often possible. Moreover, the activity of the combination is not only dependent on drug–drug combination, but also the absolute ratio of the drugs.[67]

### 12.3.1.1 Checkerboard Method

The checkerboard method involves determination of inhibition of fungal growth (relative to controls with no drug) by different combination of drugs. It is relatively easy to perform and easy to interpret and is useful for extensive screening. The results are relative and not actual measurement of drug combination efficacy.[67] Limitations of the checkerboard method include failure to detect changes in antimicrobial tolerance over time and changes in susceptibility end points that may affect interpretation of synergism or antagonism.[66] Combinations with amphotericin B (AmB) are often complicated with MIC clustering, which can affect discrimination of small differences over time. The checkerboard titration system is more suitable for drugs that have similar linear dose-response curves and time course of activity. Drug combinations such as AmB-azole where the in vitro activity of the azoles against *Candida* and cryptococcal species is initiated more slowly than the polyenes, may fail to detect synergistic or antagonistic activity. The checkerboard assay also may not correlate with other methods such as the time-kill or E-test assays.[68] Thus, this method is often used for screening followed by further analysis such as the fractional inhibitory concentration index (FICI) to assess combination antifungal activity.

The FICI is defined by the following equation:
$$FICI = FIC_A + FIC_B = \frac{MIC_A \text{ in combination}}{MIC_A \text{ tested}} + \frac{MIC_B \text{ in combination}}{MIC_B \text{ tested}}$$

where $MIC_A$ and $MIC_B$ are the MICs of drugs A and B, respectively. It has been proposed that tan FICI of $<0.5$ should represent synergy, an FICI $> 4$ should be assessed as antagonism, and an FICI of 0.5 to 4 should be considered indifferent or

12.3 Fungal Infections and Combination Therapy 341

no interaction.[69] Although FICI is easy to perform and is not very labor-intensive (it is often the preferred method to assess drug–drug interaction), there are significant disadvantages. The FICI does not assess the possible variability of interpretation according to drug concentrations in the checkerboard; dilution-based MICs determination may lead to inter-experimental errors; with some antifungal combination, the MIC endpoint is unclear and leads to errors in calculating the FICI; also, it is not amenable to statistical analysis.[66]

### 12.3.1.2 Time-Kill Method

Time-kill methods have been commonly used to assess bactericidal activity, and recently has been applied to antifungal activity and testing combination of antifungals. In this method, a standardized cell suspension ($5 \times 10^5$ cells/ml) is incubated with different concentrations of drug combinations for different time intervals up to 24–48 h. At specified time intervals, cells are plated onto agar medium to assess quantitative growth (CFU/ml) at each time point to obtain "time-kill" curves for each drug combination. Drug interactions by time-kill method are considered synergistic for $\geq 2$ $\log_{10}$ decrease in CFU/ml compared to the most active agent; antagonistic for $\geq 2$ $\log_{10}$ increase in CFU/ml compared to the least active agent; additive for $<2$ but $>1$ $\log_{10}$ decrease in CFU/ml compared to the most active agent; and indifferent for $<2$ log but $>1$ log increase in CFU/ml compared to the least active agent.[66] Although time-kill assays provide effect of combination over time by growth kinetics, it is laborious to perform and mainly applicable to single cell forms (yeast cells) and difficult to interpret with aggregates of cells and filaments (molds).

### 12.3.1.3 Epsilometer Strip (E-test)

The E-test can also be used to assess antifungal susceptibility and combination interaction. MICs are determined by using a calibrated strip impregnated with a gradient of antimicrobial concentration placed on an agar plate seeded with the isolate being tested, and measuring the point of intersection of a growth inhibition zone. Good correlation has been found with the E-test and broth macro- and microdilution methods for single antifungal agents. Recently, this method has been applied to antifungal combination testing. The manufacture (AB Bioddisk, Solna, Switzerland) guidelines for interpretation are: synergy is defined as a decrease of $\geq 3$ dilutions in the MIC; antagonism is defined as $\geq 3$ dilution increase for the antifungal combination; additivity is defined as decrease $>2$ dilutions but $<3$ dilutions; and indifference as decrease of $<2$ dilutions for the antifungal combination. In one study of drug combination interaction for *Candida* species, the E-test method had good agreement with the checkerboard and time-kill methods.[68]

The E-test is simple to perform and would be suitable for most clinical laboratories but drawbacks include nonuniformity of fungal growth lawn in some cases; feathered or trailing growth edge (MIC endpoint ambiguous); lack of extensive testing of different organisms and different antifungals; and species variation in *Candida* MIC correlation with other methods (especially *C. glabrata* and *C. tropicalis*).[70]

## 12.3.2 Antifungal Combinations for Candida species

### 12.3.2.1 In Vitro Studies

In vitro studies of amphotericin B (AmB) and fluconazole (FLU) combination against *Candida* species have shown wide variation in results. In some studies, additive effect was found, others occasionally synergistic effect and mostly indifference, depending on the methods and species.[66] At least two studies noted sequential addition of FLU followed by AmB can result in significant antagonism in vitro and in vivo.[71,72] Subsequent investigation of the interaction between AmB and FLU against *Candida* cells demonstrated that preexposure of *C. albicans* to the azole leads to transient protection against subsequent exposure to AmB.[73]

Since azoles (inhibit ergosterol biosynthesis and depletes sterol in the cell membrane) and 5-fluorocytosine (5FC, inhibits protein synthesis) act by different mechanisms on fungal cells, synergism with the combination is possible. FLU plus 5FC interaction has been tested against 27 *Candida* strains including *C. albicans* ($N = 9$), *C. glabrata* ($N = 9$), and *C. krusei* ($N = 9$).[74] Synergism was noted for five and antagonism for four *C. albicans* isolates; for *C. krusei* synergism in one and antagonism for eight isolates: and the combination was antagonistic for all *C. glabrata* isolates.[74] In this study, AmB–5FC demonstrated variable results depending on species of *Candida*.

Using time-kill analysis combination of AmB and 5FC against three isolates of *C. albicans* and *Cryptococcus neoformans* (with low dose and high-dose combinations) demonstrated no antagonism or additive effects, but drug–drug interactions were indifferent.[75] Others have used different techniques, microdilution plate assay to describe growth-inhibitory interaction of two or three antifungal drug combinations over a wide range of drug concentrations.[67] They found that AmB plus 5FC or FLU-5FC had indifferent effect on both species (3 isolates each). This study also noted the AmB-FLU had additive effect against *C. albicans* over wide range of drug concentrations, but were indifferent on the inhibitory effect of *C. neoformans*.[67]

Newer antifungal agents such as voriconazole (VORI) and caspofungin (CAS) have been tested in combination with older antifungal agents (5FC and AmB) against various *Candida* species. Results of several studies were variable with some strains exhibiting synergism, others antagonism or indifference depending on the drug combination and species.[66]

### 12.3.2.2 In Vivo Studies of *Candida* species

Animal models of invasive candidiasis in mice with normal immune system and immunocompromised have assessed monotherapy versus combination of AmB and FLU on mortality and reduction in fungal tissue burden.[76] Combination therapy in both models was not antagonistic but was not superior to AmB alone (indifferent) although superior to fluconazole alone.[76] In another study of invasive candidiasis using the same drugs in neutropenic mice and infective endocarditis in rabbits, similar findings with no antagonism but no augmentation of AmB activity was reported.[77] Using the murine model of systemic candidiasis, other investigators have examined the benefit of FLU plus AmB in fluconazole-sensitive, mid-resistant (MIC 64–128 µg/ml) and highly resistant (MIC = 512 µg/ml) *C. albicans* strains.[78] For FLU-susceptible and mid-resistant strains, the combination was antagonistic, but not for the FLU-highly resistant strains which showed additive effect.[78] AmB plus saperconazole in murine-disseminated candidiasis is also no more effective than AmB alone (indifferent).[79]

Although combination of an early echinocandin (cilofungin) and AmB showed improved cure rate versus monotherapy in murine invasive candidiasis,[80] caspofungin did not improve outcome with FLU in a similar model.[81] However, sequential therapy of caspofungin followed by FLU was as effective as caspofungin alone.[82] For azole resistant or non-*albicans Candida* AmB plus caspofungin or micafungin in experimental candidiasis demonstrated some benefit of the combination compared to monotherapy.[83,84]

Combination of standard antifungal agent combined with immunotherapy has also been examined in a few experimental studies of invasive candidiasis. Neutropenic mice with disseminated candidiasis shows synergistic effect with AmB combined with soluble IL-4 receptor (sIL4R), which was superior to FLU-sIL4R.[85] Recombinant IL-12 (rIL-12) only partially increased the efficacy of AmB, but combined with FLU dramatically improved survival.[85] Synergy between granulocyte colony stimulating factor (G-CSF) and itraconazole or FLU has also been reported in non-neutropenic mice with candidiasis.[86]

Clinical experience with combination of antifungals in disseminated candidiasis is very limited. The only prospective, randomized study to date on this issue compared FLU (800 mg/day) monotherapy to FLU plus AmB (0.7 mg/kg/day), with the AmB administered only for the first 5–6 days.[87] This was a multicenter-blinded trial with a total of 219 non-neutropenic patients with candidemia (*C. albicans* [62%], *C. glabrata* [18%]), with major risk factors being central venous catheters (94%), broad-spectrum antibiotics (96.5%), major surgery (42.9%), corticosteroids (25%), parenteral hyperalimentation (57.5%), and cancer (18.7%). Success at 30 days was not significantly different between the two groups (57% vs 69% AmB-FLU, $p = 0.08$). Persistent candidiasis after 5 days of therapy was greater (17%) in the monotherapy group versus 6% in the combined groups ($p = 0.02$). However, overall success was only slightly better in the FLU-AmB arm (69%) than the FLU arm (56%), $p = 0.02$. Renal dysfunction was greater in the combination (23%) compared to the monotherapy arm (3%), $p < 0.001$. Mortality rate at 90 days was similar (39% and 40%).

This trial has not proved the superiority of FLU-AmB over FLU monotherapy and monotherapy should remain the standard care for invasive candidiasis for routine cases. The situations where combination antifungal agents may show the greatest benefit (severe neutropenia and candida endocarditis) have not been adequately studied in clinical trials. A novel approach with promising results for invasive candidiasis is the use of human recombinant monoclonal antibody targeting heat shock protein 90 (hsp90), Myograb (Neutec Pharma) combined with standard antifungal agent.[88] This pharmaceutical sponsored pilot multicenter randomized, blinded trial compared lipid formulation of AmB (LFAB) versus LFAB plus Myograb (the latter for 5 days) in 117 patients with invasive candidiasis and assessed mycological and clinical response by day 10. Although the results appeared impressive in favor of Myograb combination (clinical response 86% vs 52%, $p < 0.001$; mycological response (89% vs 54%, $p < 0.001$) and Candida-attributable mortality (4% vs 18%, $p < 0.025$), there are some limitations of the trial.[88] Only 68 (58%) of the patients had candidemia, although mortality rate at 12 days was nearly one-half in the Myograb arm (5 [15%] of 33 patients) compared to the monotherapy arm (10 [29%] of 35 patients) on day 12, this difference narrowed by day 33 (39% vs 43%) for those with candidemia. Future trials with Myograb should be performed in larger groups of patients with candidemia, with assessment of candida-attributable mortality at 30 days or later.

### 12.3.3 Combination Therapy for Cryptococcal Meningitis

Combination of AmB plus 5FC has been used for more than 30 years for cryptococcal meningitis and this is the only antifungal combination of proven value. In the initial trial performed in 1979 in non-AIDS subjects with cryptococcal meningitis, AmB (0.3 mg/kg/day) plus 5FC (150 mg/kg/day) for 6 weeks was superior to AmB (0.4 mg/kg/day) alone for 10 weeks.[89] Subsequently, 4 weeks combination therapy was found to be just as effective as 6 weeks treatment.[90]

In patients with AIDS-associated cryptococcal meningitis treatment with AmB (0.7 mg/kg/day) with 5-FC (100 mg/kg/day) for 2 weeks followed by 8 weeks with fluconazole was shown to be an optimal therapy for cerebrospinal fluid (CSF) sterilization and reasonably tolerable.[91] At 2 weeks of therapy, the CSF cultures were negative in 60% of patients receiving AmB-5-FU versus 51% in those on AmB alone ($p = 0.06$).[91] Since then, this regimen has become standard treatment for cryptococcal meningitis. A more recent study with the use of quantitative CSF yeast counts demonstrated that AmB plus 5-FC was more fungicidal than AmB alone, AmB plus FLU and the three-drug combination (AmB-5FC-Flu) in a randomized trial of AIDS-associated cryptococcal meningitis.[92]

Treatment of cryptococcal meningitis with AmB plus 5-FC is difficult to manage in developing countries because of the toxicity of AmB. In a randomized study of

58 patients with AIDS-associated cryptococcal meningitis in Uganda, 30 patients received FLU (200 mg/day) for 2 months plus 5-FC (150 mg/kg/day) for the first 2 weeks and 28 patients received FLU monotherapy.[93] The combination therapy increased the survival at 2 and 6 months versus monotherapy, 56% vs 36% and 32% vs 12%, respectively ($p = 0.022$), and resulted in significant decrease in headaches after 1 month compared to monotherapy ($p = 0.005$).[93] An earlier trial of this combination with an open-label design in California in 32 patients with AIDS-cryptococcal meningitis had better outcome (clinical success 63% at 10 weeks) but used a higher dose of FLU (400 mg daily).[94] This result was better than previous reports of FLU alone or AmB monotherapy (35% and 40%, respectively).[94]

In experimental models of cryptococcal meningitis AmB plus FLU have more potent activity in reducing tissue fungal burden than either agents alone,[95,96] but survival studies showed the combination was as efficacious as AmB monotherapy.[96] Immune modulation with standard antifungal therapy potentially would improve outcome in AIDS-cryptococcal meningitis. A pilot study has been performed to assess the benefit of recombinant interferon-$\gamma$ (rIFN-$\gamma$1b) as adjunctive therapy in AIDS-cryptococcal meningitis.[97] There was a trend to improved mycological and clinical success in rIFN-$\gamma$1b recipients but the number of subjects in each arm was too small. Larger clinical trials would be warranted for this novel approach.

## 12.3.4 Combination Therapy for Invasive Aspergillosis

Despite availability of newer antifungal of newer antifungal agents (voriconazole) with superior efficacy to AmB for treatment of invasive aspergillosis (53% vs 32%), this disease still carries a poor prognosis in disseminated disease in severe immunocompromised hosts (especially bone marrow transplant recipients). Thus, active research for combinations with improved efficacy is avidly being pursued.

### 12.3.4.1 In Vitro and Animal Models

Various combinations of AmB, mold-active azoles, echinocandins, 5-FC, and rifampin have been studied for invasive aspergillosis. Several in vitro studies of AmB with itraconazole (ITRA) both sequentially and concomitantly have shown antagonism,[66,98] and pre-exposure to ITRA was associated with poorer mycological efficacy and survival in mice treated sequentially with AmB for invasive pulmonary aspergillosis.[99] Different interactions between AmB and other triazoles, however, have been reported. AmB and voriconazole (VORI) have shown in vitro concentration-dependent interactions with caspofungin (CAS), synergistic at low median concentrations and antagonism at higher concentrations.[100] In experimental murine invasive aspergillosis, AmB plus posaconazole did not demonstrate any antagonism.[101] Similarly, combination of VORI and Ambisone together or sequentially in a central nervous system aspergillosis model showed no antagonistic effect but enhanced activity at lower dose of Ambisone (4 mg/kg).[102] However, at higher doses of Ambisone (10 mg/kg), the combination was not superior to Ambisome alone.

Combination of VORI and CAS has been shown to be significantly more effective than any monotherapy in sterilizing visceral organs of aspergillosis in a neutropenic guinea pig model (75% sterilization of liver, brain, lung, and kidney versus 0%–8%).[103] CAS and AmB lipid complex (ABLC) were not antagonistic or synergistic in a rodent model of invasive aspergillosis, but were not more effective than ABLC alone.[104] Micafungin (an echinocandin) combined with Nikkomycin Z (a chitin synthase inhibitor) has shown enhanced efficacy versus monotherapy in one experimental systemic murine model,[105] but no enhancement in a steroid-suppressed pulmonary murine aspergillosis model.[106] In a study of pulmonary aspergillosis in rabbits, micafungin in combination with ravuconazole (a triazole) improved survival to over 75%, compared to 25% or less with monotherapies.[107]

Although some combinations in animal experiments appear promising (i.e., newer triazoles and echinocandins), the results are variable depending on the model and types of immunosuppressor (e.g., steroid compared with cyclophosphamide) and these results cannot be directly applied to clinical situations.

### 12.3.4.2 Clinical Experience with Combination Therapy

There are limited reports of antifungal combination therapy for invasive aspergillosis in humans mainly in the form of retrospective case series. In one such report of recipients of hematopoietic stem cell transplant (HSCT) with pulmonary aspergillosis (who experienced failure of initial AmB formulations), the outcome between VORI alone was compared to VORI plus CAS.[108] The combination of VORI plus CAS ($N = 6$) was associated with improved three-month survival rate, compared to VORI alone ($N = 31$), $p < 0.048$. Multivariate analysis found that the combination was associated with reduced mortality independent of other prognostic variables.[108] Another retrospective study assessed the response of CAS with LipoAMB in 48 patients with documented ($N = 23$) or possible ($N = 25$) invasive aspergillosis refractory to prior treatment.[109] The overall response rate was 42% but the response in patients with progressive documented aspergillosis was only 18%. A similar retrospective series of refractory aspergillosis pneumonia (6 proven, 4 probable, and 20 possible) in acute leukemia, reported 15 of 20 (75%) patients had favorable response to CAS plus AmB or LipoAmB.[110]

In a multicenter, noncomparative study of CAS in combination with other antifungals as salvage therapy, 53 adults with documented invasive aspergillosis (refractory or intolerant of standard therapy) were assessed.[111] Pulmonary aspergillosis was present in 81% and 87% were refractory to prior therapy. Success at the end of therapy was 55% and at day 84 was 49%, respectively.[111] A prospective, non-randomized study of VORI plus CAS as primary therapy for invasive aspergillosis in solid organ transplant recipients was compared to historical controls treated with lipid AmB.[112] The 90-day survival was 67.5% (27/40) in the combination group compared to 51% (24/47) of control (hazard ratio 0.57, 95% CI 0.29 – 1.1), $p = 0.117$. A randomized pilot study (COMBISTRAT Trial) has recently reported preliminary results of LipoAmB (10 mg/kg/day) alone versus CAS plus LipoAmB (3 mg/kg/day) in immunocompromised patients with invasive aspergillosis.[113] This small comparative trial of 30 patients showed promising results at the end of antifungal therapy in favor of dual therapy (partial or complete response rate 67% for combination versus 27% for monotherapy, $p = 0.028$). However, a larger trial is needed to confirm these results.

Further large multicenter, prospective, randomized, blinded trial is needed in severe invasive aspergillosis using VORI monotherapy as standard treatment compared to combination such as VORI plus CAS. In the meantime, VORI monotherapy should be considered as first-line treatment, except for cases of semi-invasive (subacute necrotizing pulmonary aspergillosis) where the response and outcome to itraconazole is very good and to date, there is no evidence of superiority with VORI.

## 12.4 Viral Infections

Combination of antivirals are well established for the treatment of HIV infection (will not be reviewed in this chapter) and chronic hepatitis C infection. Although the combination of pegylated interferon-alpha (PIFNα) and ribavirin (RBV) is the treatment of first choice for chronic hepatitis C, there are some emerging issues. For patients with chronic hepatitis B, there is active research in this area of combination versus monotherapy.

### *12.4.1 Chronic Hepatitis C Infections*

Chronic hepatitis C is one of the leading causes of cirrhosis, hepatocellular carcinoma, liver failure, and the need for liver transplantation. PIFNα plus RBV is the effective and efficient treatment for hepatitis C at present. Recent health technology assessment to determine long-term clinical effectiveness, costs, and incremental cost-effectiveness ratios have concluded that this combination prolongs life, improves quality of life, and is cost-effective.[114] There is also evidence that treatment of patients with chronic hepatitis C and cirrhosis with IFNα can decrease the incidence of hepatocellular carcinoma (hazard ratio 0.65, $p = 0.03$) and improve survival in a prospective cohort followed almost 7 years.[115]

There are two formulations of PIFNα available, PIFNα 2a (Pegasys RBV, Hoffman La Roche) 180 mg subcutaneously (SC) once weekly and RBV 1,000–1,200 mg daily orally (two divided doses); and PIFN-α2b (Pegetron, Schering-Plough), 1.5 ug/kg SC once weekly and RBV 800–1,200 mg orally daily. Both these formulations are considered equivalent.

**Table 12.1** Indications for therapy for chronic HCV

- Unexplained liver disease (↑ ALT) and positive HCV RNA (without liver biopsy)
- Liver biopsy stages 2–4 with positive HCV RNA
- Irrespective of symptoms or ALT levels; subjects with cirrhosis should not be decompensated
- Absence of contraindications
- Subjects willing or likely to adhere to therapy

Liver disease stages: Stage 0: no fibrosis; stage 1: fibrous expansion of portal tracts; stage 2: periportal fibrosis; stage 3: bridging fibrosis; stage 4: cirrhosis.[115, 116]
ALT = alanine aminotransferase

**Table 12.2** Contraindications for PIFNα-Ribavirin therapy

| | |
|---|---|
| *Relative contraindications* | Major depression |
| | Major psychosis |
| | Autoimmune disease |
| | Persistent injection drug use |
| | Renal failure (including dialysis) |
| *Strong contraindications* | Continued alcohol abuse |
| | Hepatic decompensation |
| | Coronary artery disease |
| | Solid organ transplantation (except liver) |
| | Uncontrolled HIV infection with low CD4 (<200 cells/ml) |
| *Absolute contraindications* | Pregnancy |
| | Breastfeeding[116] |
| | Allergy to PIFNα or RBV |

Management of chronic hepatitis C virus (HCV) should be individualized and the risk benefit quotient should be assessed. The aim of treatment is eradication of hepatitis C virus or sustained virological response (SVR), defined as testing negative for HCV RNA (qualitative PCR) 6 months after cessation of therapy. The indications for treatment depends on multiple factors including clinical or liver biopsy evidence of significant damage (see Table 12.1), in the absence of contraindications (Table 12.2).[116–118] The predictors of treatment response to PIFNα plus RBV depends to a large degree on the infecting genotype and the host's immunity. Genotype 1 having the lowest response, genotypes 2–3 having the best response, and genotypes 4–6 fall somewhere in between. Other factors that influence achieving SVR adversely include high baseline viral load (>800,000 IU/ml),[116] HIV infection, age >40 years, body weight >75 kg, poor adherence, drug abuse, advanced liver disease (bridging fibrosis, cirrhosis, significant steatosis), and black ethnicity.[118–120] Table 12.3 summarizes the SVR with combination of

## 12.4 Viral Infections

**Table 12.3** Sustained viral response (SVR) to pegylated IFNα/Ribavirin (Compiled from data obtained from Refs.[117,120–125])

| HCV types | Normal hosts SVR | HIV-infected[†] SVR |
|---|---|---|
| **OVERALL** | 54–56% | 27–40% |
| **Genotype 1** | 42–46% | 14–29% |
| High viral titer | 30–41% | 18% |
| Low viral titer | 56% | 61% |
| **Race** | | |
| Whites | 28% | 14–29% |
| Blacks | 19–28% | NA |
| **Genotype 2 or 3** | 76–82% | 44–73% |
| High viral titer | 74% | 63% |
| Low viral titer | 81% | 61% |
| **Genotypes 4–6** | 50% | NA |

One study[124] of co-infected patients pooled results of genotypes 2, 3 and 5 together.
HCV = hepatitis C virus; IFN-α = interferon-alpha; NA = not applicable.
[†]72% of HIV co-infected patients have high HCV titers > 800,000 iu/ml (>2 million copies/ml)

PIFNα/RBV in normal hosts and subjects with HIV infection. Patients coinfected with HIV have markedly decreased SVR to P1FNα/RBV compared to normal hosts.

Standard treatment of HCV is modified according to subtypes with genotypes 1, 4–6 receiving treatment for 48 weeks and dose of ribavirin adjusted for weight (800–1,200 mg/day). Treatment is terminated for patients not achieving early viral response (EVR) at week 12 ($\geq 2$ log decline in HCV RNA) or are not aviremic (negative HCV RNA) at 24 weeks, because the likelihood of SVR is negligible.[117,118] The standard treatment for subtypes 2 or 3 is 24 weeks and the ribavirin dose is fixed at 800 mg daily. Not all patients with EVR or undetectable virus during treatment have SVR. In about 10% of patients, HCV RNA reappears later in the course of treatment and in 20%, there is a relapse after therapy is stopped.

Emerging data from recent studies have indicated that the standard duration of therapy for HCV is not optimal for many patients. Modification of the duration of therapy can be implemented depending on the viral kinetics during therapy. There is evidence that changes in viremia levels over the first few weeks of treatment correlate with the likelihood of eradication of HCV, and a rapid viral response (RVR) with undetectable virus at 4 weeks may allow discontinuation of therapy at 12–16 weeks in subjects with genotypes 2 or 3, and at 24 weeks in those with genotype 1 and low baseline levels of HCV RNA.[124]

In a multicenter, prospective, randomized, open-label trial in Italy, patients with HCV genotypes 2 or 3 were allocated to receive standard 24 weeks of PIFNα/RBV ($N = 70$), or 12 weeks for those with RVR at 4 weeks ($N = 133$), or 24 weeks for those positive for HCV RNA at 4 weeks ($N = 80$).[126] In this trial, the SVR in those with RVR treated for 12 weeks was similar to those treated for 24 weeks (87% vs 89% for genotype 2, $p = 0.13$, and 77% vs 100% for genotype 3, $p = 0.24$, respectively). It is to be noted that RBV dose was variable according to weight,

1,000 mg daily (<75 kg) or 1,200 mg daily (>75 kg).[126] This study suggested that 12 weeks PIFNα/RBV is a suitable regimen for genotypes 2 or 3 for those with aviremia at 4 weeks, and furthermore, 90% of patients with relapse after 12 weeks of treatment had a response after an additional 24-week therapy.[126] Shortening therapy by half is cost-saving and reduces substantially the total burden of adverse events.

However, enthusiasm for the shorter-course therapy is dampened by a more recent, larger, multinational trial for HCV genotype 2 or 3, which showed that the 16-week regimen was inferior to 24 weeks therapy (62% vs 70%, $p < 0.001$).[127] In this trial of 1,469 patients, the SVR in those with RVR at 4 weeks was also superior for the longer course therapy, response 387/489 (79%) versus 400/470 (85%), $p = 0.02$.[127] A significant difference between these two studies is the lower dose of ribavirin (800 mg daily) used in the more recent trial,[127] hence further study is needed to confirm the optimal dose of ribavirin for abbreviated regimens. One important observation in the latter study is that SVR decreases in inverse proportion to pretreatment viral load. Among patients with baseline viral loads of ≤400,000 IU/ml, the SVR was very similar between 16-week vs 24-week regimens (1% difference).[127] Other factors that predicted SVR in this trial include lower weight (which could reflect higher serum levels of ribavirin) and absence of bridging fibrosis or cirrhosis.[127]

Based on current knowledge, 24-weeks regimen is still the standard therapy for HCV genotype 2 or 3, however, shorter regimen (12–14 weeks) could be considered for subjects with low pretreatment viral load (≤400,000 IU/ml), absence of bridging fibrosis and cirrhosis, and using a higher weight-adjusted ribavirin dose.

Although the standard duration of treatment for HCV genotype 1 is 48 weeks, there is some evidence that optimal therapy may be shortened (24 weeks) or lengthened (72 weeks) depending on viral response at 4 weeks and 12 weeks. There is accumulatory evidence (but no large randomized trials) that a subset or subjects with HCV genotype 1 with low pretreatment viremia (≤600,000 IU/ml), no predictors of poor response (advanced fibrosis or cirrhosis, high body mass index, older age, HIV co-infection, immunosuppression, black ethnicity) can achieve optimal response with 24-week regimen, provided there is RVR (aviremia) at 4 weeks.[128–130] Similar SVR can be achieved (88–89%) with shortened course as compared to 48-week regimen in these selected patients. Patients who relapse after 24-week therapy can be retreated with the standard 48-week course.

Some patients with HCV genotype 1 achieve ≥2 log drop in HCV RNA by week 12 but do not achieve aviremia. This is now defined as partial virological response (PVR) and patients may have undetectable virus by 24 weeks, representing "slow responders." There is now increasing evidence that prolonging the duration of treatment to 72 weeks may benefit these slow responders. In a randomized, open, prospective, multicenter trial in Germany, 455 patients with HCV genotype I (treatment-naïve) were allocated 48 weeks PIFNα /RBV (800 mg daily) ($N = 230$) versus 72 weeks ($N = 225$).[131] Patients with undetectable HCV RNA levels at weeks 4 and 12 had excellent SVR rates regardless of treatment (76–84%). However, slow responders with HCV RNA positive at weeks 4 or 12 but negative at week 24, showed benefit of extended duration of therapy (SVR 29% vs 17%, $p = 0.04$).[131] A particular benefit of prolonged therapy was seen in patients with low-level viremia (<6,000 IU/ml) at week 12. Another randomized, open-label multicenter trial in Spain compared 48-weeks to 72-weeks treatment in HCV-infected subjects with detectable HCV RNA at 4 weeks.[132] The rate of SVR among HCV genotype 1-infected patients was significantly higher in patients treated for 72 weeks versus 48 weeks (44% vs 28%, $p = 0.03$). The difference in response was primarily seen in patients with baseline HCV RNA $\leq$800,000 IU/ml (51% vs 27%), and no significant difference in SVR was observed with baseline viremia >800,000 IU/ml.[132] Of note, both these two studies used a fixed dose of ribavirin (800 mg daily), which may have been inadequate to achieve SVR at 48 weeks, as previous studies have shown that 1,000–1,200 mg of ribavirin is superior to 800 mg daily in naïve genotype 1 subjects (SVR, 52% vs 41%).[133] Disconcerting features of these two trials were the high rates of early discontinuation with extended therapy (36–41% vs 18–24% with 48 weeks treatment).

Further larger trials are needed to clarify the role of extended duration of PIFN$\alpha$/RBV in HCV genotype 1 slow responders, but using a higher dose of ribavirin (1,000–1,200 mg daily). Both the risk-benefit and cost-benefit ratios need to be assessed for this prolonged therapy.

## 12.4.2 Chronic Hepatitis B Virus

Great strides have been made in the past 5 years in the treatment of chronic hepatitis B virus (HBV) infection, and management issues continue to evolve over time. The burden of chronic HBV infection is approximately 350–400 million people worldwide, and more than 70% are in Asia. Definite indications for treatment are HBV DNA levels >$10^5$ copies/ml ($\geq$20,000 IU/ml) and ALT levels >2 times the upper limit of normal, or cirrhosis with high viral load alone.[134] Liver biopsy may be considered for those with ALT levels between one and two times the upper limit of normal (especially for age >40 years), and treatment initiated if there are histological abnormalities (significant inflammation or fibrosis). The 2007 update of the American Association of the Study of Liver Diseases guidelines[135] recommend that treatment be considered for patients with intermittent or mildly elevated ALT levels; those with HBeAg-positive with high serum HBV DNA after 40 years of age; and HBeAg-negative patients with HBV DNA levels of $10^4$–$10^5$ copies/ml (2,000–20,000 IU/ml), especially with abnormal liver biopsy. The ultimate goals of therapy are to decrease the risk of progression to cirrhosis, reverse decompensated cirrhosis, and reduce the risk of hepatocellular carcinoma.

Most trials of chronic HBV infection have assessed various single agents: IFN$\alpha$, PIFN$\alpha$, lamivudine, adefovir, entecavir, and telbivudine. The major limitations of monotherapy have been low rates of a durable response or viral eradication after completion of therapy and development of resistant viral mutants. In most cases

HBV inhibitors are virustatic and viral replication restarts soon after their withdrawal, allowing liver disease to progress.[136] Duration of treatment is a contentious unresolved issue and there is argument for life-long therapy.[134,136]

Unlike HIV and HCV, there is no established combination regimen for HBV-infection. Potential benefits of combination therapy include greater potency from additive or synergistic effect, allowing SVR, and preventing resistant mutants from evolving. No additive or synergistic effect of two HBV drugs has been observed so far in vivo as compared to single agents. Various combinations have been evaluated for chronic HBV infection but none has proven superior to monotherapy in inducing a higher rate of sustained response.

There have been five large RCT with either standard IFN$\alpha$ or PIFN$\alpha$ alone or with lamivudine, or lamivudine monotherapy in chronic HBV patients.[135] Four of these trials included only HBeAg-positive subjects and one HBeAg-negative patients. All the trials demonstrated greater viral suppression on or off treatment with the combination compared to lamivudine monotherapy, but not to IFN$\alpha$ alone. The combination was associated with lower rates of lamivudine resistance compared to lamivudine monotherapy. Re-treatment of IFN$\alpha$ non-responders with this combination is also no more effective than lamivudine alone.[135]

Before the advent of nucleosides for HBV, previous trials had assessed the value of sequential combination of glucocorticosteroids and IFN$\alpha$ versus IFN$\alpha$ alone for chronic HBV (eAg +ve) infection. In a review of 13 RCTs including 790 patients, the analysis showed greater loss of Hb "e" antigen (OR 1.41, $p = 0.03$) and HBV DNA (OR 1.51, $p = 0.008$) in the sequential combination group than IFN$\alpha$ alone.[137] However, the combination was no better than monotherapy in normalization of ALT levels, loss of HBV surface antigen, seroconversion to HBV e-antibody, mortality, or adverse events.

Subjects with HBV and naïve to nucleosides have been randomized to combination of lamivudine and adefovir or lamivudine alone. Results at week 52 and week 104 showed no significant difference in HBV DNA suppression, ALT normalization, or HBeAg loss.[135,138] However, genotype resistance (YMDD motif) was less common in the combination (15%) versus lamivudine (43%) monotherapy group. In a small study of 59 patients with lamivudine-resistant HBV the combination of adefovir and lamivudine was not superior to adefovir alone.[139] Recent studies, however, indicate that for patients with lamivudine-resistant HBV it is better to add adefovir than switching to adefovir monotherapy, as this reduces the rate of adefovir resistance.[136,140]

Telbivudine, a new nucleoside with potent anti-HBV activity has been compared as monotherapy versus combination with lamivudine in HBeAg positive, nucleoside-naïve patients. Results with combination regimens were similar to those with telbivudine alone.[141] A recent large, phase 3, multicenter RCT of 1,370 patients with chronic HBV showed that telbivudine was superior to lamivudine (both monotherapy) with greater HBV DNA suppression, histologic response at 1 year, and with less resistance.[142]

Present guidelines and available drugs for therapy of HBV are outlined in Table 12.4. Although the guidelines have not listed a preferred agent of choice, based on

**Table 12.4** Approved drugs for chronic hepatitis B

| Conditions | IFN-α (PIFN-α) | Lamivudine | Adefovir | Entecavir | Telbivudine |
|---|---|---|---|---|---|
| **INDICATIONS** | | | | | |
| Hbe Ag + or − | | | | | |
| • ±Chronic hepatitis | Indicated | Indicated | Indicated | Indicated | Indicated |
| • Cirrhosis | Avoid | Indicated | Indicated | Indicated | Indicated |
| • HIV/NO ART | Indicated | Not Indicated | Indicated | Indicated ? | Not Indicated |
| **DURATION OF TREATMENT** | | | | | |
| Hbe Ag + chronic hepatitis | IFNα: 16 weeks PIFN: 48 weeks | ≥1 year* | ≥1 year* | ≥1 year* | ≥1 year* |
| Hbe Ag − chronic hepatitis | >1 year | >1 year | >1 year | >1 year | >1 year |
| Cirrhosis | – | long-term in** combination | Long term | Long term | ? Long term in** combination |
| **RESPONSE RATE** | | | | | |
| Hbe Ag seroconversion (greater than controls) | 18–21% | 16–21% | 12% | 21% | 22% |
| Durable virologic response post-therapy | 20–40% | 10–20% | 10–20% | 10–20% | 10–20% |
| Histologic improvement (HbeAg + and − Hepatitis) | 38–48% (PIFNα) | 49–66% | 53–64% | 70–72% | 65–67% |
| Undetectable HBV DNA > 48 weeks on treatment | 25–70% | 40–73% | 21–51% | 67–90% | 60–88% |
| **DRUG RESISTANCE** | | | | | |
| 1 year | – | ≈20% | 0 | <1% | 2–5% |
| 4 years | – | 70–90% | 15–20% | 0.8–1.2% | >9–22% |

The above table was compiled from data obtained from references 134, 135, 140, 142, 143, and 146

ALT, alanine aminotransferase; IFNα, interferon-alpha; PIFNα, pegylated interferon alpha; HBeAg. hepatitis Be antigen; HBV, hepatitis B virus; HIV, human immunodeficiency virus

± − HBV DNA > 20,000IU/ml; − HBV DNA > 2,000 IU/ml; ALT > 2x upper limit or <2,000 UU/ml if ALT elevated after HBeAb seroconversion

\* Minimum of 1 year or at least 6 months

\*\* Long-term will result in acceptable resistance, best used in combination with adefovir

? Cross resistance to lamivudine may occur

available data of efficacy, tolerability, and availability, and drug resistance development, entecavir appears to be the best first choice. Duration of therapy remains a contentious issue. Current guidelines recommend treatment for at least a year and at least 6 months after anti-Hbe seroconversion.[135] It has been argued that HBeAg seroconversion is an inadequate endpoint for many patients, as cirrhosis and hepatocellular carcinoma often occur despite HBeAg seroconversion, HBV DNA levels $<10^4$ copies/ml, or ALT levels $<2$ times the upper limit of normal. Therefore, it has been suggested that ideal treatment endpoints should be permanent suppression of HBV DNA to undetectable levels and reduction of ALT levels to $<0.5$ times upper limit of normal.[134] Essentially, this would mean lifetime or intermittent therapy for most chronic HBV-infected subjects and the risk-benefit and cost-benefit ratios for this strategy is unknown and may be prohibitive.[143] Furthermore, only a few patients have been treated in clinical trials for up to 5 years.

The treatment endpoints of chronic HBV infection in HIV-co-infected patients are somewhat different. The prognosis for development for severe liver disease and hepatoma are worse that in normal hosts, and the liver disease runs a more rapid course. The aims of therapy in these coinfected subjects are suppression of viral replication (absence of HBV DNA or HBeAg in serum) and improvement of liver disease.[144] Therefore, long-term therapy is needed and should include concomitant treatment for the HIV infection to maintain undetectable virus (<50 copies/ml) and restore immunity. Combination therapy specific for the HBV is preferred, which include agents active against the HIV as well (i.e., lamivudine and tenofovir, or the combination of emtricitabine-tenofovir (truvada, Gilead Sciences). These two nucleosides are given in combination with a non-nucleoside or protease inhibitor to achieve optimal anti-HIV activity. Use of a single agent effective against HBV (i.e., lamivudine-zidovudine [Combivir], which is commonly used as a nucleoside backbone for HIV infection), will lead to unacceptable resistance to lamivudine(20–25% per year and 90% after 4 years), as zidovudine has no anti-HBV activity. A randomized, controlled trial comparing tenofovir and adefovir (90% of patients also received lamivudine), showed that both are safe and efficacious in decreasing HBV DNA levels in HIV-coinfected patients.[145] However, tenofovir has more potent activity against both HBV and HIV than adefovir (at recommended dose), and furthermore, adefovir is not approved for use in HIV infection. In general, combinations effective for both HBV and HIV are initiated at the time treatment is considered appropriated for HIV in coinfected patients. On occasion however, the HIV infection may not require specific therapy (those with high CD4 T-cell count), but treatment for the HBV infection would deem necessary (high HBV DNA levels and ALT levels >2 times upper limit of normal). In this situation, patients should not receive HBV medication that have activity against HIV (lamivudine, tenofovir), as this would lead to HIV drug-resistant mutants. Instead, it is recommended to use agents with HBV activity alone, such as PIFN-α, entecavir and adefovir.[144] There is a theoretical risk of adefovir predisposing to tenofovir (structurally closely related) HIV-resistant mutants, but no resistance has been shown so far. There is a single case report of entecavir monotherapy in an HIV/HBV-coinfected patient (with no anti-HIV therapy), resulting in accumulation of HIV variants with the lamuvidine-resistant mutation, M184V.[146] Although this is a single report, it is very worrisome as it occurred soon after marketing of entecavir. Thus widespread monotherapy with this anti-HBV agent in HIV-coinfected subjects could lead to significant lamivudine/emtricitabine HIV resistance.

A recent cost-effectiveness analysis of available treatments for chronic HBV infection concluded that IFN-α was most cost-effective in health care system with limited budget, and neither lamivudine or adefovir monotherapy is cost-effective.[147] However, lamivudine with subsequent adefovir for viral resistance was highly cost-effective. This analysis did not include PIFN-α, entecavir or telbivudine and further studies on this issue should be forthcoming.

## 12.5 Parasitic Infections

Dual drug therapy has been used for several decades for the most important parasitic disease world-wide (malaria). However, this is not considered combined therapy as it represents either sequential therapy for different stages of the parasite, chloroquine, for the blood (erythrocytic schizonts) stage and primaquine for the chronic hepatic stage (*Plasmodium vivax* and *P. ovale*) or two agents acting in concert at the same site (antifolate activity of sulfadoxine and pyrimethamine [SP]). Over the past 35 years, the incidence of malaria has increased twofold to threefold. This has partly been attributed to development and spread of multidrug-resistant parasites. Combined antimalarial drugs that utilize agents with different mechanisms of action against the same stage of parasites have now become standard therapy in many parts of the world, with chloroquine-resistant *P. falciparum*. Recently, combination therapy has been applied to other parasites endemic in many tropical and sub-tropical countries.

### 12.5.1 Antimalarial Combination Therapies

Chloroquine-resistant *P. falciparum* is now prevalent (30–85%) in most malaria-endemic countries of the world, except for Central America, Caribbean (Hispaniola), and parts of the Middle East. The highest areas of resistant malaria are located in Southeast Asia (85%) and South America (66%).[148] Chloroquine-resistant *P. vivax* had emerged in New Guinea, but is confined mainly to the Indonesian Archipelago especially in the east, and sporadically in Asia and South America.[148] Recently, chloroquine-resistant *P. malariae* has been reported from southern Sumatra, Indonesia.[149]

Various combinations of antimalarial drugs, including new and old agents have been tested in the field and are available in some form for treatment of malaria. A longstanding combination of two blood-stage schizonticide agents, quinine plus tetracycline, or doxycycline has been used for chloroquine-resistant *P. falciparum* for decades and still retains its efficacy. Resistance to quinine occurs sporadically and is limited to some regions of Southeast Asia and New Guinea.[147] This combination can be used for 3–7 days, and a 7-day regimen may be more effective than a 5-day regimen, 100% vs 87% efficacy in one study from Thailand.[150] The major drawback of this combined therapy is poor adherence from side-effects: tinnitus, nausea, and vertigo (cinchonism). The rates of adherence reported varies from 71% to as low as 11–20%.[151,152]

The fixed combination of SP is inexpensive and was widely prescribed in Africa for falciparum malaria, but it is no longer recommended because of increasing resistance.[153] Combining SP with another older inexpensive antimalarial, amodiaquine, is an affordable, effective alternative for multiresistant *P. falciparum*. In a RCT performed in sub-Saharan Africa, parasitological treatment failure occurred with SP monotherapy in 26%, amodiaquine (AQ) alone 16% and 10% of those treated with SP + AQ.[154] Another study in young children in Cameroon with uncomplicated falciparum malaria showed superior results with SP + AQ compared to monotherapies of the agents separately, with 14-day treatment failure of 3.3% and no late therapeutic failure on day 28.[155] A more recent larger study in Burkina Faso of 944 cases of falciparum malaria also confirmed the high efficacy of SP + AQ.[156] Thus, this combination was more effective than monotherapies and could be the optimum low-cost alternative to more expensive combination in Africa.

In parts of Africa with low malaria transmission and low drug pressure (relatively low drug resistance), chloroquine (CQ) combined with SP (SP + CQ) is recommended to delay the development of increasing drug resistance.[157] Parasitological resistance was observed at R1 level in 10% (CQ), 18.5% (SP) and 6.9% (SP + CQ), $p = 0.37$, for patients treated for falciparum malaria with single agents or combination. A recent comparative trial of monotherapies and two combinations in Central Africa for acute uncomplicated *P. falciparum* malaria found AQ + SP slightly more effective than CQ + SP, 0% and 7.2% treatment failures, respectively, and both combinations were superior to single agents.[158]

A fixed combination of atovaquone-proguanil (AP or malarone) acts synergistically on the asexual blood stage of malaria parasites by inhibition of mitochondrial electron transport and folate metabolism, and represents true combined therapy.[148] AP is used for chemoprophylaxis and treatment of multiresistant falciparum malaria. Results of several trials have found significantly better cure rates with AP compared to mefloquine, amodiaquine, or combination of CQ + SP.[159] Summary of 10 open-label trials with AP (1,000 mg/400 mg) daily for 3 days has reported cure rate of uncomplicated falciparum malaria of 99% (514/521).[160] Malarone for therapy of multiresistant *P. falciparum* malaria is better tolerated and more cost-effective than quinine + doxycycline for 7 days. Although this combination is commonly used for malaria prophylaxis for travelers and treatment of returning tourists or residents with acute falciparum malaria in developed countries, it is not commonly used in endemic tropical countries because of the relative expense compared to other available combinations. Recently, however, resistance to AP has been reported from Africa.[161,162] Higher doses of AP (3,000 mg/1,200 mg) daily for 3 days is still highly effective (95%) for falciparum malaria in Vietnam, is well-tolerated and appears just as effective as a new four-drug combination (CV8, containing dihydroartemesinin/piperaquin, trimethoprim/primaquine) against multidrug-resistant strains.[163] Of concern is the presence of two point mutations in the parasite cytochrome b gene (associated with resistance to malarone) in treatment-naïve patients in Africa of 5–10%.[164,165]

Artemesinins (primarily artemether, artesunate, and dihydroartemesinin) is a plant extract from the weed *Artemesia annun* developed in China during the 1960s.[148] These agents are potent blood-stage schizonticides and rapidly reduce parasitemia of $10^4$ schizonts per cycle. Thus, the artemesinins can abolish a high parasite burden of $10^{12}$ with three cycles (7 days). To reduce the risk of resistant mutants and shorten duration of therapy to 3 days, the artemesinins are combined with long-acting companion schizonticides. Artemesinin-based therapies (ACTs) are the best antimalarial drugs and the World Health Organization (WHO) and leading experts in the field are recommending ACT for first-line treatment for chloroquine-resistant falciparum malaria. Several comparative trials have demonstrated the superiority of ACTs over monotherapies and other combinations. In one such two-phase study in Mozambique, artesunate (AR) + SP and AQ + AR were safe and 100% effective and superior to CQ, SP, and AQ monotherapies in children with uncomplicated falciparum malaria.[166] In a RCT in Uganda, three combinations were compared in 1,017 children with uncomplicated falciparum malaria; AQ + AR, CQ + SP and AQ + SP.[167] The 28-day clinical treatment failure was significantly lower for the ACT (AQ + AR) 2%, AQ + SP (9%), and CQ + SP (35%), $p < 0.001$.[167] A similar recent RCT in children with falciparum malaria in Uganda compared three leading combinations: AQ + SP, AQ + AR, and artemether-lumefantrine in 601 subjects.[168] Artemether-lumefantrine was the most efficacious treatment with recrudescent treatment failure of 1% (28-day treatment failure of 6.7%), compared to 4.6% for AQ + AR (28-day treatment failure of 17.4%), and 14.1% for AQ + SP (28-day treatment failure rate of 26.1%, $p < 0.05$).[166]

ACTs have been most extensively used in Asia and Southeast Asia. Since the deployment of artesunate-mefloquine combination in Western Thailand, there has been a sustained decline in the incidence of *P. falciparum* malaria with cure rate to almost 100%, and significant improvement in mefloquine resistance.[169] A major barrier to widespread distribution and utilization of ACTs for malaria in many developing, resource-poor countries is the acquisition cost. One artemesinin-based combined therapy, artemether-lumefantrine (Coartem, Novartis) wholesale price is $2.40 per adult course, as compared to 10 cents retail for chlorquine.[170] The global overall deployment of ACT has been slow since the WHO recommendation in 2001 and of 43 countries that adopted ACT by February 2005, 42% (18) implemented the policy in 2004.[171] It is estimated that the minimum global cost of ACTs would be about $500 million per year, but this is unmanageable for many countries with per capita income of $2000 per year or less.[170] One affordable combination that has a cost advantage over the other ACTs is dihydroartemisinin-piperaquine (Artekin), which could cost $1 (US) per adult treatment, making it suitable for widespread deployment in Africa.[171]

The use of ACTs occasionally leads to emergence of resistant strains, probably secondary to incomplete adherence to multiple doses (6 doses over 3 days). In vitro studies have shown reduced susceptibility to artesunate among Asian isolates[172]; and in western Cambodia where ACTs are widely used, there is diminished susceptibility to mefloquine-artesunate as compared to isolates from eastern Cambodia.[148] However, in other countries (e.g., Thailand) where ACTs have been first-line therapy since the 1990s, resistance is slow to develop and efficacy is maintained above 90%.[148] A large comparative trial on the northwest border of Thailand, where multidrug-resistant falciparum malaria is prevalent, demonstrated that combining artesunate with malarone (AR + AP) was associated with a reduced risk of failure threefold compared to malarone alone or artesunate + mefloquine; failure rate 0.9%, 2.8%, and 2.4% respectively.[173]

## 12.5.2 Filariasis Therapies

Lymphatic filariasis and onchocerciasis (river blindness) are causes of significant chronic disabilities in tropical and subtropical countries with over 120 million affected persons worldwide. Lymphatic filariasis, which causes acute lymphangitis and chronic lymphatic obstruction is transmitted by the anopheles mosquito, as the infective larval form of the filarial worms *Wuchereria bancrofti*, *Brugia malayi*, and *Brugia timori*. Lymphatic filariasis occurs throughout sub-Saharan Africa and in much of Southeast Asia.

Current antifilarial drugs are unsatisfactory and include diethylcarbamazine (in use for over 50 years) and ivermectin. Both these drugs are effective in killing circulating microfilariae in the blood stream, and can cause acute systemic inflammatory reaction by release of macrofilarial products and endosymbiotic bacteria (*Wolbachia*) into the blood.[174] Diethylcarbamazine also has partial macrofilaricidal effect on the adult worm, but this can precipitate acute inflammatory reaction resulting in heightened granulomatous process with progressive fibrosis. Moreover, in countries coendemic for onchocerciasis (Sub-Saharan West and Central Africa), diethylcarbamazine can result in irreversible damage to the eye (if infected) and is contraindicated in these instances. Thus, both these agents have limited or no benefit for the individual patient with symptomatic lymphatic obstruction. Furthermore, diethylcarbamazine is associated with frequent side-effects including dizziness, myalgias, arthralgias, hypotension, chorioretinal damage, and optic neuritis.

Humans are the main reservoir for filariasis and it is theoretically possible to break the cycle of mosquito–human–mosquito transmission, by mass treatment of populations with high endemic rate of lymphatic filariasis on a regular yearly basis to suppress microfilariae and eradicate filariasis. In lymphatic filariasis, after initial infection by the larval stage, the incubation for maturation into an adult worm in the lymphatics is about a year. Thereafter, the female worms produces microfilariae every year for about 4–6 years (period of fecundity) and the adult worm lives for about 5 to >10 years. The global program to eliminate lymphatic filariasis (sponsored by WHO), aims to interrupt transmission of filariasis by reducing the levels of circulating microfilariae in infected populations by mass treatment with diethylcarbamazine or ivermectin, both in combination with albendazole as single dose therapy for 5–6 years. Albendazole has a weak microfilaricidal activity but in combination with either ivermectin or diethylcarbamazine, there appears to be enhanced efficacy.

A recent model-based analysis of trial data on mass treatment programs against lymphatic filariasis concluded that both combinations are highly effective and can have a large impact on lymphatic filariasis transmission.[175] For diethylcarbamazine-albendazole treatment, the average microfilarial loss was about 83% and worm-productivity loss was 100%. For ivermectin-albendazole treatment, average microfilarial loss was 100% and worm productivity loss was 96%. A RCT trial in Egyptian adults with asymptomatic microfilaremia compared single dose versus multi-dose (7 days) combination of diethylcarbamazine (DEC) and albendazole. Multi-dose therapy was significantly more effective than single-dose treatment with complete clearance at 12 months in 75% versus 23.1%, or reduction in microfilariae counts of 99.6% versus 85.7%, respectively.[176]

There is some debate, however, on the value of albendazole in combination with another antifilarial drug. A recent review of the topic analyzed the results of seven RCT involving 6,997 participants (995 with detectable microfilariae).[177] The authors concluded that there was insufficient evidence to confirm or refute that albendazole coadministered with DEC or ivermectin was more effective than either antifilarial drugs alone in clearing microfilariae or killing adult worms. There is also some recent data indicating that combinations with albendazole can select for benzimidazole resistance mutations in the filarial worms and other helminth parasites as well.[178]

A discovery just over 20 years ago that filarial worms depend on an endosymbiotic rickettsial-like bacteria, *Wolbachia* species, for development, embryogenesis, fertility, and viability, have opened new avenues for treatment.[179,180] Tetracyclines (including doxycycline) target these intracellular endosymbiotic bacteria interfering with worm molting, fertility, and viability.[181] Trials of doxycycline for 6–8 weeks in lymphatic filariasis and onchocerciasis have shown reduced levels of microfilaria and *Wolbachia* species.[182,183] A recent RCT of 72 subjects with *W. bancrofti* filariasis received either doxycycline 200 mg daily for 8 weeks or placebo.[184] A more recent RCT with a smaller, sample ($N = 44$) assessed the efficacy of 3-week doxycycline course versus placebo combined with single doses of albendazole and ivermectin given at 4 months (both groups).[185] The microfilarial level was significantly reduced with doxycycline treatment at 4, 12, and 24 months. However, this shorter course of doxycycline did not significantly alter detection of adult worms, thus not curative.[185] It is not clear, however, whether the triple combination therapy is more effective than doxycycline alone, owing to the design of the study. Additional RCTs with combination of DEC plus doxycycline, ivermectin plus doxycycline versus doxycycline alone are warranted with larger sample sizes.

In a larger double-blind, RCT of 161 patients infected with *B. malayi* 6 weeks of doxycycline (100 mg daily) was given to 119 subjects and placebo to 42.[186] Four months after doxycycline therapy 62 patients were allocated single-dose placebo, and 57 single-dose DEC-albendazole; the 42 subjects initially randomized to placebo doxycycline were given single-dose DEC-albendazale. Four months after doxycycline treatment, *Wolbachia* loads were reduced by 98% (as measured by PCR). Doxycycline reduced the prevalence of microfilaremia significantly at all time points (2, 4, and 12 months); and at 1 year after initial therapy the prevalence was reduced by 77% for doxycycline alone versus 87.5% for doxycycline plus DEC-albendazole.[186] The reduction of microfilaremia in patients receiving single dose of DEC-albendazole alone was only 26.7% at 1 year. Doxycycline also significantly reduced high fever and severe adverse reactions to specific antifilarial treatment, indicating a role for *Wolbachia* in these reactions.

### 12.5.3 Leishmaniasis

Visceral leishmaniasis (kala-azar) affect more than 500,000 people annually in resource-poor countries, mainly in northeastern India, Nepal, and Bangladesh, but is endemic in East Africa, coastal region of the Mediterranean, and Brazil. The infection caused by *Leishmania donovani* and transmitted by sand flies, results in involvement of the reticuloendothelial system with fever, pancytopenia, and hepatosplenomegaly. Untreated patients usually die and current standard therapy (i.e., pentavalent antimony sodium stibogluconate, amphotericin B, or liposomal formulations) are toxic and expensive and require hospitalization. An effective oral medication, miltefosine, is now available and safer than previous parenteral therapy but it is expensive, potentially teratogenic, and has significant gastrointestinal side-effects.[187] Thus, new effective therapies or combinations that are safe and inexpensive are being sought for treatment of visceral leishmaniasis.

Paromomycin, an aminoglycoside antibiotic in use for many years orally for intestinal parasites, has been shown to have a dose response efficacy for treatment of visceral leishmaniasis by intramuscular injection for 21 days.[188] In a recent RCT, intramuscular paromomycin (11 mg/kg/day) for 21 days was shown to be just as effective as amphotericin B (11 mg/kg/2 days) for 30 days, cure rate 94.6% and 98.8%, respectively.[189] Response to first-line therapy (sodium stibogluconate) has been decreasing in the Indian subcontinent, probably due to resistance to the pentavalent antimonials. Studies to assess the benefit of combined therapy with paromomycin plus stibogluconate has been performed in India and Africa.

In India, 150 patients with visceral leishmaniasis were randomized to receive either paromomycin 12 mg/kg/day with stibogluconate 20 mg/kg daily for 21 days; or paromomycin 20 mg/kg daily with stibogluconate for 21 days; or stibogluconate alone for 30 days. Final cure rates after 180 days were 48 of 52 (92.3%) for low-dose paromomycin plus stibogluconate, 45 of 48 (93.8%) for the higher dose paromomycin combination, and 26 of 49 (53.1%) for stibogluconate monotherapy ($p < 0.001$).[189] A smaller study in Kenya of 53 patients with visceral leishmaniasis assessed paromomycin alone or combined with stibogluconate, or stibogluconate monotherapy.[190] Clinical cures were achieved in all patients at termination, but splenic aspirates revealed the best parasitological cure with combined treatment (13% failures), compared to 21% failure with paromomycin alone and 45% with stibogluconate alone. Paromomycin is relatively inexpensive and is associated with transient reversible ototoxicity (2%), and pain at the injection site (55%), with transient elevation of aspartate aminotransferase levels.[189]

These latter two studies do not prove that combined therapy is more effective than paromomycin monotherapy, which has produced a cure rate of 94.6%.[190] It does appear however, that paromomycin may be more effective than stibogluconate. Further combination trials are warranted with larger sample sizes, longer follow-up to assess cure, and include shorter duration combinations, especially with miltefosine (oral) plus paromomycin.

## 12.5.4 African Trypanosomiasis (Sleeping Sickness)

*Trypanosoma brucei gambiense* is the cause of human sleeping sickness (African trypanosomiasis) in West and Central Africa and *Trypanosoma brucei rhodiense* in East Africa. This is a late-stage, insidious, chronic disease of the brain that is usually fatal if left untreated.

Whereas in the early stage of African trypanosiomiasis, (hemolymphatic stage), pentamidine or suramin are considered first-line effective treatment, for sleeping sickness melarsoprol is the agent of first choice. Melarsoprol, a combination of trivalent organic arsenic compound and dimercaprol (heavy metal chelator), is associated with severe adverse reactions. Increased treatment failure rates with melarsoprol and primary resistance have been reported from several African countries (Angola, Uganda, and Sudan).[191–194] Eflornithine, an inhibitor of ornithine decarboxylase that depletes polyamines in trypanosomes, is an effective alternative treatment for sleeping sickness.[193] However, it is costly and of limited supply and obtainable from WHO. Nifurtimox, an S-nitrofuran, was developed and registered for therapy of Chagas disease caused by *Trypanosoma chagasi*, but has been used successfully for treatment of melarsoprol-refractory sleeping sickness.[194,195] Nifurtimox activity on trypanosomes is related to free radicals, generated by nitrofuran reduction, binding to the membrane and DNA of the parasite.[196] Open and compassionate studies have used oral nifurtimox three times a day for 14–21 days.

A few studies have assessed combination of new and existing drugs for African trypanosomiasis to optimize therapy and reduce the risk of microbial resistance and recurrence.[196]

Eflornithine for 7–14 days has previously been found effective for relapsing Gambian sleeping sickness. In a non-randomized study of melarsoprol-resistant late-stage Gambian trypanosomiasis, 42 patients were treated with a sequential combination of intravenous eflornithine for 4 days, followed by three daily injections of melarsoprol.[197] At 24 months follow-up, the cure rate was 90.4% but whether this represents additive or synergistic effect of the two drugs could not be determined.

A recent larger open randomized trial was conducted in 278 patients with second stage Gambian sleeping sickness to assess monotherapy and combination therapy of melarsoprol-nifurtimox combination.[198] A consecutive 10-day low-dose melarsoprol-nifurtimox combination was more effective than standard melarsoprol regimen or nifurtimox monotherapy. Relapses were observed with all of the monotherapy regimens but none with the combination therapy ($p = 0.01$).[198] Of the monotherapy regimens, the standard melarsoprol regimen was significantly more effective than the others ($p = 0.01$), including nifurtimox monotherapy.[198] This is the first RCT in human sleeping sickness demonstrating superiority of combination therapy compared to standard monotherapy. Nifurtimox (oral administration) as monotherapy is associated with relapse in approximately half of patients,[198] and it is associated with significant gastrointestinal and neurological side effects. The combination of nifurtimox and melarsoprol would best be suited for primary therapy of sleeping sickness, rather than as salvage therapy for melarsoprol failures, as response is likely to be less in the latter situation. Future trials should compare combination of nifurtimox and oral eflornithine to monotherapy with eflornithine and melarsoprol, and subsequently with other combinations. It should be noted that for early stage Gambian trypanosomiasis, combination of pentamidine and Suramin was not more effective than either agents alone.[199]

## 12.6 Conclusion

It is evident from this review of combination therapy that combined therapies have been proven to be more effective than monotherapies mainly in chronic persistent infectious diseases, where development of resistant mutants is the primary limitation. Table 12.5 shows a summary of infections where combinations are of proven value and those that appear promising but remain unestablished or controversial. Combination therapies are more controversial and usually not proven by RCT (often accepted standard therapy) for acute bacterial and fungal infection. These combinations of agents are commonly used to enhance activity or efficacy and may have shown benefit in animal models or in vitro studies. International collaborative efforts are pressingly needed to verify superiority of combinations over monother-

## 12.6 Conclusion

**Table 12.5** Combination anti-infective therapies

| | Comments |
|---|---|
| **A. Bacterial infections** | |
| • Mycobacterial tuberculosis complex (3–4 drugs) | Accepted standard |
| • Leprosy (2–3 drugs) | Accepted standard |
| • Invasive atypical mycobacteria | Considered standard (RCT in MAC and HIV) |
| • Human brucellosis (2 drugs) | RCT-evidence |
| • Enterococcal endocarditis (2 drugs – initial 2 weeks, then monotherapy) | Accepted standard; no RCT |
| • Q fever endocarditis (2 drugs) | Recommended, no RCT |
| • Staphylococcal PVE (2–3 drugs) | Recommended, no RCT |
| • *S. aureus* endocarditis (left-sided – 2 drugs × 5 days, then monotherapy) (right-sided – 2 drugs × 2 weeks) | Recommended, minimal benefit in RCT controversial |
| • *S. viridans* endocarditis (2 drugs × 2 weeks) | No RCT, accepted alternative for convenience |
| • Prosthetic orthopedic infection (combination with rifampicin) | Recommended 1 small RCT/ unproven |
| **B. Viral infections** | |
| • HIV (3 drugs) | Proven by RCT |
| • Hepatitis C virus (2 drugs) | Proven by RCT |
| **C. Fungal infections** | |
| • Cryptococcal meningitis (2 drugs × 2 weeks, then monotherapy) | Accepted standard, RCT-evidence |
| • Severe invasive aspergillosis (2 drugs) | unproven, awaiting RCT |
| **D. Parasitic infections** | |
| • Chloroquine-resistant *P. falciparum* (artemisin-based combination) | RCT evidence, recommended |
| • Lymphatic filariasis (2 drugs) | RCT evidence, promising |
| • Late-stage African trypanosomiasis (2 drugs) | RCT evidence, promising |

HIV = human immunodeficiency virus; PVE = prosthetic valve endocarditis; RCT = randomized controlled trial.

apy for many of these guidelines with combined therapy as recommended standard without RCTs.

Several recommendations for combination therapies are based on in vitro and animal model with limited applications to human disease. Although combined therapies may appear attractive, they carry the added risk of extra-drug toxicities, increased costs on the health care system, and the potential to predispose to greater risk of superinfection and multi-resistant strains.

For instance, adjunctive use of rifampin in combination with a beta-lactam agent, vancomycin, fluoroquinolone, or doxycycline has become common practice for the therapy for *S. aureus* or coagulase-negative staphylococcal infection (methicillin sensitive or resistant strains). Although animal studies tend to show a microbiological benefit of adding rifampin (especially in chronic osteomyelitis and foreign body infection models), see Chapters 10 and 11, few human studies have addressed the issue. In a recent review of the literature, it was concluded that although rifampin in combination appears promising for hardware infections and chronic osteomyelitis, the benefit has not been established and further larger multicenter trials are needed.[200]

## 12.7 Future Directions

Presently the treatment of hepatitis C genotype I results in modest to poor response depending largely on baseline high viral load and concomitant HIV-infection. A new class of drugs that inhibit HCV N5SB polymerase and N53-4A protease known as "specifically targeted antiviral for HCV" (STAT-C) is in development. However natural occurrence of protease inhibitor-resistant variants (although uncommon) is worrisome and forbode development of widespread resistance to these agents even in combination with pegylated interferonγ.[201] However, triple combination of peginterferon, ribavin and telapravir (a STAT C) appear to be a potent regimen for this group of patients and may have robust durability than dual therapy.[201] However, further large controlled trials are needed.

## References

1. Davies, P.D.O., Cooke, R. (2008). Mycobacterial antimicrobial resistance, In: Fong, I.W., Drlica, K. (eds). Antimicrobial resistance and implications for the 21st century. Springer, New York, pp. 161–205.
2. Martinez-Cajas, J.L., Petrella, M., Wainberg, M.A. (2008). Clinical significance and biological basis of HIV drug resistance. In: Fong, I.W., Drlica, K., (eds). Antimicrobial resistance and implications for the 21st century. Springer, New York, pp. 231–261.
3. Baird, J.K. (2005). Drug therapy: effectiveness of antimalarial drugs. *N Engl J Med* 352:1565–1577.
4. Mylonakis, E., Calderwood, S.B. (2001). Infective endocarditis in adults. *N Engl J Med* 345:318–330.
5. Le, T., Bayer, A.S. (2003). Combination antibiotic therapy for infective endocarditis. *Clin Infect Dis* 36:615–621.
6. Bayer, A.S., Morrison, J.O. (1984). Disparity between time-kill and checkerboard methods for determination of in vitro bactericidal interactions of vancomycin plus rifampicin versus methicillin-susceptible and -resistant Staphylococcus aureus. *Antimicrob Agents Chemother* 26:220–223.
7. Moellering, R.C. Jr., Wennersten, C., Medrek, T., Weinberg, A.N. (1970). Prevalence of high-level resistance to aminoglycosides in clinical isolates of enterococci. *Antimicrob Agents Chemother* 10:335–360.

8. Eliopoulos, G.M. (1993). Aminoglycoside resistant enterococcal endocarditis. *Infect Dis Clin North Am* 7:117–133.
9. Moellering, R.C. Jr., Wennersten, C., Medrek, T., Weinberg, A.N. (1991). Synergy of penicillin and gentamicin against enterococci. *J Infect Dis* 124(Suppl):S107–S204.
10. Matsumoto, J.Y., Wilson, W.R., Wright, A.J., Geraci, J.E., Washington, II,J.A. (1980). Synergy of penicillin and decreasing concentrations of aminoglycosides against enterococci from patients with infective endocarditis. *Antimicrob Agents Chemother* 18:944–947.
11. Mainardi, J.L., Gutmann, L., Acar, J.F., Goldstein, F.W. (1995). Synergistic effect of amoxicillin and cefotaxime against Enterococcus faecalis. *Antimicrob Agents Chemother* 39:1984–1987.
12. Brandt, C.M., Rouse, M.S., Lane, N.W., Stratton, C.W., Wilson, W.R., Steckelberg, J.M. (1996). Effective treatment of multidrug-resistant experimental endocarditis with combination of cell-wall active agents. *J Infect Dis* 173:909–913.
13. Gavalda, J., Torres, C., Tenorio, C., López, P., Zaragoza, M., Capdevila, J.A., Almirante, B., Ruiz, F., Borrell, N., Gomis, X., Pigrau, C., Baquero, F., Pahissa, A. (1999). Efficacy of ampicillin plus ceftriaxone in treatment of experimental endocarditis due to Enterococcus faecalis strains highly resistant to aminoglycosides. *Antimicrob Agents Chemother* 43:639–646.
14. Plastino, K.A., Connors, J.E., Spinler, S.A. (1994). Possible synergy between aminoglycosides and vancomycin in the treatment of *Staphylococcus epidermidis* endocarditis. *Ann Pharmacother* 28:737–739.
15. Yu, V.L., Zuravleff, J.J., Bornholm, J., Archer, G. (1984). In vitro synergy testing of triple antibiotic combination against *Staphylococcus epidermidis* isolates from patients with endocarditis. *J Antimicrob Chemother* 14:359–366.
16. Archer, G.L., Johnson, J.L., Vasquez, G.J., Haywood, H.B. 3rd (1983). Efficacy of antibiotic combinations including rifampin against methicillin-resistant *Staphylococcus epidermidis*: in vitro and in vivo studies. *Rev Infect Dis* 5(Suppl):S538–S542.
17. Fantin, B., Carbon, C. (1992). In vivo antibiotic synergism: contribution of animal models. *Antimicrob Agents Chemother* 36:907–912.
18. Fantin, B., Leclercq, R., Arthur, M., Duval, J., Carbon, C. (1991). Influence of low-level resistance to vancomycin on efficacy of teicoplanin and vancomycin for treatment of experimental endocarditis due to *Enterococcus faecium*. *Antimicrob Agents Chemother* 35:1570–1575.
19. Caron, F., Carbon, C., Guttman, L. (1991). Evaluation of the triple combination penicillin-vancomycin-gentamicin in an experimental endocarditis caused by moderately penicillin- and a highly glycopeptide-resistant strain of *Enterococcus faecum*. *J Infect Dis* 164:888–893.
20. Join-Lambert, O., Mainardi, J.L., Cuvelier, C., Dautrey, S., Farinotti, R., Fantin, B., Carbon, C. (1998). Critical importance of in vivo amoxicillin and cefotaxime concentration for synergy in treatment of experimental *Enterococcus faecalis* endocarditis. *Antimicrob Agents Chemother* 42:468–470.
21. Baddour, L.M., Wilson, W.R., Bayer, A.S., Fowler, V.G., Jr, Bolger, A.F., Levison, M.E., Ferrieri, P., Gerber, M.A., Tanl, L.Y., Gewitz, M.H., Tong, D.C., Steckelberg, J.M., Baltimore, R.S., Shulman, S.T., Burns, J.C., Falace, D.A., Newburger, J.W., Pallasch, J., Takahashi, M., Taubert, K.A. (2005). Infective endocarditis: diagnosis, antimicrobial therapy, and management of complications: a statement for healthcare professionals from the Committee on Rheumatic Fever Endocarditis and Kawasaki Disease Council on Cardiovascular Disease in the Young, and the Councils on Clinical Cardiovascular Surgery and Anesthesia, American Heart Association: Endorsed by the Infectious Diseases Society of America. *Circulation* 111:e394–e434. DOI:10.1161/Circulation AHA.105.165564.
22. Costerton, W., Veeh, R., Shirtliff, M., Pasmore, M., Post, C., Ehrlich, G. (2003). The application of biofilm science to the study and control of chronic bacterial infections. *J Clin Invest* 112:1466–1477.

23. Donlan, R.M., Costerton, J.W. (2003). Biofilms: survival mechanisms of clinically relevant microorganisms. *Clin Microbiol Rev* 15:167–193.
24. Kobasa, W.D., Kaye, K.L., Shapiro, T., Kaye, D. (1983). Therapy for experimental endocarditis due to *Staphylococcus epidermidis*. *Rev Infect Dis* 5(Suppl 3):S533–S537.
25. Galetto, D.W., Boscia, J.A., Kobasa, W.D., Kaye, D. (1986). Teicoplanin compared with vancomycin for treatment of experimental endocarditis due to methicillin-resistant *Staphylococcus epidermidis*. *J Infect Dis* 154:69–75.
26. Lowry, F.D., Wexler, M.A., Steigbigel, W.H., (1982). Therapy of methicillin-resistant *Staphylococcus epidermidis* experimental endocarditis. *J Lab Clin Med* 100:94–104.
27. Bayer, A.S., Lam, K. (1985). Efficacy of vancomycin plus rifampin in experimental aortic valve endocarditis due to methicillin-resistant *Staphylococcus aureus*: in vitro-in vivo correlations. *J Infect Dis* 151:157–165.
28. Perdikaris, G., Giamerellou, H., Pefanis, A., Donta, I., Karayiannakos, P. (1995). Vancomycin or vancomycin plus netilmicin for methicillin- and gentamicin resistant *Staphylococcus aureus* aortic valve experimental endocarditis. *Antimicrob Agents Chemother* 39:2289–2294.
29. Sande, M.A., and Courtney, K.B. (1976). Nafcillin-gentamicin synergism in experimental staphylococcal endocarditis. *J Lab Clin Med* 88:118–124.
30. Zak, O., Scheld, W.M., Sande, M.A. (1983). Rifampin in experimental endocarditis due to *Staphylococcus aureus* in rabbits. *Rev Infect Dis* 5:481–490.
31. Karchmer, A.W., Moellerig, R.C. Jr., Maki, D.G., Swartz, M.N. (1979). Single – antibiotic therapy for streptococcal endocarditis. *JAMA* 241:1801–1806.
32. Wilson, W.R., Thompson, R.L., Wilkowske, C.J., Washington, J.A. 2nd, Giuliani, E.R., Geraci, J.E. (1981). Short-term therapy for streptococcal infective endocarditis: combined intramuscular administration of penicillin and streptomycin. *JAMA* 245:360–363.
33. Francioli, P., Ruch, W., Stamboulian, D. (1995). Treatment of streptococcal endocarditis with a single daily dose of ceftriaxone and netilmicin for 14 days: a prospective multicenter study. *Clin Infect Dis* 21:1406–1410.
34. Sexton, D.J., Tenenbaum, M.J., Wilson, W.R., Steckelberg, J.M., Tice, AL, Gilbert, D., Dismukes, W., Drew, R.H., Durack, D.T., and the Endocarditis Treatment Consortium Group. (1998). Ceftriaxone once daily for four weeks compared with ceftriaxone plus gentamicin once daily for two weeks for treatment of endocarditis due to penicillin-susceptible streptococci. *Clin Infect Dis* 27:1470–1474.
35. Wilson, W.R., Giuliani, E.R., Geraci, J.E. (1982). Treatment of penicillin-sensitive streptococcal infective endocarditis. *Mayo Clinic Proc* 57:95–100.
36. Mandell, G.L., Kaye, D., Levison, M.E., Hook, E.W. (1990). Enterococcal endocarditis: an analysis of 38 patients observed at the New York Hospital-Cornell Medical Center. *Arch Intern Med* 125:258–264.
37. Moellering, R.C. Jr., Watson, B.K., Kunz, L.J. (1974). Endocarditis due to group D streptococci: comparison of disease caused by *Streptococcus bovis* with that produced by enterococci. *Am J Med* 57:239–250.
38. Wilson, W.R., Wilkowske, C.J., Wright, A.I., Sande, M.A., Geraci, J.E. (1984). Treatment of streptomycin-susceptible and streptomycin-resistant enterococcal endocarditis. *Ann Intern Med* 100:816–823.
39. Oliason, L., Schadewitz, K. (2002). Enterococcal endocarditis in Sweden, 1995–1999: can shorter therapy with aminoglycoside be used. *Clin Infect Dis* 34:159–166.
40. Gavalda, J., Onrubia, P.L., Martin Gómez, M.I., Gomis, X., Ramirez, J.L., Len, O., Rodriquez, D., Crespo, M., Ruiz, I., Pahissa, A. (2003). Efficacy of ampicillin combined with ceftriaxone and gentamicin in the treatment of experimental endocarditis due to *Enterococcus faecalis* with no high-level resistance to aminoglycosides. *J Antimicrob Chemother* 52:514–517.
41. Gavaldà J., Len O., Miró J.M., Muñoz P., Montejo M., Alarcón A., de la Torre-Cisneros J., Peña C., Martínez-Lacasa X., Sarria C., Bou G., Aguado J.M., Navas E., Romeu J., Marco

F., Torres C., Tomos P., Planes A., Falcó V., Almirante B., Pahissa A. (2007), Treatment of *Enterococcus faecalis* endocarditis with ampicillin plus ceftriaxone. *Ann Intern Med* 146:574–579.
42. Abramis, B., Sklaver, A., Hoffman, T., Greenman, R. (1979). Single or combination therapy of staphylococcal endocarditis in intravenous drug abusers. *Ann Intern Med* 90:789–791.
43. Chambers, H.F., Miller, T., Newman, M.D. (1998). Right-sided *Staphylococcus aureus* endocarditis in intravenous drug abusers: two-week combination therapy. *Ann Intern Med* 109:619–624.
44. Ribera, E., Gómez-Jimenez, J., Cortes, E., del Valle, O., Planes, A., Gonzalez-Alujas, Almirante, B., Ocana, I., Pahissa, A. (1996). Effectiveness of cloxacillin with and without gentamicin in short-term therapy for right-sided *Staphylococcus aureus* endocarditis. *Ann Intern Med* 125:969–974.
45. Fontún, J., Navas, E., Martinez-Beltran, J., Pérez-Molina, J., Martin-Dávila, P., Guerrero, A., Moreno, S. (2001). Short-term therapy for right-sided endocarditis due to *Staphylococcus aureus* in drug abusers: cloxacillin versus glycopeptides in combination with gentamicin. *Clin Infect Dis* 33:120–125.
46. Heldman, A.W., Hartert, T.V., Ray, S.C., Daoud, E.G., Kowalski, T.E., Pompili, V.J., Sisson, S.D., Tidmore, W.C., vom Eigen, K.A., Goodman, S.N., Lietman, P.S., Petty, B. G., Flexner, C. (1996). Oral antibiotic treatment of right-sided staphylococcal endocarditis in injection drug users: prospective randomized comparison with parenteral therapy. *Am J Med* 101:68–76.
47. Dworkin, R.J., Lee, B.L., Sande, M.A., Chambers, H.F. (1989). Treatment of right-sided staphylococcal endocarditis in intravenous drug users with ciprofloxacin and rifampin. *Lancet* ii:1071–1073.
48. Korzeniowski, O., Sande, M.A., and the National Collaborative Endocarditis Study Group. (1982). Combination antimicrobial therapy for *Staphylococcus aureus* endocarditis in patients addicted to parenteral drugs and in non-addicts. *Ann Intern Med* 97:496–503.
49. Falagas, M.E., Matthaiou, D.K., Bliziotis, I.A. (2006). The role of aminoglycoside in combination with a β-lactam for the treatment of bacterial endocarditis: a meta-analysis of comparative trials. *J Antimicrob Chemother* 57:639–647.
50. Braun, S., Casabe, J., Morris, A., Corey, G.R., Cabell, C.H. International Collaboration on Endocarditis – Prospective Cohort Study Investigators (2007), Contemporary clinical profile and outcome of prosthetic valve endocarditis. *JAMA* 297:1354–1361.
51. Lalani, T., Kanafani, Z.A., Chu, V.H., Moore, L., Corey, C.K., Pappas, P., Woods, C.W., Cabell, C.H., Hoen, B., Selton-Suty, C., Doco-Lecompte, T., Chirouze, C., Raoult, D., Miro, J.M., Mestres, C.A., Olaison, L., Eykyn, S., Abrutyn, D., Fowler, V.G., Jr. The International Collaboration on Endocarditis Merged Database Study Group, (2006). Prosthetic valve endocarditis due to coagulase-negative staphylococci: findings from the International Collaboration on Endocarditis Merged Database. *Eur J Clin Microbiol Infect Dis* 25:365–368.
52. Karchmer, A.W., Archer, G.L., Dismukes, W.E. (1983). *Staphylococcus epidermidis* causing prosthetic valve endocarditis: microbiologic and clinical observations as guides to therapy. *Ann Intern Med* 98:447–455.
53. Karchmer, A.W., Archer, G.L., National Collaborative Endocarditis Study Group. (1984). Methicillin-resistant *Staphylococcus epidermidis* prosthetic valve endocarditis: a therapeutic trial. 24th Interci Conf. Antimicrob Agents Chemother (abstr # 476); also reference in Karchmer, A.W. (2000). Infections of prosthetic heart valves; in: Infections Associated with Indwelling Medical Devices, 3rd ed., Waldvogel, F.A., Bisno, A.L. (eds), *ASM Press, Washington, DC*, pp. 145–172.
54. Lucet, J.C., Hermann, M., Rohner, P., Auckenthaler, R., Waldvogel, F.A., Lew, D.P. (1990). Treatment of experimental foreign-body infection caused by methicillin-resistant *Staphylococcus aureus*. *Antimicrob Agents Chemother* 34:2312–2317.
55. Chaud, C., Herrmann, M., Vaudaux, P., Waldvogel, F.A., Lew, D.P. (1991). Successful therapy of experimental chronic foreign-body infection due to methicillin-resistant

*Staphylococcus aureus* by antimicrobial combinations. *Antimicrob Agents Chemother* 35:2611–2616.
56. Bliziotis, I.A., Samonis, G., Vardakas, K.Z., Chrysanthopoulou, S., Falagas, M.E. (2005). Effect of aminoglycoside and β-lactam combination therapy versus β-lactam monotherapy on the emergence of antimicrobial resistance: a meta-analysis of randomized, controlled trials. *Clin Infect Dis* 41:149–158.
57. Paul, M., Silbigar, I., Grozinsky, S., Soores-Weizer, K., Leibovici, L. (2006). Beta-lactam antibiotic monotherapy versus beta-lactam-aminoglycoside combination therapy for sepsis. *Cochrane Database of Systemic Rev* (1):CD003344.
58. Safdar, N., Handelsman, J., Maki, D.G. (2005). Does combination antimicrobial therapy reduce mortality in gram-negative bacteremia. A meta-analysis. *Lancet Infect Dis* 5:192–193.
59. Garnacho-Montero, J., Sa-Borges, M., Sole-Violan, J., Barcenilla, F., Escoresca-Ortega, A., Ochoa, M., Cayuela, A., Rello, J. (2000). Optimal management therapy for *Pseudomonas aeruginosa* ventilator-associated pneumonia: an observational multicenter study comparing monotherapy with combination antibiotic therapy. *Crit Care Med* 35:1888–1895.
60. Waterer, G.W. (2005). Monotherapy vs combination antimicrobial therapy for pneumococcal pneumonia. *Curr Opin Infec Dis,* 18:151–153.
61. Weiss, K., Tillotson, G. (2005). The controversy of combination vs monotherapy in the treatment of hospitalized community-acquired pneumonia. *Chest* 128: 940–946.
62. Baddour, L.M., Yu, V.L., Klugman, K.P., Felman, C., Ortquist, A., Rello, J., Morris, A.J., Luna, C.M., Snydman, D.R., Ko, W.C., Chedid, M.B.F., Hui, D.S., Andremont, A., Chiou, C. C., International Pneumococcal Study Group. (2004). Combination therapy lowers mortality among severely ill patients with pneumococcal bacteremia. *Am J Resp Crit Care Med* 170:440–444.
63. Rex, J.H., Pfaller, M.A., Walsh, T.J., Chaturvedi, V., Espinel-Ingroff, A., Ghannoum, M.A., Gosey, L.L., Odds, F.C., Rinaldi, M.G., Sheehan, D.J., Warnock, D.W. (2001). Antifungal susceptibility testing: practical aspects and current challenges. *Clin Microbiol Rev* 14:643–658.
64. NCCLS, (2003). Reference method for broth dilution antifungal susceptibility testing of yeasts: approved standard, 2nd ed. NCCLS document M27-A2. NCCLS, Wayne, PA.
65. Espinel-Ingroff, A., Chaturvedi, V., Fothergill, A., Rinaldi, M.G. (2002). Optimal testing conditions for determining MICs and minimum fungicidal concentrations of new and established antifungal agents for uncommon molds: NCCLS collaborative study. *J Clin Microbiol* 40: 3776–3781.
66. Mukherjee, P.K., Sheehan, D.J., Hitchcock, C.A., Ghannoum, M.A. (2005). Combination treatment of invasive fungal infections. *Clin Microbiol Rev* 18:163–194.
67. Ghannoum, M.A., Fu, Y., Ibrahim, A.S., Mortara, L.A., Shafiq, M.C., Edwards, J.E.J., Criddle, R.S. (1995). In vitro determination of optimal antifungal combinations against *Cryptococcus neoformans* and *Candida albicans*. *Antimicrob Agent Chemother* 39:2459–2465.
68. Lewis, R.E., Dickema, D.J., Messer, S.A., Pfaller, M.A., Klepser, M.E. (2001). Comparison of E. test, checkerboard dilution and time-kill studies for detection of synergy or antagonism between antifungal agents tested against Candida species. *J Antimicrob Chemother* 49: 345–351.
69. Odds, F.C. (2003). Synergy, antagonism and what the checkerboard puts between them. *J Antimicrob Chemother* 52:1.
70. Sewell, D.L., Pfaller, M.A., Barry, A.L. (1994). Comparison of broth macrodilution, broth microdilution, and E-test antifungal susceptibility tests for fluconazole. *J Clin Microbiol* 32:2099–2102.
71. Lewis, R.E., Lund, B.C., Klepser, M.E., Ernst, E.J., Pfaller, M.A. (1998). Assessment of antifungal activities of fluconazole and amphotericin B administered alone and in combina-

tion against Candida albicans by using a dynamic in vitro mycotic infection model. *Antimicrob Agents Chemother* 42: 382–1386.
72. Louie, A., Kaw, P, Banerjee, P., Liu, W., Chen, G., Miller, M.H. (2001). Impact of the order of initiation of fluconazole and amphotericin B in sequential or combination therapy on killing of *Candida albicans* in vitro and in a rabbit model of endocarditis and pyelonephritis. *Antimicrob Agents Chemother* 40:2511–2516.
73. Vasquez, J.A., Arganoza, M.T, Vaishampayan, J.K., Atkin, R.A. (1996). In vitro interaction between amphotericin B and azoles in *Candida albicans*. *Antimicrob Agents Chemother* 40: 2511–2516.
74. Te, Dorsthorst, D.T., Verweij, P.E., Meletiadis, J., Bergervoet, M., Punt, N.C., Meis, J.F., Mouton, J.W. (2002). In vitro interaction of flucytosine combined with amphotericin B or fluconazole against thirty-five yeast isolates determined by both fractional inhibitory concentration index and the response surface approach. *Antimicrob Agents Chemother* 46:2982–2989.
75. Keele, D.J., DeLallo, V.C., Lewis, R.F., Ernst, E.J., Klepser, M.E. (2001). Evaluation of amphotericin B and flucytosine in combination against *Candida albicans* and *Cryptococcus neoformans* using time-kill methodology. *Diagn Microbiol Infect Dis* 41:121–126.
76. Sugar, A.M., Hitchcock, C.A., Troke, P.F., Picard, M. (1995). Combination therapy of murine invasive candidiasis with fluconazole and amphotericin B. *Antimicrob Agents Chemother* 39:598–601.
77. Sanati, H., Ramos, C.F., Bayer, A.S., Ghannoum, M.A. (1997). Combination therapy with amphotericin B and fluconazole against invasive candidiasis in neutropenic-mouse and infective-endocarditis rabbit models. *Antimicrob Agents Chemother* 41:1345–1348.
78. Louie, A. Banerjee, P., Drussano, G.H., Shayegani, M., Miller, M.H. (1999). Interaction between fluconazole and amphotericin B in mice with systemic infection due to fluconazole-susceptible or – resistant strains of *Candida albicans*. *Antimicrob Agents Chemother* 43:2841–2847.
79. Sugar, A.M., Saliban, M., Goldani, L.Z. (1994). Saperconazole therapy of murine disseminated candidiasis: efficacy and interactions with amphotericin B. *Antimicrob Agents Chemother* 35:371–373.
80. Hanson, L.H., Perlman, A.M., Clemons, K.V., Stevens, D.A. (1991). Synergy between cilofungin and amphotericin B in a murine model of candidiasis. *Antimicrob Agents Chemother* 35: 1334–1337.
81. Graybill, J.R., Bocanegra, R., Najvar, L.V., Hernandez, S., Larsen, R.A. (2003). Addition of caspofungin to fluconazole does not improve outcome in murine candidiasis. *Antimicrob Agents Chemother* 47:2373–2375.
82. Barchiesi, F., Spreghini, E., Baldassarri, I., Margigliano, A., Arzeni, D., Giannini, D., Scalise, G. (2004). Sequential therapy with caspofungin and fluconazole for Candida albicans infection. *Antimicrob Agents Chemother* 48:4056–4058.
83. Hossain, M.A., Reyes, G.H., Long, L.A., Mukherjee, P.K., Ghannoum, M.A. (2003). Efficacy of caspofungin combined with amphotericin B against azole-resistant *Candida albicans*. *J Antimicrob Chemother* 51:1427–1429.
84. Olson, J.A., Adler-Moore, J.P., Smith, P.J., Proffitt, R.T. (2005). Treatment of *Candida glabrata* infection in immunosuppressed mice by using a combination of liposomal amphotericin B with caspofungin or micafungin. *Antimicrob Agents Chemother* 49:4895–4902.
85. Menacacci, A., Cenci, E., Bacci, A., Bistoni, F., Romani, L. (2000). Host immune reactivity determines the efficacy of combination immunotherapy and antifungal chemotherapy in candidiasis. *J Infect Dis* 181.686–694.
86. Yamamoto, Y., Nehida, K., Klein, T.W. Friedman, H., Yamaguchi, H. (1992). Immunomodulators and fungal infections: use of antifungal drugs in combination with G-CSF. In: Friedman, H., Klein, T.W., Yamaguchi, H., (eds). Microbial infections. New York, Plenum Press, pp. 231–241.

87. Rex, J.H., Pappas, P.G., Karchmer, A.W., Sobel, I., Edwards, J.H., Hadley, S., Brass, Vasquez, J.A., Chapman, S.W., Horowitz, H.W., Zervos, M., McKinsey, D., Lee, J., Babinchak, T., Bradsher, R.W., Cleary, J.D., Cohen, D.M., Danziger, L., Golman, M., Goodman, J., Hilton, E., Hyslop, N.E., Kett, D.H., Lutz, J., Rubin, R.H., Scheld, W.M., Schister, M., Simmons, B., Stein, D.K., Washburn, R.G., Mautner, L., Chu, T.-C., Panzer, H., Rosenstein, R.B., Booth, J, for the National Institute of Allergy and Infectious Diseases Mycoses Study Group (2003). A randomized and blinded multicenter trial of high dose fluconazole plus placebo versus fluconazole plus amphotericin B as therapy for candidemia and its consequences in non-neutropenic subjects. *Clin Infect Dis* 36:1221–1228.
88. Pachl, J., Svoboda, P., Jacobs, Vanderwoude, K., van der Hoven, B., Spronk, P., Masterson, G., Malbrain, M., Aoun, M., Garbino, J., Takala, J., Drgona, L., Bunie, J., Matthews, R., for the Myograb Invasive Candidiasis study group (2006). A randomized, blinded, multicenter trial of lipid-associated amphotericin B alone versus combination with an antibody-based inhibitor of heat shock protein 90 in patients with invasive candidiasis. *Clin Infect Dis* 42:1404–1413.
89. Bennett, J.E., Dismukes, W.E., Duma, R.J., Medoff, G., Sande, M.A., Gallis, H., Leonard, J., Fields, B.T., Bradshaw, M., Haywood, H., McGee, Z.A., Cate, TR, Cobbs, C.G., Warner, J. F., Alling, D.W. (1979). A comparison of amphotericin B alone and combined with flucytosine in the treatment of crytococcal meningitis. *N Engl J Med* 301:126–131.
90. Dismukes, W.E., Cloud., G., Gallis, H.A., Kerkering, T.M., Medoff, G., Craven, P.C., Kaplowitze, L.G., Fisher, J.F., Gregg, G.R., Bowles, G.A. (1987). Treatment of cryptococcal meningitis with a combination of amphotericin B and flucytosine for four compared with 6 weeks. *N Engl J Med* 317:334–341.
91. van der Horst, C.M., Saag, M.S., Cloud, G.A., Hamill, R.J., Graybill, J.R., Sobel, J.D., Johnson, P.C., Tuazon, C.H., Kerkering, T.M., Moskovitz, B.L., Powderly, W.G., Dismukes, W.E. (1997). Treatment of cryptococcal meningitis associated with the acquired immunodeficiency syndrome. *National Institute of Allergy and Infectious Diseases Mycoses Study Group and AIDS Clinical Trials Group*. *N Engl J Med* 337:15–21.
92. Brouwer, A.E., Rajanuwong, A., Chierakul, W., Griffin, G.E., Larson, R.A., White, N.J., Harrison, T.S. (2004). Combination antifungal therapies for HIV-associated cryptococcal meningitis: a randomized trial. *Lancet* 363:1764–1767.
93. Mayanya-Kizza, H., Oishi, K., Mitarai, S., Yamashita, H., Nalorgo, K., Watanabe, K., Izumi, T., Jungala, O., Augustine, K., Mugerwa, R., Nagatake, T., Mitsumoto, K. (1998). Combination therapy with fluconazole and flucytosine for cryptococcal meningitis in Ugandan patients with AIDS. *Clin Infect Dis* 26:1362–1366.
94. Larsen, R.A., Bozzette, S.A., Jones, B.E., Haghighat, P., Leal, M.A., Forthal, D., Bauer, M., Tilles, J.G., McCutchan, J.A., Leedom, J.A. (1994). Fluconazole combined with flucytosine for the treatment of cryptococcal meningitis in patients with AIDS. *Clin Infect Dis* 19:741–745.
95. Larsen, R.A., Bauer, M., Thomas, A.M., Graybill, J.R. (2004). Amphotericin B and fluconazole, a potent combination therapy for cryptococcal meningitis. *Antimicrob Agents Chemother* 48:985–991.
96. Barchiesi, F.A., Schimizzi, A.M., Caselli, F., Novelli, A., Fallani, S., Giannini, D., Arzeni, D., Di Cesare, S., Di Francesco, L. F., Fortuna, M., Giacometti, A., Carle, F., Mazzei, T., Sealize, G. (2000). Interactions between triazole and amphotericin B against *Cryptococcus neoformans*. *Antimicrob Agents Chemother* 44:2435–2441.
97. Pappas, P.G., Bustamante, B., Ticona, E., Hamil, R.J., Johnson, P.C., Reboli, A., Aberg, J., Hasbun, R., Hsu, H.H. (2004). Recombinant interferon γ1b as adjunctive therapy for AIDS-related acute cryptococcal meningitis. *J Infect Dis* 189:2185–2191.
98. Segal, B.H., Steinbach, W.J. (2007). Combination antifungals: an update. *Expert Rev Anti-Infect Ther* 5:883–892.

99. Lewis, R.E., Prince, R.A., Chi, J., Kontogiannis, D.P. (2002). Itraconazole preexposure attenuates the efficacy of subsequent amphotericin B therapy in murine model of acute invasive pulmonary aspergillosis. *Antimicrob Agents Chemother* 46:3208–3214.
100. O'Shaughnessy, E.M., Meletiadis, J., Sterigiopoulou, T., Demchok, J.P., Walsh, T.J. (2006). Antifungal interactions within the triple combination of amphotericin B, caspofungin and voriconazole against Aspergillosis species. J Antimicrob Chemother PMID: 17071635.
101. Najvar, L.K., Cacciapuoti, A., Hernandez, S., Halpern, J., Bocanegra, R., Gurnani, M., Menzel, F., Loebenberg, D. Graybill, J.R. (2004). Activity of posaconazole combined with amphotericin B against *Aspergillus flavus* infection in mice: comparative studies in two laboratories. *J Antimicrob Chemother* 47:1376–1381.
102. Clemons K.V., Espiritu, M., Parmar, R., Stevens, D.A. (2005). Comparative efficacies of conventional amphotericin B, lipsomal amphotericin B (Ambisome), caspofungin, micafungin, and voriconazole alone and in combination against experimental murine central nervous system aspergillosis. *J Antimicrob Chemothe* 49:4867–4875.
103. Kirkpatrick, W.R., Perea, S, Coco, B.J., Patterson, T.F. (2002). Efficacy of caspofungin alone and in combination with voriconazole in a guinea pig model of invasive aspergillosis. *J Antimicrob Chemothe* 46:2564–2568.
104. Sivak, O., Bartlett, K., Risovic, V., Choo, E., Marra, F., Batty, D.S., Jr., Wasan, K.M. (2004). Assessing the antifungal activity and toxicity profile of amphotericin B lipid complex (ABLC:Abelcet ®) in combination with caspofungin in experimental systemic aspergillosis. *J Pharm Sci* 93:1382–1389.
105. Capilla-Lugue, J., Clemons, K.V., Stevens, D.A. (2003). Efficacy of micafungin alone or in combination against systemic murine aspergillosis. *Antimicrob Agents Chemother,* 41:1452–1455.
106. Clemons, K.V., Stevens, D.A. (2006). Efficacy of micafungin alone or in combination against experimental pulmonary aspergillosis. *Med Mycol* 44:69–73.
107. Petraitis, V., Petvaitiene, R., Sarafandi, A.A., Kelaher, A.M., Lyman, C.A., Casler, H.E., Sein, T., Groll, A.H., Bacher, J., Avila, N.A., Walsh, T.J. (2003). Combination therapy in treatment of experimental pulmonary aspergillosis: synergistic interaction between an antifungal triazole and an echinocandin. *J Infect Dis* 187:1834–1843.
108. Marr, K.A. Boechk, M., Carter, R.A., Kim, H.W., Corey, L. (2004). Combination antifungal therapy for invasive aspergillosis. *Clin Infect Dis* 39:797–802.
109. Kontoyiannnis, D.P., Hachem, R., Lewis, R.E., Rivero, G.A., Torres, H.A., Thomby, J., Champlin, R., Kantarjian, H., Bodey, G.H., Raad, II. (2003). Efficacy and toxicity of caspofungin in combination with liposomal amphotericin B as primary or salvage treatment of invasive aspergillosis in patients with hematologic malignancies. *Cancer* 98:292–299.
110. Aliff, T.B., Maslak, P.G., Juric, J.G., Heaney, M.L., Cathcart, K.N., Sepkowitz, K.A., Weiss, M.A. (2003), Refractory Aspergillus pneumonia in patients with acute leukemia: successful therapy with combination caspofungin and liposomal amphotericin. *Cancer* 47: 1025–1032.
111. Maertens, J., Glasmacher, A., Hebrecht, R., Thiebaut, A., Cordonnier, C., Segal, B.H., Killor, J., Taylor, A., Kartsonis, N., Patterson, T.F., Aoun, M., Sable, C., Caspofungin Combination Therapy Study Group, (2006). Multicenter noncomparative study of caspofungin in combination with other antifungals as salvage therapy in adults with invasive aspergillosis. *Cancer* 107:2888–2897.
112. Singh, N., Limaye, A.P., Forrest, G., Safdar, N., Munoz, P., Pursell, K., Houston, S., Rosso, F., Montoya, J.G., Patten, P., Del Busto, R., Aguado, J.M., Fisher, R.A., Klintmalm, G.B., Miller, R., Wagener, M.M., Lewis, R.E., Kontoyiannis, D.P., Hussain, S. (2006). Combination of voriconazole and caspofungin as primary therapy for invasive aspergillosis in solid organ transplant recipients: a prospective multicenter, observational study. *Transplantation* 81:320–326.
113. Caillot, D., Thiebaut, A., Herbrecht, R., de Botton, S., Pigneux, A., Bernard, F., Larche, J., Monchecourt F., Alfandari, S., Mahi, L. (2007). Liposomal amphotericin B in combination

with caspofungin for invasisve aspergillosis in patients with hematological malignancies. A randomized pilot study (Combistrat Trial). *Cancer* 110:2740–2746.
114. Siebert, U., Sroczynski, G. German Hepatitis C Model GEHMO Group. HTA Expert Panel on Hepatitis C. (2005). Effectiveness and cost-effectiveness of initial combination therapy with interferon/peginterferon plus ribavirin in patients with chronic hepatitis C in Germany: a health technology assessment commissioned by the German Federal Ministry of Health and Social Security. *Internat J. Techn Assess Health Care* 21:55–65.
115. Shiratori, Y., Ito, Y., Yokosuka, O., Imazeki, F., Nakata, R., Tanaka, N., Arakawa, Y., Hashimoto, E., Hirota, K., Yoshida, H., Ohashi, Y., Omata, M., for the Tokyo-Chiba Hepatitis Research Group, (2005). Antiviral therapy for chronic hepatitis C: association with reduced hepatocellular carcinoma development and improved survival. *Ann Intern Med* 142:105–114.
116. Scott, J.D., Gretch, D.R. (2007). Molecular diagnostics of hepatitis C virus infection. A systematic review. *JAMA* 297:724–732.
117. Sherman, M., Shafran, S., Burak, K., Doucette, K., Wong, W., Girgrah, N., Yoshida, E., Renner, E., Wong, D., Deschenes, M. (2007). Management of chronic hepatitis C: consensus guidelines. *Can J Gastroenterol* 21(Suppl C):25C–34C.
118. Yee, H.S., Currie, S.L., Darling, J.M., Wright, T.L. (2006). Management and treatment of hepatitis C viral infection: recommendations from the Department of Veterans Affairs Hepatitis C Resource Center Program and the National Hepatitis C Program office. *Am J Gastroenterol* 101:2360–2378.
119. Strader, D.B., Wright, T., Thomas, D.L., Seeff, L.B. (2004) Diagnosis, management, and treatment of hepatitis C. *Hepatology* 39:1147–1171.
120. Dienstag, J.L., McHutchinson, J.G. (2006). American Gastroenterology Association medical position statement on the management of hepatitis C., *Gastroenterology* 130:225–230.
121. Shire, N.J., Sherman, K.E., (2005). Clinical trials of treatment for hepatitis C virus infection in HIV-infected patients: past, present and future. *Clin Infect Dis,* 41(Suppl I):*s63–s68.*
122. Chung, R.T., Andersen, J., Volberding, P., Robbins, G.K., Liu, T., Sherman, K.E., Peters, M. G., Koziel, M.J., Bhan, A.K., Alston, B., Colquhoun, D., Nevin, T., Harb, G., van der Horst, C., for the AIDS Clinical Trials Group A5071 Study Team, (2004). Peginterferon alfa-2a plus ribavirin versus interferon alfa-2a plus ribavirin for chronic hepatitis C in HIV-coinfected persons. *N Engl J Med* 351:451–459.
123. Torriani, F.J., Rodriguez-Torres, M., Rochstroh, J.K., Lissen, E., Gonzalez-Garcia, J., Lazzarin, A., Carosi, G., Sasadeusz, J., Katlama, C., Montaner, J., Sette, H. Jr., Passe, S., De Pamphilis, J., Duff, F., Schrenk, U.M., Dieterich, D.T., for the APRICOT Study Group. (2004). Peginterferon alfa-2a plus ribavirin for chronic hepatitis C virus infection in HIV-infected patients. *N Engl J Med* 351:438–450.
124. Hoofnagle, J.H., Seef, L.B. (2006). Peginterferon and ribavirin for chronic hepatitis C. *N Engl J Med* 355:2444–2451.
125. Carrat F, Bani-Sadr F, Pol S, Rosenthal, E., Lunel-Fabiani, F., Benzerkri A, Morand P, Goujard, C., Pialoux, G., Piroth L, Salmon-Ceron, D., Degott, C., Cacoub, P., Peronne, C., for the ANRS HCO2 RIBAVIC Study Team. (2004). Pegylated interferon alfa-2b vs standard interferon alfa-2b, plus ribavirin, for chronic hepatitis C in HIV-infected patients: a randomized controlled trial. *JAMA* 117:120–125.
126. Mangia, A. Santoro R, Minerva N, Ricci GL, Carretta V, Persico M, Vinelli.F, Scotto, G., Bacca, D., Annese, M., Romano, M., Zechini, F., Sogari, F., Spirito, F., Andriulli, A. (2005). Peginterferon alfa-2b and ribavirin for 12 vs. 24 weeks in HCV genotype 2 or 3. *N Engl J Med* 352:2609–2617.
127. Shiffman, M.L., Suter, F., Bacon, B.R., Nelson, D., Harley, H., Solá, R., Shafran, S.D., Barrange, K., Lin, A., Soman, A., Zeuzem, S., for the ACCELERATE Investigators. (2007). Peginterferon alfa-2a and ribavirin for 16 or 24 weeks in HCV genotype 2 or 3, *N Engl J Med* 357:124–134.

128. Ferenci, P., Fried, M.W., Shiffman, M.L., Smith, C.I., Marinos, G., Goncales, F.L., Jr., Häussinger, D., Diago, M., Carosi, G., Dhumeaux, D., Craxi, A., Chaneac, M., Reddy, K.R. (2005). Predicting sustained virological responses in chronic hepatitis C patients treated with peginterferon alfa-2A(40KD)/ribavirin. *J Hepatol* 43:425–433.
129. Jensen, D.M., Morgan, T.R., Marcellin, P., Pockros, P.J., Reddy, K.R., Hadziyannis, S.J., Ferenci, P., Ackrill, A.M., Willems, B. (2006). Early identification of HCV genotype I patients responding to 24 weeks peginterferon alpha-2a (40KD)/ribavirin therapy. *Hepatology* 43:954–960. (Erratum in 2006; 43:1410).
130. Zeuzem, S., Buti, M., Ferneci, P., Sperl, J., Horsmans, Y., Cianciara, J., Ibranyi, E., Weiland, O., Noviello, S., Brass, C., Albrecht, J. (2006). Efficacy of 24 weeks treatment with peginterferon alfa-2b plus ribavirin in patients with chronic hepatitis C infected with genotype I and low pretreatment viremia. *J Hepatol* 44:97–103.
131. Berg, T., von Wagner, M., Nasser, S., Sarrazin, C., Heintges, T., Gerlach, T., Buggisch, P., Goeser, T., Rasenack, T, Pape, G.R., Schmidt, W.E., Kallinowski, B., Klinker, H., Spengler, U., Martus, P., Alshuth, U., Zenzem, S. (2006). Extended treatment duration for hepatitis C virus type I: comparing 48 versus 72 weeks of peginterferon alfa-2a plus ribavirin. *Gastroenterology* 130:1086–1097.
132. Sánchez-Tapias J.M., Diago M., Escartín P., Enríquez J., Romero-Gómez M., Bárcena R., Crespo J., Andrade R., Martínez-Bauer E., Pérez R., Testillano M., Planas R., Solá R., García-Bengoechea M., Garcia-Samaniego J., Muñoz-Sánchez M., Moreno-Otero R. for the TeraViC-4 Study Group. (2006) Peginterferon-alfa2a plus ribavirin for 48 versus 72 weeks in patients with detectable hepatitis C virus RNA at week 4 of treatment. *Gastroenterology* 131:451–460.
133. Hadziyannis S.J., Sette H. Jr., Morgan T.R., Balan V., Diago M., Marcellin P., Ramadori G., Bodenheimer H. Jr., Bernstein D, Rizzetto M, Zeuzem S, Pockros PJ, Lin A, Ackrill AM for the PEGASYS International Study Group, (2004). Peginterferon-a2a and ribavirin combination therapy in chronic hepatitis C. *Ann Intern Med* 140:346–355.
134. Lai , C.-F., Yuen, M.-F. (2007). The natural history and treatment of chronic hepatitis B: a critical evaluation of standard treatment criteria and end points *Ann Intern Med* 147:58–61.
135. Lok A.S., McMahon B.J. (2007). Chronic hepatitis B. *Hepatology* 45:507–539.
136. Pawlotsky, J.M., (2008). Hepatitis virus resistance, in: Fong, I.W., Drlica, K., (eds). Antimicrobial Resistance and Implications for the twenty-first century. Springer, New York, pp. 291–323.
137. Mellerup M.T., Krogsgaard K., Mathurin P., Gluud C., Poynard T. (2002). Sequential combination of glucocorticosteroids and alfa interferon versus alfa interferon alone. Cochrane Database Syst Rev (2):CD000345.
138. Sung, J.J., Zeuzem, S., Chow, W.C., Heathcote, E.J., Perrillo, R., Brosgart, T.C., Woessner, M., Scott, S.A., Campbell, F.M., (2003). A randomized double-blind phase II study of lamivudine compared to lamivudine plus adefovir dipivoxil for treatment of naïve patients with chronic hepatitis B: 52 week analysis. *J Hepatol* 38:25A.
139. Peters, M G., Hann, H.H., Martin, P., Heathcote, E.J., Buggisch, P., Rubin, R., Bourlierre, M., Kowdley, K., Trepo, C., Gray, D., Sullivan, M., Kleber, I., Ebrahimi, R., Xiong, S., Brusgart, C.L. (2004). Adefovir dipivoxil alone or in combination with lamivudine in patients with lamivudine-resistant chronic hepatitis B. Gastroenterology 343–347.
140. Fung, S.K., Chae, H.B., Fontana, R.J., Conjeevaram, H., Marrero, J., Oberhelman, K., Hussain, M., Lok, A.S.F. (2006). Virologic response and resistance to adefovir in patients with chronic hepatitis B. *J Hepatol* 44:283–290.
141. Lai, C.-L., Leung, N., Teo, E.-K., Tong, M., Wong, F., Hann, H.W., Han, S., Poynard, T., Myers, M., Chao,G., Lloyd, D., Brown, N.A., and the Telbivudine Phase II Investigator Group, (2005). A 1-year trial of telbivudine, lamivudine, and the combination in patients with hepatitis B e antigen-positive chronic hepatitis B. *Gastroenterology* 129:528–536.
142. Lai, C.-L., Gane, E., Liaw, Y.-F., Hsu, C.W., Thongsawat, S., Wang, Y., Chen, Y., Heathcote, E.J., Rasenack, J., Bzowej, N., Naoumov, N.V., Di Bisceglie, A.D., Zeuzem, S., Moon

Y.M., Goodman, Z., Chao, G., Constance, B.F., Brown, N.A., for the Globe Study Group, (2007). Telbivudine versus lamivudine in patients with chronic hepatitis B. *N Engl J Med* 357:2576–2588.
143. Degertekin, B., Lok, A.S.F. (2007). When to start and stop hepatitis B treatment: can one set of criteria apply to all patients regardless of age at infection? (Editorial). *Ann Intern Med* 147:62–64.
144. Koziel, M.J., Peters, M.G. (2007). Viral hepatitis in HIV infection (Current Concepts). *N Engl J Med* 356:1445–1454.
145. Peters, M.G., Anderson, J., Lynch, P., Liu, T., Alston-Smith, B., Brosgart, C.L., Jacobson, J.M., Johnson, V.A., Pollard, R.B., Rooney, J.F., Sherman, K.E., Swindells, S., Polsky, B., for the ACTG Protocol LA5127 Team, (2006). Randomized controlled study of tenofovir and adefovir in chronic hepatitis B virus and HIV infection: ACTG A5127. *Hepatology* 44:1110–1116.
146. McMahon, M.A., Jilek, B.L., Brennan, T.P., Shen, L., Zhou, Y., Wind-Rotolo, M.,, Xing, S., Bhat, S., Hale, B., Hegarty, R., Chong, C.R., Phil, M., Liu, J.O., Siciliano, R., Thio, C.L. (2007). The HBV drug entecavir – effects on HIV-1 replication and resistance. *N Engl J Med* 356:2614–2621.
147. Kanwal, F., Gralnek, IM., Martin, P., Dulai, G.S., Farid, M., Spiegel, B.M.R. (2005). Treatment alternatives for chronic hepatitis B virus infection: a cost-effectiveness analysis. *Ann Intern Med* 142:821–831.
148. Baird, J.K. (2005). Effectiveness of antimalarial drugs. *N Engl J Med* 352:1565–1577.
149. Maguire, J.D., Sumawinata, I.W., Masbar, S., Laksana, B., Prodjodipuro, P., Susanti, I., Sismadi, P., Mahmud, N., Bangs, M.J., Baird, J.K. (2002). Chloroquine-resistant Plasmodium malariae in south Sumatra, Indonesia. *Lancet* 360:58–60.
150. Bunnag, D., Karbwang, J., Na-Bangchang, K., Thanavibul A., Chittamas, S., Harinasuta,T. (1996). Quinine-tetracycline for multidrug resistant falciparum malaria. *Southeast Asian J Trop Med Public Health* 27:15–18.
151. Fungladda, W., Honrado, E.R., Thimasarn, K., Kitayaporn, D., Karbwang, J., Kamolratanakul, P., Masngammueng, R. (1998). Compliance with artesunate and quinine + tetracycline for treatment of uncomplicated falciparum malaria in Thailand. *Bull World Health Organ* 76 (Suppl I): 59–66.
152. Denis, M.B. (1998). Improving compliance with quinine + tetracycline for treatment of malaria: evaluation of health education interventions in Cambodian villages. *Bull World Health Organ* 76(Suppl I):43–49.
153. Roper, C., Pearce, R., Bredenkamp, B., Gumede, J., Drakeley, C., Mosha, F., Chandramohan, D., Sharp, B. (2003). Antifolate antimalarial resistance in southeast Africa: a population-based analysis. *Lancet* 361:1174–1181.
154. Staedke, S.G., Kamya, M.R., Dorsey, G., Gasasira, A., Ndeezi, G., Charlebois, E.D., Rosenthal, P.J. (2001). Amodiaquine, sulfadoxine/pyrimethamine, and combination therapy for treatment of uncomplicated falciparum malaria in Kampala, Uganda: a randomized trial. *Lancet* 358:368–374.
155. Basco, L.K., Same-Ekobo, A., Ngane, V.F., Ndvunga, M., Metoh, T., Ringwald, P., Soula, G. (2002). Therapeutic efficacy of sulfadoxine-pyrimethamine, amodiaquine, and the sulfadoxine-pyrimethamine-amodiaquine combination against uncomplicated Plasmodium falciparum malaria in children in Cameroon. Bull. *World Health Organ* 80:538–545.
156. Zongo, I., Dorsey, G., Rouamba, N., Dokomajilar, C., Lankoande, M., Ouedraogo, J-B, Rosenthal, P.J. (2005). Amodiaquine, sulfadoxine-pyrimethamine, and combination therapy for uncomplicated falciparum malaria: a randomized controlled trial from Burkina Faso. *Am J Trop Med Hyg* 73:826–832.
157. Ndyomugyemi, R., Magnussen, P., Clarke, S. (2004). The efficacy of chloroquine, sulfadoxine-pyrimethamine and a combination of both for the treatment of uncomplicated Plasmodium falciparum malaria in an area of low transmission in Western Uganda. *Trop Med Internat Health* 9:47–52.

158. Menard, D., Madji, N., Manirakiza, A., Djalle, D., Koula, M.R., Talarmin, A. (2005). Efficacy of chloroquine, amodiaquine, sulfadoxine-pyrimethamine, chloroquine-sulfadoxine-pyrimethamine combination and amodiaquine-sulfadoxine-pyrimethamine combination in Central African children with noncomplicated malaria. *Am J Trop Med Hyg* 72:581–585.
159. Loutfy, M.R., Kain, K.C. (2003). Drug-resistant malaria; in: Fong, I.W., Drlica, K. (eds). Reemergence of established pathogens in the 21st century. Kluwer Academic/Plenum Publishing, New York, pp.335–360.
160. Kremser, P.G., Looareesuwan, S., Chulay, J.D. (1999). Atovaquone and proguanil hydrochloride for treatment of malaria. *J Travel Med* 6(Suppl I): S18–S20.
161. Muehlen, M., Schreiber, J., Ehrhardt, S., Otchwemah, R., Jelinek, T., Bienzle, U., Mockenhaupt, F.P. (2004). Short communication: prevalence of mutations associated with resistance to atovaquone and to the antifolate effect of proguanil in Plasmodium falciparum isolates from northern Ghana. *Trop Med Int Health,* 9:361–363.
162. Musset, L., Bouchard, O., Matheron, L., Le Bras, J. (2006). Clinical atovaquone-proguanil resistance of Plasmodium falciparum associated with cytochrome b codon 268 mutations. *Microbes Infect* 8:2599–2604.
163. Giao, P.T., de Vries, P.J., Hung Le, Q, Binh, T.Q., Nam, N.V., Kager, P.A. (2004). CV8, a new combination of dihydroartemisinin, piperaquine, trimethoprim and primaquine, compared with atovaquone-proguanil against falciparum malaria. *Tropical Med Int Health* 9:209–216.
164. Gebru, T., Hailu, A., Kremsner, P.G., Kun., J.F., Grobusch, M.P. (2006). Molecular surveillance of mutations in the cytochrome b gene of Plasmodium falciparum in Gabon and Ethiopia. *Malar J* 5:112.
165. Happi, C.T., Gbotosho, G.O., Folarin, O.A., Milner, D., Sarr, O., Sowunmi, A., Kyle, D.E., Milhous, W.K., Wirth, D.F., Odoula, A.M.J. (2006). Confirmation of emergence of mutations associated with atovaquone-proguanil resistance in unexposed Plasmodium falciparum isolates from Africa. *Malar J* 5:82.
166. Abacassamo, F., Enrosse, S., Aponte, J.J., Gomez-Olive, F.X., Quinto, L., Mabunda, S., Barreto, A., Magnussen, P., Ronn, A.M., Thompson, R., Alonso, P.L. (2004). Efficacy of chloroquine, amodiaquine, sulfadoxine-pyrimethamine, and combination therapy with artesunate in Mozambican children with non-complicated malaria. *Trop Med Int Health* 9: 200–208.
167. Staedke, S.G., Mpimbaza, A., Kamya, M.R., Nzarubara, B.K., Dorsey, G., Rosenthal, P.J. (2004). Combination treatments for uncomplicated falciparum malaria in Kampala, Uganda: randomized clinical trial. *Lancet* 364:1950–1957.
168. Dorsey, G., Staedke, S., Clark, T.D., Njama-Meya, D., Nzarubara, B., Maiteki-Sebuguzi, C., Dokomaijilar, C Kamya, M.R., Rosenthal, P.J., (2007). Combination therapy for uncomplicated falciparum malaria in Ugandan children: a randomized trial. *JAMA* 297:2210–2219.
169. Nosten, F., van Vugt, M., Price, R., Luxemburger, C., Thway, K.L., Brockman, A., McGready, R., ter Kuile, F., Looareesuwan, S., White, N.J. (2000). Effects of artesunate-mefloquine combination on incidence of *Plasmodium falciparum* malaria and mefloquine resistance in western Thailand: a prospective study. *Lancet* 356: 297–302.
170. Arrow, K.J., Gelband, H., Jamison, D.T. (2005). Making antimalarial agents available in Africa. *N Engl J Med* 353:333–335.
171. Mutabingwa, T.K. (2005). Artemisin-based combination therapies (ACTs): best hope for malaria treatment but inaccessible to the needy. *Acta Tropica* 95:305–315.
172. Pickard, A.L., Wongsrichanalai, C., Purfield, A., Kamwendo, D., Emery, K., Zalewski, C., Kawamoto, F., Miller, R.S., Meshnick, S.R. (2003). Resistance to antimalarials in Southeast Asia and genetic polymorphisms in pfmdr1. *Antimicrob Agents Chemother* 47:2418–2423.
173. van Vugt, M., Leonardi, E., Phaipun, L., Slight, T., Thway, K.L., McGready, R, Brockman, A., Villegas, L., Looareesuwan, S., White, N.J., Nosten, F. (2002). Treatment of uncomplicated multidrug-resistant falciparum malaria with artesunate-atovaquone-proguanil. *Clin Infect Dis* 35:1498–1504.

174. Cross, H.F., Haarbrink, M., Egerton, G., Yazdanbakhsh, M. Taylor, M.J. (2001). Severe reactions to filarial chemotherapy and released of Wolbachia endosymbionts into blood. *Lancet* 358:1873–1875.
175. de Kraker, M.E., Stolk, W.A., van Oortmarssen, G.J., Habbema, J.D. (2006). Model- based analysis of trial data: microfilaria and worm-productivity loss after diethylcarbamazine-albendazole or ivermectin-albendazole combination therapy against *Wuchereria bancrofti*. *Trop Med Inter Health* 11:718–728.
176. El Setouchy, M, Ramzy, M.R., Ahmed, E.S., Kandil, A.M., Hussain, O., Farid, H., Helmy, H., Weil, G.J. (2004). A randomized clinical trial comparing single and multi-dose combination therapy with diethylcarbamazine and albendazole for treatment of bancroftian filariasis. *Am J Trop Med Hyg* 70:191–196.
177. Critchley, J., Addis, D., Gamble, C., Garner, P., Gelband, H., Ejere, H., (International Filariasis Review Group). (2005). Albendazole for lymphatic filariasis (Review). Cochrane Database Syst Rev CD003753.
178. Schwab, A.E., Boakye, D.A., Kyelem, D., Pritchard, A.K. (2005). Detection of benzimidazole resistance-associated mutations in the filarial nematode Wuchereria bancrofti and evidence for selection by albendazole and ivermectin combination treatment. *Am J Trop Med Hyg* 73:234–238.
179. McLaren, D.J., Worms, M.J., Laurence, B.R., Simpson, M.G. (1975). Microorganisms in filarial larvae (Nematoda). *Trans R Soc Trop Med Hyg* 69:509–514.
180. Kozek, W.J. (1977). Transovarially-transmitted intracellular microorganisms in adult and larvae stages of Brugia malayi. *J Parasitol* 63:992–1000.
181. Lammie, P.J. (2006). The promise of Wolbachia-targeted chemotherapy as a public health intervention for lymphatic filariasis and onchocerciasis. *Clin Infec Dis* 42:1090–1092.
182. Hoerauf, A., Mand., S., Adjei, O., Fleischer, B., Büttner, D.W. (2001). Depletion of Wolbachia endobacteria in Onchocercia volvulus by doxycycline and microfilaridemia after ivermectin treatment. *Lancet* 357:1415–1416.
183. Hoerauf, A., Mand, S., Fisher, K., Kruppa, T., Marfo-Debrekyei, Y., Debrah, A.Y., Pfarr, K. M., Adjei, O., Buttner, D.W. (2003). Doxycycline as a novel strategy against bancroftian filariasis-depletion of Wolbachia endosymbionts from Wuchereria bancrofti and stop of microfilaria production. *Med Microbiol Immunol (Berl)* 192:211–216.
184. Taylor, M.J., Mokunde, W.H., McGarry, H.F., Turner, J.D., Mand, S., Hoerauf, A. (2005). Macrofilaricidal activity after doxycycline treatment of Wuchereria bancrofti: a double blind randomized placebo-controlled trial. *Lancet* 365:2116–2121.
185. Turner, J.D., Mand, S., Debrah, A.Y., Muehlfield, K., Pfarr, K.F., McGarry, H.F., Adjei, O., Taylor, M.J., Hoerauf, A. (2006). A randomized, double-blind clinical trial of a 3-week course of doxycycline plus albendazole and ivermectin for the treatment of *Wuchereria bancrofti* infection. *Clin Infect Dis* 42:1081–1089.
186. Supali, T., Djuardi, Y., Pfarr, K.M., Wibowo, H., Taylor, M.J., Hoerauf, A., Houwing-Duistermaat, J.J., Yazdanbakhsh, M., Sartono, E. (2008). Doxycycline treatment of Brugia malayi-infected persons reduces microfilaremia and adverse reactions after diethylcarbamazine and albendazole treatment. *Clin Infect Dis* 46:1835–1393.
187. Sundar, S., Jha, T.K., Thakur, C.P., Engel, J., Sindermann, H., Fisher, C., Junge, K., Brycesan, A., Berman, J. (2002). Oral miltefosine for Indian visceral leishmaniasis. *N Engl J Med* 347:1739–1746.
188. Thakur, C.P., Kanyok, T.P., Pandey, A.K., Sinha, G.P., Messick, C., Olliaro, P. (2002). Treatment of visceral leishmaniasis with injectable paromomycin (aminosidine): an open-label randomized phase II clinical study. *Trans R Soc Trop Med Hyg* 94:432–433.
189. Thakur, C.P., Kanyok, T.P., Pandey, A.K., Sinha, G.P., Zaniewski, A.E., Houlihan, H.H., Oliaro, P. (2000). A prospective randomized, comparative, open-label trial of the safety and efficacy of paromomycin (aminosidine) plus sodium stibogluconate versus sodium stibogluconate alone for the treatment of visceral leishmaniasis. *Trans R Soc Trop Med Hyg* 94: 429–431.

190. Chunge, C.N., Owate, J., Pamba, H.O., Donno, L. (1990). Treatment of visceral leishmaniasis in Kenya by aminosidine alone or combined with sodium stibogluconate. *Trans R Soc Trop Med Hyg* 84:221–225.
191. Legros, D., Evans, S., Maiso, F., Enyaru, J.C.K., Mbulamberi, D. (1999). Risk factors for treatment failure after melarsoprol for Trypanosoma brucei gambiense trypanosomiasis in Uganda. *Trans R Soc Trop Med Hyg* 93:439–442.
192. Stanghellini, A., Josenando, T. (2001). The situation of sleeping sickness in Angola: a calamity. *Trop Med Int Health* 6:330–334.
193. Leyros, D., Ollivieri, G., Gastellu-Etchgorry, M., Paquet, C., Burri, C., Jennin, J., Büscher, P. (2002). Treatment of human African trypanosomiasis – present situation and needs for research and development. *Lancet Infect Dis* 2:437–440.
194. Pepin, J., Milord, F., Mpia, B., Meurice, F., Ethier, L., DeGroof, D., Bruneel, H. (1989). An open clinical trial of nifurtimox for arseno-resistant Trypanosoma brucei gambiense sleeping sickness in central Zaire. *Trans R Soc Trop Med Hyg* 83:514–517.
195. Pepin, J., Milord, F., Meurice, F., Ethier, L., Loko, L., Mpia, B. (1992). High-dose nifurtimox for arseno-resistant Trypanosoma brucei gambiense sleeping sickness: an open trial in central Zaire. *Trans R Soc Trop Med Hyg* 86:254–256.
196. Fairlamb, A.H. (1990). Future prospects for the chemotherapy of human trypanosomiasis. I. Novel approaches to the chemotherapy of trypanosomiasis. *Trans R Soc Trop Med Hyg* 83:613–617.
197. Mpia, B., Pepin, J. (2002). Combination of eflornithine and melarsoprol for melarsoprol-resistant Gambian trypanosomiasis. *Trop Med Int Health* 7:775–779.
198. Bisser, S., N'Siesi, F.X., Lejon, V., Preux, P.-M., Nieuwenhove, S.V., Mia Bilenge, C.M., Büscher, P. (2007). Equivalence trial of melarsoprol and nifurtimox monotherapy for the second-stage Trypanosoma brucei gambiense sleeping sickness. *J Infect Dis* 195:322–329.
199. Pepin, J., Rhonde, N. (1996). Relapses following treatment of early-stage Trypanosoma brucei gambiense sleeping sickness with combination of pentamidine and suramin. *Trans R Soc Trop Med Hyg* 90:183–186.
200. Perlroth, J., Kuo, M., Tan, J., Bayer, A.S., Miller, L.G.l. (2008). Adjunctive use of rifampin for the treatment of *Staphylococcus aureus* infections. A systemic review of the literature. *Arch Intern Med* 168:805–819.
201. Bartels, D.J., Zhou, M., Zhang, E.Z., Marcial, M., Byrn, R.A., Pfeiffer, T. Tigges, A.M., Adiwijaya, B.S., Lin, C., Kwong, A.D., Kieffer, T.L., (2008). Natural prevalence of hepatitis C virus variants with decreased sensitivity to NS 3-4 A protease inhibitors in treatment-naïve subjects. *J Infect Dis* 198:800–807.

# Index

## A

Acute otitis media (AOM)
  clinical practice guidelines, 40–41
  diagnosis, 37–38
    management algorithm, 41–42
    middle-ear effusion and pathogenesis, 36–37
    treatment
      acute sinusitis, 28–30
      antibacterial therapy, 38
      antibiotics, 39, 40
      symptomatic therapy, 39
Acute respiratory distress syndrome (ARDS)
  characteristics, 140–141
  genetic polymorphism, 151
  immune cell apoptosis, 136
  neutropenia, 132
  pathogenic process, 141
  ventilation management, 148–149
Acute sinusitis
  definition, 28
  symptoms and signs, CT, 29
  treatment, 32–35
Adjunctive therapy
  fungal meningitis
    clinical features, 18
    management, IDSA guidelines, 19–20
    treatment, 19
  pulmonary exacerbation
    hypertonic saline inhalation, 90–91
    ibuprofen, 91–92
    recombinant human DNAse, 91
    simvastatin and glutathione, 92
  sepsis syndrome, 149
  tuberculous meningitis
    incidence, 15–16
    pathogenesis and clinical features, 16
    treatment, 17–18
African trypanosomiasis, 361–362
Amodiaquine (AQ), 356
Amphotericin B (AmB), 342
Antibiotic cement (AC), 310
Antibiotic prophylaxis, VAP
  chlorhexidine and oral decontamination, 62–63
  selective decontamination of the digestive tract (SDD), 61
Antibiotic therapy, febrile neutropenia
  low-risk factors, 170
  oral out-patient management, 169–170
  scoring, 171
Antibiotic-associated diarrhea (AAD)
  CDAD, 195–196
  probiotics
    *Candida difficile* diarrhea, 239–240
    prevention of, 239
Antibiotic-associated hemorrhagic colitis, 196
Antifungal prophylaxis, febrile neutropenia
  amphotericin B, 180
  fluconazole, 179
  itraconazole and posaconazole, 179–180
Antimalarial combination therapies
  ACTs use of, 357–358
  atovaquone-proguanil (AP), 356

379

sulfadoxine and pyrimethamine (SP) combination, 356
Artemesinin-based therapies (ACTs), 357

## B

Bacterial infective endocarditis (IE), combination therapy
  animal models
    cell wall active agents combinations, 331
    CoNS, 331
    vancomycin-gentamicin-rifampin, 331–332
  enterococcal endocarditis, 333–334
  in vitro synergistic effect testing
    definition, 329
    enterococci and streptococci, 329–330
    mechanism for, 329
    penicillin, 330
  prosthetic valve endocarditis (PVE), 336–337
  staphylococcal endocarditis, 334–335
  streptococcal endocarditis, 332–333
Bacterial meningitis
  CT scan misconception, 5–6
  dexamethasone therapy
    adults, 11–15
    childrens, 9–11
  fever and altered mental status, 4–5
  lumbar puncture, antibiotics
    clinical features and outcomes, 7
    CT scan criteria, 6–7
    drawbacks, 7–8
  pathophysiology
    bacterial pathogens, 3
    clinical features, 4
    invasion, 3–4
Bacterial sinusitis. *See also* Sinusitis
  diagnostic issues
    acute sinusitis, 28–30
    chronic sinusitis, 30
  pathophysiology, 28
  treatment, 32–35
Bacterial vaginosis (BV), 245–246
Biofilm antibiotic resistance, 265–266

Bloodstream infections (BSI)
  antibiotic lock therapy (ALT), 273–274
  coagulase-negative Staphylococcus (CoNS), 272
  diagnosis of, 270–271
  issues in, 272–273
  management, 271–272
  mechanism
    adherence and colonization, 269
    catheter infection routes, 268
    contaminated fluid infusion, 269
  rates of, 268
*Bordetella pertussis* infection, pertussis
  booster vaccination, 121
  components, 115
  epidemiology, 117
  immunity
    cell-mediated immunity, 116
    IgG and IgA antibody response, 115–116
  infection and genomics, 114–115
  maternal antibodies, 120–121
  prevention, 120
  virulence factors, 114

## C

*Candida* species, antifungal combinations
  in vitro studies, 342
  in vivo studies
    AmB and FLU, 343–344
    Myograb combination, 344
Candidiasis, neonates, 246
Carbapenems, 174
Cardiovascular device infectious
  cardiac devices and infections, 277
  pacemakers
    and ICD infection, 280–283
    LVAD, 283–285
  prosthetic valve endocarditis (PVE)
    definite and late PVE, 277, 278
    health care-associated, 278
    infective endocarditis (IE), 279
    management, 278
    prevention of, 280
    *S. aureus,* 279, 280
    surgical therapy, 278–280
Caspofungin (CAS), 346–347

Cefepime, 173
Ceftazidime, 173
Central nervous system infections.
    *See* Meningitis
Central venous catheters (CVCs), 267
Chlorhexidine, VAP, 62–63
Chloroquine (CQ), 356
Chronic sinusitis
    anaerobe prevalence, 31
    bacterial infection, 31–32
    definition, 30
    etiology, 30–31
    management, 35–36
Clinical pulmonary infection score
        (CPIS), 50
*Clostridium difficile*-associated
        diarrhea (CDAD)
    active immunization, 213
    adhesion blocking, 213
    algorithm, 210–212
    antibiotic-associated diarrhea, 195–196
    asymptomatic infection, 194
    celecoxib, 213
    diagnosis, 194, 199–200
    hamster model, 212–213
    micro-organism, 189–190
    monoclonal antibodies, 212
    pathogenesis
        A and B toxins, 191–192
        actin cytoskeleton, 192
        binary toxin and hypervirulent strains,
            192–194
        interferon-gamma IFN-g deficiency,
            192
        pathogenicity locus (PaLoc), 191
        protection mechanism, 190–191
        toxin-variant strain, 191
    prevention
        aminoacid administration, 210
        dietary manipulation, 210
        environmental disinfectant, 209
        restrictive antibiotic policy, 209
    ramoplanin, 212
    recurrences
        bacteriotherapy, 208–209
        hypervirulent strain, 204–205
        passive immunotherapy, 207–208
        pragmatic approach, 205
        prevalence, 204
        probiotics, 206
        repeated/continued antibiotics, 204
        vancomycin, 206–207
    rifalazil, 212
    risk factors
        antimicrobials, 197–198
        comorbidities, 198–199
        $H_2$-receptors antagonists ($H_2$ RAS),
            198
        proton pumps inhibitors (PPI),
            198–199
    screening antigen immunoassay, 214
    specific therapy
        asymptomatic carrier, 202
        decompression colonoscopy, 204
        intravenous metronidazole
            monotherapy, 203
        intravenous vancomycin, 203–204
        metronidazole fecal concentration, 201
        nitazoxanide, 203
        pseudomembranous colitis, 202
        rifampin and tolevamer, 203
        vancomycin-resistant enterococci
            (VRE) colonization, 201
    toxin immunoenzymatic A/B assay, 214
Coagulase-negative staphylococcus (CoNS),
        272
Coagulation dysfunction
    activated protein C (APC), 138–139
    fibrinolytic system, 138
    plasminogen activator inhibitor type I
        (PAI-1), 139
Colonocyte-binding protein, 192
Colony-stimulating factors (CSF),
        178–179
Combination antimicrobial therapies
    bacterial infective endocarditis (IE)
        animal models, 330–332
        enterococcal endocarditis, 333–334
        in vitro synergistic effect testing,
            329–330
        prosthetic valve endocarditis (PVE),
            336–337
        staphylococcal endocarditis, 334–335
        streptococcal endocarditis, 332–333
    combination anti-infective therapies, 363
    community-acquired pneumonia, 338

fungal infections
    Candida species, 342–344
    checkerboard method, 340–341
    cryptococcal meningitis, 344–345
    epsilometer strip (E-test), 341–342
    invasive aspergillosis, 345–347
    target sites, 338–339
    time-kill methods, 341
gram-negative bacterial infections, 337
Mycobacterium tuberculosis and HIV
    infection, 327
parasitic infections
    African trypanosomiasis, 361–362
    antimalarial combination therapies,
        355–358
    filariasis therapies, 358–360
    leishmaniasis, 360–361
specifically targeted antiviral for
    HCV (STAT-C), 364
viral infections
    hepatitis B virus (HBV), 351–355
    hepatitis C infections, 347–351
Continuous lateral rotational
    therapy (CLRT), VAP, 61
Corticosteroids
    corticotrophin, 146
    hydrocortisone and fludrocortisone,
        145–146
Cryptococcal meningitis, 344–345
    clinical features, 18
    management, IDSA guidelines, 19–20
    treatment, 19
Culture cytotoxicity neutralization assay for
    toxin B (CCNA), 199–200
Cystic fibrosis transmembrane
    conductance regulator (CFTR)
    mutation
    bacterial clearance, 77–78
    defective chloride transport, 77
    gene location, 75
    immunity and mucin defects, 78
    mechanism, 76
    protienomics and gene therapy, 92–93
Cystic fibrosis, pulmonary infections
    Alcaligenes xylosoxidans
        infection, 81
        treatment, 89
    Aspergillus spp, 82–83

Burkholderia cepacia
    antimicrobial resistance and
        transmissibility, 81
    genomovars, 80
filamentous fungi, 83
management
    antipseudomonal therapy, 84–85
    antistaphylococcal antibiotic
        therapy, infants, 84
    maintenance therapy, 85–87
    mycobacteria species, 81–82
pathobiology, CFTR mutation
    bacterial clearance, 77–78
    defective chloride transport, 77
    gene location, 75
    immunity and mucin defects, 78
    mechanism, 76
Pseudomonas aeruginosa
    biofilm formation, 79–80
    micro-colonies, 79
pulmonary exacerbation
    adjunctive therapy, 90–92
    treatment, 87–88
Stentotrophomonas maltophilia
    infection, 81
    treatment, 89
viral infections, 83

D
Device-related infections
    and infections risk, 262
    bacterial communication system, 288
    cardiovascular device infections
        cardiac devices and infections, 277
        ICD, LVAD and pacemakers
            infections, 280–285
        prosthetic valve endocarditis (PVE),
            277–280
    central vs. vascular catheter infections
        prevention
        infectious complications, 274–275
        mupirocin therapy, 275–276
        prevention evidence-based procedures,
            275
    intravascular devices (IVDs) and BSI
        antibiotic lock therapy (ALT), 273–274
        diagnosis of, 270–271

Index 383

issues in, 272–273
management, 271–272
mechanism, 268–270
nosocomial infections, 261
pathogenesis
  antimicrobial agents resistance, 265–267
  biofilms and planktonic bacteria, 263, 266
  local defence impairment, 264–265
  slime role in, 264
vascular grafts
  aortic grafts infection, 286–287
  endovascular grafts, 287
  femoropopliteal graft infection, 285
  surgical intervention, 286–287
Dexamethasone therapy, bacterial meningitis
adults
  diagnosis and management algorithm, 14
  meningococcal meningitis, 13
  outcomes, 11
  penicillin susceptibility, 15
  RCT-assessment, 12
children, 9–11

# E

Empiric antifungal therapy, neutropenia
  amphotericin B, 175–176
  caspofungin, 177
  fluconazole, 176
  itraconazole and voriconazole, 176
Endocytic pattern-recognition receptors, 129
Entrococcal endocarditis
  *Enterococcus faecalis*, 334
  penicillin G combination, 333
Enzyme immunoassay (EIA), 199
Extended-spectrum beta-lactamases (ESBL), 59–60

# F

Febrile neutropenia
  definition, 167
  directed antifungal therapy, 181

empiric antifungal therapy
  amphotericin B, 175–176
  caspofungin, 177
  fluconazole, 176
  itraconazole and voriconazole, 176
granulocyte-colony-stimulating factors, 181
micro-organism and etiology
  high-risk patients, 171–172
  initial antibiotic therapy, 169–171
  monotherapy, 173–174
monoclonal antibodies, 180–181
mortality rate, 168
pathogenesis
  cytotoxic agents and MBL deficiency, 167
  mechanisms, 166
  risk and severity, 166–167
prevention
  antifungal prophylaxis, 179–180
  colony-stimulating factors (CSF), 178–179
  prophylactic antibiotics, 177–178
  therapy duration, 174–175
Filariasis, combination therapy
  diethylcarbamazine, 358–359
  doxycycline, 359–360
  ivermectin-albendazole treatment, 359
  *Wolbachia* species, 359
Fluconazole (FLU), 342
Fluoroquinolone prophylaxis, 177–178
Foreign-body-related infection. *See* Device-related infections
Fractional inhibitory concentration index (FICI), 340–341
Fungal infections, combination antimicrobial therapies
  *Candida* species, 342–344
  checkerboard method, 340–341
  cryptococcal meningitis, 344–345
  epsilometer strip (E-test), 341–342
  invasive aspergillosis, 345–347
  target sites in, 338–339
  time-kill methods, 341
Fungal meningitis
  clinical features, 18
  management, IDSA guidelines, 19–20
  treatment, 19

## G

Glycoprotein 96 (gp96), 192
Granulocyte-colony-stimulating factor (G-CSF), sepsis, 150
Guanosine triphosphatase (GTPase), 192

## H

$H_2$-receptors antagonists ($H_2$ RAS), 198
Head and neck infections. *See* Acute otitis media (AOM); Sinusitis
*Helicobacter pylori* infection, 247
Hepatitis B virus (HBV), combination therapy
   and HIV infection, 354
   drugs for, 353
   entecavir and adefovir, 354–355
   nucleosides for, 352
   PIFNα and lamivudine, 352
Hepatitis C virus
   contraindications for, 348
   genotype, 350
   indications for treatment, 348
   PIFNα/RBV, 349–351
   rapid viral response (RVR), 349–350
   sustained viral response (SVR), 349, 350

## I

Immumochromatography assay for toxins A and B (ICTAB), 199–200
Immune response, sepsis
   cytokines and adaptive immune response, 130
   innate immune system, 128–129
   pattern recognition receptors, 129
   toll-like receptors (TLRs), 129–130
Immunotherapy, sepsis
   granulocyte-colony-stimulating factor (G-CSF), 150
   intravenous immunoglobulins (IVIG), 149–150
Implantable cardioverter defibrillator (ICD), 280–283

Infective endocarditis (IE), 279.
   *See also* Bacterial infective endocarditis (IE), combination therapy
Intensive insulin therapy, sepsis, 146
Interleukin-6 (1 L-6), 303
Intravascular devices (IVDs) and BSI
   antibiotic lock therapy (ALT), 273–274
   coagulase-negative Staphylococcus (CoNS), 272
   diagnosis of, 270–271
   issues in, 272–273
   management, 271–272
   mechanism
      adherence and colonization, 269
      catheter infection routes, 268
      contaminated fluid infusion, 269
      rates of, 268
Intravenous drug abuse (IVDA), 334–335
Invasive aspergillosis
   in vitro and animal models, 345–346
   voriconazole (VORI) and caspofungin (CAS), 346–347

## L

Left ventricular assist device (LVAD), pacemakers, 283–285
Leishmaniasis, 360–361

## M

Meningitis
   bacterial meningitis
      CT scan misconception, 5–6
      dexamethasone therapy, 9–15
      fever and altered mental status, 4–5
      lumbar puncture, antibiotics, 6–8
      pathophysiology, 3–4
   fungal meningitis
      clinical features, 18
      management, IDSA guidelines, 19–20
      treatment, 19
   tuberculous meningitis
      incidence, 15–16
      pathogenesis and clinical features, 16
      treatment, 17–18

Methicillin-resistant *S. epidermidis* (MRSE), 306–307
Microbiological techniques, VAP
  blind-protected telescoping catheter (PTC), 52
  diagnosis
    criteria, 55
    gold standard, 52–54
  endobronchial aspiration (EA), 51
  protected specimen brush (PSB), 51–52
Mitogen-activated protein (MAP) kinases, 192
Monotherapy, febrile neutropenia
  carbapenems, 174
  ceftazidime and cefepime, 173
  piperacillin/tazobactam, 173–174

# N

Necrotizing enterocolitis (NEC), 235–236
Newborns and children, probiotics
  infectious diarrheas
    day-care setting, 238
    nosocomial diarrhea, 237–238
  necrotizing enterocolitis, 235–236
Noninvasive positive-pressure ventilation (NPPV), 60
Nosocomial Infection Surveillance (NNIS) system, 304

# O

Orthopedic implants and prosthetic joint infections
  clinical presentation
    early and delayed infections, 304
    risk factors, 304–305
  diagnosis
    histopathological examination, 303
    imaging techniques, 302–303
    magnetic resonance imaging (MRI), 303
  management
    antimicrobial choices, 315
    antimicrobial therapy issues, 313–316
    debridement and prosthesis retention criteria, 313
    matrix metalloproteinases (MMP), 316
    medical therapy, 305–307
    one-stage direct exchange criteria, 314
    oral therapy, 314
    quinolones in, 307
    rifampin combinations, 306, 307
    tetracyclines, 314–316
    treatment algorithm, 312–313
  microbiological aspects
    coagulase negative staphylococci (CoNS), 300
    limitations of, 301–302
    polymerase chain reaction (PCR), 300–301
    sensitivity, 300
    sonication method, 301
  multicenter, randomized trials, 318
  prevention, 316–318
  prophylaxis for, 317
  surgical management principles
    debridement approach, 308
    direct exchange, 310–311
    fracture-fixation devices, 311
    limitation of, 309
    one-stage *vs.* two-stage arthroplasties, 309–310
    *S. aureus* and CoNS, 308–309
    spinal implant infection, 311
  titanium, 318

# P

Pacemakers
  and ICD infection
    electrode extraction, 282–283
    endocarditis management, 282
    pocket infection, 281–282
  LVAD, 283–285
Parasitic infections, combination therapy
  African trypanosomiasis, 361–362
  antimalarial combination therapies, 355–358
  filariasis therapies
    diethylcarbamazine, 358–359
    doxycycline, 359–360
    ivermectin-albendazole treatment, 359
    *Wolbachia* species, 359

leishmaniasis, 360–361
Pegylated interferon-alpha (PIFNa), 347–350
Penicillin, bactericidal synergy, 330
Pertussis, adults
  diagnosis and management
    antibiotics, 119
    nasopharyngeal secretion, PCR, 118–119
  epidemiology
    prevalence, 116–117
    whole-cell pertussis vaccination, 117–118
  immunity
    cell-mediated immunity, 116
    IgG and IgA antibody response, 115–116
    micro-organism and pathogenesis, 114–115
Piperacillin/tazobactam monotherapy, 173–174
Plasma membrane-binding protein, 192
Plasminogen activator inhibitor type I (PAI-1), sepsis, 139
Probiotics, infectious diseases
  action mechanisms
    bacterial translocation, 234–235
    cell-mediated immunity, 233–234
    colonization resistance, 231–232
    immunomodulation, 232–234
    luminal factors, 229
    microbial toxins inactivation, 232
    mucosal integrity, 229–230
  adverse effects, 250
  antibiotic-associated diarrhea (AAD)
    *C. difficile* diarrhea, 239–240
    prevention of, 239
  candidiasis, neonates, 246
  food additives, 249–250
  gastrointestinal tract (GI), 228
  *Helicobacter pylori* infection, 247
  history of, 228
  infants, 227
  newborns and children
    infectious diarrheas, 236–238
    necrotizing enterocolitis, 235–236
  parasitic infections, 248–249
  resident microbial flora, 227
  surgical-related infections
    bacterial infections, 248
    hemorrhagic pancreatitis, 247
  urogenital infections
    animal studies, 242
    clinical utility in, 243–245
    microbiological studies, 243
    urinary tract infection (UTI), 241–242
    vaginitis, 245–246
Prophylactic antibiotics, febrile neutropenia
  fluoroquinolone prophylaxis, 177–178
  trimethoprim–sulfamethoxazole, 177
Prosthetic valve endocarditis (PVE), 331, 336–337
Proton pumps inhibitors (PPI), 198
*Pseudomonas aeruginosa*
  aerolized dextran and macrolides, 93
  antipseudomonal therapy
    antibiotics, 84–85
    DNA genotyping, 85
  biofilm formation, 79–80
  flagella vaccine, 90
  infection mechanism, 76–77
  maintenance therapy
    aerolized antimicrobials inhalation, 85–86
    antibiotics inhalation, 86–87
    oral antibiotics and microlides, 87
  micro-colonies, 79
  pulmonary exacerbation, 88
  *vs.* mycobacterial colonization, 82

# R

Recurrent CDAD (RCDD)
  bacteriotherapy, 208–209
  passive immunotherapy, 207–208
  probiotics, 206
  vancomycin, 206–207
Respiratory syncytial virus (RSV) infection
  epidemiology
    immunosuppressed subjects, 106–107
    prevalence and manifestations, 105
    pulmonary disease and influenza A, 106
  formalin-inactivated RSV vaccine, 104
  IgE homocytotropic antibodies, 104

immunity
  cell-mediated immunity, 105
  IgM and IgG response, 104–105
infectivity and pathogenicity, 103–104
management
  molecular diagnosis, 107
  palivizumab, 108
  ribavirin and polyclonal
    immunoglobulin, 107–108
  preventative strategies, 108–109
  recombinant RSV subunit vaccine, 109
RSV isolates, 103
Ribavirin (RBV), 347–350

## S

Secreted pattern-recognition molecules, 129
Sepsis syndrome. *See also* Systemic inflammatory response syndrome (SIRS)
  activated protein C (APC), 144–145
  adjunctive therapy, 149
  antimicrobial therapy, 142–144
  blood transfusion, 147–148
  corticosteroids, 145–146
  definition, 128
  early goal directed therapy, 141–142
  genetics
    polymorphisms, 150–151
    predisposition, 151
  immune response
    cytokines and adaptive immune response, 130
    innate immune system, 128–129
    pattern recognition receptors, 129
    toll-like receptors (TLRs), 129–130
  immunomodulatory agents, 151–152
  immunotherapy
    granulocyte-colony-stimulating factor (G-CSF), 150
    intravenous immunoglobulins (IVIG), 149–150
  intensive insulin therapy, 146
  management, 141
  mechanical ventilation management, 148–149
  pathogenesis
    acute respiratory distress syndrome (ARDS), 140–141
    coagulation dysfunction, 138–139
    complement system, 139–140
    hemodynamics, 132–133
    high mobility group box-1 (HMGB1) protein, 131–132
    immune cell apoptosis, 135–136
    immunoparalysis, 136–137
    macrophage inhibitory factor (MIF), 131
    macrophages and neutrophils, 130–131
    mechanism, 133–135
    neutrophils and TREM-1, 132
    nuclear factor (NF)-kB and interferon-γ (IFN-γ), 131
    tissue oxygenation, 137–138
  thiazolidinediones, 153
  thymosin α1 and ulinastatin, 153
  vasopressin and vasopressors, 147
Sinusitis
  acute sinusitis
    definition, 28
    symptoms and signs, CT, 29
    treatment, 32–35
  chronic sinusitis
    anaerobe prevalence, 31
    bacterial infection, 31–32
    definition, 30
    etiology, 30–31
    management, 35–36
  micro-organism, 30–32
  pathophysiology
    allergy, 27–28
    clinical symptoms, 28
    paranasal sinuses, 27
Sleeping sickness. *See* African trypanosomiasis
Soluble triggering receptor expressed on myeloid cells (sTREM-1), 55–56
Staphylococcal endocarditis
  combination therapy role, 335
  *S. aureus,* 334–335
Streptococcal endocarditis, 332–333

Sulfadoxine and pyrimethamine (SP), 356
Systemic inflammatory response syndrome (SIRS)
ARDS, 141
definition, 128
immune response, 128
pathogenesis, 130

## T

Tuberculous meningitis
incidence, 15–16
pathogenesis and clinical features, 16
treatment, 17–18

## U

Urinary tract infection (UTI), 241–242
Urogenital infections, probiotics
animal studies, 242
clinical utility
recurrence of, 244
spinal cord injury, 244–245
microbiological studies, 243
prevention of, 240–241
urinary tract infection (UTI)
coliform bacteria, 241
recurrent UTI, 241–242
vaginitis
bacterial vaginosis (BV), 245–246
yeast vulvovaginitis, 245

## V

Vancomycin-resistant enterococci (VRE)
colonization, 201
Vasopressin, sepsis, 147
Ventilator-associated pneumonia (VAP)
clarithromycin, 67
diagnostic issues
clinical criteria, CPIS, 49–50
microbiological techniques, 51–55
TREM-1 measurement, 55–56
direct E-test, 66–67
microbial etiology, 56–57
prevention
antibiotic prophylaxis, 61–63
aspiration reduction, 64–65
continuous lateral rotational therapy (CLRT), 61
gastric acidity maintenance, 63
noninvasive positive-pressure ventilation (NPPV), 60
rotational therapy, 60–61
ventilator circuit, 65
treatment issues
antibiotic selection, 57–58
empiric and combination therapy, 58
endotoxin assay, 57
extended-spectrum beta-lactamases (ESBL), 59–60
therapy duration, 58–59
tobramycin and cefazolin, 59
Voriconazole (VORI), 346–347

## W

Whooping cough, adults
diagnosis and management
antibiotics, 119
nasopharyngeal secretion, PCR, 118–119
epidemiology
prevalence, 116–117
whole-cell pertussis vaccination, 117–118
immunity
cell-mediated immunity, 116
IgG and IgA antibody response, 115–116
micro-organism and pathogenesis, 114–115

## Y

Yeast vulvovaginitis, 245

Printed in the United States of America